Imaging of the Temporomandibular Joint

Ingrid Rozylo-Kalinowska · Kaan Orhan
Editors

Imaging of the Temporomandibular Joint

Springer

Editors
Ingrid Rozylo-Kalinowska
Independent Unit of Propaedeutics of Dentomaxillofacial Radiology
Medical University of Lublin
Lublin, Poland

Kaan Orhan
Faculty of Dentistry
Department of Dentomaxillofacial Radiology
Ankara University
Ankara, Turkey

ISBN 978-3-319-99467-3 ISBN 978-3-319-99468-0 (eBook)
https://doi.org/10.1007/978-3-319-99468-0

Library of Congress Control Number: 2018963841

This Springer imprint is published by the registered company Springer Nature Switzerland AG
The registered company address is: Gewerbestrasse 11, 6330 Cham, Switzerland

To my wife, Ayşe Işıl, and to my son, Alp, for their unconditional love and untiring efforts to help me achieve both my personal and professional goals; to my mother, father, and sister, Kadriye, Ibrahim, and Buket, for their continuous support in every step of my life

—Kaan Orhan

To my family for their enormous patience and support each day of my life

—Ingrid Różyło-Kalinowska

Preface

Imaging of temporomandibular joint (TMJ) provides practical clinical examples of studies performed with different imaging modalities and offers a unique learning experience for imaging specialists in training as well as for experienced radiologists and clinicians wishing to be updated on the current state of the art and the latest developments in the fields of imaging and image-guided interventions. In this book, conventional imaging to advanced imaging of TMJ will be covered.

This book offers a comprehensive, detailed, up-to-date review of our current knowledge in the TMJ imaging. The eminently readable text is complemented by numerous and superb illustrations. The authors of the individual chapters were invited to contribute because of their outstanding personal experience in the dento-maxillofacial imaging and their major contributions to the radiological literature on the topic.

The authors, internationally renowned experts in their field, have contributed chapters that are disease oriented and cover all relevant imaging modalities, including magnetic resonance imaging, cone beam computed tomography, and nuclear medicine, as well as image-guided interventions.

Detailed imaging findings are given in each chapter to demonstrate the level of detail required for image interpretation with insightful "pearls and pitfalls," all designed to provide novice as well as experienced readers a brief but concise summary of the advantages and limitations of using this technology in the clinical setting. Chapters 2–3 cover basics of TMJ including anatomy and histology, while Chap. 4 covers fundamentals of radiology and radiation protection before discussing any imaging modality. From Chaps. 5–18, topics cover a spectrum of various imaging modalities and clinical applications in TMJ diseases. Finally, Chaps. 19 and 20 cover topics about micro-CT application in TMJ bone research and genetic approaches for TMJ diseases.

As a result, this book offers a comprehensive review of the state of the art in dentomaxillofacial imaging. Moreover, this book will be of great interest for not only maxillofacial radiologists and specialized neuro- or head and neck radiologists.

Ankara, Turkey — Kaan Orhan
Lublin, Poland — Ingrid Różyło-Kalinowska

Contents

Introduction

The discovery of X-rays approximately 120 years ago changed dramatically the diagnostic capabilities. Since then, there have been many advances in medicine, which have had more of an impact on modern healthcare. Radiology offers the best way of thinking about different diseases of patients and the suitable methods to understanding what is "real" diagnosis; moreover, it gives opportunity to understand how we see, smell, hear, feel, taste, touch, and more ultimately see how sick or how healthy we all are. Recently, with the use of CBCT, MRI, and ultrasonography, radiology is becoming integral to diagnose maxillofacial diseases accurately.

As the world's population and that of the world age increase, healthcare costs would increase in part because of increasing prevalence of chronic diseases. New technologies treat diseases that were once considered fatal, thus prolonging lives. Improvements in imaging studies and investigations allow us and patients to know beforehand what could possibly be the diagnosis of the diseases. The growing demand for dentomaxillofacial radiology allows us to jump in another level of diagnosis together with influential research on imaging.

It should be emphasized that success is measured by the people's impact on their community, and that is the goal, we as the editors of this book would like to achieve with the publication of this book. I would like to remember that good healthcare is a team effort from the physicians, to the nurses, to the radiologists, and while the radiologists may not be the star striker, we are certainly taking one for the team. For these reasons and goals, this book should be regarded as a stage in learning and understanding the TMJ imaging that will stimulate both radiologists and students to seek a more in-depth appreciation of the subject and its contribution to the scientific community of dentomaxillofacial radiology.

Ankara, Turkey — Kaan Orhan

Introduction to TMJ Imaging 1

Kaan Orhan

1.1 Introduction

The correct diagnosis has an important place in the treatment of temporomandibular joint (TMJ) pathology, with radiographic imaging being an important element in the diagnosis. Because of the anatomic complexity of the TMJ and its proximity to the temporal bone, mastoid air cells, and auditory structures, imaging of the joint structures can be problematic. With respect to the TMJ this involves assessment of the integrity and relationships of the hard and soft tissues, including the mandibular condyle, the glenoid fossa and articular eminence of the temporal bone, and the articular disk and its attachments [1].

The petrous and tympanic parts of the temporal bone lie in close proximity to the joint. To avoid superimposition of these parts, various projection techniques have been applied in the quest for usable images. Over the years, when radiologists were limited to the use of conventional radiographic imaging, different oblique projections were used, each one of them with shortcomings in their depiction of the joint [2]. Several imaging techniques now being used for TMJ viewing are conventional radiography, plain and panoramic radiography, computerized tomography (CT) scanning, cone beam CT (CBCT), arthrography, magnetic resonance imaging (MRI), axiography, and ultrasonography [3–11].

TMJ problems are common and affect up to one-third of all adults at some stage in their lives, as well as affecting children and adolescents. In epidemiological studies, subgroups of temporomandibular disorders (TMDs) are often evaluated only through clinical examination of the population investigated [12, 13]. However, when assessing the prevalence of joint pathology, the difference between objective diagnosis and subjective patient-reported pain can pose a challenge in terms of

K. Orhan
Department of Dentomaxillofacial Radiology, Ankara University, Faculty of Dentistry, Ankara, Turkey

I. Rozylo-Kalinowska, K. Orhan (eds.), *Imaging of the Temporomandibular Joint*, https://doi.org/10.1007/978-3-319-99468-0_1

making a diagnosis. Moreover, for scientific studies, an objective diagnosis using imaging techniques must be reproducible [14]. Although we have several criteria for TMDs, there are still unclear correlations between clinical signs and symptoms and the imaging findings in all TMD patient groups [15].

This brings about the need for close collaboration between clinicians and radiologists, and personal communication between these practitioners can improve patient care. The workflow of radiologists has changed dramatically in recent years. Commonly, using Picture Archiving and Communication System (PACS) solutions has led radiologists to interpret the images most often with a lack of clinical information. Close collaboration can be the way to change the radiology workflow to either include face-to-face meetings or provide a way for radiologists and referring physicians to collaborate in real time; this will improve patient care, especially in pathologies such as TMD. Because of the anatomic complexity of the TMJ and its proximity to the temporal bone, mastoid air cells, and auditory structures, imaging of the joint structures should also be investigated. Therefore, careful clinical and radiological examinations are essential for the evaluation of the TMJ. In this book, TMJ anatomy, imaging methods, radiological techniques, and the classification of various pathologies are discussed.

1.2 What Does the Clinician Need in Terms of TMJ Imaging?

TMDs comprise a large number of articular and/or muscular conditions in the orofacial region. The main articular alterations in TMDs are disc displacements and degenerative changes in both the soft and hard tissues of the TMJ. These features are mostly characterized by symptoms such as pain, joint sounds, and limited jaw opening, either singly or in combination [16], with TMJ pain being the major reason for patients to refer to a clinic for treatment [17]. The etiology of pain in TMD patients has not been clearly understood. There are several possible sources of TMJ pain, such as inflammatory changes in the synovial membrane, including the production of fluid resulting in joint effusion; alterations in the bone marrow of the mandibular condyle; and impingement and compression [18]. TMJ sound is considered a pathologic sign of TMD, and is commonly recognized as a sign of internal derangement; its recording is required to make a diagnosis of disc displacement, with a consequent reduction of clinical examinations. Although patients without TMD may demonstrate TMJ sound symptoms [19–21], the treatment of these patients can be challenging, since the exact diagnosis is of utmost importance.

Several guidelines have been released regarding TMJ and TMD and the need for imaging [22–24]. The American Academy of Orofacial Pain (AAOP) released its first guideline in 1990; this focused solely on the diagnosis and management of TMDs. In 2013, they updated their guidelines and expanded the number of clinical orofacial pain-related disorders [22, 23]. However, for TMD, the AAOP uses the expanded taxonomy developed with the International RDC/TMD Consortium Network and Orofacial Pain Special Interest Group. The expanded taxonomy is, however, a compilation of all types of TMD and hence it includes both painful and non-painful conditions [24]. In this guideline, TMDs are classified into four major groups: TMJ disorders, masticatory muscle disorders, headache, and disorders of associated structures [22, 24]. The current guidelines, which are widely used, are the Research Diagnostic Criteria for Temporomandibular Disease (RDC-TMD) to Diagnostic Criteria for Temporomandibular Disorders (DC/TMD) and the expanded TMD Taxonomy [24]. The first version of the RDC-TMD was published in 1992 as a dual-axis assessment protocol with operationalized diagnostic algorithms for the most common TMDs [25]. Currently, the RDC-TMD guidelines are regarded as a reference protocol for TMD research and this has led to the protocol's translation into more than 20 languages [25, 26].

Clinicians should perform the clinical examination and then refer the patient to the radiologist for imaging. The most important part of the patient's referral is to provide as much clinical information as possible to the radiologist; this allows both sets of practitioners to make a proposed diagnosis in a realistic way and it also avoids any medico-legal implications.

1.3 How Does the Clinician Decide What Kind of TMJ Imaging is Required?

As stated above, there are several guidelines for the evaluation of clinical history and examination for the diagnosis of TMD. However, the methods of diagnostic imaging of the TMJ that measure the degree of integrity of its components should be carried out along with consideration of the clinical findings, especially for evaluation in cases of trauma; occlusal changes; and limited mouth opening; and in the presence of joint noises, systemic joint diseases, infection, and failure of conservative treatment.

For bone imaging, the conventional diagnostic tool of the two-dimensional (2D) radiograph has shown various advantages, such as the low radiation dose and its low cost; further, the procedure is simple and quick and non-invasive. The appearance of new digital 2D systems with numerous features of image enhancement, in addition to the above-mentioned advantages, means that digital 2D radiography may be a simple and acceptable modality in this field as well.

However, 2D radiographs have several drawbacks, including errors that are classified as "errors of projection" and "errors of identification". Errors of projection are due to the 2D feature, which causes a shadow of the 3D object. As a result, this distortion and differential magnification may lead to errors of identification and reduced measurement accuracy [27–29]. For example, on 2D radiographs, the TMJ and the borders of the mandible condyle sometimes show artifacts that are due to magnification differences between the patient's left and right sides, depending on proximity to the image receptor. New technological advances have been made in craniofacial imaging to resolve these errors, and these methods are becoming increasingly popular for orthodontic diagnosis and assessment of treatment. For example, 3D computerized tomography (CT) avoids the superimposition and problems due to magnification and offers visualization of the craniofacial structures with more precision than the 2D method [29]. At first, medical CT (MDCT) was used for this purpose. MDCT studies showed that 3D CT analysis could provide accurate and reliable assessments for orthodontic and maxillofacial applications [30, 31]. However, despite these advantages, the effective dose of MDCT is much higher than that of the conventional cephalometric radiograph. This renders its use for routine cephalometric analysis and growth assessment unjustifiable. Besides, MDCT is also an expensive procedure and the scanners are not easily accessible by dentists. In the past decade, a technique called cone beam computerized tomography (CBCT) was proposed for maxillofacial imaging [4, 18–24], as first reported in the literature by Mozzo et al. [32]. A CBCT scan uses a different type of acquisition than traditional MDCTs. The X-ray source produces a cone-shaped X-ray beam and this makes it possible to capture the image in a single shot, rather than capturing slices separately, as in MDCT. The resultant volume can be reformatted to provide multiple reconstructed images with perspectives such as sagittal, coronal, and axial images, similar to traditional MDCT images. The advantages of this imaging modality are a lower radiation dose than MDCT and the possibility that individualized overlap-free reconstructions and Digital Imaging and Communications in Medicine (DICOM) data can be imported and exported for other applications that use routine TMJ imaging, especially for bone structures [29]. Low-dose high-resolution 3D scans such as CBCT images might provide more accurate diagnostic data for certain purposes and conditions, such as surgical intervention and anatomic variations.

For soft-tissue imaging, MRI can be another alternative, with ultrasonography for the visualization of soft tissues. The etiology of TMJ pain is not clear, but internal derangements and bone degenerative changes, such as osteoarthritis, effusion, and bone marrow edema, can be considerable [33]. MRI is an advanced imaging technique that provides excellent contrast in soft tissues without radiation or surgical invasion [34]. MRI is currently considered to be the optimum modality for imaging the TMJ. Therefore, MRI is widely used in the region of the TMJ, particularly to examine disk position and configuration, posterior disk attachment, and mandibular marrow status, and to assess the presence of joint effusion. MRI of the TMJ has resulted in better understanding of the TMJ and a better comprehension of its disorders [35].

MRI has become the gold standard in diagnosing articular disc displacement. MRI findings of disc displacements and osteoarthritis (OA) are significantly related to clinical signs and symptoms of TMD, although MRI features of OA and disc displacement have been observed in asymptomatic TMJs. TMJ effusion and condylar bone marrow edema, which typically appear as bright signals on MR images, have been traditionally investigated as markers of inflammation [36]. Ultrasonography is a quite sensitive aid in the diagnosis of TMJ disorders. It has become one of the most commonly recommended methods in recent decades because of its noninvasive nature and inexpensiveness, and its use for evaluating the integrity and correlation of the hard and soft tissues of the TMJ through static and dynamic assessments [37–39].

However, there are some disadvantages in using ultrasonography, as the interpretation of the images is highly dependent on the operator, because the images can be foggy and not clear. Difficulty in visualizing the articular disc is one of the limitations of ultrasonography. The disc is visualized only through the small gap between the zygomatic process of the temporal bone and the head of the condyle. It is difficult to acquire satisfactory images, especially when the condyle rotates and translates from the mouth-closed position to the mouth-open position. Therefore only the lateral part of the TMJ can be reached, while the medial part remains hidden by the above-mentioned structures [37].

As many different kinds of imaging modalities such as CT, CBCT, USG, MRI, Nuclear medicine can be used for the TMJ, a thorough understanding of the characteristics of each imaging modality is important. Ferreira et al. [22] classified information on different examination techniques for TMJ imaging types, based on their indications and risks (Table 1.1). The various chapters in this book elaborate in detail how best to visualize the TMJ and its pathologies, thus indicating to clinicians which examinations to ask for.

Table 1.1 Indications for TMJ Imaging (derived from Ferreira et al. [22])

	Disorders	Signs	Indications for imaging
Congenital or developmental disorders	Aplasia	No structure	CBCT, CT, radiographic exams
	Hypoplasia	Size reduction	CBCT, CT, radiographic exams
	Hyperplasia	Dimensional increase	CBCT, CT, radiographic exams
	Dysplasia	Structural change	CBCT, nuclear medicine, CT, radiographic exams
Acquired disorders	Neoplasm	Formation/bone destruction	CBCT, nuclear medicine, CT, MRI
		Growth of soft tissue	CBCT, nuclear medicine, MRI, US
		Metastasis	Nuclear medicine
Disc displacement (DD)	DD with reduction	Disc recapture	MRI, US
	DD without reduction	No disc recapture	MRI, US
TMJ dislocation		Open lock	Clinical diagnosis, radiographic exams, CT, CBCT
Inflammatory disorders	Synovitis/ capsulitis	Effusion, inflammation, pain	MRI, US
	Polyarthritis	Remodeling	CBCT, CT, MRI, radiographic exams
Non-Inflammatory disorders	Primary osteoarthritis Secondary osteoarthritis	Uni/bilateral cortical alteration, remodeling	CBCT, CT, MRI, radiographic exams
Ankylosis		Bone formation/ compromised movement	CBCT, CT, MRI, radiographic exams
Fracture (condyle)		Asymmetry, fracture	CBCT, CT, radiographic exams

TMJ temporomandibular joint, *CBCT* cone beam computerized tomography, *CT* computerized tomography, *MRI* magnetic resonance imaging, *US* ultrasonography

1.4 Conclusions

Temporomandibular joint pain is mostly related to internal derangement, degenerative changes, joint effusion, and bone marrow edema in the joint, but the imaging findings cannot be regarded as unique and dominant factors in defining the occurrence of TMDs. There should be close collaboration between clinicians and radiologists to ensure that a correct diagnosis is made; moreover, standardized terminology and evidence-based guidelines must be taken into consideration for the correlation of clinical symptoms and imaging findings.

References

1. Brooks SL, Brand JW, Gibbs SJ, Hollender L, Lurie AG, Omnell KA, Westesson PL, White SC. Imaging of the temporomandibular joint: a position paper of the American Academy of Oral and Maxillofacial Radiology Review. Oral Surg Oral Med Oral Pathol Oral Radiol Endod. 1997;83(5):609–18.
2. Isberg A. Temporomandibular joint dysfunction: a practitioner's Guide. 1st ed. London: Martin Dunitz Publishers; 2002. p. 173–96.
3. Okeson JP. Assessment of orofacial pain disorders. In: Okeson JP, editor. Orofacial pain: Guidelines for assessment, diagnosis, and management. Chicago: Quintessence; 1996. p. 19–44.
4. Dworkin SF, LeResche L. Research diagnostic criteria for temporo-mandibular disorders: review, examinations and specifications, critique. J Craniomandib Disord. 1992;6:301–55.
5. Okeson JP. History and examination for temporomandibular disorders. In: Okeson JP, editor. Management of temporomandibular disorders and occlusion. 4th ed. St. Louis: Mosby; 1998. p. 234–309.
6. Kaplan AS. Plain, tomographic, and panoramic radiography and radionuclide imaging. In: Kaplan AS, Assael LA, editors. Temporomandibular disorders, diagnosis and treatment. Philadelphia: W.B. Saunders; 1991. p. 312–36.
7. Danielson PA. Arthrography. In: Kaplan AS, Assael LA, editors. Temporomandibular disorders, diagnosis and treatment. Philadelphia: W.B. Saunders; 1991. p. 337–52.
8. Milbauer DL. Magnetic resonange imaging and computerized tomography. In: Kaplan AS, Assael LA, editors. Temporomandibular disorders, diagnosis and treatment. Philadelphia: W.B. Saunders; 1991. p. 353–70.
9. Christiansen EL, Thompson JR. Radiographic evaluation of the TMJ. In: Pertes RA, Gross SG, editors. Clinical management of temporomandibular disorders and orofacial pain. Chicago: Quintessence; 1995. p. 161–74.
10. Westesson PL. Magnetic resonance imaging of the temporomandibular joint. In: Pertes RA, Gross SG, editors. Clinical management of temporomandibular disorders and orofacial pain. Chicago: Quintessence; 1995. p. 175–96.
11. Pharoah MJ. The prescription of diagnostic images for temporomandibular joint disorders. J Orofac Pain. 1999;13:251–4.
12. Heffez L, Jordan S. A classification of temporomandibular joint disc morphology. Oral Surg Oral Med Oral Pathol. 1989;67:11–9.
13. Jensen U, Ruf S. Longitudinal changes in temporomandibular disorders in young adults: indication for systematic temporomandibular joint screening. J Orofac Orthop. 2007;68: 501–9.
14. Abou-Atme YS, Zawawi KH, Melis M. Prevalence, intensity, and correlation of different TMJ symptoms in Lebanese and Italian subpopulations. J Contemp Dent Pract. 2006;7:71–8.

15. Dijkgraaf LC, De Bont LGM, Boering G. Three-dimensional visualisation of the temporomandibular joint: a computerised multisectional autopsy study of disc position and configuration. J Oral Maxillofac Surg. 1992;50:2–10.
16. Campos MI, Campos PS, Cangussu MC, Guimarães RC, Line SR. Analysis of magnetic resonance imaging characteristics and pain in temporomandibular joints with and without degenerative changes of the condyle. Int J Oral Maxillofac Surg. 2008;37(6):529–34.
17. Limchaichana N, Nilsson H, Ekberg E, Nilner M, Petersson A. Clinical diagnoses and MRI findings in patients with TMD pain. J Oral Rehabil. 2007;34(4):237–45.
18. Park HN, Kim KA, Koh KJ. Relationship between pain and effusion on magnetic resonance imaging in temporomandibular disorder patients. Imaging Sci Dent. 2014;44(4):293–9.
19. Manfredini D, Basso D, Salmaso L, Guarda-Nardini L. Temporomandibular joint click sound and magnetic resonance-depicted disk position: which relationship? J Dent. 2008;36(4):256–60.
20. Eren H, Kolsuz ME, Orhan K. An overall look for temporomandibular joint pathologies and imaging. Int J Orthop. 2015;2(6):452–61.
21. American Academy of Craniofacial Pain. Craniofacial pain: a handbook for assessment, diagnosis and management. Chattanooga: Chroma, Inc.; 2009.
22. Ferreira LA, Grossmann E, Januzzi E, de Paula MV, Carvalho AC. Diagnosis of temporomandibular joint disorders: indication of imaging exams. Braz J Otorhinolaryngol. 2016;82(3):341–52. https://doi.org/10.1016/j.bjorl.2015.06.010.
23. De Leeuw R, Klasser GD. Orofacial pain: guidelines for ssessment, diagnosis, and management. Chicago: Quintessence; 2013.
24. Klasser GD, Goulet J-P, De Laat A, Manfredini D. In: Farah CS, Balasubramaniam R, McCullough MJ, editors. Classification of orofacial pain: Contemporary oral medicine a comprehensive approach to clinical practice. Berlin: Springer; 2017.
25. Dworkin SF, LeResche L. Research diagnostic criteria for temporomandibular disorders: review, criteria, examinations and specifications, critique. J Craniomandib Disord. 1992;6(4):301–55.
26. International RDC/TMD Consortium Network. International consensus workshop: convergence on an orofacial pain taxonomy [Internet] [cited 2018 April 25]. https://ubwp.buffalo.edu/rdc-tmdinternational.
27. Baumrind S, Frantz RC. The reliability of head film measurements. 1. Landmark identification. Am J Orthod. 1971 Aug;60(2):111–27.
28. Baumrind S, Frantz RC. The reliability of head film measurements. 2. Conventional angular and linear measures. Am J Orthod. 1971;60(5):505–17.
29. Oz U, Orhan K, Abe N. Comparison of linear and angular measurements using two-dimensional conventional methods and three-dimensional cone beam CT images reconstructed from a volumetric rendering program in vivo. Dentomaxillofac Radiol. 2011;40(8):492–500.
30. Swennen GR, Schutyser F, Barth EL, De Groeve P, De Mey A. A new method of 3-D cephalometry Part I: the anatomic Cartesian 3-D reference system. J Craniofac Surg. 2006;17(2):314–25.
31. Swennen GRJ, Barth EL, Schutyser F, De Groeve P, Lemaitre A. Three-dimensional (3-D) cephalometry, the basics for virtual planning. J Cranio Maxillofac Surg. 2004;32(Suppl 1):135.
32. Mozzo P, Procacci C, Tacconi A, Martini PT, Bergamo IA. A new volumetric CT machine for dental imaging based on the cone-beam technique: preliminary results. Eur Radiol. 1998;8:1558–64.
33. Ogura I. Magnetic resonance imaging characteristics of temporomandibular joint pain during opening and biting in patients with disc displacement. Oral Surg Oral Med Oral Pathol Oral Radiol Endodontol. 2006;102(5):669–72.
34. Manfredini D, Basso D, Arboretti R, Guarda-Nardini L. Association between magnetic resonance signs of temporomandibular joint effusion and disk displacement. Oral Surg Oral Med Oral Pathol Oral Radiol Endodontol. 2009;107(2):266–71.
35. Tasali N, Cubuk R, Aricak M, Ozarar M, Saydam B, Nur H, et al. Temporomandibular joint (TMJ) pain revisited with dynamic contrast-enhanced magnetic resonance imaging (DCE-MRI). Eur J Radiol. 2012;81(3):603–8.

36. Schmitter M, Gabbert O, Ohlmann B, Hassel A, Wolff D, Rammelsberg P, et al. Assessment of the reliability and validity of panoramic imaging for assessment of mandibular condyle morphology using both MRI and clinical examination as the gold standard. Oral Surg Oral Med Oral Pathol Oral Radiol Endodontol. 2006;102(2):220–4.
37. Emshoff R, Jank S, Bertram S, Rudisch A, Bodner G. Disk displacement of the temporomandibular joint: Sonography versus MR imaging. Am J Roentgenol. 2002;178:1557–62.
38. Ongole R, Panjrath N, Ahsan A, Pai MK. Temporomandibular joint arthrography an overview. Pakistan Oral Dent Jr. 2002;22(1):67–9.
39. Orhan K, Seki U, Rozylo-Kalinowska I. Diagnostic accuracy of magnetic resonance imaging and clinical signs of temporomandibular joint disorders: a 10-year research update review. Oral Radiol. 2017;33:81–91.

Anatomy of the Temporomandibular Joint

2

B. Ufuk Sakul, Burak Bilecenoglu, and Mert Ocak

2.1 Development of the Temporomandibular Joint

2.1.1 Ossification and Development of the Temporomandibular Joint

During the process of their development, the bones comprise a cartilaginous tissue or connective tissue (mesenchymal condensations, blastemas). There are two types of ossification. The desmal (intramembranous) ossification occurs via the transformation of the mesenchymal cells of the connective tissue into osteoprogenitor cells and osteoblasts directly (direct bone formation). In endochondral ossification, mesenchymal cells first differentiate into chondroblasts at sites which will become bones in the future and form the cartilage model, which is then replaced by the bony tissue in time (indirect bone formation) [1].

Osteogenesis (bone formation) includes the processes of immature (woven bone, fibrous bone, primary bone) and mature (lamellar bone, secondary bone) bone formation and the processes at the sites of bone growth. However, osteogenesis does not happen at every site on the skeleton simultaneously. It begins with the clavicula on the 2nd month of the embryologic development and ends with the closure of the epiphyseal plates of the long bones nearly at the age of 20 [1].

Electronic Supplementary Material The online version of this chapter (doi:10.1007/978-3-319-99468-0_2) contains supplementary material, which is available to authorized users.

B. U. Sakul
Medipol University, Faculty of Medicine, Department of Anatomy, Istanbul, Turkey

B. Bilecenoglu (✉)
Ankara University, Faculty of Dentistry, Department of Anatomy, Ankara, Turkey

M. Ocak
Hacettepe University, Faculty of Medicine, Department of Anatomy, Ankara, Turkey

I. Rozylo-Kalinowska, K. Orhan (eds.), *Imaging of the Temporomandibular Joint*, https://doi.org/10.1007/978-3-319-99468-0_2

Development of the skeletal system originates from paraxial mesoderm, somatic mesoderm, and neural crest. When the notochord and neural tube are formed, intraembryonic mesoderm located laterally to these structures thickens and forms paraxial mesoderm in two columns [2, 3]. At the end of the third week, paraxial mesoderm blocks become segmented, and these blocks are called somitomeres in the head region and somites from the occipital region toward the caudal region. Anteromedial part of a somite is called sclerotome, and dorsolateral part is called dermatomyotome [2, 3].

At the end of the 4th week, mesodermal cells generate the connective tissue called mesenchyme. Sclerotome cells are structures that are also capable of forming the mesenchyme. Mesenchymal cells can migrate and can transform into fibroblasts, chondroblasts, or osteoblasts. The majority of the mesoderm that gives shape to the bones in the cranium originates from neural crest and makes the bony and connective tissue components there. However, occipital somites and somitomeres constitute the majority of the roof of the cranium and the base [3].

Flat bones of the cranium are shaped by the direct differentiation of the mesenchyme at the dermis into the bone (intramembranous ossification). However, a significant majority of the bones are formed via the formation of hyaline cartilage by the mesenchymal cells and then the ossification of these models through endochondral ossification [3].

Temporomandibular joint (TMJ) is composed via adjoining of two joints. It is composed of a growth line between the mandible and os temporale and a secondary cartilage (developed from two distinct blastemas: temporal blastema and condylar blastema). The shape of the joint is directly affected by teeth development. Teeth development begins around the 40th day of the embryonic life, with the invagination of the epithelium of the oral cavity to the mesenchyme underneath it. Thus, epithelial bands in the shape of a "U" arise in the upper and lower jaws. These structures are generic dental bands. This close relation between two different embryonic tissues triggers a complex gradual genetic interaction and, as a result, enables tooth formation. In addition, not only the presence of teeth but also the biting pattern and occlusion affect the shape of the joint. TMJ is the last joint to begin its development in the 7th to 10th intrauterine week. At 12th week of intrauterine life, temporal blastema ossifies to form the mandibular fossa, and condylar blastema becomes the articular cartilage of the condyle forming two separate joint cavities [1].

2.1.2 Development of the Mandible

Viscerocranium, which comprises facial bones, develops from the first two pharyngeal arches. Original mesenchymes derive from the mesoderm, followed by the migration of the neural crest cells to the arches, which are the fundamental source of the connective tissue elements including the ligaments of the facial and oral regions and the cartilage and bone [2]. From the dorsal segment of the first pharyngeal arch, maxillary prominence arises. This prominence gives rise to the maxilla, zygomatic bone, and a portion of the temporal bone. The ventral portion of the first arch is known as the mandibular prominence and includes Meckel's cartilage. The mesenchyme surrounding this cartilage condenses and ossifies via membranous ossification, forming the mandible. This cartilage is lost after a period of time except for the sphenomandibular ligament. The muscles originating from the first pharyngeal arch (e.g., masticatory muscles) are innervated by the mandibular branch of the trigeminal nerve [3].

2.1.3 Development of the Joint Spaces

Joint development begins at week 6 and before the end of the 8th week; joints acquire the properties of the joints of an adult [2]. The limb buds come from a mesenchymal blastema consisting of the paraxial mesoderm on the trunk wall (somatopleura). The cells condense (precartilaginous blastema), giving rise to a premature skeleton with a cartilaginous structure [1]. In regions that will be transformed into joints, cells cluster more densely. During this process, joints arise in two forms, segmented and localized joints. Segmented joints are formed by making a gap in a preformed part of the skeleton. Localized joints are formed by the extension of two preformed pieces of skeleton toward each other. In the parts where they come into contact, initially, a mucosal sac is formed, which transforms into a joint space in time. In some joints, articular disc develops. TMJ is the best example of this kind of joint development [1, 4].

2.2 Anatomy of the Temporomandibular Joint

2.2.1 Classification and General Features of Joints

Joints are formed by the congregation of two or more bones, hold the bones together, and enable the muscle movement. Joint types can be classified into three main groups. In the fibrous and cartilaginous type of joints, space between adjacent bones is filled with solid connective tissue either fibrous tissue or cartilage. In fibrous joints (synarthrosis), which are known as immovable joints, connective tissue fills the gaps between the bones and tightly fixes the bones with no joint cavity. In cartilaginous joints (amphiarthroses), which are known as partially movable joints, the hyaline cartilaginous tissue is found between the articular surfaces. In some of the joints found in this group, the cartilaginous tissue between the articular surfaces can become ossified in time due to aging, and thus, these joints become immovable. Again, in joints of the symphysis group, which is a subgroup of this type of joints, a fibrocartilaginous articular disc is found, similar to some movable joints. The examples are pubic symphysis and intervertebral symphysis. The last group is the movable joints, synovial joints (diarthrosis) [5].

In synovial joints, articular surfaces contact each other but do not show structural continuity. Articular capsule surrounds articular surfaces and articular cavities, holding the articular surfaces together. This capsule structurally and functionally comprises two layers, which are an outer fibrous layer and inner synovial layer (synovial membrane). Fibrous layer is made of fibrous connective tissue and protects the joint from extraneous effects. Synovial layer lines the inner surface of the fibrous layer and is attached to it via loose connective tissue. However, it does not cover articular cartilage and articular disc or meniscus if present. The primary role of this membrane is to secrete synovial fluid and ensure its reabsorption. The articular cavity (joint space) is the potential cavity between the articular surfaces. There is a negative intra-articular pressure inside the articular cavity, which is the strongest factor that holds the joint together. The structures that connect the adjacent bones and maintain stability in the joints are called ligaments, and they are divided into two groups, extracapsular ligaments (external ligaments of the joint) and intracapsular ligaments (internal ligaments of the joint), depending on their relationship with the articular capsule. In some of the synovial-type joints, auxiliary structures called articular discs, meniscus, and labrum, which enable the compatibility of the articular surfaces, can be found. Articular disc is a fibrocartilaginous structure that is attached to the articular capsule and partially or completely divides articular cavity in two. In general, its middle part is thin, while its edges are thick and disc-shaped [6].

2.2.2 Temporomandibular Joint

TMJ is located on each side of the cranium. It is located anterior to the external acoustic meatus and posterosuperior to the masseter muscle. It is located between the mandible's condyle and the mandibular fossa and articular eminence of the temporal bone. This joint allows the mobility of the mandible for speech and mastication and is found in the skull base [4, 7–9]. TMJ takes role in food intake and breakdown and producing sound [1].

TMJ has some common features with the other joints in the human body. TMJ includes an articular disc that could be seen in some other joints in the human body. TMJ has bony articular surfaces, articular capsule, synovial membrane, and ligaments just like other joints. But TMJ has differences that make it special among other joints in the body. TMJ of each side is connected with a single mandible that necessitates the harmonic and coordinated function of each TMJ. Articular surfaces of TMJ are covered by fibrocartilage, while many other joints have hyaline cartilage. TMJ is the only joint in the human body to have a rigid endpoint of closure with the dental arches on each jaw contacting each other that is called occlusion. TMJ is the last joint to begin its development in the 7th to 10th intrauterine week from two distinct blastemas [4, 10, 11].

2.2.2.1 Bony Structures of the Temporomandibular Joint

Temporal Bone

Mandibular Fossa

Mandibular fossa in temporal bone has a concave shape, and its articular surface is larger than the condyle. Its deepest part is as thin as paper and is generally semitransparent, and this shows that although the fossa is an important bony structure involved in the TMJ, it is not a functionally stress-bearing part of the joint [1, 4]. Mandibular fossa is not totally involved in the TMJ. The articular surface of the mandibular fossa is located on the inferior aspect of the squamous part of temporal bone just anterior to the tympanic plate. The anterior part of the petrosquamous and petrotympanic fissures of the mandibular fossa participates in the joint. These two fissures thus create a ridge at the posterior border of the articular surface of the mandibular fossa known as the posterior articular ridge. The lateral pole of this posterior articular ridge is evident just anterior to the external acoustic meatus and is called as the postglenoid process. Medial border of the fossa narrows slightly and is bounded by a bony wall that is known as the entoglenoid process. Articular eminence, which has a convex structure, is found on the anterior of the mandibular fossa just at the lower edge of the zygomatic arch [4, 12, 13].

Articular Eminence

Articular eminence is the entire transverse bony bar that forms the root of the zygoma, which has a convex structure and is found on the anterior of the mandibular fossa [4, 12, 13]. This articular surface is traveled by the condyle and disc as they glide forward and backward in normal jaw movements. It forms an articular surface with a downward course, which is also called the slope of the eminence. The cartilage layer on articular eminence is especially thick, and here transmission of vectoral forces occurs via articular disc [1]. The articular eminence sometimes includes air-filled cavities called cellulae, just like the mastoid process of the temporal bone. While the degree of convexity of this prominence varies, it is important for the perpendicularity of the forward movement of the mandible [13]. Mandibular fossa and articular eminence form an articular surface in the shape of the letter S. The horizontal articular surface continuing anteriorly from the tip of the articular eminence is called as the preglenoid plane [1, 14].

Mandible

Mandibular Condyle

The part of the mandible that participates in the TMJ is mandibular condyle. From the anterior point of view, the condyle has a bipolar structure, comprising medial and lateral poles. The medial pole of the condyle is directed more posteriorly. Thus if the long axes of two condyles are extended medially, they meet at approximately in front of the foramen magnum forming an angle ranging between 145° and 160°. The articular surface of the condyle lies mostly on its anterosuperior aspect, facing the posterior slope of the articular eminence.

While the articular surface of the mandibular condyle is convex in all directions, it is wider mediolaterally (15–20 mm) than anteroposteriorly (8–10 mm) [13].

Other Mandibular Structures Related to the Temporomandibular Joint

Bone structure of the mandible and the robustness of os temporale compensate the load that arises during the joint movements. However, the primary structure that tolerates the load is the oblique line of the mandible, which is located at the anterior edge of mandibular ramus and arises from just underneath the coronoid process. The strain that arises due to the reciprocating contact of the teeth during mastication is conducted underneath to mandibular body and oblique line. Thus, the strain is distributed, and putting excessive load on the condyle is prevented [11].

2.2.2.2 Cartilage Structures of the Temporomandibular Joint

Articular Cartilage

In synovial joints, articular surfaces contact each other but do not show structural continuity. Articular surfaces are usually covered with a 2–5-mm-thick hyaline cartilage. This cartilage is called articular cartilage. If an articular disc is present between the articular surfaces, articular faces are generally covered with a fibrous cartilage rather than a hyaline cartilage. In general, all of the joints in the human body have a hyaline articular cartilage except sternoclavicular joint, acromioclavicular joint, and TMJ. Articular cartilage does not contain any blood vessels and nerves [10, 11].

Articular Disc

In some of the synovial-type joints, auxiliary cartilage structures called articular discs, meniscus, or labrum, which enable the compatibility of the articular surfaces, can be found. Articular disc is a fibrocartilaginous structure that is attached to the articular capsule and partially or completely divides articular cavity in two [11].

The disc is the most important anatomic structure of the TMJ, and it is a biconcave oval fibrous structure with a thin intermediate zone (avascular) and thick borders that prevent displacement of the disc during translation [6]. The disc is not a regular structure; anterior portion of the disc is approximately 2 mm thick, while the posterior portion is 3 mm thick. The intermediate portion of the disc is the thinnest part nearly 1 mm. The anterior part of articular disc attaches to the capsule with collagen fibers. Anterior to this attachment site, from the outer side of the capsule, tendinous fibers of superior head of the lateral pterygoid muscle attach [11]. The remaining large part of the muscle called as the inferior head of the lateral pterygoid muscle attaches to the pterygoid fovea of the mandible. Therefore, during the pulling forward of the mandibula by the lateral pterygoid muscle, the articular disc is pulled forward alongside the articular capsule [5]. The posterior band continues as the bilaminar zone (before the cartilaginous part of the external acoustic meatus; the part which the connective tissue is divided into two as upper and lower parts) and connects the disc to the capsule posteriorly [1, 15].

The disc acts as a cushion to absorb stress in the TMJ and divides the TMJ into two separate and functionally different cavities. So, if the contraction of the masticatory muscles increases (like in spasm), pressure acting on the disc will increase too. As a result of the increased pressure, integrity or structure of the disc could be destroyed. Or the disc will respond to this increased pressure by changing its position, which is called disc displacement. As a result of disc displacement, proper movement of the TMJ is affected that will result in temporomandibular disorders [4, 11].

Bilaminar Zone and Retrodiscal Tissue

The disc is connected to a region which shows dense vein and nerve terminations posteriorly and comprises loose connective tissue. This region is known as the retrodiscal tissue (retroarticular tissue). Superiorly and inferiorly, disc attaches to the retrodiscal tissue via two laminas, known as superior retrodiscal lamina and inferior retrodiscal lamina [11].

Superior retrodiscal lamina of the retrodiscal tissue is made of dense elastic fibers composed of elastin and extends from disc toward the back of the mandibular fossa and connects it to the tympanic part of temporal bone known as the postglenoid process. Superior retrodiscal lamina prevents slipping of the disc during excessive mouth opening [11, 13].

The inferior retrodiscal lamina is made of collagen fibers and connects the inferior edge of the disc to the condylar process of the mandible via the articular surface [11, 13]. Inferior retrodiscal lamina of the bilaminar zone attaches to the mandibular neck region with articular capsule and constitutes the posterior border of the inferior joint cavity. This region, which is made of tight collagen fibers, continues toward the posterior as a well-vascularized retroarticular plexus between each lamina. Due to the intra-articular negative pressure, venous plexus creates a pump mechanism as the mouth opens and closes, and this mechanism is important as it feeds the joint. Inferior retrodiscal lamina prevents excessive rotation of the disc over the condyle [1, 4].

When the mouth opens, inferior retrodiscal lamina relaxes, and superior retrodiscal lamina stretches. This process is reversed when the mouth closes [1].

Capsule

Capsule surrounds articular surfaces and articular cavities, holding the articular surfaces together. This capsule structurally and functionally comprises two layers, which are a fibrous membrane and synovial membrane. The fibrous membrane is made of fibrous connective tissue and protects the joint from extraneous effects. The synovial membrane covers all the intra-articular surfaces except the disc and articular cartilage and is attached to it via loose connective tissue [4].

The large superior part of the capsule, which is found in the loose connective tissue structure, is attached laterally to the articular surface of the mandibular fossa, anterolaterally to the articular eminence, and anteriorly to the preglenoid plane as the anterior pole and to the postglenoid process and posterior articular ridge as the posterior pole. The narrow inferior part adheres to the mandibular neck, to the superior part of the pterygoid fovea. The capsule is rather wider than the articular surfaces. This situation allows the mandibular condyle to slide forward easily during protraction [1, 5, 8, 16]. Posterior part of the capsule is longer and includes more elastic fibers than the other parts. Therefore, it does not restrict the forward movement of the condyle by extending while opening the jaw. This elasticity also helps to restore the mandibular condyle to its original position when closing the jaw

[14, 17]. On the anterior part of the capsule, there is an orifice which the superior head of the lateral pterygoid muscle passes to attach the anterior pole of the disc. The main task of the capsule is to limit the forward translation of the condyle and resist outward, inward, and downward tractions, which can lead to the dislocation of the joint [11]. The temporomandibular ligament (aka lateral ligament) reinforces the capsule from the lateral side. Capsule neighbors with the facial nerve laterally and auriculotemporal nerve medially [16]. Articular disc is connected to capsule both anteromedially and laterally [1].

Synovial Membrane and Synovial Fluid

Just like other joints in the human body, synovial membrane lines the inner surface of the fibrous membrane and is attached to it via loose connective tissue. However, it does not cover the articular cartilage and articular disc. The primary role of this membrane is to secrete synovial fluid and ensure its reabsorption. While most of the synovial fluid in the joint space comes from plasma by dialysis, a very small amount of synovial fluid (0.05 ml) is secreted by type A and B synoviocytes. Composition of the synovial fluid is nearly the same in all joints, with highly viscous hyaluronic acid and some free cells including mostly macrophages [1, 4, 10].

As the articular cavity is divided by the disc into two separate cavities, there are two synovial membranes: synovial membrane of the superior joint cavity and the synovial membrane of the inferior joint cavity. The former lines the fibrous membrane superior to the disc, and the latter lines the fibrous membrane inferior to the disc [17, 18]. The superior joint cavity contains an average of 1.2 ml, and the lower joint cavity contains 0.5–0.9 ml synovial fluid. Synovial fluid's role is to nourish the avascular tissues in the joint, lubricate the articular surfaces, and clear the tissue debris caused by normal wear and tear of the articulating surfaces. The amount of the synovial fluid is important for the arthroscopic examination of the joint [4, 15].

2.2.2.3 Ligaments of the Temporomandibular Joint

The structures that connect the bones are called ligaments, and they are divided into two groups, extracapsular ligaments (external ligaments of the joint) and intracapsular ligaments (internal ligaments of the joint), depending on their relationship with the capsule [11].

TMJ has three ligaments other than the joint capsule. These ligaments hold the joint together and restrict its movements [5]. The ligaments of the TMJ consist of collagen connective tissue, which is not elastic. They are structures that maintain the position of the mandible and play a passive role in the restriction of the movements of the joint [11, 13]. When the anatomical terminology is considered, TMJ has three ligaments: temporomandibular ligament, stylomandibular ligament, and sphenomandibular ligament. But when it comes to dental terminology, it is used to divide the ligaments of the TMJ as functional ligaments and accessory ligaments. Functional ligaments comprise the temporomandibular ligament, capsular ligament, and collateral ligaments, while the stylomandibular ligament, sphenomandibular ligament, and variable retinacular ligament are counted as accessory ligaments. And in the literature, a discomallear ligament and an anterior mallear ligament are considered as other ligaments of the TMJ [11, 13].

Temporomandibular Ligament (Lateral Ligament)

The temporomandibular ligament is attached to zygomatic arch and articular eminence superiorly. It narrows as it extends downward and posteriorly and adheres to the outer surface and posterior edge of the mandibular neck. It supports the capsule externally. The ligament's outer surface neighbors the parotid gland, and its inner surface neighbors the joint capsule [1, 4, 5, 19]. This protects the external acoustic meatus by preventing the mandibular condyle from going backward [16]. Temporomandibular ligament comprises two parts, outer oblique and inner horizontal [11].

The outer oblique part begins from the external surface of the articular eminence and zygomatic process of the temporal bone and extends posteriorly and downward to the mandibular neck via the inferior part of the condyle. The outer oblique part restricts the movement of the opening of the jaw, which is performed in the rotational direction, by inhibiting the excessive forward movement of the condyle [11, 13, 15].

The inner horizontal part is narrower and shorter, begins from the outer surface of articular eminence and zygomatic process of the temporal bone and extends horizontally toward the back, and is attached laterally to the condyle. It prevents the posterior movement of the condyle and articular disc, preventing the retrodiscal tissue from trauma [4, 15, 18, 20]. The inner horizontal part also functions to prevent the extension and stretching of the lateral pterygoid muscle [13].

Sphenomandibular Ligament

Sphenomandibular ligament remains medial to the capsule and is detached from the articular capsule [4, 16, 18]. This ligament, derived from the perichondrium of Meckel's cartilage of the first pharyngeal arch, is attached superiorly to the spine of the sphenoid bone (spina ossis sphenoidalis) that is lateral to the spinous foramen, expands while extending downward, and adheres to the lingula of the mandible. Its outer surface neighbors the lateral pterygoid muscle, and inner surface neighbors the medial pterygoid muscle [5, 17–19]. It is crossed by chorda tympani at the region close to its superior tip [16]. Between the sphenomandibular ligament and neck of the mandible, maxillary artery, maxillary vein, and inferior alveolar neurovascular bundle pass [5, 16]. The main function of this ligament is to prevent the effect of an extra pressure during the opening and closing of the jaw on the inferior alveolar neurovascular bundle that passes through the mandibular canal [20]. Moreover, throughout its course, this ligament is perforated by the mylohyoid neurovascular bundle. Although the tonus of the masticatory muscles carries the weight of the mandible with an active support, this ligament also provides primary passive support to the mandible [16]. Although it does not have a direct connection to the capsule, due to its position, this ligament restricts the extent of jaw opening [1, 4]. This ligament is connected to the anterior mallear ligament, which is another remnant of Meckel's cartilage [4, 8].

Stylomandibular Ligament

It is a segment of deep cervical fascia, thickened into a band shape. It extends from styloid process to the inferior of the posterior edge of the mandibular ramus and mandibular angle. Stylomandibular ligament passes between the masseter muscle and medial pterygoid muscle throughout its course. Moreover, it is found between the parotid gland and submandibular gland [4, 5, 17–19]. Stylomandibular ligament restricts the excessive protrusive movement of the mandible and supports the temporomandibular ligament [13, 15].

Other Ligaments Related to the Temporomandibular Joint

A medial ligament, which is a variation, extends from the inner edge of te mandibular fossa to the neck of the mandible and supports the joint capsule from the inner side if present [1, 12]. It is considerably weaker and much thinner than the temporomandibular ligament. As it has fused well with joint capsule, it can sometimes go unnoticed [17].

In addition to the ligaments listed above, another ligament related to TMJ has been defined in the literature. Another variable ligament, which is named as retinacular ligament, is approximately 5 cm long and 2 cm wide, is between the parotid gland and mandibular ramus, and extends from the top to the bottom. Actually, it is defined as a thickening of the fascia of the masseter muscle. Its course begins in the superior by adhering to the anterior and posterior surfaces of the articular eminence, cartilaginous part of the external acoustic meatus, posterior tip of the lateral pterygoid muscle, outer segment of the temporomandibular ligament, mandibular condyle, and retrodiscal tissue at the posterior side and becomes narrower as it descends and ends when it attaches to the fascia of the masseter muscle at the level of mandibular angle. Retinacular ligament conducts the strain generated during the contraction of the masseter muscle to the retrodiscal tissue and TMJ [11, 21].

Besides these ligaments, in the dental literature, the joint capsule itself is named as a capsular ligament and collateral ligaments are present. Collateral (discal) ligaments are the ligaments between lateral and medial borders of the disc and poles of the mandibular condyle. These are short collagen fibers that restrict rotational movements in lower joint space, and these ligaments ensure that the disc and condyle move together in protraction and retraction [11].

2.2.2.4 Muscles Related to Temporomandibular Joint Function

Muscles of the masticatory system are the masseter muscle, temporal muscle, pterygoid muscles (medial pterygoid muscle and lateral pterygoid muscle), suprahyoid muscles (digastric muscle, mylohyoid muscle, stylohyoid muscle), and some other head and neck muscles. Head and neck muscles are not directly related to the chewing function [22].

Masticatory muscles derive from the second pharyngeal arch and named as masseter muscle, temporalis muscle, lateral pterygoid muscle, and medial pterygoid muscle. All these masticatory muscles are innervated by the mandibular nerve and its branches. In addition to these muscles, suprahyoid muscles, infrahyoid muscles, sternocleidomastoid muscle, and posterior neck muscles play roles in the stabilization of the mandible and control of mandibular movements, although they do not have direct roles in the chewing function [11].

The masseter muscle is a rectangle-shaped muscle that mainly originates from the zygomatic arch and adheres to the lateral part of the inferior edge of the mandibula. It has superficial and deep fibers. While the superficial fibers extend downward and slightly to the posterior, deep fibers extend vertically. When the masseter muscle contracts, it lifts the mandibula upward and is a strong muscle that provides the required strength for efficient chewing. Its superficial branch also helps the protrusion of the mandible [7, 13, 23].

Temporal muscle is a fan-shaped, broad muscle. It originates from the temporal fossa and lateral surface of the skull and passes through the zygomatic arch and adheres to the coronoid process. Depending on the direction of the fibers, it is classified into three parts: anterior, medial, and posterior parts. When the temporal muscle contracts as a whole, it lifts the mandibula upward. When the anterior part is contracted, the mandibula lifts up vertically; when the medial part is contracted, the mandibula moves upward and backward; and when the posterior part is contracted, the mandible moves backward (retrusion) [13, 20].

Medial pterygoid muscle originates from the inner surface of the lateral pterygoid plate and adheres to the pterygoid tuberosity at the medial surface of the mandibular angle. When it contracts, it protrudes the mandible and lifts the mandibula upward. Unilateral contraction of this muscle brings the mandible into a mediotrusive position [13, 20].

Lateral pterygoid muscle has two heads as inferior head and superior head with two different functions. Inferior head starts from the outer surface of the lateral pterygoid plate and adheres to the condyle neck [4]. When contracted bilaterally, condyles are pulled downward, toward articular eminence, and the mandible becomes protruded. Unilateral contraction causes the condyle to move mediotrusively and the mandibula to move laterally in the opposite direction. When this muscle contracts together with the depressor muscles, the mandibula moves downward, and condyles move forward and downward on the articular eminence; thus lateral pterygoid muscle is highlighted as the only muscle that opens the jaw [11].

The superior head is smaller than the inferior head. It starts from the infratemporal surface of the sphenoid bone and adheres to the joint capsule, disc, and condyle. When this muscle contracts, it pulls the disc anteromedially. It is inactive during the downward movement of the mandible, which is the opening of the jaw. It is active when it contracts together with the elevator muscles, particularly when power is exerted as the teeth are closing, so it helps joint stability during closure [13, 20].

2.2.2.5 Blood Supply and Innervation of the Temporomandibular Joint

The blood supply to the TMJ is only responsible for superficial structures of the joint, and there is no blood supply inside the capsule. The avascular structures inside the capsule are supplied by the synovial fluid. The arteries that supply the

TMJ mainly derive from the superficial temporal artery and maxillary artery, which are the terminal branches of the external carotid artery [5, 8]. The main artery of the joint is the articular branch of the superficial temporal artery. In addition to this artery, TMJ is supplied by the ascending pharyngeal branch of the external carotid artery; deep auricular, anterior tympanic, and middle temporal branches of the maxillary artery; and transverse facial branch of the superficial temporal artery. The veins of the TMJ are named the same as the arteries [1, 11, 15]. A special venous structure called retroauricular plexus assists the drainage of the veins [1]. Lymphatic vessels of the TMJ drain to superficial and deep parotid nodes [4, 11].

While considering the innervation of any joint in the human body, "Hilton's law" is accepted as a rule. "Hilton's law" is the principle that the nerve supplying a joint also supplies both the muscles that move the joint and the skin covering the articular insertion of those muscles. Therefore the TMJ is mainly innervated by the auriculotemporal nerve and masseteric nerve, which are the branches of mandibular branch of the trigeminal nerve [4, 5, 8, 17, 24, 25]. The TMJ is mainly innervated by the articular branch of the auriculotemporal nerve [11]. Auriculotemporal nerve, its articular branch, and masseteric nerve innervate the joint capsule laterally, dorsally, and medially. Deep temporal nerves and articular branches that arise from the nerve to lateral pterygoid innervate the joint capsule from the anterior, whereas the branches of facial nerve innervate the temporomandibular ligament. Articular branches of the otic ganglion found just below the oval foramen are responsible for the parasympathetic innervation of the synovial membrane and its synovial fluid secretion [1, 4]. Capsule, temporomandibular ligament, and retrodiscal tissue include mechanoreceptors (Ruffini corpuscles and Pacinian corpuscles) and nociceptors (free nerve endings) that are highly sensitive. Ruffini corpuscles and Pacinian corpuscles are limited to the capsule, and these mechanoreceptors are related to the position of the mandible and acceleration of mandibular movements during reflexes. Golgi tendon organs are confined to the ligaments and responsible for the sense of proprioception from the joint. Impulses originated from all these receptors help to control the dynamic and static balance, posture, and movements of the mandible [4].

Temporomandibular ligament and the tissue surrounding the joint are innervated very well. In young individuals, the entire disc has sensory innervation, while in older individuals, only the parts that adhere to the joint capsule are innervated. This is the main cause of the severe pain that arises in the functional disorders of the TMJ in young individuals [1].

2.2.2.6 Relations of the Temporomandibular Joint

The thin roof of the mandibular fossa is as thin as paper (0.2–4 mm) and neighbors the middle cranial fossa at the superior. The course of the maxillary artery and its proximal branches is found just medial to the joint capsule. This part of the maxillary artery is named as the mandibular part of the artery and has four branches here: deep auricular artery, anterior tympanic artery, middle meningeal artery, and inferior alveolar artery. Its most important branch here is the middle meningeal artery which is just located in the medial part of the joint [4]. Auriculotemporal nerve and chorda tympani are also medial to the joint capsule. The masseteric artery from the second part of the maxillary artery passes through the mandibular notch in front of the mandibular neck, below the articular eminence. The frontal and zygomatic branches of the facial nerve which innervate the muscles of facial expression in the superior aspect of the face, auriculotemporal nerve, and superficial temporal vessels are located laterally to the joint capsule and are important in the surgery of the TMJ. Superior part of the infratemporal fossa, which includes both heads of the lateral pterygoid muscle, is anteromedial to the mandibular condyle. In the posterior part, the condyle is in close relationship with the parotid gland and external acoustic meatus. Between these two lies a well-vascularized retrodiscal tissue [10, 11].

2.2.2.7 Anatomy-Related Disorders of the Temporomandibular Joint

Of course, the following chapters will give detailed information about temporomandibular disorders (TMDs). But here, we will give a brief summary of only the anatomy-related disorders of the TMJ [13].

TMDs, as defined by the American Academy of Orofacial Pain, is a term that includes the problems caused by joints and masticatory muscles and all of the functional disorders of the masticatory system [13]. This term describes musculoarticular disorders that are characterized by the symptoms such as pain in the orofacial area, restriction in mouth opening, sense of fatigue in the masticatory muscles, and sounds in TMJ [26]. While TMDs are observed at least once in the three-fourths of the population, only 34% of these are reported [27, 28]. TMDs are more commonly observed in women [15].

TMDs have many inexplicable causes. The joint properties should be recognized more extensively so that the etiology of these disorders can be explained. Anatomically detailed examination of the joint structure will be of great benefit in the design of surgical procedures and implants to be used in the treatment [27, 28].

In occlusion defects, in cases where lower and upper jaw incompatibility is detected or there is tooth loss, inappropriate vectoral forces could affect the TMJ. In these cases, degeneration of the joint cartilage and disc can be frequently observed. These degenerative changes (osteoarthrosis) are often accompanied by defects (perforations) in the lateral region of the articular disc. The causes of osteoarthritis include physiological abrasion, trauma, and bruxism, and the clinical appearance may change from mild to severe [1, 13].

The TMJ can also be affected by all diseases that have symptoms regarding joints, such as rheumatic diseases. For example, half of the patients with rheumatoid arthritis have symptoms related to TMJ. For this reason, the TMDs should be evaluated for the diagnosis of rheumatic diseases [13].

Especially in elderly individuals, central fracture of mandibular fossa toward the middle cranial fossa may occur. In all of the diseases related to the TMJ, pain is frequently reflected to the external ear [1, 15, 29]. Some authors mention that if the patient has unilateral pain, it is often originated from the ear diseases, and if the patient has bilateral pain, it is often originated from the joint [12].

In individuals with laxity in TMJ ligaments and capsule or low articular eminence, excessive contraction of the lateral pterygoid muscle causes the joint heads to slide away from the articular eminence resulting in a dislocation. The same thing could also occur when the mouth is opened excessively during yawning and biting [1, 10, 30]. When the joint dislocations are examined, in dislocations of the mandibular condyle toward the anterior direction, the disc slides forward with the condyle and gets ahead of the articular eminence [12, 19]. In these cases, the patient's mouth remains open to the full extent and cannot be closed even if the patient wants to [10, 15, 19]. This could occur in other cases like retroarticular hematoma due to falling on the lower jaw or getting stuck at the lower jaw or infections of the parotid gland [1]. It can also be caused by the excessive opening of the jaw during tooth extraction. It is often bilateral [14]. The most common dislocation of TMJ occurs on the side of the strike, as a result of the pressure from the lateral side when the mouth is in the open position. The TMJ dislocations may also be associated with mandibular fractures. These types of dislocations usually appear as the dislocation of the jaw in the lateral direction. Posterior dislocation of the TMJ is not seen because of the anatomical structure of the temporomandibular ligament and mandibular fossa [10, 12, 18, 19]. As a result of falling on the jaw or direct trauma to the jaw, usually, fracture of the mandibular neck is seen before the dislocation occurs. In these cases, due to the bleeding from the venous plexus in the retromandibular tissue, mouth opening is restricted [1]. Care should be taken during surgical interventions because of the close relation of the facial nerve and the auriculotemporal nerve with the joint, and the anatomy of the region should be well known. In addition, in dislocations of the TMJ and in ruptures of the articular capsule or temporomandibular ligament, as a result of the damage to the fibers of the auriculotemporal nerve related to the joint, laxity and weakness could be seen [10, 14, 18].

The shape of articular surfaces; the shape, position, and integrity of the teeth; occlusion; and masticatory muscles and their innervation comprise the craniomandibular system. This system also affects movements in the joint. Missing teeth or malocclusion defects in this system cause movement disorders in the TMJ [1].

In cases of arthritis of the TMJ, anatomical problems such as malocclusion or sounds in the joint may be observed as a result of the functional disorder of the TMJ. Sounds heard from the joint are especially the results from the altered relation between the disc and condyle when opening and closing the mouth [10, 12, 18, 30]. The radiological appearance of the first stage of the TMJ disease is reduced joint cavity without any changes in bones. In the late stage, narrowed joint cavity is observed together with the bone changes, which possibly include ankylosis [15].

The congenital anomalies affecting the TMJ include the hypoplasia of the condyle, as well as hypertrophia of the coronoid process or hyperplasia of the mandibular condyle. In the coronoid process hypertrophies, if this process is compressed under zygomatic arch, this may restrict jaw movements [29].

2.3 Biomechanics of the Temporomandibular Joint

Biomechanics of the TMJ comprises a complex combination activity. In order to maintain a perfect movement, both joints on each side must function together. Another issue about the TMJ is that there are two different joints (mentioned below) in one joint system. As will be described later, while the opening of the jaw until interincisal distance is up to 20–25 mm, only rotational movement occurs in the inferior joint cavity (discomandibular joint). Especially when opening the jaw more than 25 mm of interincisal distance, the condyle must leave the mandibular fossa to front over the articular eminence. This movement of the joint is called translation, and it occurs in the superior joint cavity (discotemporal joint) [1, 11].

2.3.1 Condyle Position

Since the coordinated movement of the condyle and disc together complicates the movement of the TMJ, an axis of movement in this joint cannot be mentioned. If the jaw is pulled excessively forward, the condyle is aligned below the articular eminence at the front. Thus, since the jaw will be pushed as low as the height of the eminence, it can be opened slightly more. However, in order to open the jaw completely, hyoid muscles should also contract [1, 11, 17].

2.3.2 Effect of Occlusion to the Temporomandibular Joint

The way the teeth fit together directly affects the TMJ and related components. When all teeth are present and there is a stable occlusion between them, maximum necessary support is maintained for muscles and mastication and TMJ. If there is missing teeth or poor occlusion, different and asymmetrical vectoral forces could be exerted to the TMJ leading to instability, damage, degeneration, or TMDs [13].

2.3.3 Force Vectors

During the mandibular movements, the joint disc placed between the glenoid fossa and condyle plays an important role as a stress absorber, reducing the stress in the joint and causing it to be redistributed [11].

Even when maximum chewing pressure is applied on the occlusal surfaces, not a lot of load is placed on TMJ within the mandibular fossa. This is because the load, created by occlusal forces, is transferred from teeth to the cranium [1].

Although the stability of the TMJ is maintained by many factors, TMJ displacement is not a rare condition. Stability of the TMJ is maintained by masticatory muscles (active stabilization of the TMJ is maintained by masticatory muscles), occlusion, ligaments related with the TMJ (passive stabilization of the TMJ is maintained by sphenomandibular ligament), and the position of the disc and condyle with the intra-articular pressure as the most important factor [1, 11].

2.3.4 Physiology of Jaw Motion

The mandible can move upward (elevation), downward (depression), forward (protraction), and backward (retraction). In addition to those movements, the condyle makes a rotational movement on the inferior surface of the disc [5, 15]. This movement is made around the longitudinal axis passing through the center of the condyle [8]. During the opening of the jaw, the condyle slides forward together with the disc and reaches the lower level of the articular eminence. While the forward sliding movement continues, the condyle also rotates at the bottom surface of the disc [5].

TMJ allows movement in all three axes. Because of its shape, it is a bicondylar type of joint between two condyles of the mandible and temporal bones of each side [1]. So actually there are two TMJs on each side, working in unison. On the other hand, the mandible is the only bone in the body that is not capable of independent movement on one end [11].

In general bicondylar type of synovial joints has only two examples in the body: one is the TMJ and the other is knee joint. In this type of joints, the main action in the joint is flexion and extension, while these joints are capable of rotational movements [16].

TMJ can be considered as two distinct joints, one located between the disc and temporal bone (discotemporal joint, superior joint) and the other located between the disc and condyle (discomandibular joint, inferior joint). Usually, the discotemporal joint is involved in sliding movement, whereas discomandibular joint is involved in slight opening and closing movement around the transverse axis [1, 11, 17, 20]. Since the mandible is a single bone, joints of both sides cannot move independently (biomechanical connection). This allows very complicated movements to be made [1, 11].

During the opening of the jaw, the movement is first observed in the discomandibular joint. Then, the function of discotemporal joint begins as the disc slides forward together with the condyle. The disc moves forward until the posterosuperior fibroelastic fibers reach their limit. When the jaw is closed, these fibroelastic fibers are responsible for pulling the disc back to its original position. When the disc reaches the anterior edge of articular eminence, it starts to go forward and downward. In this position, the jaw is excessively open. When the disc is pulled forward, the joint capsule also moves with it. Loose connective tissue (retrodiscal tissue) located between the capsule and external auditory meatus fills the arising cavity [4, 10, 11].

The masticatory muscle that plays the main role in the forward movement of the condyle with the disc is the lateral pterygoid muscle. So, when the lateral pterygoid muscle initiates the opening movement of the jaw, the jaw is actually opened by inhibition of other masticatory muscles, gravity, and help of some other muscles (geniohyoid muscle, mylohyoid muscle, anterior belly of digastric muscle, and platysma) [11, 18, 19, 24]. The axis of this movement passes through the mandibular foramen. This is why the inferior alveolar neurovascular bundle is never affected by so many mandibular movements [1]. During rest, the teeth in the upper and lower jaws are located slightly away from each other. They come into contact with each other when the jaw is closed (occlusion). The closing of the jaw is enabled by contractions of temporal muscle, masseter muscle, and medial pterygoid muscle against gravity and inhibitions of the muscles related to jaw opening. Especially during the withdrawal of the jaw to mandibular fossa, anterior fibers of temporal muscle are contracted in particular and ensure that the condyle is fully settled into the mandibular fossa [11].

When inferior heads of lateral pterygoid muscles of each side contract, this results in total movement of mandible anteriorly with the sliding of condyles of each side over articular eminence. This type of motion is called protrusion, while the reverse is called retrusion. Retrusion of the mandible is mainly made by contractions of the middle and posterior fibers of the temporal muscle supported by deep part of the masseter muscle and geniohyoid and digastric muscles [1, 13].

In addition to these movements, the mandible makes rotational movements to right and left, which is known as the lateral excursions (grinding movement). In this movement, while the joint of one side makes forward sliding movement, the joint of the other side makes a rotational movement around the vertical axis. These movements continue by alternating the sides. In lateral excursions, inferior head of the lateral pterygoid muscle is active in particular, and middle and posterior fibers of the temporal muscle are also active during lateral excursions [1, 4].

During biting with incisors, some of the muscular strain is transferred on the incisors, while some are transferred on the condyle. However, during chewing using molars, the majority of the strain is on the teeth. Here, the condyle only acts as a guide to regulate the movement [11, 17].

All these movements that arise due to the function of the masticatory muscles are known as mastication [16]. Mastication is made of asymmetrical movements, combined translational and rotational movements. Protraction and retraction movements of the mandible begin at discotemporal part of the TMJ and are managed by the dental arches. For this reason, dental deformities and occlusion defects affect the course of movement in the TMJ. Mediotrusion and laterotrusion (translational movements toward the medial and lateral) movements are also managed by dental arches. The condyle of one side rotates around a vertical axis within the mandibular fossa, the condyle of the opposite side moves forward on the articular eminence, and the opposing semiarches on this side are separated from each other [1].

Mastication begins at the side of the rotation (active side, laterotrusion side) with the movement of mandible against the maxilla. The other side of the mandible that moves together is contralateral balance side (mediotrusion side). In this side, the translational movements of the condyle are observed [1].

2.3.5 Age-Related Anatomic Changes in the Temporomandibular Joint

As in all structures in the human body, age-related changes occur in the TMJ. As the age increases, the condyle becomes more flattened, the capsule becomes thicker, the structure of the disc changes, and sometimes osteoporosis of the underlying bone is seen. The disc of the TMJ becomes thinner, and internal changes are seen in the histologic structure. In addition, as the age increases, nerves of the TMJ decrease in number [11].

These age-related changes lead to a decrease in synovial fluid formation and decrease the resilience during mastication and structural changes in the cartilage tissue [4].

2.4 Dissection of the Temporomandibular Joint

Figure 2.1 a/b
Figure 2.2 a/b
Figure 2.3 a/b
Figure 2.4 a/b/c/d
Figure 2.5 a/b
Figure 2.6 a/b
Figure 2.7 a/b
Figure 2.8 a/b
Figure 2.9 a/b
Figure 2.10 a/b
Figure 2.11 a/b
Figure 2.12 a/b
Figure 2.13 a/b

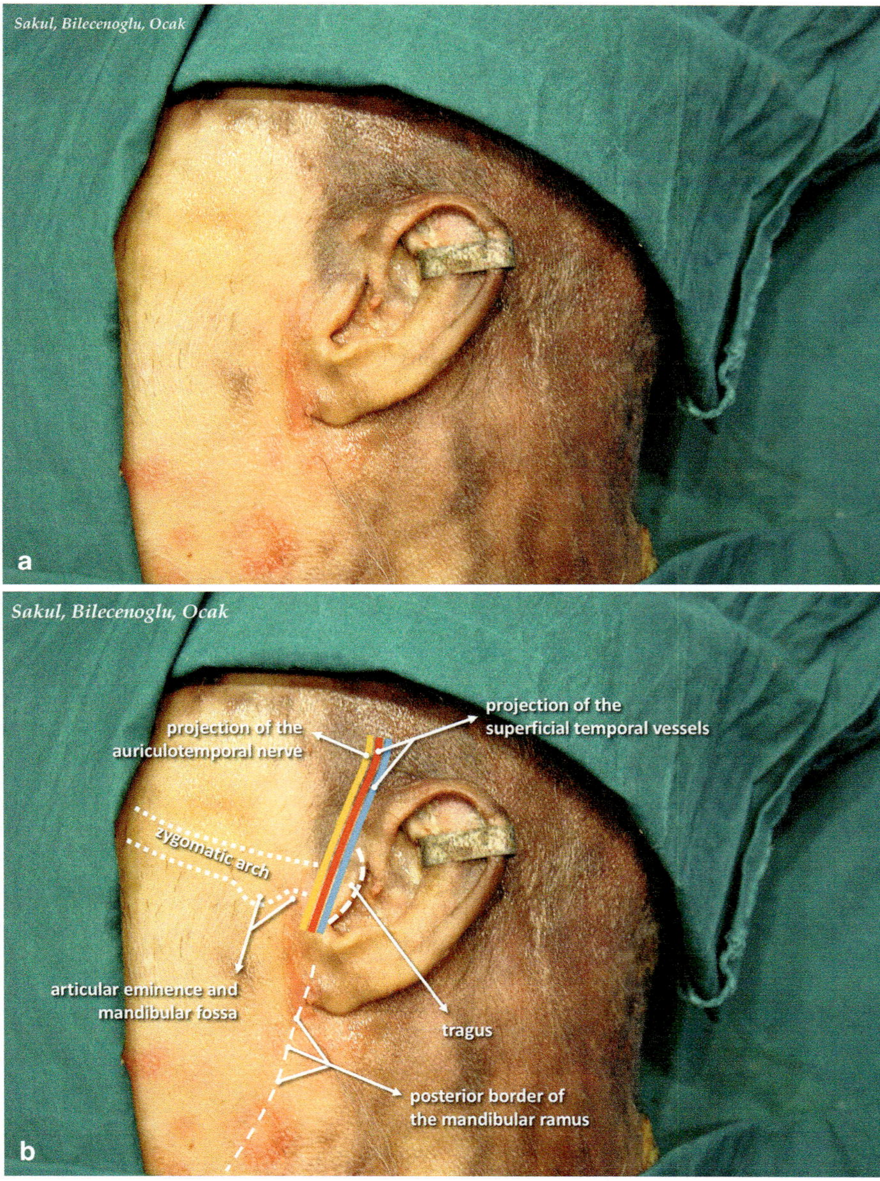

Fig. 2.1 (**a**) Left side of 67-year-old male cadaver before dissection. (**b**) Main landmarks about the TMJ

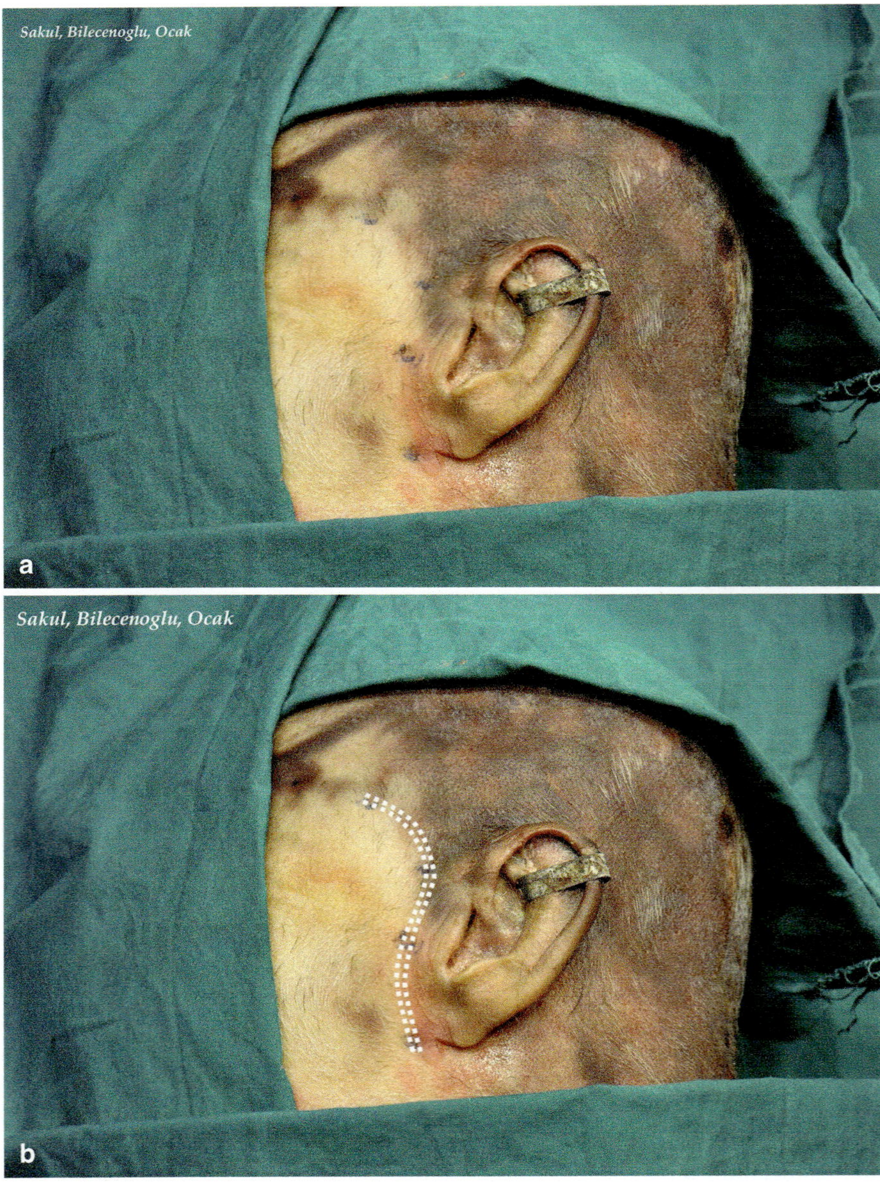

Fig. 2.2 Guide for surgical incision

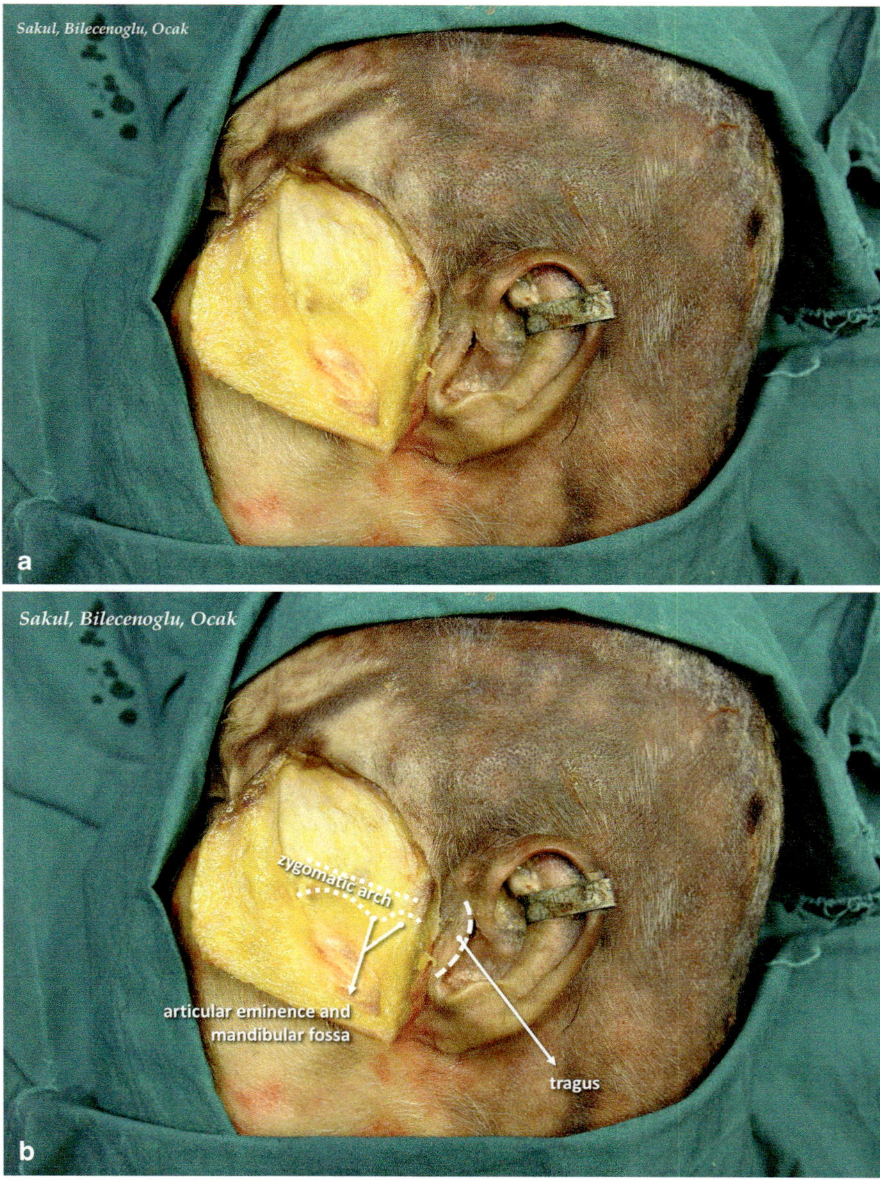

Fig. 2.3 (**a**) Left side after first incision. (**b**) Tragus and projection of some anatomic landmarks after the first incision

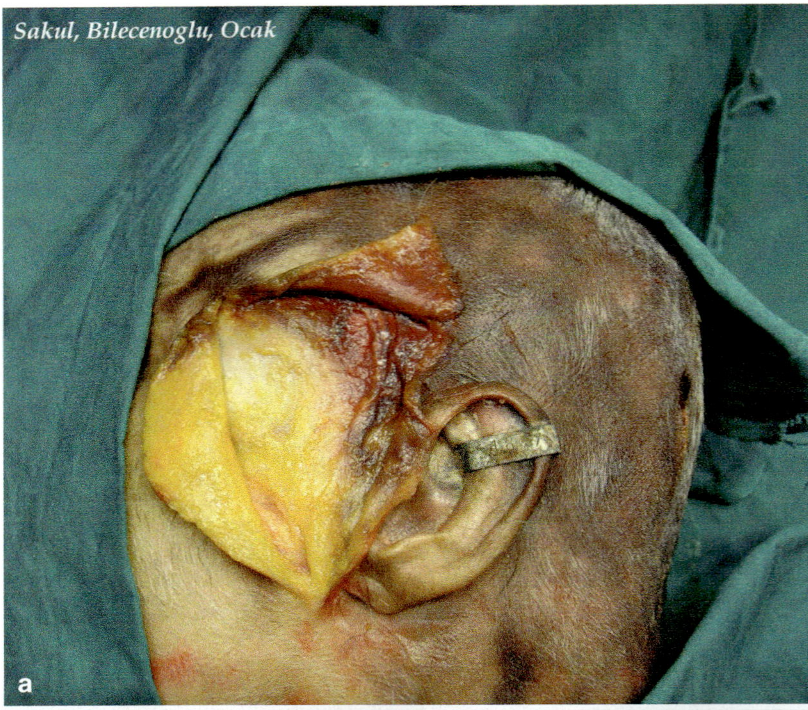

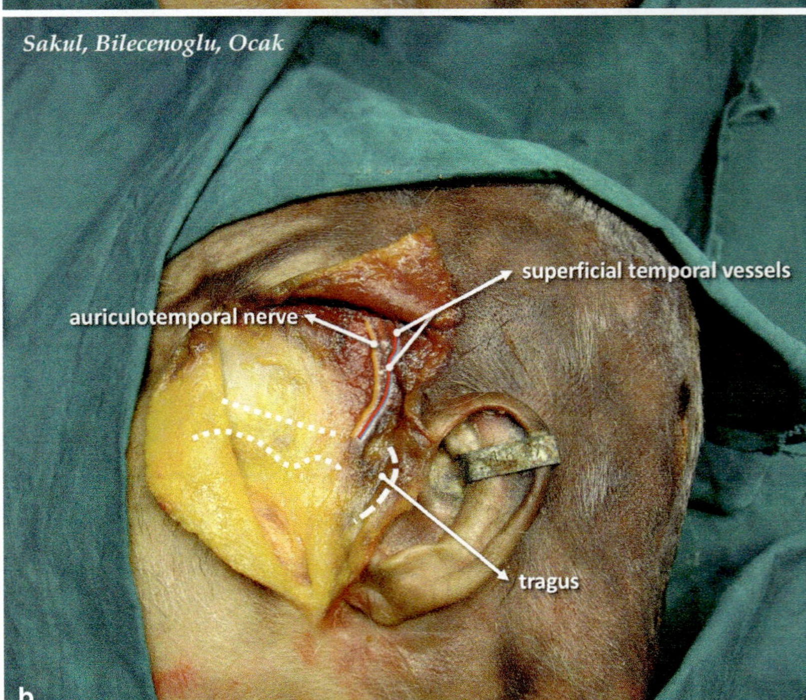

Fig. 2.4 (**a**, **b**) Left side after the additional incisions to point out the auriculotemporal nerve and the superficial temporal vessels, tragus is tilted posteriorly for a better view. (**c**, **d**) Auriculotemporal nerve and superficial temporal vessels are highlighted

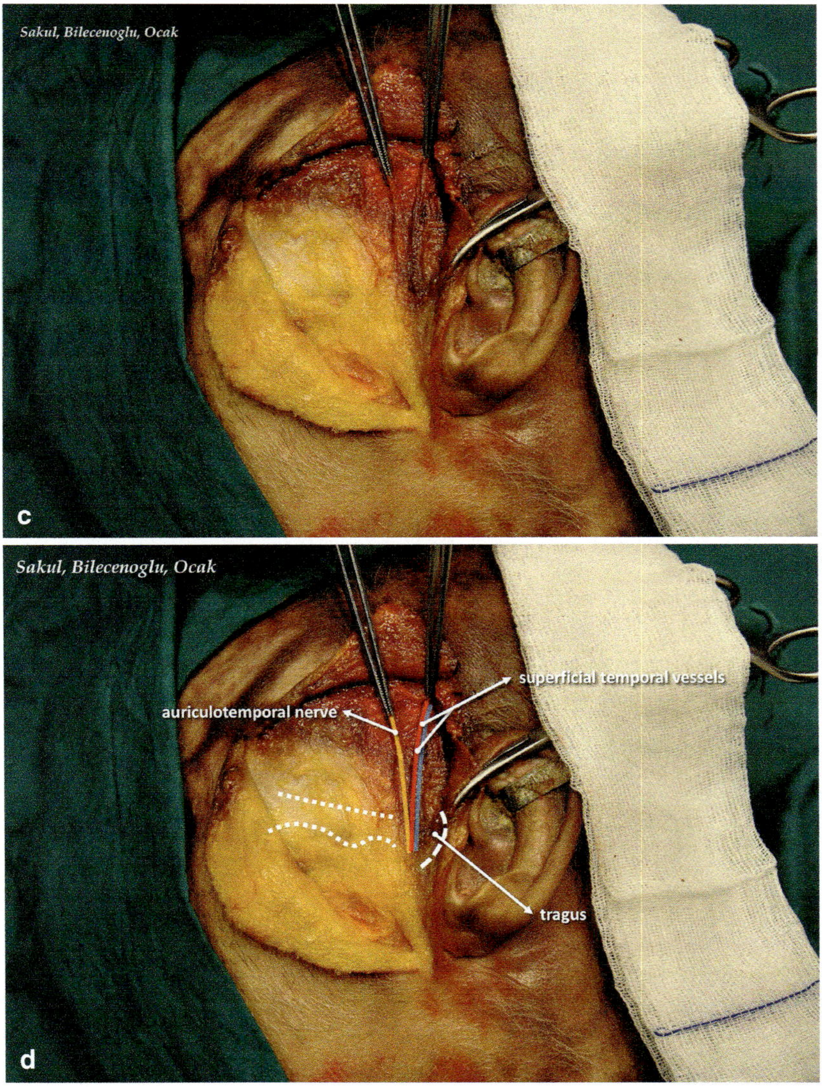

Fig. 2.4 (continued)

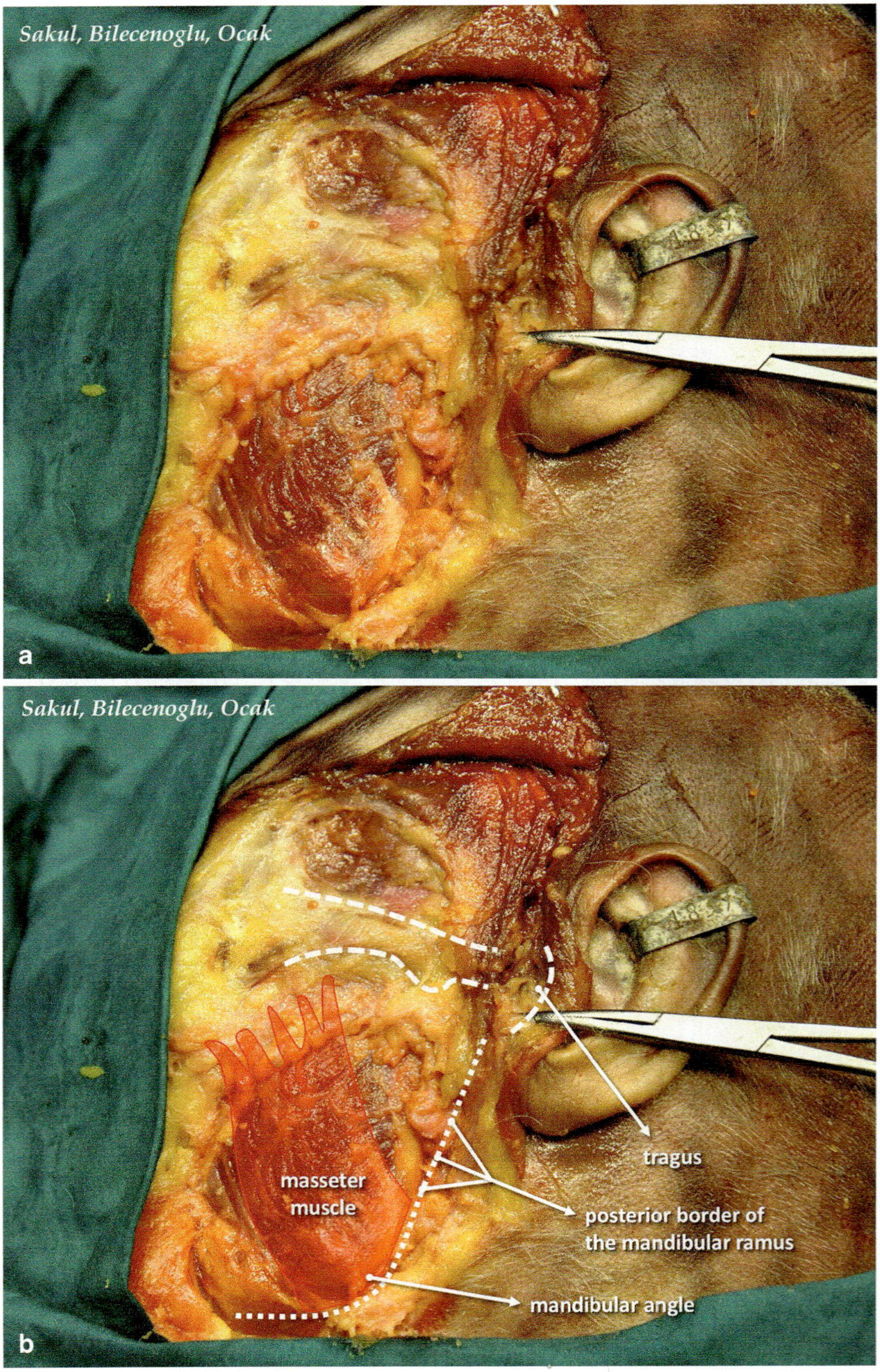

Fig. 2.5 (**a**) Left side after extended dissection, parotid gland is removed to reveal the masseter muscle. (**b**) Landmarks in this layer

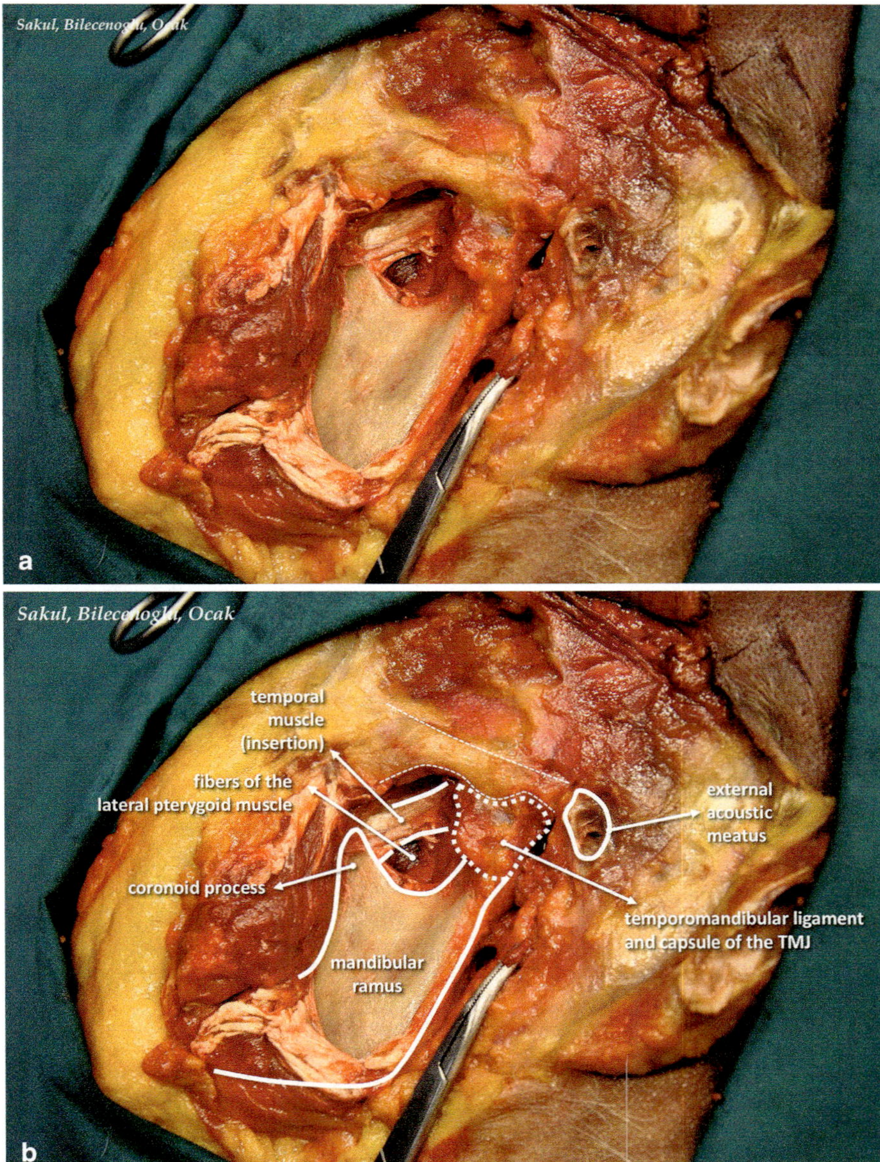

Fig. 2.6 (**a**) Left side after deeper dissection, the masseter muscle is removed to reveal the mandible, and the auricle is flipped backward for a better view. (**b**) Anatomic structures in this layer

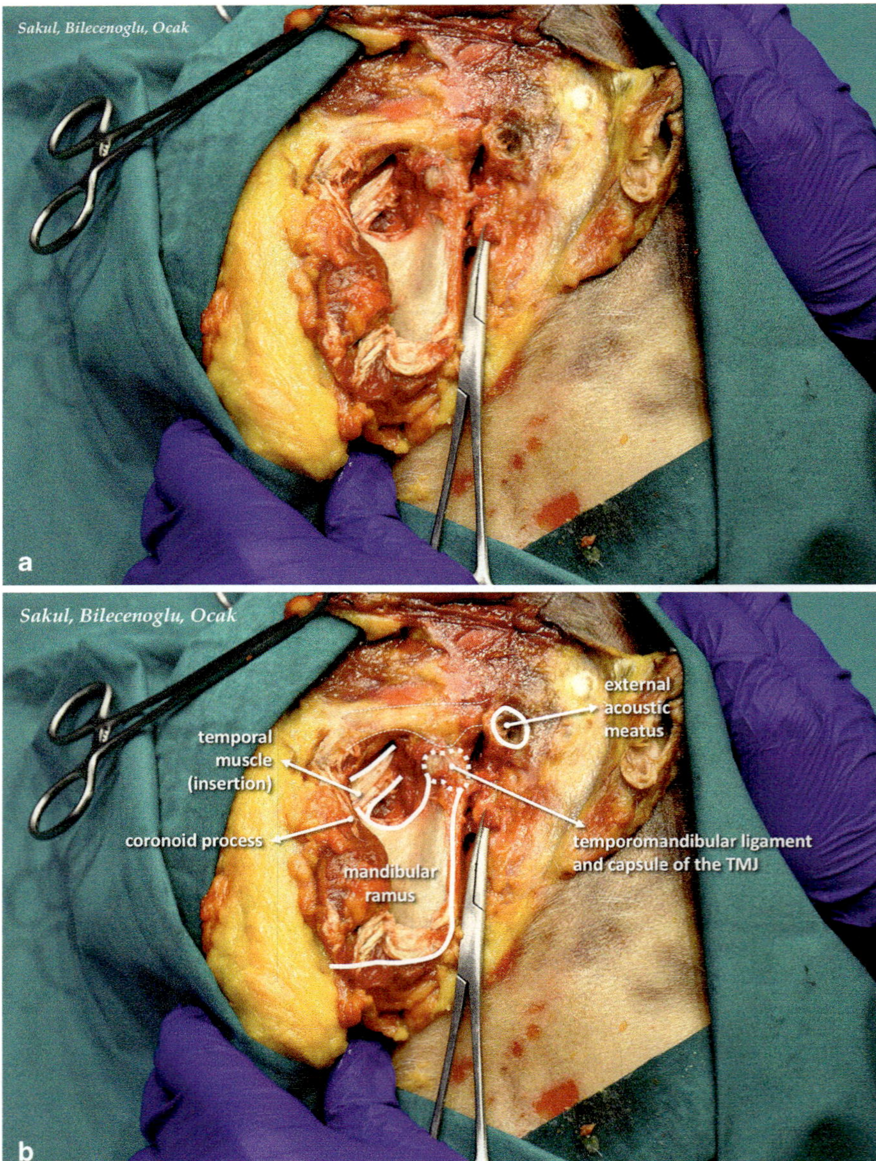

Fig. 2.7 (**a**) The same plane of Fig. 2.6, left side after deeper dissection, mouth opened. (**b**) Anatomic structures in this layer

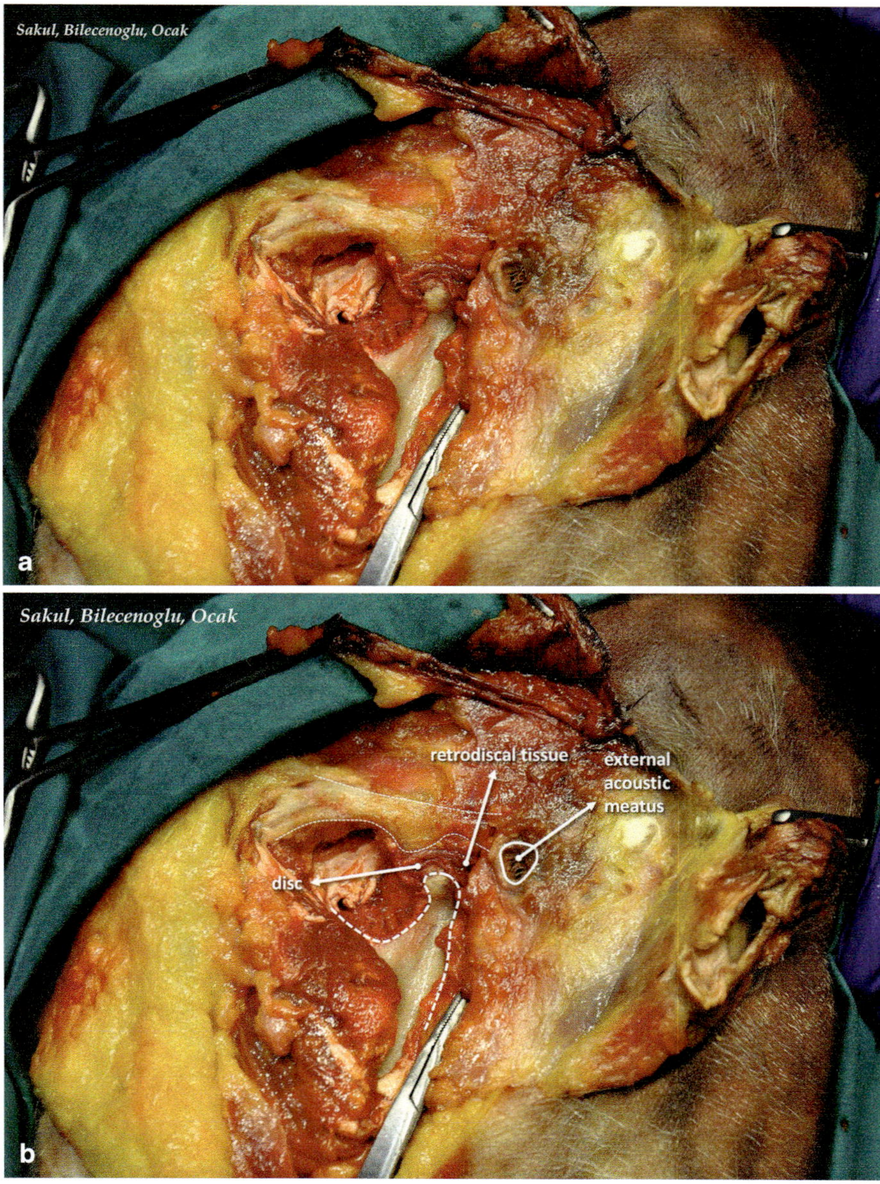

Fig. 2.8 (**a**) External view of the TMJ after the temporomandibular ligament and capsule removed. (**b**) Anatomic structures in this layer

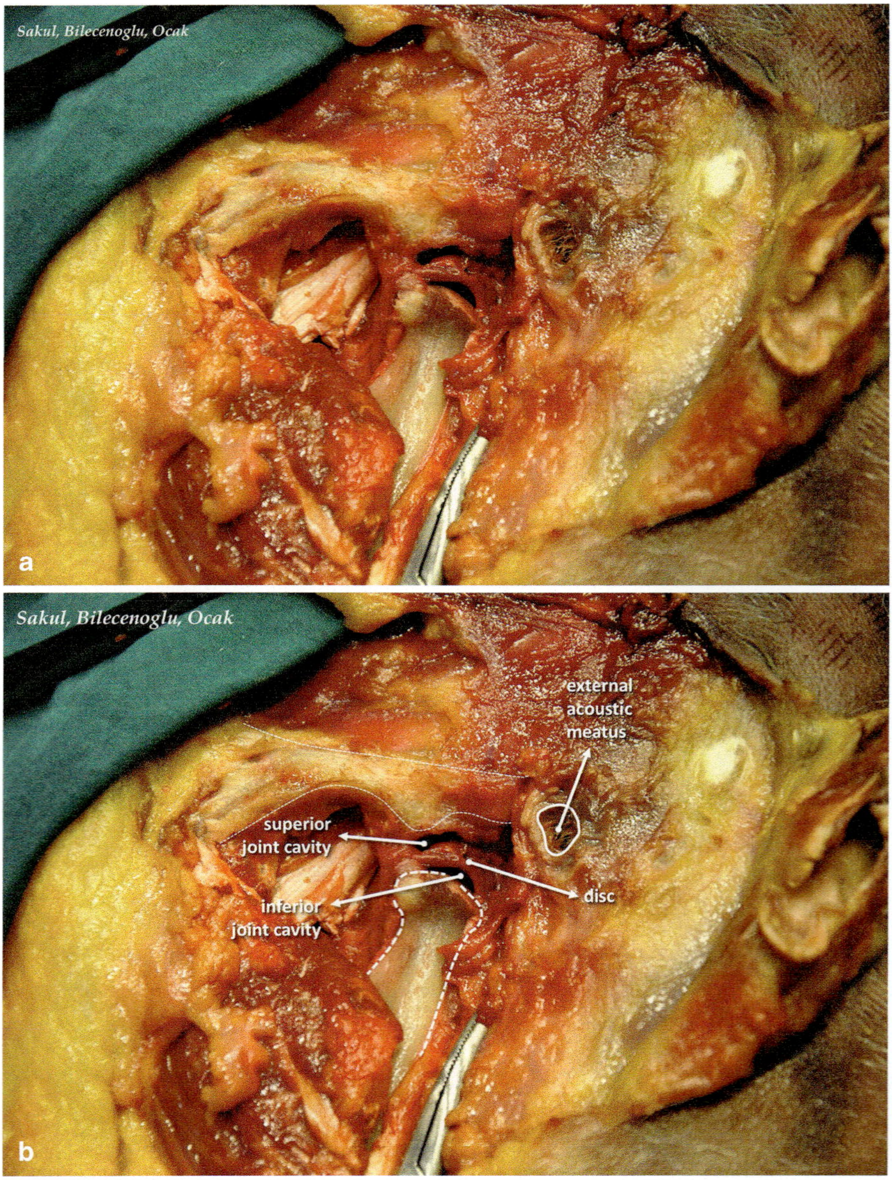

Fig. 2.9 (**a**) External view of the TMJ after the temporomandibular ligament and capsule removed, showing joint spaces. (**b**) Anatomic structures in this layer

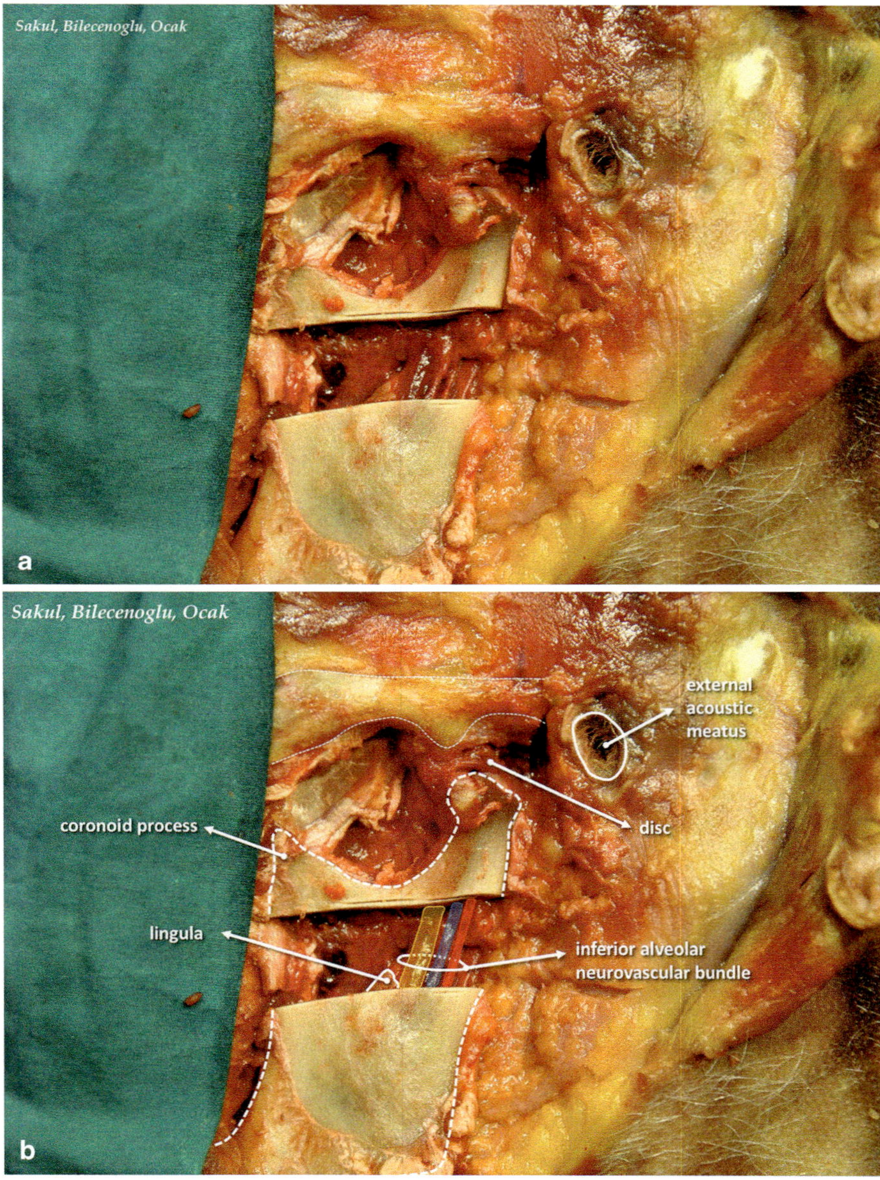

Fig. 2.10 (**a**) External view of the deeper level, mouth opened. A window through the mandibular ramus is opened to reveal some contents of the infratemporal fossa. (**b**) Anatomic structures in this layer

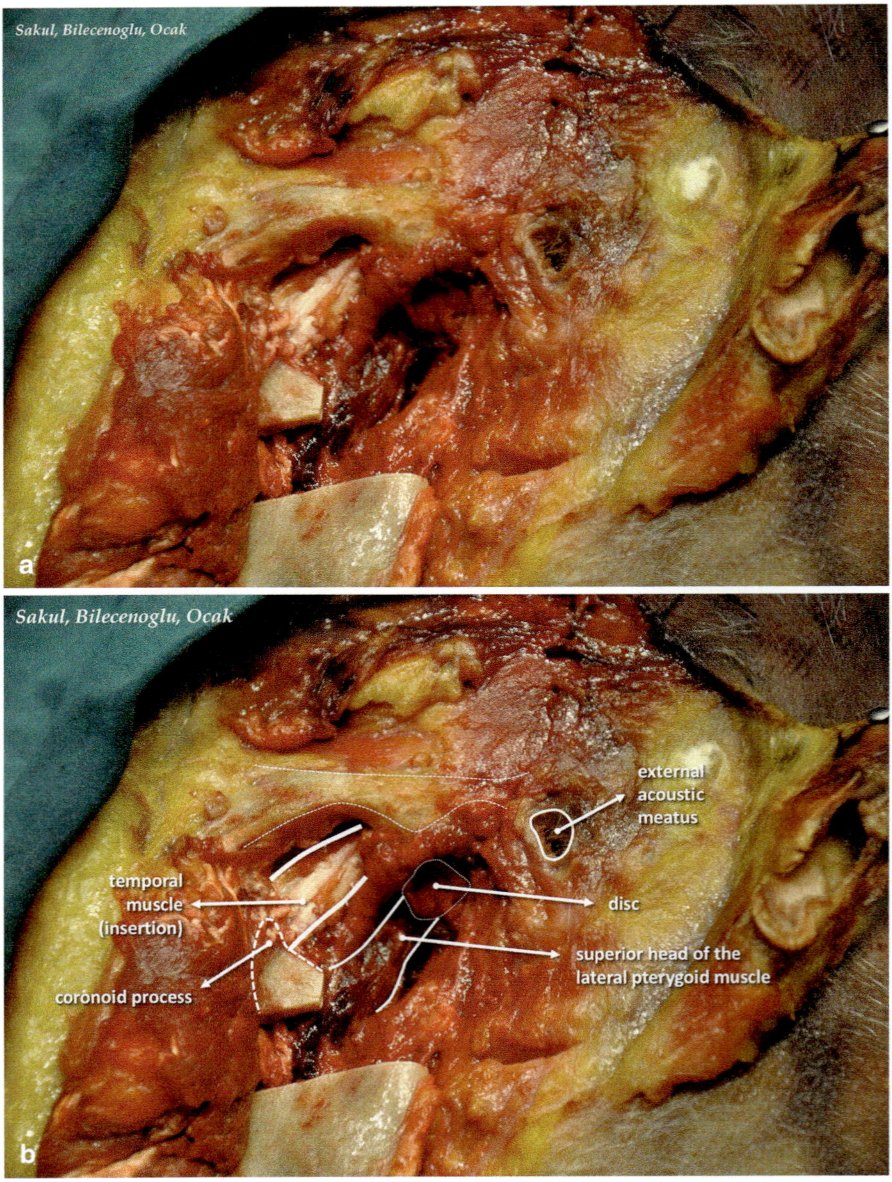

Fig. 2.11 (**a**) External view of the same level with Fig. 2.10, mouth opened. The condyle is removed to reveal the superior head of lateral pterygoid muscle and its connection to the disc. (**b**) Anatomic structures in this layer

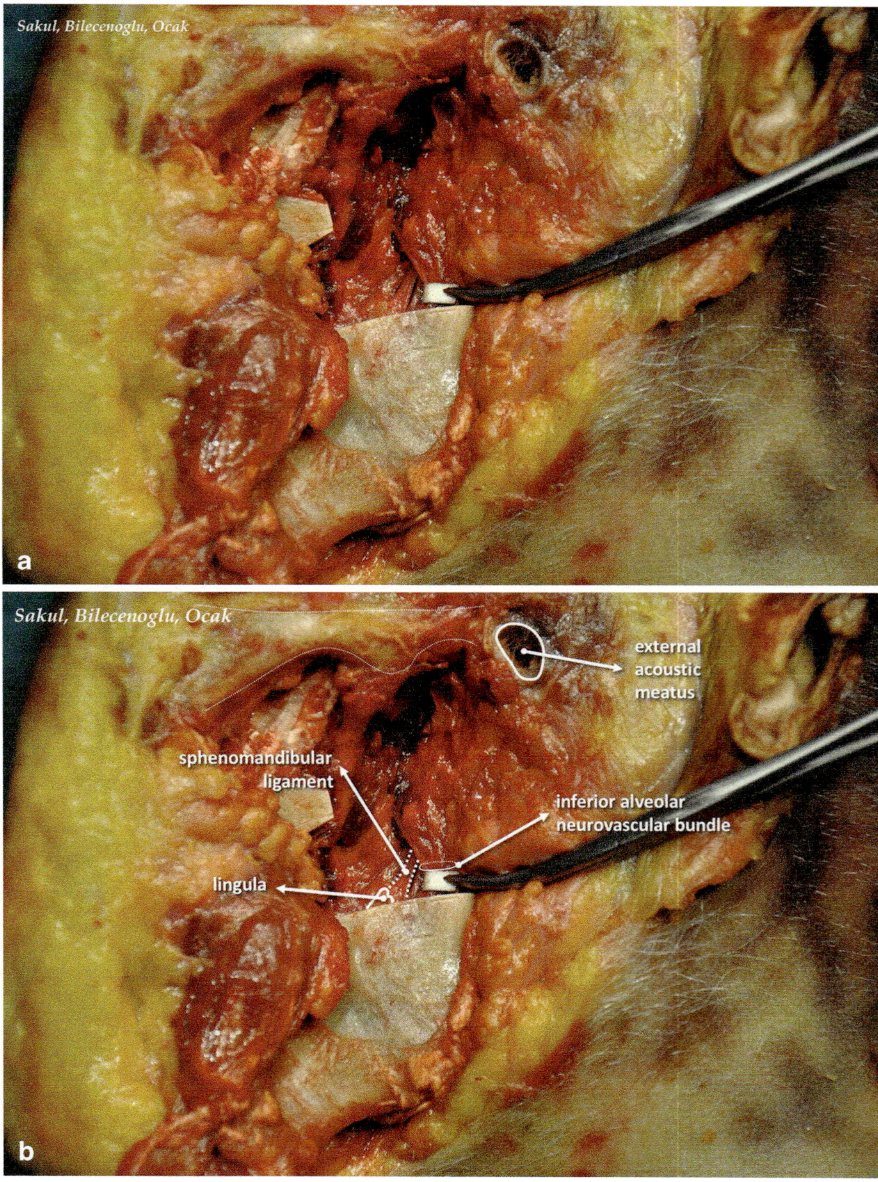

Fig. 2.12 (**a**) External view of the same level with Fig. 2.10, mouth opened. The inferior alveolar neurovascular bundle is retracted backward to reveal the sphenomandibular ligament. (**b**) Anatomic structures in this layer

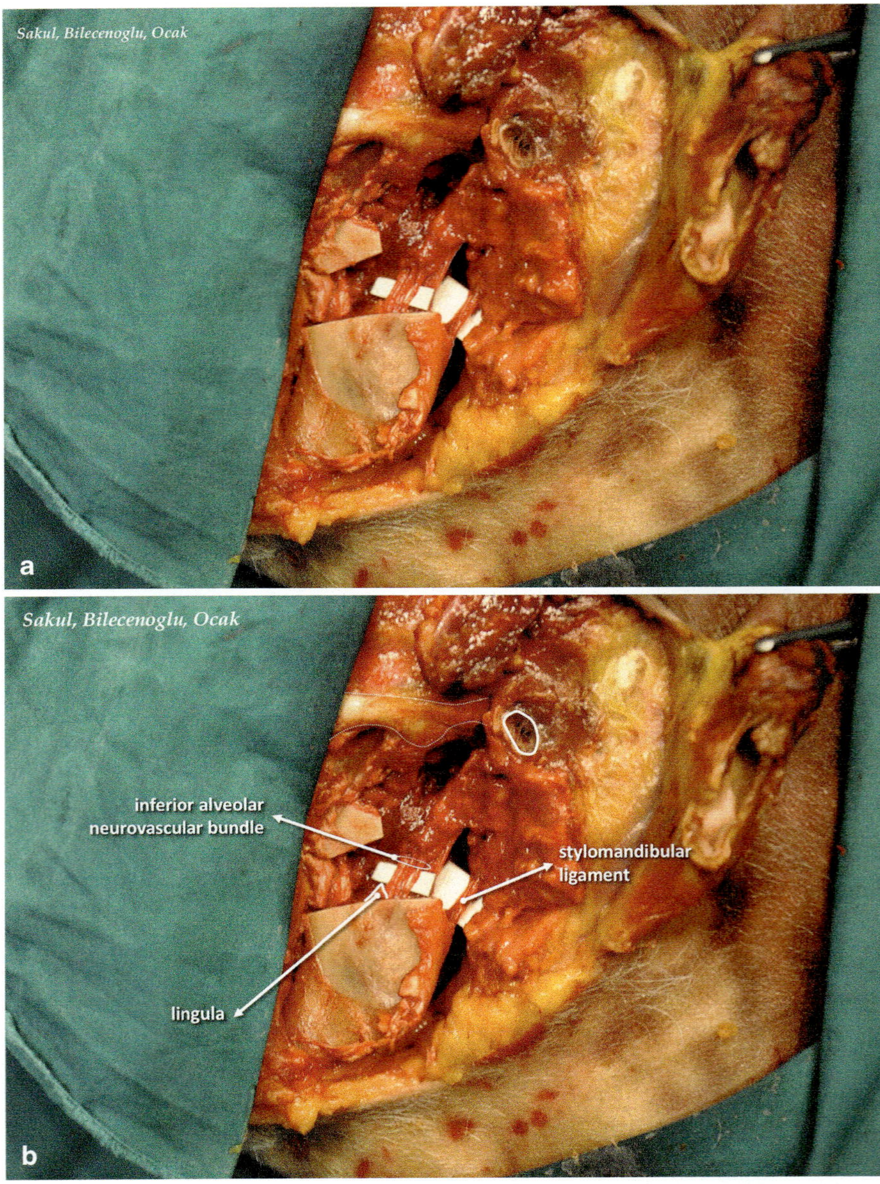

Fig. 2.13 (**a**) External view of the same level with Fig. 2.10, mouth opened. The inferior alveolar neurovascular bundle is in its original position; retromandibular tissue is removed to reveal the stylomandibular ligament. (**b**) Anatomic structures in this layer

References

1. Winkler S, Dalkowski K, Mair J, Klebe S, Waschke J, Böckers TM, et al. Sobotta lehrbuch anatomie. Berlin: Elsevier; 2015.
2. Moore K, Persaud T, Torchia M. The developing human: clinically oriented embryology. 8th ed. Philadelphia: Saunders/Elsevier; 2008.
3. Sadler T. Langman's medikal embriyoloji. Ankara: Palme yayıncılık; 1996.
4. Standring S. Gray's anatomy: the anatomical basis of clinical practice. 41st ed. New York: Elsevier; 2016.
5. Sargon MF. Anatomi akıl notları. Ankara: Güneş Tıp Kitapevleri; 2016.
6. Taner D, Sancak B, Akşit D, Cumhur M, İlgi S, Kural E, et al. Fonksiyonel anatomi ekstremiteler ve sırt bölgesi. Ankara: Metu Press; 2000.
7. Janfaza P, Nadol J. Surgical anatomy of the head and neck. Cambridge: Harvard University Press; 2011.
8. Sancak B, Cumhur M. Fonksiyonel anatomi baş boyun ve İç organlar. 4th ed. Ankara: ODTÜ Yayıncılık; 2008.
9. Türker M, Yücetaş Ş. Ağız, diş, çene hastalıkları ve cerrahisi. 3rd ed. İstanbul: Özyurt Matbaacılık; 2015.
10. Moore KL, Dalley AF, Agur AM. Clinically oriented anatomy. 7th ed. Philadelphia: Lippincott Williams & Wilkins; 2014.
11. Şakul B, Bilecenoğlu B. Baş ve boynun klinik bölgesel anatomisi. Ankara: Özkan Matbaacılık; 2009.
12. Gökmen F. Sistematik anatomi. İzmir: Güven Kitabevi; 2003.
13. Okeson JP. Management of temporomandibular disorders and occlusion. 6th ed. St. Louis: Elsevier; 2008.
14. Dere F. Anatomi Atlası ve Ders Kitabı Cilt 2. In: Baskı, Ozefagus Anatomisi. 4th ed. Istanbul: Nobel Tıp Kitabevi; 1999.
15. Norton N. Netter'in diş hekimleri için baş ve boyun anatomisi. Ankara: Güneş Tıp Kitapevleri; 2013.
16. Ozan H. Ozan anatomi premium. 3rd ed. Ankara: Klinisyen Kitapevi; 2014.
17. Arıncı K, Elhan A. Anatomi 1. Cilt. 5th ed. Ankara: Güneş Kitapevi; 2014.
18. Snell RS. Clinical anatomy by regions. 9th ed. Philadelphia: Lippincott Williams & Wilkins; 2012.
19. Tortora GJ, Petti K. Principles of human anatomy. Hoboken: Wiley; 2002.
20. Yalçın S, Aktaş İ. Diş hekimliğinde temporomandibular eklem hastalıklarına yaklaşım. 2nd ed. İstanbul: Vesta Yayın Grubu; 2015.
21. Shiraishi Y, Hayakawa M, Hoshino T, Tanaka S. A new retinacular ligament and vein of the human temporomandibular joint. Clin Anat. 1995;8(3):208–13.
22. Dos Santos J. Occlusion: principles and treatment. Chicago: Quintessence Publishing; 2007.
23. Dawson PE. Functional occlusion: from TMJ to smile design. New York: Elsevier; 2007.
24. Cumhur M, Sargon MF, Sürücü HS, İlgi S, Sancak B, Taner D, et al. Fonksiyonel nöroanatomi. Ankara: ODTÜ Geliştirme Vakfı; 2007.
25. McMinn RM. Last's anatomy: regional and applied. 9th ed. London: Churchill Livingstone; 1994.
26. Carlsson GE, Magnusson T. Management of temporomandibular disorders in the general practice. Chicago: Quintessence Publishing; 1999.
27. Ingawalé S, Goswami T. Temporomandibular joint: disorders, treatments, and biomechanics. Ann Biomed Eng. 2009;37(5):976–96.
28. Ueki K, Marukawa K, Nakagawa K, Yamamoto E. Condylar and temporomandibular joint disc positions after mandibular osteotomy for prognathism. J Oral Maxillofac Surg. 2002;60(12):1424–32.
29. Mathes SJ. Plastic surgery. In: The Head & Neck, vol. 3. 3rd ed. Philadelphia: Saunders; 2006.
30. Pansky B, Gest TR. Lippincott açıklamalı İnsan anatomisi atlası: baş & boyun. Philadelphia: Lippincott Williams & Wilkins; 2015.

Growth, Development, and Ossification of Mandible and Temporomandibular Joint

3

Beyza Karadede, Berşan Karadede, and Mehmet İrfan Karadede

Jaw joint has been the subject of a variety of basic biological researches because of its importance on mandibular development and growth as well as mammalian phylogeny. The problems associated with temporomandibular joint (TMJ) dysfunction syndrome and growth-functional adaptation's clinical significance have greatly increased today [1].

The role of the mandibular condyle's secondary cartilage center on the development and growth of the joint is one of the discussion topics. The idea that it is an independent primer growth center such as the epiphyseal growth plate is still sort of a dominant idea today. It is also accepted that condyle cartilage may be compatible with functional or other various factors and can affect the development of jaw-face-related functional changes during growth [1].

Phylogenesis: the lower jaw shows radical changes in mammalian history. In this process a new jaw joint evolves. The lower jaw of the reptile consists of many membrane bones around a cartilage branch (Meckel cartilage). The back of this cartilage becomes ossified and transforms into the joint tip. In intermediate types, the membranous part that carries the teeth joins to the condyle formation together with the Meckel cartilage. With the mammalian transition, the Meckel cartilage separates from the lower jaw and is limited to the development of the auditory ossicles only. The lower jaw becomes one piece and forms the jaw joint with the temporal bone at the posterior end.

The development of the face is regulated by a large number of genes expressed in specific models temporally and spatially. While significant progress has been made in the characterization of the genes that act in the oral cavity region, the regulators of the development of the aboral (lateral) region are largely unknown [2].

Mandibular condyle has versatile growth capacity, while the growth of long bones is unidirectional [3]. Compared to the joints of long bones, the genes that regulate the development and growth of TMJ are quite difficult to understand. It can

B. Karadede · B. Karadede · M. İ. Karadede (✉)
İzmir Katip Çelebi University, Faculty of Dentistry, Çiğli İZMİR, Turkey

I. Rozylo-Kalinowska, K. Orhan (eds.), *Imaging of the Temporomandibular Joint*, https://doi.org/10.1007/978-3-319-99468-0_3

be assumed that the genetic control of TMJ development differs from the cartilages of long bones, since the morphogenesis of the secondary cartilage and other intraarticular structures in the TMJ is later and distinctly different from the legs. However, studies of specific genes that regulate TMJ morphogenesis and growth have only begun to appear in the literature in the last decade. Studies conducted up to now using knockout and overexpression of candidate genes show that there is a developmental hierarchy of joints with the condyle development primer. There is also a gene expression hierarchy: the expression of Runx2 and Sox9 is critical for capillary cartilage formation. Many of the other genes discussed in this report can regulate TMJ morphogenesis by affecting the expression of Sox9 and Runx2 and controlling the IHH-PTHrP axis through these genes [4].

TMJ is regulated by some of the same genes that are important in extremity joints, but others have specific or different effects on TMJ. Members of Runx2, Sox9, and TGF-β/BMP family are critical factors in chondrogenic cartilage morphogenesis, and it is important for Indian hedgehog (Ihh) articular disc and cavitation formation [5]. Osterix (Osx) is a critical regulator of endochondral bone formation during postnatal TMJ development [5]. Clearly, some genes have critical importance for a chondrogenic pathway specification for MCC precursor-blastic cells [6]. In mice without Runx2, Sox9, BMPr1a, and TGFBr2, the condylar cartilage never develops or shapes. Yet other genes act downstream of this "fate-determining" gene, which presumably regulates the proper multiplication and differentiation of MCC cells and also governs the formation of joint conditioning and the formation of interzone upper and lower joint spaces between the developing condyle and the mandibular fossa [6].

TMJ development is long-lasting and is completed toward the end of fetal life and depends on the formation of two separate blastemas and their subsequent growth. TMJ is an evolutionarily new joint formed between the malleus and incus [7]. TMJ is the last joint formed in the human body, and its embryological development is quite different from other synovial joints, consisting of a single blast [7, 8]. Both TMJs act as a single unit during articulation due to mandibular movements and occlusion [7].

During the normal embryological development of TMJ from the first pharyngeal bone, there are three stages: the blastemic phase, the cavitation phase, and finally the maturation phase [9]. The development of the temporal bone and the mandible are different from each other but are related to each other in terms of TMJ development [9].

Mandibular condylar cartilage is defined as secondary cartilage in embryology [10–12]. Secondary cartilages, unlike primary skeletal cartilages, are seen in the late embryonic period, their origins are different, and finally the released matrix components and growth factors are different [12, 13]. Temporal connections are differentiated temporally and spatially later from condylar structures [14].

The secondary cartilage of the condyle consists of four layers [15]:

1. Fibrous connective tissue region
2. Differentiated connective tissue cell region

3. Reproduction area of cells
4. Endochondral ossification region

Other structures [15]:

5. Eminence
6. Disc
7. Condyle

The development of mandibular condyle cartilage begins with the condensation of mesenchymal cells from cranial neural crest cells [12, 16]. From the 5th week of intrauterine life, skeletal elements are formed by the condensation of mesenchymal cells, transforming into chondroblasts and cartilage cell precursors [8]. The mandible develops from the deep part of the 1st pharyngeal arch (Fig. 3.1 [17]). First, Meckel cartilage, which is a primitive mandibular stalk, appears. Meckel cartilage shows a close relationship with the 1st pharyngeal arch nerve—mandibular nerve—and with its branches in this stage of development and forms the skeletal support of these. In the area where the inferior alveolar nerve is divided into mental and incisive branches from the lateral edges of the Meckel cartilage, indications of first ossification for the mandible appears at the 6th week of the intrauterine period [8].

First, a cartilage arm (Meckel cartilage) appears in the mandibular arch and extends to front and middle from the developing ear capsule cartilage. It thickens at the back end. Between this tip and the ear capsule, cartilage streaks of os incus and os malleus of the middle ear are revealed. Meckel cartilage and incus cartilage grow, shape, and adapt to each other. A large number of membrane bones develop at 6th week. The mandible is derived from these membranous concentrations at the bifurcation point of the mandibular nerve in both sides. In the meantime, another membrane bone appears near the back end of the Meckel cartilage. This bone fragment

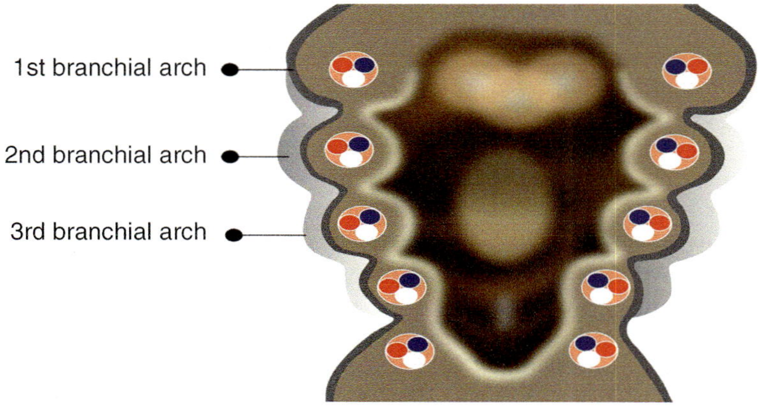

Fig. 3.1 Branchial arches during the 4th week of embryologic development (Modified from Sadler [17])

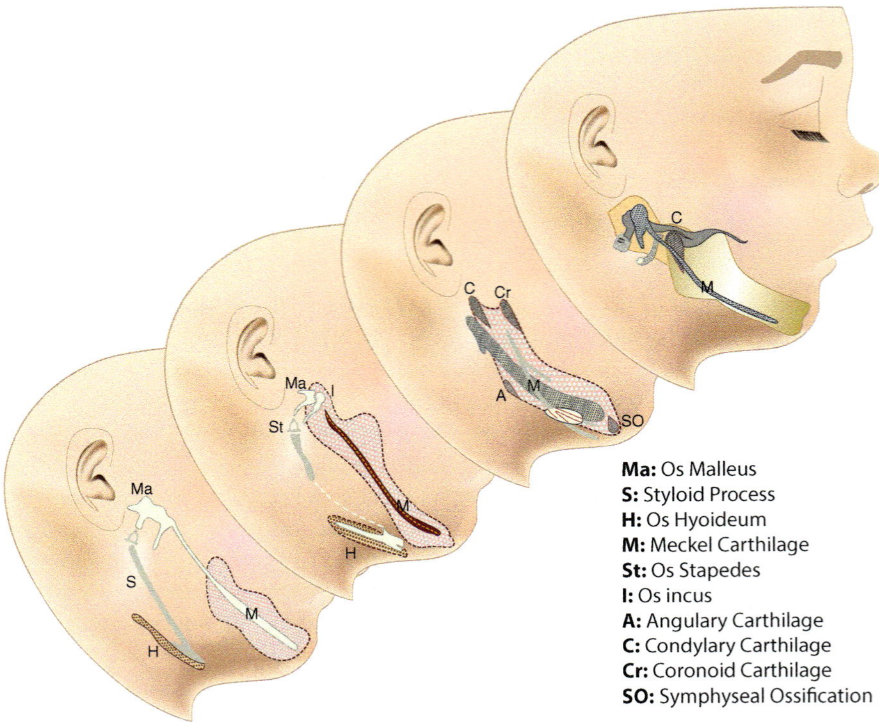

Fig. 3.2 Lateral view of the head and face of embryologic development stages (Modified from Sadler [17])

is shaped into the tympanic bone and, with an extension of the temporal bone, limits the middle ear around the developing ear bones [1] (Fig. 3.2 [17, 18]).

It gets the most advanced shape in 15 mm embryo at 6th week. It widens backward and forward, extending from the cartilaginous ear capsule to the midline in one arm. In the midline, both ventral tips tied with mesenchyme turn upward. It is wrapped around from one end to the other with a thick fibrous tissue. Dorsal tips make the hammer bone (os malleus) in the ear; the remaining part forms a temporary draft to the mandible. Membranous bone formation, even in small amounts, is seen in the lateral regions of the Meckel cartilage in a 6.5-week embryo [19].

During the development of TMJ, the first structure observed is the articular fossa in 7th–8th week of embryonic period [20, 21]. Mesenchymal condensation is observed in the temporomandibular connective area on the mandibular ramus to be formed at the 7th week [20, 22]. The joint cavity begins to appear as homogeneous intermediate cells after 7th week [8]. This condensation is an indicator of condyle formation. Condyle formation is associated with masseteric and auriculotemporal nerves. The auriculotemporal nerve passes through the condyle and Meckel cartilage to be formed [22]. Homogeneous intermediate cells degenerate at 8th week, and the joint cavity forms. The first indication of TMJ development is seen at week 8, with the condensation of mesenchymal cells starting from neural crest cells in the dorsal region of the mandible. Within the next 2 weeks, these cells proliferate and differentiate into condyle cartilage. Vascularization of all the components and active bone formation are seen in the condylar and glenoid fossa regions in the postnatal period compared to the prenatal period [8].

In most synovial joints, the development of synovial spaces is completed at approximately week 7, but TMJ does not occur in this phase. However, extremity joints take the adult shape directly with the formation of TMJ cavities, within a single blastema in which both adjacent endochondral bones are developed. TMJ first develops from temporal and processus (proc) condylaris mesenchymas, which are initially far apart from each other, developing toward each side. Fossa articularis and articular surface of tuberculum articulare become more fibrous and less vascular as the age progresses. During embryological development, TMJ disc has a relationship with the mandible and the masticatory muscles, especially m. pterygoideus lateralis and m. massetericus. The TMJ disc develops from the first branchial arch muscles and mesenchyme. A large part of the TMJ disc is derived from a mesenchymal layer, and this layer is a structure that extends from m. pterygoideus, passes over proc. condylaris, and attaches to developing malleus [9].

Van Der Linden et al. said that the disc was formed by mesenchymal condensation of the future TMJ region [23]. The investigations reported that the first TMJ structures were the lower bond spacings following the lower part of the disc [24]. Jaw movement is an important mechanical factor for the prenatal development of the condyle cartilage of the mandible [25]. The ligaments of the lateral pterygoid muscle are located parallel to the developing disc [24]. During the intrauterine life, the first mouth opening is at 7.5 weeks [25]. Mouth closure is activated after 11th week, while it is passive in the first time [26]. Initial formations of the lower cavity, the lower part of the disc, and the upper cavity are observed during the activation stage of mouth opening [24]. On the other hand, Giambartolomei et al. reported that the neuromuscular capacity to achieve mandibular movements (opening and closing) before birth starts at 14–15 weeks of prenatal development and gets completed at approximately 20 weeks [27].

At approximately 8 weeks, the primitive joint within the Meckel cartilage is like a simple jaw joint before the malleus and incus are formed [20]. At 8 weeks of age, the membranous bone grows anteroposteriorly and superoinferiorly [19]. At week 8, intramembranous ossification occurs of the zygomatic process of the squamous part of the temporal bone. The intramembranous ossification of the mandibular ramus extends to the base of the condyle to be formed. In the craniolateral regions of the condyle to be formed, there is a mesenchymal condensation that forms articular disc [22].

The lower joint space develops as small gaps or cracks between the articular disc and the mandibular condyle at 9th week [28]. Intramembranous ossification of the squamous part of the temporal bone continues, and no cartilage area is observed. In this period, cartilage formation occurs at the center of the blastema. Lateral pterygoid muscle enters the condyle-disc complex at this week [22].

The seconder cartilage of the condyle is formed from condylar blastema via histodifferantiation at the 10th week of the fetus [29]. The condylar blastema is located in the region of the dorsal extrusions of the mandibular body [29]. It is thought that both glenoid and condylar ligaments originate from the same blastema [29]. In both half jaws, secondary cartilage occurs mainly at three points. The first and largest one of these cartilages plays an important role in the development of the mandible and jaw joint. One side of the condyle extensions merges with the bone and the other side with fibrous cover on top edge. In the sagittal section of 32-mm-long fetus, the condylar blastema center was observed to be at the lower part of the external pterygoid muscle [29]. The glenoid blastema center of 35-mm-long fetus was seen in the coronal region [29]. The backward growth of the mandibular ramus is observed as the settlement of bone body from mandibular hole to backward and upward. From this area, the mandible moves away from Meckel cartilage. This piece begins as a fibrous condensation, as if it were at the body, and then quickly becomes ossified. At week 10 (40 mm), the coronoidal and condylar extensions are massively ossified. The development of these extensions is then transformed by the appearance of secondary cartilage. Secondary cartilages develop independently of the main cartilage skeleton or Meckel cartilage at different points in the membrane bone formation place. For this reason, these are called secondary cartilage focuses. These are the result of metamorphosis and proliferation of cells in thick fibrous covers.

The condyle is initially cartilaginous but between the 10th and 11th weeks develops by the coming together of the mesenchymal cells lining laterally of the Meckel cartilage, and the articular fossa begins to ossify [21, 30]. Endochondral ossification proceeds by forming a bony fusion with the mandibular body [30]. At the 10th week of embryological development, the lower joint cavity is formed, and the condensation of the intercellular cells which will form the condyle at the upper part of the bone nucleus of the membranous bone is observed [19, 22]. But there is no sign of the upper joint cavity. At this week, the blood vessels are observed in the lateral regions of the joint capsule entering the external portion of the articular disc, and the upper joint space begins to form at about 11th week [22, 28]. Approximately at the 12th week, it begins to develop with the lower jaw and middle ear. At this stage in a 10-week aged fetus, lateral pterygoid tendon continues to the malleus through the petrotympanic fissure after providing the disc formation [31]. In Yuodellis' work on 10-week-old fetuses, it is reported that the lateral pterygoid does not contribute to the formation of the disc or malleus, unlike what is known [32]. Moffett reported that the connection of the lateral pterygoid tendon with the malleus was lost in the 18-week fetus [33]. It is thought that the medial part of the disc is formed by the lateral pterygoid tendon and the lateral part is formed by the condensation of the mesenchyme [32].

The anterior part of the mandible completely encloses the Meckel cartilage, from the mental nerve foramen through the posterior part of the ending of it. This part of the cartilage is first surrounded by a bone extension from the middle plane; then cartilage tissue is gradually disintegrated, and the surrounding membranous bone arms fill its place. They can be observed as one or two nodules in the symphysis connective tissue at the end of the latest fetal period. Meckel cartilage disappears completely except the fibrous covering of it. This covering then turns into sphenomandibular and sphenomalleolar ligaments. Only the most dorsal tip ossifies to make os malleus, which is attached to the sphenoid bone with the sphenomandibular ligament [1].

The lower part of the temporomandibular joint capsule was completely formed in the 11th–12th-week fetus [23]. There is a primordium disc composed of mesenchymal tissue between the lower and upper regions of the articular disc [19]. Membrane bones grow and gradually gain their original shape. At this stage there is a wide range of mandibular and temporal joint elements. Then secondary cartilage occurs at the condyle projection. It appears (embryo size 50 mm) in the 12th week. Condylar blastoma is not observed at the level of the external auditory canal at the coronal segment of 50 mm [29]. The differentiation of the condyle head was found to be in sections of 55 mm [15]. Augier reported that the temporal squama began to ossify from the 32 mm fetal zygomatic region and formed the temporal elements of the articulation [15]. In the 12th–14th week, the condyle extends back toward the zygomatic process of the temporal bone. As an intermediate tissue, only a dense tissue liner remains on the upper surface of the condyle. These tissue conditions appear with tissue condensation attached to the lateral pterygoid muscle and form the joint disc. Intermediate mesenchyme is shaped and shaped by two clefts in the tissue when the joint spaces are near and above the contour of the condyle temporal. Between 65 and 75 mm embryo periods, the formation of upper and lower joint spaces was completed. Articular disc primarily occurs 12th–14th week of prenatal life [19]. Condylar growth at week 14 occurs with interstitial and apical growth of cartilage. The first endochondral bone growth is seen this week [19]. The superior or temporal region of the other part of the articular disc is composed of the same projection after 14 weeks. At week 11, an upper articular cavity was formed between the squamous piece of the temporal bone and the articular disc, and at 14 weeks, all TMJ structures, including the upper cavity and the vesicle capsule, were observed to form [19, 22].

From the 15th week onward, the chondrocytes were sufficiently differentiated, and in this stage, cartilage shows the properties of the postnatal structure. According to Van Der Linden et al. [22], the TMJ disc develops from an embryonic mesenchymal cell block called the "developmental space" that intervenes between the continuously developing temporal bone and process condyle. Some researchers have studied the connection between TMJ disc, malleus, and Meckel cartilage [30]:

1. There is no direct continuity from the posterior region of TMJ disc to the malleus and sphenomandibular ligament [30].
2. The mesenchyme cells attached to Meckel cartilage in a human fetus of 13.5 weeks are continuous with the region between the TMJ disc and the articular space [30].

At the 16th week, the mandibular condyle cartilage and Meckel cartilage are formed [14]. Between 12th and 17th week, whole TMJ system is formed at the same time as condyle growth and intramembranous bone formation in the temporal region [19, 22]. The middle part of the joint disc originates from the tendon of the lateral pterygoid tendon. This tendon passes over the condyle and is attached to the posterior process of the Meckel cartilage with its side projection. Then it takes the precise position behind the joint capsule in 21st week. At this time, the perichondrium of the Meckel cartilage extends from the mandible to the skull and converts to sphenomandibular ligament. The lateral part of TMJ disc originates from mesenchyme extending from between masseter and lateral pterygoid muscle to posterior region of the condyle. The joint protrusion is difficult to recognize at birth and typically takes shape only after the deciduous teeth has been completed.

At the age of 22 weeks, the glenoid fossa was formed. When permanent teeth enter the occlusion during the growth period, the glenoid fossa is formed. In younger individuals, the glenoid fossa is shallow, and the joint process is smaller. It maintains its maturation in two different forms and in two separate ways. This determines the degree of strain in the mandibular movement and occlusion.

At the first form, the occlusion deepens and "overbite" appears at the front. The lower fibers of the lateral pterygoid muscles, which undergo condylar translational movement, are highly developed. Lateral movements are restricted. The other form of maturation is characterized by a tête-à-tête occlusion. The glenoid fossa is shallow. The joint process (tuberculum articulare) is less inclination.

The lateral movement of the mandible is facilitated. Upper fibers in the lower part of the lateral pterygoid muscles have developed. On the other hand, tooth loss and bruxism cause the glenoid fossa to become shallow, and the inclination of joint tubercle decreases. Temporomandibular joints are typically completely different at 25th and 26th weeks of pregnancy [21]. At week 34, the anterior malleolar and sphenomandibular ligaments are composed of Meckel cartilage [32]. Meckel cartilage residues were found in the region of anterior malleolar and sphenomandibular ligament junctions in adult individuals [32]. Rees [34] mentioned that the adult disc and the ligament extensions present in the retrodissected region of the capsule are composed of discomalleolar ligament residues in the fetuses. According to Harpman and Woollard, only the median part of the disc is composed of lateral pterygoid tendon [35]. It becomes increasingly tapered with newly added cells in this region. Condylar extensions scroll down and extend forward from the ramus to the mandibular canal. The first part of the formation is endochondral ossification. This lasts until the fifth month of fetal life. In the fifth month of fetal life, previous cartilage left its place largely in bone trabeculae. The thickness of the cartilage gradually decreases in this period, and eventually it becomes completely ossified outside the joint surface.

The mandible appears as a dense fibrous strip laterally of the nerves of the lower central and incisor teeth. In this tissue, ossification starts into the angle that forms between the mental and central nerves at the 7th week (17–18 mm). This corresponds to the mental canal area in adult individuals. Bone formation from this point continues under the mental nerve and backward from the lateral side of the lower central nerve. Jaws develop in the form of a groove as a connective tissue. In this region, synosterisis is completed before the end of the first year. The lateral and internal bone plates grow on central nerve and convert the bone to the canal. A similar bony structure develops backward in the form of a plaque along the lateral aspect of the mandibular nerve which later turns into a groove and then into a channel. Thus, primary ossification center behind, mandibular channel ahead, grows to the as far as the symphysis. While it surrounds to the lower central and lateral nerves, the mandibular body forms.

Another secondary cartilage is called coronoid cartilage and forms a strip along the top and the front edge of the coronoid process. When the coronoid process first occurs, the embryo is 80 mm. The outer face is wrapped with a fibrous sheath. It is located on the bone membrane. It disappears completely before birth. The third secondary cartilage appears in the connective tissue at the symphysis end of both jaws when the embryo is 100 mm. They are separated from each other by the connective tissue, and wherein the cells are made additions to the cartilage surface. The symphysis cartilaginous is completely independent from perichondrium with the Meckel cartilage which disappears during the start of jaw ossification.

3.1 Histo-anatomy of Mandibular Condyle

The TMJ consists of the mandibular condyle, mandibular fossa, and fibrocartilaginous [36] disc [37, 38]. Articular disc has a fibrocartilaginous structure. The central portion of the disc is approximately 1–2 mm thinner than in peripheral region [38]. The joint surfaces are covered with fibrous connective tissue. The presence of fibrous tissue on the articular surfaces provides less degenerative changes and more repair forces against harmful agents. There is no hyaline cartilage as in other synovial joints. The temporomandibular joint disc is located on the apex of the condyle, while the mouth is in closed position, and joint disc is composed of biconcave fibrous tissue. Temporomandibular joint disc divided into two main parts as lower and upper part. The lower joint space is localized between the mandible and the articular disc [39]. The upper joint space is localized between the temporal bone and the articular disc. All of the temporomandibular joint is encapsulated with synovial membrane [39]. Joint chondrocytes are present throughout postnatal life, and their biological properties remain unchanged [40]. TMJ is separated from other joints in many ways. It is a synovial type of joint. It has movements that do not match the existing rules in other joints [41]. TMJ disc has a biconcave morphology of fibrocartilaginous nature. The dorsum anterior and posterior of disc are called anterior and posterior bands. The anteroposterior dimension is larger than in the mediolateral dimension. In retrodiscal posterior band in the region of space known as bilaminary region that joined with highly vascularized and loose connective tissue [37], Kantomaa [42] reported that the enzyme activity of TMJ shows changes in anteroposterior and lateromedial directions with the concentration of the surface thickness, and although the exchange of multipotential mesenchymal cells is the main source of new cells in the condylar cartilage, the absence of equilibrium in all areas of the condylar is due to environmental diversity and stimuli. Mandibular condyle, compared to other joints in the body, has some differences with its histomorphology and growth aspects. It grows and develops by way of endochondral ossification

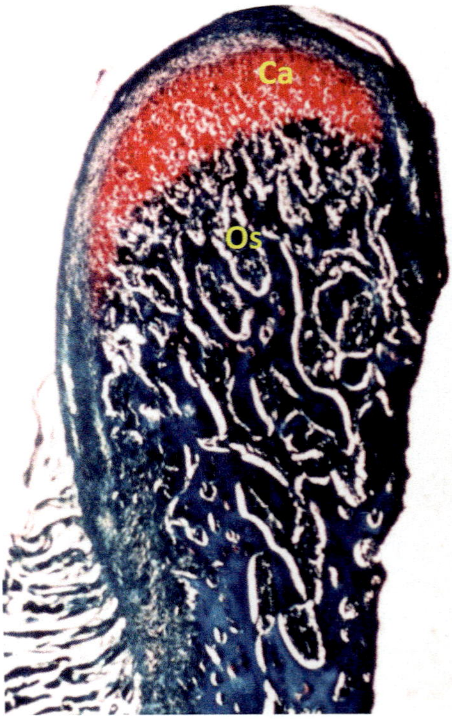

Fig. 3.3 Direction of the mandibular growth

(Fig. 3.3). The endochondral ossification layers of the mandibular condyle were divided into four groups by Girdler [43] and eight groups by Luder [44], Bloom and Fawcett [45], Bosshardt-Luehrs, Merida-Velasco et al. [46], and Luder [47]. Karadede [47] has studied the mandibular condyle in more detail by dividing the endochondral ossification layers into seven layers:

1. Fibrous layer: This layer, which is anteriorly and marginally thin and thicker in the posterior region, is resistant to mastication pressures and lacks veins and nerves (Fig. 3.4).
2. Proliferative layer (composed of mesenchymal cells): It is composed of mesenchymal cells that lead to chondroblasts, where the mitosis is abundant, thin in the beginning of anterior parts, very thick in the central region, and wide in the posterior (Fig. 3.4).
3. Upper hypertrophic layer: The thickness of this layer is almost invisible in the marginal parts of the anterior, the largest in the central, and broad in the posterior; besides, there are chondroblasts with young cartilage cells (Fig. 3.4).
4. Lower hypertrophic layer: In terms of thickness, the posterior aspect is wider, the central part is lager, and the anterior part is thinner; besides this layer contains chondrocytes with mature cartilage cells (Fig. 3.4).
5. Erosion layer: In this layer, the matrix of degenerated chondrocytes showed calcification, and vessel migration began. In other words, chondrocytes are

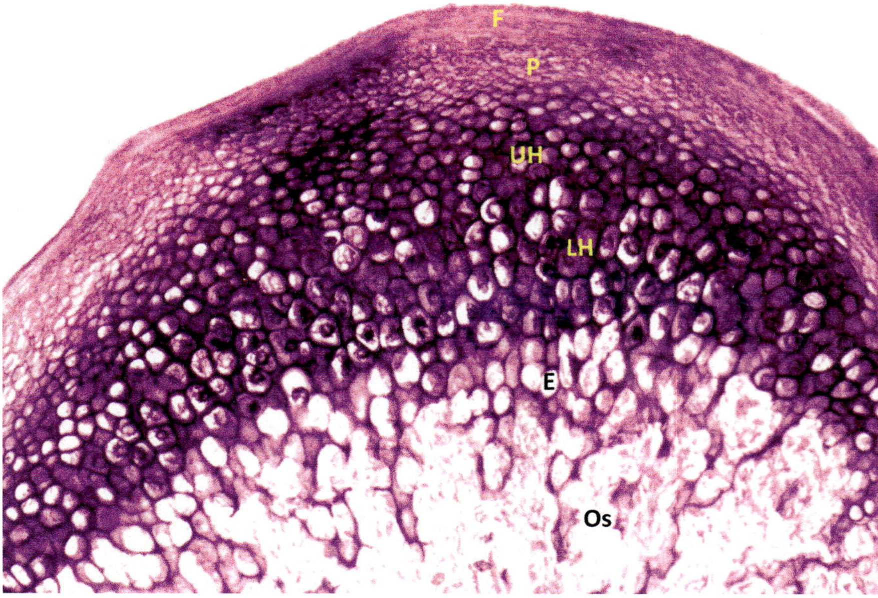

Fig. 3.4 Mandibular condyle. *Ca* cartilages layer, *Os* ossification layer, Mallory-Azan ×10

degenerated and removed from the zone. This function is through phagocytes and blood vessels. These cells, which show chondrogenic character, are intertwined with bone cells and cover large areas of the bone marrow (Fig. 3.5).

6. The ossification layer: Cells with chondrogenic character are significantly reduced. Bone trabeculae have begun to be observed. In an amount of the bone marrow, it is also observed a significant reduction (Fig. 3.5).
7. Bone (collum mandibularis) layer: Osteocytes are observed in the trabecular bone structure below the ossification layer. Cells with chondrogenic characters can no longer be observed (Fig. 3.5).

The fibrous layer, which forms the joint surface of the condyle, has come from the connective tissue and is devoid of vascularity. Karadede [48] and Girdler [43] defend that the fibrous and proliferative layer does not exhibit chondrogenic properties. Kantomaa [42] defend that the fibrous layer is slightly orthochromatic and argued that the orthochromatic and intercellular matrix of the proliferative layer was slightly metachromatic and this argument is partially compatible with Karadede [48]. Kantomaa [42], Karadede [48], and Girdler [43] reported that the hypertrophic layer carries a chondrogenic character. The proliferative layer beneath the fibrous layer was found to be a polymorphic cell area, and it contained progenitor (precursor) cells and showed intense cell division in this layer [48, 49].

In the mandibular condyle, the fibrous layer, the proliferative layer, and the upper and lower hypertrophic layers are thin in the anterior region, the posterior areas are wide, and the central areas are wider. The thinness of the anterior thickness of the

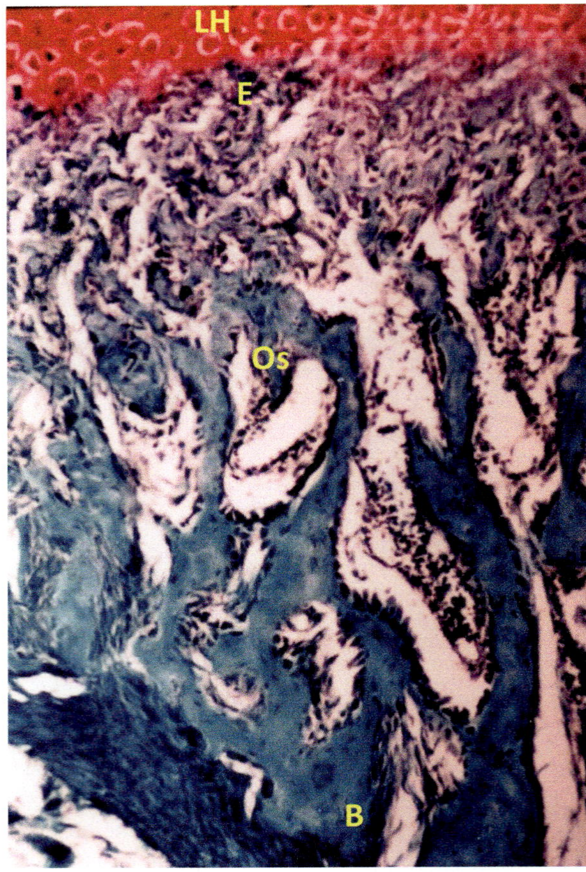

Fig. 3.5 The endochondral ossification layers of the mandibular condyle. *F* fibrous layer, *P* proliferative layer, *UH* upper hypertrophic layer, *LH* lower hypertrophic layer, *E* erosion layer, *Os* ossification layer, Mallory-Azan ×20

condylar cartilage and the observation of the proliferative cell layer by immature chondroblasts show the dysfunction of the anterior region [48].

The progenitor cells in the middle and posterior areas of the mandibular condyle (where mesenchymal cells producing mitochondrial chondroblasts are present) are larger. The rate of transformation of these cells into chondroblasts and chondrocytes is the same in the middle and back areas. These cells are larger than the cells in the anterior region, and their extracellular matrix is wider too. For this reason, the resorptive activities in the middle and back subchondral areas are higher in terms of loss of degenerated chondrocytes. And as a result, this shows that the condyle grows up and down [44, 48].

Experimental studies show that differentiation of mesenchymal cells into chondroblasts is driven by functional forces [42]. Experimental studies have also shown that functional factors play an important role in regulating the growth of mandibular condyles [50]. Hatipoglu et al. [41] shows that the base of the fossa mandibularis is thin and the fibrous ligament covering the joint face (pit) is quite thin. This indicates that the pit is not a functional part of the joint; at least it has been shown that the pit

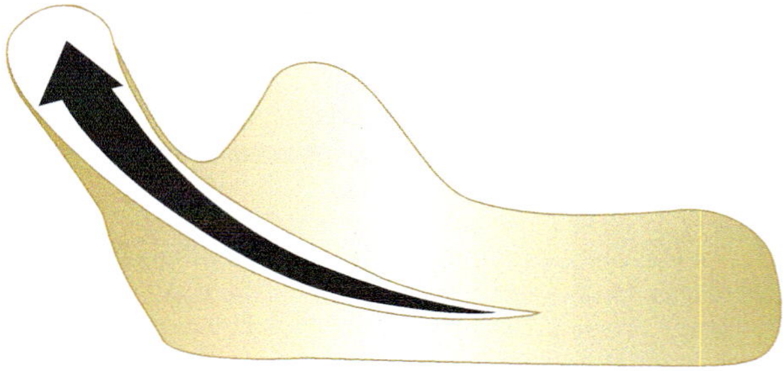

Fig. 3.6 The chondrocytes are degenerated and removed from the zone. Bone trabeculae have begun to be observed. *LH* lower hypertrophic layer, *E* erosion layer, *Os* ossification layer, *B* bone, Mallory-Azan ×40

does not fully participate in the function. The thinness of the anterior thickness of the condylar cartilage and the observation of the proliferative cell layer by immature chondroblasts show the dysfunction of the anterior region. The investigations reported that growth pattern of posterior cartilage depends on metabolic differentiation, excess mitosis, and different chewing pressures [42, 44, 51].

In conclusion, during the endochondral ossification of the mandibular condyle, seven layers which have different features were noted in the condyle. It is stated from the thickness of the condyle cartilage is thin in the front region, wide in the back region, and wider in the middle. Mandibular condylar cartilage has been reported to be thicker in the regions involved in the chewing function. It has also been observed that the condyle grows upward and backward (Fig. 3.6).

References

1. Soydan N. Gelişim ve Büyüme: Diş Hekimleri İçin. Istanbul: İstanbul Diş Hekimliği Fakültesi; 1993.
2. Cesariojeffry M, Almaidhan AA, Jeong J. Expression of fork Headbox transcription factor genes Foxp1 and Foxp2 during jaw development. New York: Elsevier; 2016.
3. Owtad P, Park JH, Shen G, Potres Z, Darendeliler MA. The biology of Tmj growth modification. J Dent Res. 2013;92(4):315–21.
4. Hinton RJ. Genes that regulate morphogenesis and growth of the temporomandibular joint: a review. Dev Dyn. 2014;243(7):864–74.
5. Hinton RJ, Jing J, Feng JQ. Current topics in developmental biology, vol. 115, chap. 4. New York: Elsevier Inc.; 2015. p. 85–86.
6. Gu S, Wu W, Liu C, Yang L, Sun C, Ye W, et al. Bmpr1a mediated signaling is essential for temporomandibular joint development İn mice. PLoS One. 2014;9(8):E101000.
7. Keith DA. Development of the human temporomandibular joint. Br J Oral Surg. 1982;20(3):217–24.
8. Osborn JW. Dental anatomy and embryology. In: Rowe AHR, Johns RB, editors. A companion to dental studies. Oxford: Blackwell Scientific Publications; 1981.
9. Bender ME, Rosa LB, Steven GL. Development of the pediatric temporomandibular joint. Oral Maxillofac Surg Clin N Am. 2018;30(1):1–9.
10. Proffit WR. Concept of growth and development. In: Proffit WR, Fields HW, Sarver DH, editors. Contemporary orthodontics. 5th ed. St Louis: Mosby; 2013. p. 20–65.

11. Chai Y, Jiang X, Ito Y, Bringas P Jr, Han J, Rowitch DH, Soriano P, Mcmahon AP, Sucov HM. Fate of the mammalian cranial neural crest during tooth and mandibular morphogenesis. Development. 2000;127(8):1671–9.
12. Fujikawa K, Yokohama-Tamaki T, Morita T, Baba O, Qin C, Shibata S. An in situ hybridization study of perlecan, Dmp1, and Mepe in developing condylar cartilage of the Fetal mouse mandible and limb bud cartilage. Eur J Histochem. 2015;59(3):2553.
13. Shibata S, Morita T, Yokohama-Tamaki T, Murakami G, Cho BH. An Immunohistochemical study of matrix components in early-stage vascular canals within mandibular condylar cartilage in midterm human fetuses. Anat Rec. 2015;298(9):1560–71.
14. Augier M. Squelette Cephalique: Morphogenese, Morphologie, Craniometrie. In: Poirier P, Charpy A, editors. Traite D'anatomie Humaine; 1931.
15. Bumann A, Lotzmann U. Tmj disorders and orofacial pain: the role of dentistry in a multidisciplinary diagnostic approach. Stuttgart: Thieme; 2002.
16. Jahan E, Matsumoto A, Rafiq AM, Hashimoto R, Inoue T, Udagawa J, Sekine J, Otani H. Fetal jaw movement affects Ihh signaling in mandibular condylar cartilage development: the possible role of Ihh as mechanotransduction mediator. Arch Oral Biol. 2014;59(10):1108–18.
17. Sadler TW. Langman's medical embryology. 8th ed. Philadelphia: Lippincott Williams & Wilkins; 2011.
18. Chaya MD, Elavarasi P. Functional anatomy and biomechanics of temporomandibular joint and the far-reaching effects of its disorders. J Adv Clin Res Insights. 2016; https://doi.org/10.15713/ins.jcri.115.
19. Furstman L. The early development of the human temporomandibular joint. Am J Orthod. 1963;49(9):672–82.
20. Sperber GH. Craniofacial embryology. 4th ed. Cambridge: Great Britain at The University Press; 1993.
21. Çil AS, Bozkurt M, Bozkurt DK. Intrauterine temporomandibular joint dislocation: prenatal sonographic evaluation. Clin Med Res. 2014;12(1–2):58–60.
22. Merida-Velasco JR, Rodriguez-Vazquez JF, Merida-Velasco JA, Sanchez-Montesinos I, Espin-Ferra J, Jimenez-Collado J. Development of the human temporomandibular joint. Anat Rec. 1999;255(1):20–33.
23. Van Der Linden EJ, Burdi AR, De Jongh HJ. Critical periods in the prenatal morphogenesis of the human lateral pterygoid muscle, the mandibular condyle, the articular disc and medial articular capsule. Am J Orthod Dentofac Orthop. 1987;91(1):22–8.
24. Öğütcen-Toller M, Juniper RP. The embryologic development of the human lateral pterygoid muscle and İts relationships with the temporomandibular joint disc and Meckel's cartilage. J Oral Maxillofac Surg. 1993;51(7):772–8.
25. Enomoto A, Watahiki J, Nampo T, Iri T, Ichikawa Y, Tachikawa T, Koutaro M. Mastication markedly affects mandibular condylar cartilage growth, gene expression, and morphology. Am J Orthod Dentofac Orthop. 2014;146(3):355–63.
26. Sperger GH. Craniofacial embryology. 3rd ed. Bristol: Wright; 1981. p. 32.
27. Giambartolomei LA, Brunotto MN, De Ferraris MEG. Human temporomandibular joint disc: anatomy and measurements in prenatal development. Acta Odontol Latinoam. 2011;24(1):98–103.
28. Carvalho De Moraes LO, Tedesco RC, Arraéz-Aybar LA, Klein O, Mérida-Velasco JR, Alonso LG, et al. Eur J Histochem. 2015;59(4):2569.
29. Baume LJ, Holz J. Ontogenesis of the human temporomandibular joint: 2. Development of the temporal components. J Dent Res. 2015;49(4):864–75.
30. Kumar GS. Temporomandibular joint (Chapter 15). In: Orban's oral histology & embryology. 13th ed; 2011. p. 361.
31. Coleman RD. Temporomandibular joint: relation of the retrodiskal zone to Meckel's cartilage and lateral pterygoid muscle. J Dent Res. 2015;49(3):626–30.
32. Yuodellis RA. The morphogenesis of the human temporomandibular joint and its associated structures. J Dent Res. 1966;45(1):182–91.

33. Moffett BC. The prenatal development of the human temporomandibular joint. Contrib Embryol. 1957;36:21–8.
34. Rees LA. The structure and function of the mandibular joint. Br Dent J. 1954;96:125–33.
35. Harpman JA, Woollard HH. The tendon of the lateral pterygoid muscle. J Anat. 1938;73(Pt 1):112–5.
36. Hill A, Duran J, Purcell P. Lubricin protects the temporomandibular joint surfaces from degeneration. PLoS One. 2014;9(9):e106497.
37. Gabriela Granja Porto GG, Vasconcelos BVE, Andrade ESS, Silva-Junior VA. Comparison between human and rat TMJ: anatomic and histopathologic features. Acta Cir Bras. 2010;25(3):290–3.
38. Choukas NC, Sicher H. The structure of the temporomandibular joint. Oral Surg Oral Med Oral Pathol. 1960;13:1203–13.
39. Balı RK, Chandra S, Chandra S, Chandra M, Chandra N. Texbook of dental and oral histology *with embryology and multiple choice questions*. New Delhi: Jaypee; 2007. p. 257–62.
40. Shen G, Darendeliler MA. The adaptive remodeling of condylar cartilage: a transition from chondrogenesis to osteogenesis. J Dent Res. 2005;84:691–9.
41. Hatipoglu MT, Delilbasi L, Anil A. Temporomandibular Eklem. A.I.T.1.A. No: 199, Ankara, 1982.
42. Kantomaa T. New aspects of the histology of the mandibular condyle in the rat. Acta Anat. 1986;126:218–22.
43. Girdler NM. The behaviour of mandibular condylar cartilage in cell culture. J Oral Maxillofac Surg. 1993;22:178–84.
44. Luder HU. Structure and growth activities of the mandibular condyle in monkeys (Macaca fascicularis): I. İntracondylar variations. Am J Anat. 1983;166:223–35.
45. Bloom W, Fawcett D. A textbook of histology. 9th ed. Philadelphia: Saunders; 1968.
46. Merida-Velasco JR, Rodiguez-Vazquez JF, Merida-Velasco JA, Sanchez-Montesinos I, Espın-Ferra J, Jimenez-Collado J. Development of the human tempromandibular joint. Anat Rec. 1999;255(1):20–33.
47. Bosshardt-Luehrs CPB, Luder HU. Cartilage matrix production and chondrocyte enlargement as contributors to mandibular condylar growth in monkeys (Macaca fasccicularis). Am J Orthod Dentofac Orthop. 1991;100(4):362–9.
48. Karadede Mİ. Mandıbular Kondil Hısto-Anatomisinin Ratlarda İncelenmesi, Dicle Üniversitesi Diş Hekimliği Fakültesi Dergisi, Cilt 6, Sayı 1,2,3, Ocak-Mayıs-Eylül, 1995.
49. Matsumato F, Miyamato Y, Nagayama M. Light and electron-microscopic observations on the mandibular condylar cartilages in growing rats on a low-calcium diet. Acta Anat. 1991;142:41–8.
50. Copray CVM, et al. Growth and growth pressure of mandibular condylar and some primary cartilages of the rat in vitro. Am J Orthod Dentofac Orthop. 1986;90(1):19–46.
51. Kantomaa T, et al. Weaning and the histology of the mandibular condyle in the rat. Acta Anat. 1992;144:311–5.

Radiation Protection

4

Ruben Pauwels

4.1 Effects of Ionizing Radiation

Two types of effects of ionizing radiation on living tissue can be distinguished:

- Stochastic, comprising cancer and genetic (i.e., heritable) effects due to irreversible cell damage, usually to the DNA.
- Deterministic effects (i.e. tissue reactions), caused by the death of populations of cells due to high-dose exposure. The nature of the effect depends on the tissue, e.g., skin erythema, hair loss, cataract, infertility, and effects to the vascular, hematopoietic, and gastroenterological systems.

4.1.1 Stochastic Effects

4.1.1.1 The Linear-Non-Threshold Model

The exact relationship between radiation dose and stochastic effects has been under scrutiny ever since the first long-term effects from ionizing radiation were discovered. The most generally accepted model to predict stochastic effects is the linear-non-threshold (LNT) model (Fig. 4.1), which is based on the following principles:

- Cancer and genetic effects follow a random model. In other words, the effect is expressed as a *probability*.
- The probability of a stochastic effect (but not its severity) is *linearly* proportional to the radiation dose.
- There is no dose at which the attributable risk is zero. In other words, there is *no threshold* dose below which there is no additional risk for stochastic effects.

R. Pauwels
Mechanical Engineering Department, KU Leuven, Leuven, Belgium

Department of Radiology, Faculty of Dentistry, Chulalongkorn University, Bangkok, Thailand

I. Rozylo-Kalinowska, K. Orhan (eds.), *Imaging of the Temporomandibular Joint*, https://doi.org/10.1007/978-3-319-99468-0_4

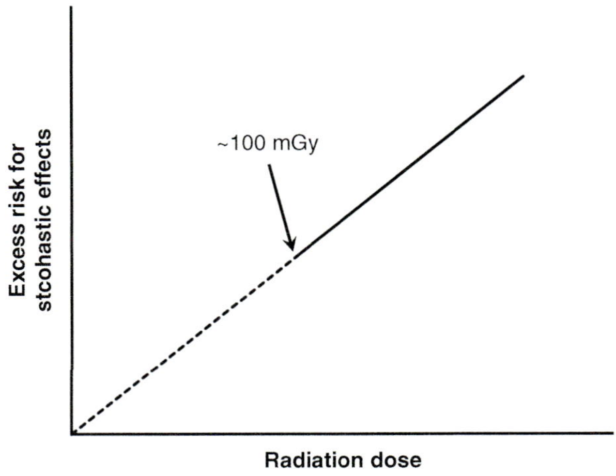

Fig. 4.1 Simplified representation of the linear-non-threshold model. Whereas this model is generally accepted at dose levels of 100 mGy or above, the exact relation between dose and effect is uncertain at typical doses found in diagnostic radiology

The validity of a linear dose-effect model has been demonstrated at doses above 100 mGy, using epidemiological data (e.g., the life span study of atomic bombing survivors) and experimental data [1]. However, at lower doses, the uncertainty of the estimated risk can be several orders of magnitude larger than the actual risk. This is why the LNT model is still considered as a hypothesis, until it is either confirmed through additional, conclusive data or until sufficient evidence for an alternative model has been found. In practice, radiation protection principles assume that the LNT model is valid [1]. Therefore, any exposure should adhere to the justification and optimization principles described in this chapter. Should at any given time a consensus be reached regarding the applicability of alternative models (e.g., linear quadratic, supralinear, hormesis), these protection principles may change accordingly.

4.1.1.2 Effect of Age and Gender on Stochastic Risk

Aside from the random nature of stochastic effects, there are several factors (e.g., cell division rate) that affect the probability of these effects at the level of tissues, individuals, or populations. The dependence of the stochastic risk on the sensitivity of tissues and organs is taken into account in the calculation of the effective dose, described further in this chapter. Differences between age- and gender-matched individual can be caused, for example, by their genetic makeup and the presence or absence or other risk factors. At a population level, the risk for stochastic effects is highly dependent on the age at the time of exposure and, mainly at younger ages, the gender of the exposed individual. According to the BEIR VII model, for all cancers combined, there is an inverse nonlinear relation between age and risk [2]. In terms of gender, for all cancer combined, females are at a higher risk than males; the absolute difference in risks between females and males is higher at younger ages (Fig. 4.2).

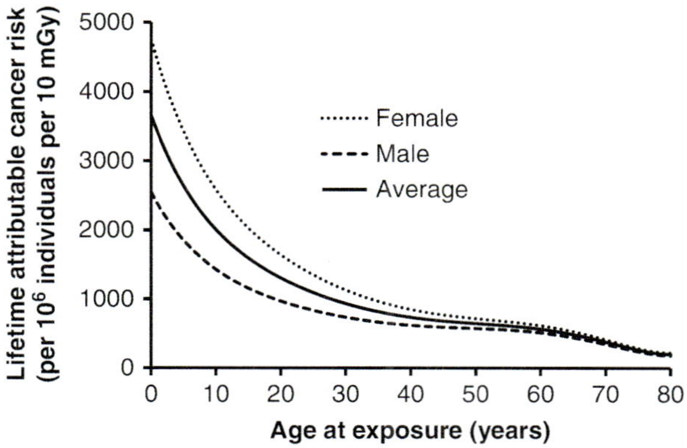

Fig. 4.2 Estimated lifetime Estimated lifetime attributable cancer incidence attributable cancer incidence risk from radiation, for all cancers combined, as a function of age at exposure, normalized to a dose of 10 mGy (Derived from the BEIR VII report [2])

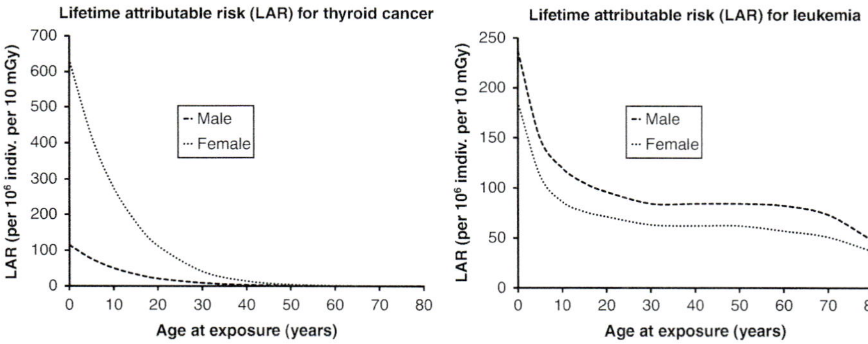

Fig. 4.3 Estimated lifetime attributable cancer risk from radiation, for thyroid cancer (left) and leukemia (right), as a function of age at exposure, normalized to a dose of 10 mGy (Derived from the BEIR VII report [2])

However, when looking at the effect of age and gender on the risk for stochastic effects to specific organs, a few important observations can be made (Fig. 4.3), for example:

- Thyroid cancer incidence is more strongly connected to age and gender than that of other cancers. While the risk for thyroid cancer is highest at birth, the risk is negligible at ages over 40. Females are at a much higher risk (4–5×, depending on the age) than males of the same age.
- Leukemia shows a similar relation to age as the total cancer risk. However, the risk is 30–40% higher risk for males.
- Several cancers are grouped as "other" in the BEIR VII report; these include a few organs that are exposed in TMJ imaging such as the salivary glands, brain, and skin. These "other" cancers show a similar age distribution compared with that of the total cancer risk, but the risk for females is only slightly higher within this group.

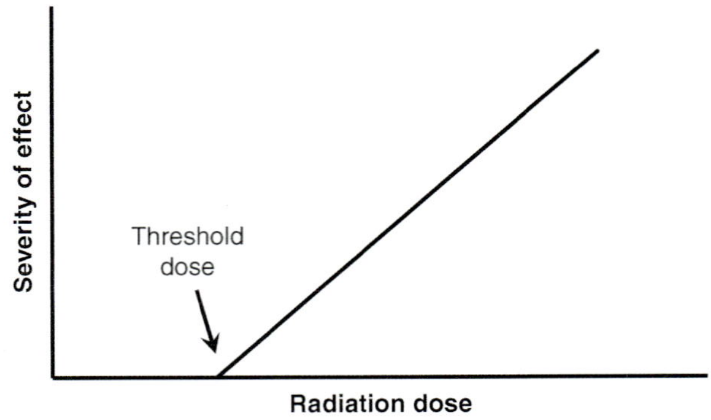

Fig. 4.4 Simplified representation of the dose-effect relation for deterministic effects

4.1.2 Deterministic Effects

The dose-effect relationship is considerably different between stochastic and deterministic effects. First of all, deterministic effects are predicted using a threshold dose (Fig. 4.4), which is defined as the dose level at which the incidence of tissue reactions is 1% [1]. Different thresholds have been determined for tissues that are prone to deterministic effects; also, separate threshold values have been determined for single and fractioned exposures, as the latter type of exposure allows for a healing period. For a single exposure, the current threshold for cataract, depression of hematopoiesis, and circulatory disease is 500 mGy. As described further in this chapter, absorbed doses from TMJ examinations are much lower than thresholds for deterministic effects; therefore, unlike stochastic effects, deterministic effects are not taken under consideration when making decisions regarding the appropriate use of these examinations, except in the rare case that they take place in the same time period as other high-dose exposures (e.g., radiotherapy in the head and neck region).

4.2 Radiation Dose: Definitions

The radiation dose of a medical exposure can be expressed using different quantities and units. This subsection will define absorbed dose, equivalent dose, and effective dose, which are complementary metrics to express the dose to a patient (or the dose to workers and public). Other quantities (e.g., computed tomography dose index, dose-area product) are used for practical applications such as dose tracking, quality assurance, and research.

The term "kerma" is occasionally used instead of "dose." Kerma refers to the transferred energy from photons to electrons, whereas dose refers to the deposited energy from secondary electrons to matter. However, although strictly speaking "kerma" and "dose" are not interchangeable, the difference between them is negligible at X-ray energies used in diagnostic radiology [3].

The quantities and units in this subsection adhere to the International Commission on Radiological Protection [1, 4], the International Commission on Radiation Units and Measurements (ICRU) as well as the International System of Units (SI).

4.2.1 Absorbed Dose

The absorbed dose, D, is defined as:

$$D = \frac{\Delta\bar{\varepsilon}}{\Delta m} \tag{4.1}$$

where $\Delta\bar{\varepsilon}$ is the mean energy imparted to matter of mass Δm by ionizing radiation. The SI unit for absorbed dose is gray (Gy), equal to joule per kilogram (J kg^{-1}).

4.2.2 Equivalent Dose (Radiation Weighted Dose)

The equivalent dose, H_T, is defined as:

$$H_T = \sum_R w_R D_{T,R} \tag{4.2}$$

where $D_{T,R}$ is the mean absorbed dose from radiation type R in a tissue or organ T and w_R is the radiation weighting factor for radiation type R. The SI unit for equivalent dose is sievert (Sv), which is equal to joule per kilogram.

The distinction between absorbed dose and equivalent dose is needed because different types of radiation (e.g., X-rays, neutrons, α particles) have varying biological effectiveness. However, for X-rays, the value of w_R is 1, implying that the numerical value of absorbed dose and equivalent dose is the same for medical exposures; only the unit is different.

4.2.3 Effective Dose

The effective dose, E, was introduced to take into account that different tissues and organs in the human body have a wide variation in sensitivity to ionizing radiation, in terms of probability and detriment of stochastic effects. The effective dose is a weighted sum of the equivalent doses in all radiosensitive tissues and organs of the body:

$$E = \sum_T w_T H_T \tag{4.3}$$

where H_T is the equivalent dose in a tissue or organ, T, and w_T is the tissue weighting factor. The unit for the effective dose is the same as equivalent dose, sievert (Sv).

The tissue weighting factors represent the relative contribution of each tissue or organ to the total health detriment from radiation exposure [1]. The sum of all w_T

Table 4.1 ICRP 103 tissue weighting factors [1]

Tissue	w_T	Σw_T
Bone marrow (red), colon, lung, stomach, breast, remainder tissues[a]	0.12	0.72
Gonads	0.08	0.08
Bladder, esophagus, liver, thyroid	0.04	0.16
Bone surface, brain, salivary glands, skin	0.01	0.04
	Total	1.00

[a]Remainder tissues: adrenals, extrathoracic (ET) region, gallbladder, heart, kidneys, lymphatic nodes, muscle, oral mucosa, pancreas, prostate (♂), small intestine, spleen, thymus, uterus/cervix (♀)

values is 1, but the individual weighting factors are periodically reviewed by the ICRP. Table 4.1 lists the most recent weighting factors from ICRP Publication 103 [1]. It can be seen that several organs or tissues in the list receive no or marginal exposure from dental examinations. For dental exposures, only the following organs have a notable contribution to the effective dose: the red bone marrow, esophagus, thyroid, bone surface, brain, salivary glands, skin, and several remainder tissues (extrathoracic region, lymphatic nodes, muscle, oral mucosa). Organs in the thorax (lung, heart, thymus, breast) or located more caudally receive a negligible dose from dental exposures, with the possible exception of maxillary occlusal radiographs.

Despite the common use of the effective dose to express radiation risk of medical exposures, there are several limitations to it. The weighting factors in Table 4.1 are rounded considerably compared with the relative detriment to each tissue [5]. They are also based on epidemiological data with a high level of uncertainty and are therefore expected to be revised as new data becomes available. They are also age- and gender-averaged and therefore can only be used as a risk estimate for standard populations, not for individuals or subpopulations [1].

4.3 Radiation Dose and Risk in TMJ Imaging

4.3.1 Patient Dose

The radiation dose to patients undergoing different types of TMJ examinations is not nearly as well-described as that of dental imaging. Furthermore, older dosimetric data may have limited current relevance, due to the increased digitization in 2D radiography (incl. panoramic radiography) as well as recent development in CT imaging allowing for (ultra)low-dose scanning. Therefore, this section will be limited to recently published dosimetric data and will exclude data pertaining to dental, ear, or other head examinations (unless the exposed region and exposure parameters are considered to be identical to TMJ imaging).

Projectional Radiography Recent dosimetric evidence regarding planar radiography for TMJ imaging is scarce. Matsuo et al. [6] estimated an effective dose of 12–25 μSv for orbitoramus projection and 5–27 μSv for Schuller's view, depending

Table 4.2 Effective dose from panoramic radiography (published since 2013)

	Effective dose (μSv)[a]
Chinem et al. [7]	27
Granlund et al. [9]	19–75
Lee et al. [10]	7
Signorelli et al. [8]	22
Davis et al. [11]	8–11
Shin et al. [12]	6
Han et al. [13]	10–26
Lee et al. [14]	9–38

Note that methodology can differ considerably between studies (e.g., radiographic unit, exposure parameters, phantom, number/location/calibration of dosimeters)
[a]Rounded to 1 μSv

on the collimation of the X-ray beam. Effective doses of skull radiographs acquired with modern cephalometric equipment are below 10 μSv [7, 8].

Panoramic Radiography Effective doses for panoramic radiography reported in literature since 2013 are listed in Table 4.2, ranging between 6 and 75 μSv but generally being below 30 μSv.

Diagnostic Cone Beam Computed Tomography Kadesjö et al. [15] estimated the effective dose for a dual-TMJ CBCT scan at 184 μSv for a non-optimized and 92 μSv for an optimized protocol. For two single-TMJ scans using a small field of view (FOV), Lukat et al. [16] estimated an effective dose of 10, 14, and 21 μSv for pediatric, adolescent, and adult protocols, respectively. As these studies comprise 2 CBCT units from the >50 units in clinical use worldwide, which exhibit a wide variability in FOV size, tube voltage, tube current, exposure time, and other parameters, it can be expected that TMJ imaging using CBCT has a wide dose range, similar to the dose range found in dental CBCT. Pauwels et al. [17] showed a 19-fold effective dose range on 14 dental CBCT models. In a systematic review, Al-Okshi et al. [18] reported median effective doses of 28.5 μSv for dental CBCT scans with FOV heights ≤5 cm, 69.9 μSv for FOV heights of 5.1–10.0 cm, and 114.0 μSv for FOV heights >10 cm.

Diagnostic Computed Tomography The doses from CT examinations have evolved considerably in recent years, owing to the availability of new detector systems as well as iterative reconstruction algorithms. Whereas it was estimated by Boeddinghaus and Whyte [19] that an effective dose of 1.2 mSv can be reached for TMJ examinations, an optimized CT protocol by Kadesjö et al. [15] resulted in an effective dose of 124 μSv, which is well within the dose range for CBCT. Widmann et al. [20] explored the use of an ultralow-dose CT protocol for orbital imaging, achieving a computed tomography dose index (CTDI) value as low as 2.64 mGy; the corresponding effective dose can be estimated at approx. 30 μSv per 5 cm scan length [21]. For craniofacial bone imaging, the same authors noticed no significant difference between a scan acquired at a CTDI of 0.82 mGy (~9.4 μSv per 5 cm scan length) using model-based iterative reconstruction and a reference scan at a CTDI of 30.48 mGy [22]. For imaging of the paranasal sinuses, effective doses of 131 μSv [23] and 19 μSv [24] have been achieved in clinical practice at diagnostically acceptable image quality levels.

Interventional Computed Tomography Acord et al. [25] found an average dose-area product (DAP) for C-arm pediatric CT acquired for joint injections of 21.4 mGy cm^2; although dedicated conversion factors from DAP to effective dose are lacking, it can be roughly estimated that this value corresponds to an effective dose below 10 μSv [12]. Zhu et al. [26] implemented a low-dose pediatric protocol for interventional C-arm CT, yielding a CTDI value of 0.3–0.4 mGy compared with 4.8 mGy using default settings and 0.6 mGy for conventional CT; the corresponding effective dose for the optimized C-arm CT exposure would be approx. 3–4 μSv per 5 cm scan length (or FOV height) vs. ~7 μSv per 5 cm scan length for conventional CT.

4.3.2 Comparative Risk

Due to the increasing information (and sometimes misinformation) spread regarding cancer risks of medical exposures, it is important that referrers as well as end users are aware of the radiation-induced cancer risk and are able to communicate this issue to their patients. Typically, rather than providing the patient with absolute estimates of dose, risk, or detriment for their planned procedure, the risks are put into perspective in order to explain to the patient that the expected benefit of the procedure outweighs the risk.

A first comparison that can be made is with other imaging modalities. For CBCT and CT, one can express the dose in terms of "x" radiographs, as the patient will be already familiar with these imaging techniques at this point. However, there are several limitations to this approach. First, effective dose reported for 2D radiography are variable, as shown above. Second, certain patients may require a relatively high-dose CBCT or CT exposure equivalent to 20 or more panoramic radiographs, in which case they may be deterred by this comparison. In this case, the practitioner must carefully clarify to the patient what the added value from the planned scan is compared to lower-dose alternatives and how this may impact the diagnosis and treatment outcome.

A second comparison is with the natural background radiation. Whereas background radiation is highly variable throughout the world as well, the worldwide average (3.0 mSv per year or ~8.2 μSv per day) can be used. Based on an estimate of the effective dose of the radiograph or scan, the equivalent radiation time can be provided to the patient. For radiographs and low-dose scans, the effective dose typically corresponds to only a few days of natural background radiation, whereas for high-dose scans, a dose equal to several months of background radiation is received.

Table 4.3 Radiation dose received during airplane travel, calculated using the European Program Package for the Calculation of Aviation Route Doses (EPCARD; http://www.helmholtz-muenchen.de/en/epcard-portal/epcard-home/index.html)

From	To	Effective dose (μSv)
Paris	Tokyo	35
London	New York	40
Los Angeles	New York	35

Somewhat similar, the dose of medical exposures can be expressed in relation to doses received during air travel; for long-distance flights, typical effective doses of 35–40 μSv are received, similar to a low-dose CBCT scan or a high-dose panoramic radiograph (Table 4.3).

4.4 Principles of Radiation Protection

4.4.1 Justification

The first fundamental principle of radiation protection, commonly referred to as the justification principle, states that:

> Any decision that alters the radiation exposure situation should do more good than harm [1]

In other words, a referral should only be done if the "good" (e.g., improved diagnostic confidence, improved treatment planning and treatment outcome) outweighs the "harm" (i.e., the risk for stochastic effects). Despite the simplicity of this principle, its application in daily practice is far from straightforward. Especially on a case-by-case basis, it is impossible to determine either the benefit or the potential harm with reasonable accuracy. Nonetheless, each exposure should be accompanied by a referral [27], which takes into account:

- The appropriateness of the request
- The urgency of the radiological procedure
- The characteristics of the medical exposure
- The characteristics of the individual patient
- Relevant information from the patient's previous radiological procedures

To help the practitioner in making informed decisions regarding justification, guidelines and referral criteria are produced. As their name implies, these documents should not be interpreted as regulations but have been designed to assist the clinician in their decision process, assuring good practice according to individual patient needs.

Making recommendations regarding justification for particular clinical tasks is beyond the scope of this chapter; the reader is referred to the chapters dealing with varying clinical applications in order to understand the (potential) benefit and drawbacks of each imaging technique, as well as typical indications for which each technique is used. This book and any other document dealing with justification of TMJ imaging should be considered as a guideline; decisions regarding the most appropriate imaging technique should always be made on a case-by-case basis.

4.4.2 Optimization of Exposures

4.4.2.1 Field of View Collimation

The collimation of the field of view (FOV) to the region of interest for diagnosis and/or treatment planning can be considered as the most effective strategy for radiation dose optimization. Whereas TMJ imaging may sometimes require the depiction of the entire maxillofacial region, for many applications an image containing only the joint suffices. For dental CBCT, the effective dose can be reduced by over 80% through FOV collimation alone (Fig. 4.5) [28]; similar dose reduction can be expected for TMJ imaging. Similarly, collimation of projection radiographs [6], panoramic radiographs [11], and CT [29] can be pivotal dose reduction strategies, especially for smaller patients.

Reducing the FOV size has benefits in terms of image quality as well. The use of a smaller active detector area results in a reduced amount of detected X-ray scatter, resulting in an improved projection image [30]. Furthermore, in CBCT in particular, large FOVs require the use of correspondingly large voxel sizes for practical reasons

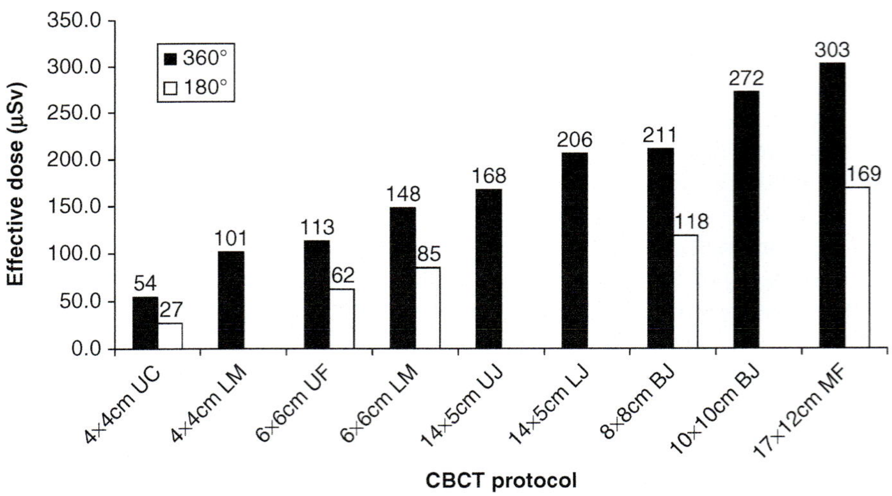

Fig. 4.5 Effective dose vs. field of view size and position, for the 3D Accuitomo 170 (J. Morita, Kyoto, Japan) at 90 kV, 87.5 mAs (360° rotational scan) and 45 mAs (180° rotational scan). Dose increases with increasing diameter and/or height of the FOV and is higher for mandibular than maxillary scans. *BJ* both jaws, *CBCT* cone-beam computed tomography, *LJ* lower jaw, *LM* lower molar, *MF* maxillofacial, *UC* upper canine, *UF* upper frontal, *UJ* upper jaw. Reproduced from Pauwels et al. [28] under the British Institute of Radiology's License to Publish

(i.e., reconstruction time, data size, available random access memory), whereas small FOVs can be reconstructed at smaller voxel sizes. For example, a 4 × 4 cm FOV reconstructed at a voxel size of 0.075 mm (16-bit, uncompressed DICOM) would be approx. 289 MB in size, whereas an 8 × 8 cm FOV at the same voxel size would be 2.3 GB in size, and a 15 × 15 cm FOV at the same voxel size would be 14.9 GB in size. When the voxel size is necessarily increased for larger FOVs to ensure that they can be visualized, processed, and stored using current-generation hardware, the true spatial resolution is no longer determined by other technical factors (e.g., number of projections, detector pixel size, focal spot); instead, the voxel size serves as a limiting factor for spatial resolution.

4.4.2.2 Tube Voltage Selection

The tube voltage (kV) is a rather complex exposure parameter because of its multi-fold effect on the X-ray spectrum, which in turn affects the amount and nature of X-ray attenuation by the patient. An increased kV results in a higher mean and maximum X-ray energy; in addition, the number of produced X-rays is increased at each energy level. Seeing that the probability of photoelectric absorption and Compton and Rayleigh scatter is dependent on X-ray energy, as well as the angular distribution of X-ray scatter, the kV has a pronounced effect on both radiation dose and image quality.

Investigations regarding the optimal kV for hard tissue imaging in the dentomaxillofacial region, at which the image quality is maximized at a certain dose level (or the dose is minimized at a certain image quality level), have been quite scarce. One reason for this is that the majority of radiographic and CBCT units operate at a fixed kV or within a limited voltage range. Two studies on a CBCT unit with a tube voltage selectable between 60 and 90 kV revealed that the highest kV value was the most dose-efficient [31], regardless of patient head size [32]. It remains to be seen whether tube voltage values above 90 kV are optimal for TMJ imaging, due to the vicinity of the temporal bone. Pending further investigation, a recommendation can be made to users of CBCT units with selectable kV to use the highest available kV and to adapt the mAs according to patient size and image quality requirements (see next section).

4.4.2.3 Tube Current and Exposure Time Selection

The tube current (mA) and exposure time (s) are often combined into a single parameter (i.e., the tube current-exposure time product or mAs) because of their similar effect on image quality and radiation dose. In CBCT they are best considered separately because of the possible link between exposure time and voxel size (see below).

The mA and exposure time are both linearly proportionate to the radiation dose (e.g., an increase of the mAs by 50% increases the patient dose by 50% when all other factors are constant). The main effect on image quality is in terms of image noise; the relationship typically follows a hyperbolic trend, implying that, at low mA levels, an increase in mAs by a certain step size will have a more pronounced effect on image noise than the same step size at high mA levels. Another potential effect in CBCT or CT is the presence of aliasing (undersampling) artefacts, manifested as radial streaks, when the number of projections, which dictates the total exposure time is insufficient. A final factor to consider is that the exposure time for most CBCT models is linked to the reconstructed voxel size. In this case, not only image noise will be affected but spatial resolution as well. It is also possible that the FOV size affects the voxel size, as mentioned above [33].

Based on these considerations, the user of any radiographic equipment should select the mA value at which image quality (in terms of noise and/or sharpness) is acceptable for a given patient size and diagnostic task. In digital imaging, above-optimal mAs will not deteriorate image quality as long as the saturation level for the detector is not reached, but this does not adhere to the optimization principle because the patient will have received a radiation dose that is higher than necessary.

Previous research regarding mA adaptation have indicated several practical considerations as well as limitations:

- It is possible to considerably reduce the mAs for smaller patients without any loss in image quality. It has been demonstrated on nonclinical CBCT scans that, to achieve a constant noise level, an average 5-year-old male can undergo scanning at a 30% lower mAs than an average adult male. Furthermore, adult females can be exposed at 10% lower mAs than males, on average [32]. Automatic exposure control, which is widespread in CT [34] and modern panoramic radiography units [11] but not yet common in CBCT, would address this issue by automatically adjusting the tube current according to patient size.
- Depending on the diagnostic task, the definition of "acceptable" image quality (as well as the mAs needed to reach this acceptable level) can vary considerably. Specific indications for TMJ imaging may differ in terms of the required sharpness and/or contrast.
- The optimal mAs for a given radiographic modality, patient and diagnostic task is, to a large extent, specific to the unit (i.e. model of radiographic equipment) under consideration [35]. This is mainly obvious in CBCT imaging; due to the range in kV used by different models, as well as differences in terms of imaging hardware and software, it is not possible to determine a universally applicable optimal mA level.

4.4.2.4 Shielding of Patients

Quite soon after the discovery of X-rays, adverse effects to workers dealing with ionizing radiation were found, leading to the use of shielding as one of the main protective strategies for workers and public (see Sect. 4.4.3). However, the use of shielding can be of benefit for patients as well, under the right conditions. Different types of personal shielding can be considered, primarily thyroid collars/shields, aprons, and glasses, containing an X-ray blocker such as lead.

The use of patient shielding in radiography or scanning of the head and neck is an ongoing topic of debate, and the following considerations should be taken into account:

- Shielding is almost exclusively blocking primary radiation, which originates from the X-ray tube and enters the patients from the outside. For scattered radiation generated and distributed inside the patient (i.e., internal scatter), the shielding will block any scatter that exits the body, but this has no effect on patient dose. There is, however, a fraction X-ray scatter generated in the anterior mandible which is deflected in a caudal-posterior manner and which may thus temporarily exit the patient below their chin and reenter the patient more caudally, for example, at the thyroid level. For this relative small fraction of "external" scatter, shielding may result in dose reduction even if it is placed outside the primary X-ray beam area.

- Shielding should be used with care when partially blocking the primary X-ray beam, as the blocking of X-rays leads to obscuration (in 2D imaging) or severe metal artefacts (in 3D iamging) at the level of the shielding. For example, whereas a thyroid collar would not interfere with the visualization of the hard tissues of the dentomaxillofacial region (as it is located sufficiently caudal to those tissues), for certain clinical applications such as airway evaluation, the use of thyroid shielding would lead to a nondiagnostic image.
- The presence of shielding materials may lead to an adverse reaction of an AEC system, resulting in a boost in the tube output which eventually would increase patient dose compared with a non-shielded scan [36]. Depending on the type of AEC used, shielding should be placed after acquisition of the scout images (for CT or CBCT), or should not be placed near the primary beam.
- Thyroid shielding can be considered as the most effective type of patient shielding in dental imaging, showing an average reduction in absorbed dose to the thyroid of ~45% when using a tightly fitted thyroid collar with a lead-equivalent thickness of at least 0.25 mm [37–41]. However, its efficacy for TMJ imaging is more limited due to the relatively large distance to the region of interest. Nonetheless, due to the relatively high contribution of the thyroid to the effective dose and stochastic risk from head and neck examinations, as well as the pronounced effect of age on risk for radiation-induced thyroid cancer, it can be recommended that thyroid shielding should be routine practice for pediatric examinations (unless counter-indicated due to the abovementioned issues regarding artefacts and AEC).
- Lead-/bismuth-doped glasses are currently not considered to have a significant benefit for dentomaxillofacial imaging, since deterministic effects to the eye lens do not occur at these dose levels (see above). Nonetheless, the use of such glasses can reduce the dose to the eye lens by more than 60% [37, 42]. However, they may cause artefacts interfering with image interpretation in TMJ imaging, as the shielding is at the same axial level as the region of interest.
- Whereas doses below the neck are extremely low for dentomaxillofacial examinations, two recent studies has shown significantly lower doses to sensitive organs such as breasts and gonads when using a lead apron in CBCT [43] and panoramic radiography [44], whereas another study showed no significant effect of lead apron shielding [45]. Unless counter-indicated, an apron can be considered for female patients, particularly pregnant patients for whom the examination cannot be postponed or patients who have explicitly expressed concern regarding the radiation risk.

4.4.2.5 Diagnostic Reference Levels (DRLs)

Diagnostic reference levels (DRLs) are a tool for optimization, required by the IAEA [27]. DRLs are based on estimations of typical patient doses for a given radiographic procedure within a defined geographical area (e.g., a country or region); they are typically defined as the rounded 75th percentile of the dose distribution from a representative sample of radiographic units. X-ray facilities should compare their own dose estimates with corresponding DRL values and review their optimization process if unusual deviations are found. As DRL values are expected to fluctuate over time (e.g., due to technological advancements), they should be periodically reviewed through collaborative efforts between X-ray facilities, professional bodies, the health authority, and the regulatory body. Note that DRLs are not dose limits, as the latter cannot be applied to patients.

Table 4.4 shows recently (≥2010) established diagnostic reference levels for panoramic radiography. Different dose indices have been used to define these DRLs: entrance surface dose (ESD), dose-width product (DWP), and dose-area product (DAP).

For AP or PA skull radiographs, in Europe, DRLs ranging between 2.5 and 5 mGy (ESD) and between 600 and 1000 mGy cm^2 (DAP) have been reported [53]. For CT and especially CBCT, dedicated DRLs for TMJ imaging are lacking; for head CT, in Europe, DRLs, ranging between 760 and 1300 mGy.cm (dose-length product, DLP) or between 50 and 75 mGy (computed tomography dose index, CTDI), have been determined [53]. However, for sinus CT, DRLs were much lower (DLP, 140–350 mGy.cm; CTDI, 15–25 mGy); for TMJ imaging, similar dose levels should be attainable. Readers are suggested to always contact their local health authority to retrieve relevant DRLs, if available.

Table 4.4 Diagnostic reference levels for panoramic radiography

Dose index	Country	Protocol	Image receptor	DRL	Reference
ESD (mGy)	Greece	Adult	All	4.1	Manousaridis et al. [46]
			DR	3.5	
			CR	4.2	
			Film	3.7	
		Small adult/ female	All	3.3	
		Child	All	2.2	
DWP (mGy mm)	Ireland	Adult	N/A	60	Walker and van der Putten [47]
	South Korea		All	60.1	Lee et al. [48]
	UK	Adult	All	74	HPA [49]
		Child	All	49	
DAP (mGy cm^2)	South Korea	Child	All	95.9	Kim et al. [50]
		Adult	All	120.3	Han et al. [51]
	UK	Adult	All	93	HPA [49]
		Child	All	67	
	USA		All	100	NCRP [52]

4.4.3 Application of Dose Limits (Protection of Workers and Public)

During radiographic examinations, people in the vicinity of the equipment are subjected to radiation exposure. The main source of exposure is scattered radiation coming from the patient during image acquisition; a small amount of leaked radiation from the X-ray tube could also occur. Protection of workers and public is assured through adherence to the principle of application of dose limits of the ICRP [1]:

> …the total dose to any individual from regulated sources in planned exposure situations other than medical exposure of patients should not exceed the appropriate limits specified by the Commission

Along with this principle, dose limits to workers and publics have been proposed by the ICRP, most recently in ICRP Publication 103 (2007) [1], except for the eye lens for which a lower dose limit for occupational exposure was proposed in 2011 [54] (Table 4.5). These limits are usually adopted by other organizations and implemented in national and regional legislation as such.

Apart from these general dose limits, the concept of dose constraints has been introduced. These dose constraints are specific to each type of radiation exposure and are determined to represent good practice rather than a hard cut-off between an acceptable and unacceptable dose. Clinics or hospitals operating above this constraint can be recommended, without legal obligation, to evaluate whether dose-reduction techniques specifically aimed at workers and public can be implemented.

Whereas the implementation of dose reduction techniques for patients typically leads to a proportional dose reduction to workers and public as well, additional considerations are needed to ensure that doses are below the abovementioned dose limits or dose constraints (and, regardless, as low as possible):

Table 4.5 Dose limits for occupational and public exposure, according to ICRP Publication 103 [1] and ICRP's Statement on Tissue Reactions [54]

Type of limit	Occupational	Public
Annual effective dose	20 mSv[a,b]	1 mSv[c]
Annual equivalent dose to:		
Eye lens	20 mSv[a]	15 mSv
Skin[d]	500 mSv	50 mSv
Hands and feet	500 mSv	–

[a]Averaged over 5 years, with no single year exceeding 50 mSv

[b]Additional restrictions apply for pregnant women; after a worker declares a pregnancy, the dose to the embryo/fetus should not exceed about 1 mSv during the remainder of the pregnancy

[c]Similar to the occupational dose, a higher annual dose could be allowed in a single year in special circumstances, providing that the average over 5 years does not exceed 1 mSv/year

[d]Averaged over 1 cm^2, regardless of the area exposed

- *Distance*. The importance of adequate distance to the radiation source can be shown using the inverse square law, which states that the radiation dose in a point surrounding a radiation source decreases proportionally to the square of the distance to that source. In other words, a distance of 2 m to the source reduces the dose with a factor 4 compared with a distance of 1 m and a distance of 3 m with a factor 9. Note that the source of radiation in this case is the patient, not the X-ray tube. Also note that the scattering of radiation stops as soon as the image acquisition has ended and that there is no need for additional protective measures after wards (unlike in nuclear medicine).
- *Shielding*. The use of shielding in strategic locations (e.g., walls and windows), or the use of mobile barriers, can assure that the majority of scattered and leaked radiation is absorbed before reaching workers and public. Shielding is especially important if adequate distance is not feasible, for example, due to limited available space. Although high-density metals (typically lead and leaded glass) are often used, an equivalent thickness of concrete or other building materials can be considered instead. Personal shielding such as lead aprons and collars can also be used, although room-based shielding is preferred and more convenient.
- *Time*. The cumulative time in which a worker is subjected to radiation exposure should be limited as much as possible.

The data on scatter doses around equipment used in TMJ imaging is somewhat limited. For CBCT, doses of 4–47 μSv/scan have been measured at 1 m of the isocenter, with a median of 7.4 μSv [55]. For (low-dose) CT, similar amounts of scatter can be expected, albeit with a different spatial distribution due to the supine position of the patient. In comparison, for intraoral and panoramic radiography, doses at 1 m of less than 1 μSv have been reported [56, 57]. Therefore, when a CBCT or CT unit is placed in a hospital or clinic, special consideration is needed regarding the layout of the room(s), and the need for shielding to assure compliance with dose limits or dose constraints should be evaluated. This often requires a case-by-case approach, as the amount of scattered dose can vary considerably depending on the CT/CBCT model as well as its relative location compared to workers and public. A qualified medical physicist is typically involved to measure (or estimate) the dose in the vicinity of the unit and to provide guidance on proper installation and shielding requirements.

References

1. ICRP, International Commission on Radiological Protection. The 2007 recommendations of the international commission on radiological protection. ICRP publication 103. Ann ICRP. 2007;37:1–332.
2. NRC, National Research Council of the National Academies. Health risks from exposure to low levels of ionizing radiation: BEIR VII – phase 2. Washington, DC: The National Academies Press; 2006.
3. Hendee WR, Ritenour ER. Medical imaging physics. 4th ed. New York: Wiley-Liss; 2002.

4. ICRP, International Commission on Radiological Protection. Recommendations of the ICRP. ICRP Publication 26. Ann ICRP. 1977;1:1–53.
5. Martin CJ. Effective dose: how should it be applied to medical exposures? Br J Radiol. 2007;80:639–47.
6. Matsuo A, Okano T, Gotoh K, Yokoi M, Hirukawa A, Okumura S, Koyama S. Absorbed dose and the effective dose of panoramic temporo mandibular joint radiography. Nihon Hoshasen Gijutsu Gakkai Zasshi. 2011;67:1275–83. [Article in Japanese].
7. Chinem LA, Vilella BDS, Maurício CL, Canevaro LV, Deluiz LF, Vilella ODV. Digital orthodontic radiographic set versus cone-beam computed tomography: an evaluation of the effective dose. Dental Press J Orthod. 2016;21:66–72.
8. Signorelli L, Patcas R, Peltomäki T, Schätzle M. Radiation dose of cone-beam computed tomography compared to conventional radiographs in orthodontics. J Orofac Orthop. 2016;77:9–15.
9. Granlund C, Thilander-Klang A, Ylhan B, Lofthag-Hansen S, Ekestubbe A. Absorbed organ and effective doses from digital intra-oral and panoramic radiography applying the ICRP 103 recommendations for effective dose estimations. Br J Radiol. 2016;89:20151052.
10. Lee C, Lee SS, Kim JE, Huh KH, Yi WJ, Heo MS, Choi SC. Comparison of dosimetry methods for panoramic radiography: thermoluminescent dosimeter measurement versus personal computer-based Monte Carlo method calculation. Oral Surg Oral Med Oral Pathol Oral Radiol. 2016;121:322–9.
11. Davis AT, Safi H, Maddison SM. The reduction of dose in paediatric panoramic radiography: the impact of collimator height and programme selection. Dentomaxillofac Radiol. 2015;44:20140223.
12. Shin HS, Nam KC, Park H, Choi HU, Kim HY, Park CS. Effective doses from panoramic radiography and CBCT (cone beam CT) using dose area product (DAP) in dentistry. Dentomaxillofac Radiol. 2014;43:20130439.
13. Han GS, Cheng JG, Li G, Ma XC. Shielding effect of thyroid collar for digital panoramic radiography. Dentomaxillofac Radiol. 2013;42:20130265.
14. Lee GS, Kim JS, Seo YS, Kim JD. Effective dose from direct and indirect digital panoramic units. Imaging Sci Dent. 2013;43:77–84.
15. Kadesjö N, Benchimol D, Falahat B, Näsström K, Shi XQ. Evaluation of the effective dose of cone beam CT and multislice CT for temporomandibular joint examinations at optimized exposure levels. Dentomaxillofac Radiol. 2015;44:20150041.
16. Lukat TD, Wong JC, Lam EW. Small field of view cone beam CT temporomandibular joint imaging dosimetry. Dentomaxillofac Radiol. 2013;42:20130082.
17. Pauwels R, Beinsberger J, Collaert B, Theodorakou C, Rogers J, Walker A, Cockmartin L, Bosmans H, Jacobs R, Bogaerts R, Horner K, SEDENTEXCT Project Consortium. Effective dose range for dental cone beam computed tomography scanners. Eur J Radiol. 2012;81:267–71.
18. Al-Okshi A, Lindh C, Salé H, Gunnarsson M, Rohlin M. Effective dose of cone beam CT (CBCT) of the facial skeleton: a systematic review. Br J Radiol. 2015;88:20140658.
19. Boeddinghaus R, Whyte A. Computed tomography of the temporomandibular joint. J Med Imaging Radiat Oncol. 2013;57:448–54.
20. Widmann G, Juranek D, Waldenberger F, Schullian P, Dennhardt A, Hoermann R, Steurer M, Gassner EM, Puelacher W. Influence of ultra-low-dose and iterative reconstructions on the visualization of orbital soft tissues on maxillofacial CT. AJNR Am J Neuroradiol. 2017;38:1630–5.
21. Huda W, Ogden KM, Khorasani MR. Converting dose-length product to effective dose at CT. Radiology. 2008;248:995–1003.
22. Widmann G, Schullian P, Gassner EM, Hoermann R, Bale R, Puelacher W. Ultralow-dose CT of the craniofacial bone for navigated surgery using adaptive statistical iterative reconstruction and model-based iterative reconstruction: 2D and 3D image quality. AJR Am J Roentgenol. 2015;204:563–9.

23. Bang M, Choi SH, Park J, Kang BS, Kwon WJ, Lee TH, Nam JG. Radiation dose reduction in paranasal sinus CT: with feasibility of iterative reconstruction technique. Otolaryngol Head Neck Surg. 2016;155:982–7.
24. Aksoy EA, Özden SU, Karaarslan E, Ünal ÖF, Tanyeri H. Reliability of high-pitch ultra-low-dose paranasal sinus computed tomography for evaluating paranasal sinus anatomy and sinus disease. J Craniofac Surg. 2014;25:1801–4.
25. Acord M, Shellikeri S, Vatsky S, Srinivasan A, Krishnamurthy G, Keller MS, Cahill AM. Reduced-dose C-arm computed tomography applications at a pediatric institution. Pediatr Radiol. 2017;47:1817–24.
26. Zhu X, Felice M, Johnson L, Sarmiento M, Cahill AM. Developing low-dose C-arm CT imaging for temporomandibular joint (TMJ) disorder in interventional radiology. Pediatr Radiol. 2011;41:476–82.
27. IAEA, International Atomic Energy Agency. Radiation protection and safety of radiation sources: international basic safety standards. In: General safety requirements part 3. Vienna: IAEA; 2014. Available at https://www-pub.iaea.org/MTCD/publications/PDF/Pub1578_web-57265295.pdf.
28. Pauwels R, Zhang G, Theodorakou C, Walker A, Bosmans H, Jacobs R, Bogaerts R, Horner K, SEDENTEXCT Project Consortium. Effective radiation dose and eye lens dose in dental cone beam CT: effect of field of view and angle of rotation. Br J Radiol. 2014b;87:20130654.
29. Christner JA, Zavaletta VA, Eusemann CD, Walz-Flannigan AI, McCollough CH. Dose reduction in helical CT: dynamically adjustable z-axis X-ray beam collimation. AJR Am J Roentgenol. 2010;194:49–55.
30. Pauwels R, Jacobs R, Bogaerts R, Bosmans H, Panmekiate S. Reduction of scatter-induced image noise in cone beam computed tomography: effect of field of view size and position. Oral Surg Oral Med Oral Pathol Oral Radiol. 2016;121:188–95.
31. Pauwels R, Silkosessak O, Jacobs R, Bogaerts R, Bosmans H, Panmekiate S. A pragmatic approach to determine the optimal kVp in cone beam CT: balancing contrast-to-noise ratio and radiation dose. Dentomaxillofac Radiol. 2014a;43:20140059.
32. Pauwels R, Jacobs R, Bogaerts R, Bosmans H, Panmekiate S. Determination of size-specific exposure settings in dental cone-beam CT. Eur Radiol. 2017;27:279–85.
33. Librizzi ZT, Tadinada AS, Valiyaparambil JV, Lurie AG, Mallya SM. Cone-beam computed tomography to detect erosions of the temporomandibular joint: effect of field of view and voxel size on diagnostic efficacy and effective dose. Am J Orthod Dentofac Orthop. 2011;140:e25–30.
34. Alibek S, Brand M, Suess C, Wuest W, Uder M, Greess H. Dose reduction in pediatric computed tomography with automated exposure control. Acad Radiol. 2011;18:690–3.
35. Pauwels R, Seynaeve L, Henriques JC, de Oliveira-Santos C, Souza PC, Westphalen FH, Rubira-Bullen IR, Ribeiro-Rotta RF, Rockenbach MI, Haiter-Neto F, Pittayapat P, Bosmans H, Bogaerts R, Jacobs R. Optimization of dental CBCT exposures through mAs reduction. Dentomaxillofac Radiol. 2015;44:20150108.
36. Kaplan S, Magill D, Felice MA, Xiao R, Ali S, Zhu X. Female gonadal shielding with automatic exposure control increases radiation risks. Pediatr Radiol. 2018;48(2):227–34.
37. Goren AD, Prins RD, Dauer LT, Quinn B, Al-Najjar A, Faber RD, Patchell G, Branets I, Colosi DC. Effect of leaded glasses and thyroid shielding on cone beam CT radiation dose in an adult female phantom. Dentomaxillofac Radiol. 2013;42:20120260.
38. Hidalgo A, Davies J, Horner K, Theodorakou C. Effectiveness of thyroid gland shielding in dental CBCT using a paediatric anthropomorphic phantom. Dentomaxillofac Radiol. 2015;44:20140285.
39. Qu X, Li G, Zhang Z, Ma X. Thyroid shields for radiation dose reduction during cone beam computed tomography scanning for different oral and maxillofacial regions. Eur J Radiol. 2012b;81:e376–80.
40. Qu XM, Li G, Sanderink GC, Zhang ZY, Ma XC. Dose reduction of cone beam CT scanning for the entire oral and maxillofacial regions with thyroid collars. Dentomaxillofac Radiol. 2012a;41:373–8.

41. Tsiklakis K, Donta C, Gavala S, Karayianni K, Kamenopoulou V, Hourdakis CJ. Dose reduction in maxillofacial imaging using low dose Cone Beam CT. Eur J Radiol. 2005;56:413–7.
42. Prins R, Dauer LT, Colosi DC, Quinn B, Kleiman NJ, Bohle GC, Holohan B, Al-Najjar A, Fernandez T, Bonvento M, Faber RD, Ching H, Goren AD. Significant reduction in dental cone beam computed tomography (CBCT) eye dose through the use of leaded glasses. Oral Surg Oral Med Oral Pathol Oral Radiol Endod. 2011;112:502–7.
43. Schulze RKW, Sazgar M, Karle H, de Las Heras Gala H. Influence of a commercial lead apron on patient skin dose delivered during oral and maxillofacial examinations under cone beam computed tomography (CBCT). Health Phys. 2017;113:129–34.
44. Schulze RKW, Cremers C, Karle H, de Las Heras Gala H. Skin entrance dose with and without lead apron in digital panoramic radiography for selected sensitive body regions. Clin Oral Investig. 2017;21:1327–33.
45. Rottke D, Patzelt S, Poxleitner P, Schulze D. Effective dose span of ten different cone beam CT devices. Dentomaxillofac Radiol. 2013;42:20120417.
46. Manousaridis G, Koukorava C, Hourdakis CJ, Kamenopoulou V, Yakoumakis E, Tsiklakis K. Establishment of diagnostic reference levels for dental panoramic radiography in Greece. Radiat Prot Dosim. 2015;165:111–4.
47. Walker C, van der Putten W. Patient dosimetry and a novel approach to establishing Diagnostic Reference Levels in dental radiology. Phys Med. 2012;28:7–12.
48. Lee JS, Kim YH, Yoon SJ, Kang BC. Reference dose levels for dental panoramic radiography in Gwangju, South Korea. Radiat Prot Dosim. 2010;142:184–90.
49. HPA, Health Protection Agency. HPA-CRCE-034: doses to patients from radiographic and fluoroscopic x-ray imaging procedures in the UK (2010 review). Chilton: HPA; 2010.
50. Kim YH, Yang BE, Yoon SJ, Kang BC, Lee JS. Diagnostic reference levels for panoramic and lateral cephalometric radiography of Korean children. Health Phys. 2014;107:111–6.
51. Han S, Lee B, Shin G, Choi J, Kim J, Park C, Park H, Lee K, Kim Y. Dose area product measurement for diagnostic reference levels and analysis of patient dose in dental radiography. Radiat Prot Dosim. 2012;150:523–31.
52. NCRP, National Council on Radiation Protection and Measurements. Reference levels and achievable doses in medical and dental imaging: recommendations for the United States, NCRP Report No. 172. Bethesda: NCRP; 2012.
53. EC, European Comission. Radiation protection N° 180. Diagnostic reference levels in thirty-six European countries. Luxembourg: Publications Office of the European Union; 2012.
54. ICRP, International Commission on Radiological Protection. ICRP statement on tissue reactions and early and late effects of radiation in normal tissues and organs - threshold doses for tissue reactions in a radiation protection context. ICRP publication 118. Ann ICRP. 2012;41:1–322.
55. SEDENTEXCT. Deliverable 2.2: Completion of scatter dose measurements around CBCTs and recommendations for protective measures and positioning of CBCT units in dental offices. 2010. Available on http://www.sedentexct.eu/system/files/SEDENTEXCT%20D2.2%20v1%20FINAL_0.pdf. Accessed 18 Mar 2018.
56. Gijbels F, Jacobs R, Debaveye D, Bogaerts R, Verlinden S, Sanderink G. Dosimetry of digital panoramic imaging. Part II: occupational exposure. Dentomaxillofac Radiol. 2005;34:150–3.
57. Sutton DG, Williams JR. Radiation shielding for diagnostic X-rays: report of a Joint BIR/IPEM Working Party. London: British Institute of Radiology; 2000.

Conventional Radiography in TMJ Imaging

5

Keith Horner and David MacDonald

5.1 Introduction

Conventional radiography (also known as "plain" radiography) is the oldest form of medical imaging. The TMJ presents a particular challenge because of its location; obtaining a plain radiographic image free of significant superimposition by other parts of the cranium, in particular the dense base of skull, is impossible. In simple terms, the normal bony anatomy of the TMJ consists essentially of an ellipsoid condylar head positioned within a concave articular fossa, with a space separating these two components. The bony anatomy of the joint also means that no single radiographic projection provides complete topographical information. The outline of these irregularly shaped structures on plain radiographic images is governed by the particular profile to which the X-ray beam was tangential. Minor positioning and angulation differences will change this relationship and the resulting image. These limitations help to explain the plethora of projections that have been described for imaging the component parts of the joint (Table 5.1). The development of cross-sectional imaging, initially by tomography but later by CT, has steadily reduced the perceived value of many of the plain radiographic methods of imaging the TMJ. Panoramic radiography, often available in primary dental care facilities, remains widely used and is included in this chapter under the heading of "conventional" radiography.

K. Horner (✉)
Division of Dentistry, School of Medical Sciences, Faculty of Biology, Medicine and Health, The University of Manchester, Manchester, UK
e-mail: keith.horner@manchester.ac.uk

D. MacDonald
Division of Oral & Maxillofacial Radiology, Department of Oral, Biological and Medical Sciences, Faculty of Dentistry, University of British Columbia, Vancouver, BC, Canada
e-mail: dmacdon@dentistry.ubc.ca

I. Rozylo-Kalinowska, K. Orhan (eds.), *Imaging of the Temporomandibular Joint*, https://doi.org/10.1007/978-3-319-99468-0_5

Table 5.1 Conventional radiographic projections which have been used for imaging of the temporomandibular joint (TMJ)

Projection	Example	Technique	TMJ structure(s) imaged
Transcranial oblique lateral ("modified Stenver's view")	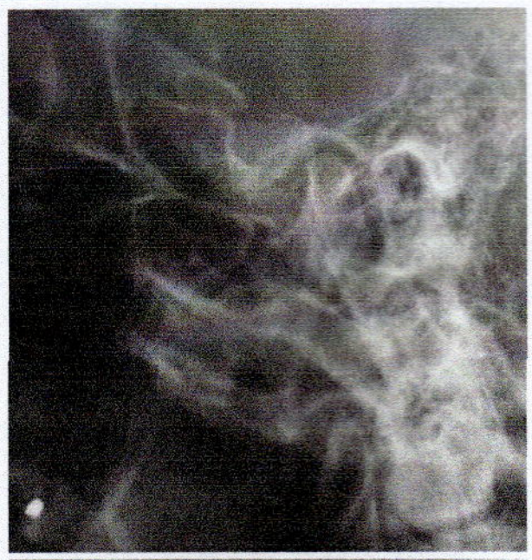 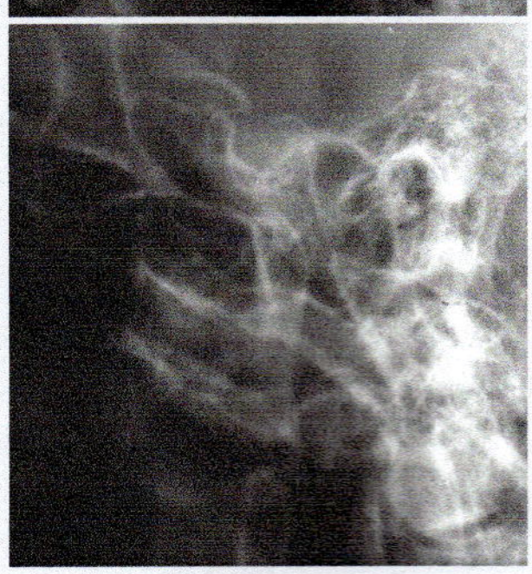	*Position of patient and image receptor* Sagittal plane of head parallel to the image receptor Joint of interest next to the image receptor Views with patient's mouth closed and then opened *Direction and location of the X-ray beam* Central ray angled 25° caudally and centred at a point 5 cm superior to the joint furthest from the image receptor	Condylar head Articular fossa Joint space (closed view)
Transpharyngeal ("Parma view", "McQueen view", "Toller's view")	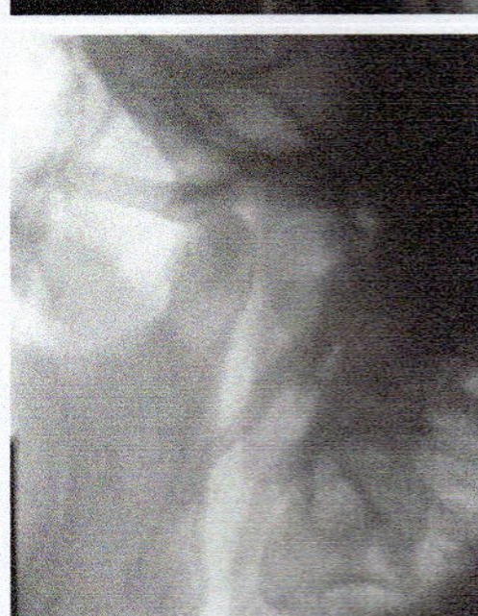	*Position of patient and image receptor* Sagittal plane of head parallel to the image receptor Joint of interest next to the image receptor Patient opens mouth as much as possible *Direction and location of the X-ray beam* Central ray angled 5–10° cranially and 5–10° posteriorly, with the central ray directed through the sigmoid notch of the mandible closest to the X-ray source towards the TMJ closest to the image receptor	Condylar neck and head

Table 5.1 (continued)

Projection	Example	Technique	TMJ structure(s) imaged
Transorbital ("Zimmer's view")	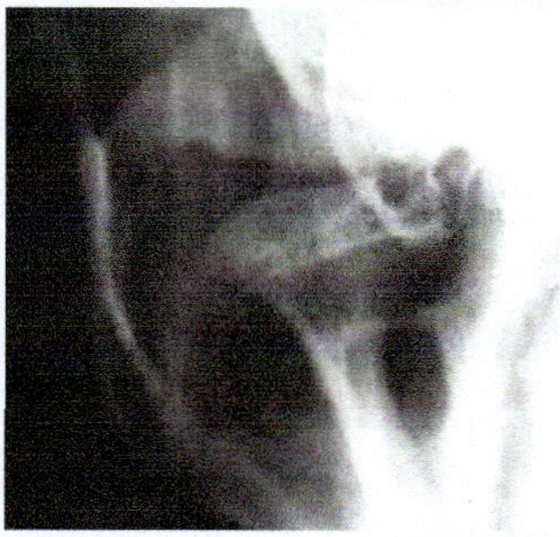	*Position of patient and image receptor* Image receptor at the back of the head and with the patient facing the X-ray source, with the axial plane horizontal and with the sagittal plane turned c. 30° towards the side of interest Patient opens mouth as much as possible *Direction and location of the X-ray beam* The central beam directed through the ipsilateral orbit towards the TMJ	Condylar neck and head
Submento-vertical	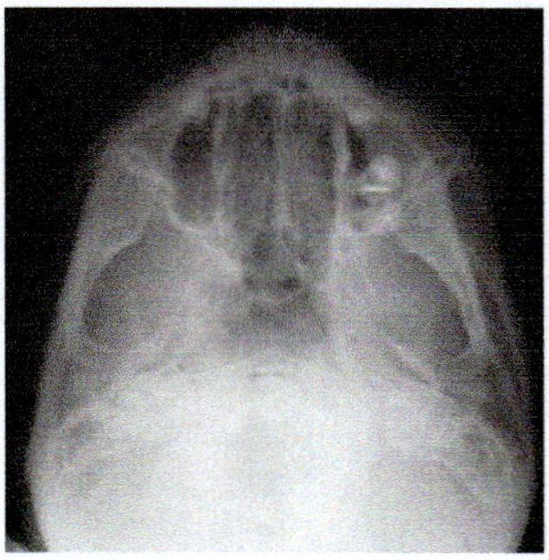	*Position of patient and image receptor* Patient faces the X-ray source and then extends neck maximally so that the orbito-meatal plane is near as possible to be parallel to the image receptor *Direction and location of the X-ray beam* Central beam directed perpendicular to the orbito-meatal plane and parallel to the sagittal plane in the midline, at the level of the TMJs	Condylar head
PA facial bones ("reverse Towne's view")	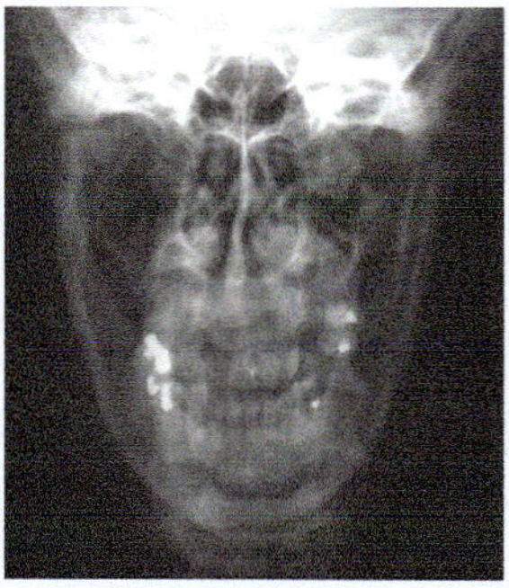	*Position of patient and image receptor* Sagittal plane of head perpendicular to the image receptor Patient facing the image receptor Patient opens mouth as much as possible *Direction and location of the X-ray beam* Cranial 10–30° angulation of the beam Centre of the beam positioned to pass through the condylar necks	Condylar neck and head

(continued)

Table 5.1 (continued)

Projection	Example	Technique	TMJ structure(s) imaged
Lateral cephalogram	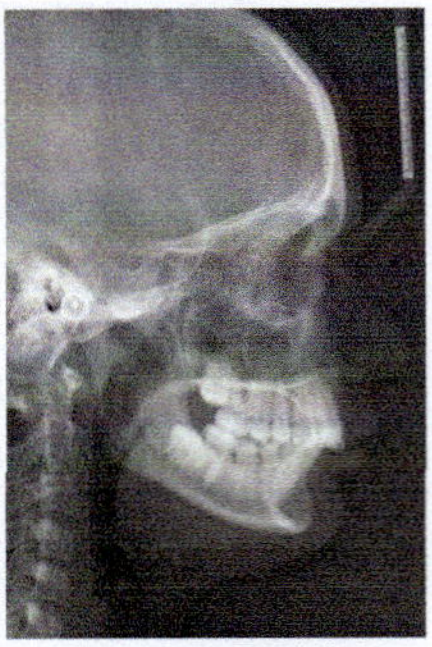	*Position of patient and image receptor* Head in cephalostat with sagittal plane of head parallel with the image receptor and in a natural head position with teeth in occlusion *Direction and location of the X-ray beam* Perpendicular to the sagittal plane and image receptor and centred over the external auditory meatus	Not applicable
PA cephalogram	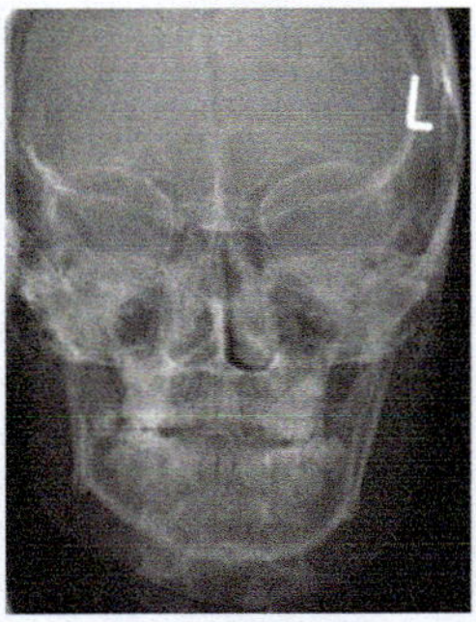	*Position of patient and image receptor* Head in cephalostat with sagittal plane and the Frankfort plane that are perpendicular to the image receptor and in a natural head position with teeth in occlusion *Direction and location of the X-ray beam* Perpendicular to the image receptor and centred over the bridge of the nose	Not applicable

Most are of historical interest only. The names of views and details of the radiographic techniques are inconsistent in the literature, and those used are consistent with the authors' preference and practice. Note that the imaging of the listed structures is limited to the two-dimensional profile of those structures as determined by the patient's anatomy, patient position and X-ray beam angulation. The transpharyngeal view was traditionally taken using a dental X-ray set, using a short focus-to-skin distance

It is important to remember that conventional radiography only provides images of the bony components of the TMJ. This is the most clinically relevant limitation of its use, bearing in mind that the most prevalent of TMJ pathoses (myalgia/ myofascial pain, internal disc derangement) only or principally affect the soft tissues. For the assessment of internal derangements, the availability of arthrography and especially MR imaging has reduced the indications for conventional radiography dramatically.

Thus, most plain radiographic examinations are only of historical interest and can reasonably be described as obsolete. In his 2010 review, Petersson [1] highlighted their limitations and applauded the absence of plain radiographs from the research diagnostic criteria for temporomandibular disorders (RDC/TMD) [2]. Recent reviews and textbooks do not mention plain radiography, apart from panoramic radiography, as part of the imaging strategy for the TMJ [3–7].

Of those plain radiographs listed in Table 5.1, only the reverse Towne's view might currently be taken, in cases of suspected fracture involving the mandibular condyle or the condylar neck, although current practice increasingly favours the use of cross-sectional imaging in such cases (see Sect. 5.3). Cephalograms (lateral and/or postero-anterior projections) are used for the imaging assessment of some conditions related to the TMJ which result in facial growth anomalies, such as condylar hypoplasia and hyperplasia, but do not provide detailed information about the TMJs themselves because of superimpositions. Apart from these exceptions, therefore, for the overwhelming majority of patients with clinical signs or symptoms related to the TMJ, the only conventional radiographic examination would be the panoramic radiograph.

5.2 Panoramic Radiography: Technical Aspects

Several different names have been given to this technique, including dental panoramic tomography, pantomography and panoral, along with various manufacturers' names which have incorrectly used as general terms for equipment. The term panoramic radiography is preferred here. Traditionally, panoramic radiographs provide an image of the complete mandible and maxilla. This includes the bony components of the TMJ (Fig. 5.1).

Excellent textbook descriptions of the principles of panoramic radiographic image formation are available [5, 8], and only a summary is given here. Panoramic radiography is generally considered to be a form of tomography in which a layer within the patient's face is imaged. As with any radiographic tomography, there is a rotation of the X-ray source and image receptor around the patient's head. With panoramic radiography, a rather complex motion with a continuously moving centre of rotation is set up to image a curved layer within the patient (also known as the image layer, focal plane or focal trough) corresponding to the patient's teeth and jaws. Another important aspect of the method is that a vertical slit X-ray beam is used. For film-based or indirect (phosphor plate) digital systems, a coordinated horizontal movement of the image receptor means that the slit beam scans across it during the exposure, building the image data. Direct digital systems use a tall, narrow, vertical detector aligned with the slit beam to capture the attenuated X-ray beam.

The image layer is designed to accommodate the shape of the dental arch and jaws. It is narrower anteriorly but becomes progressively broader posteriorly to

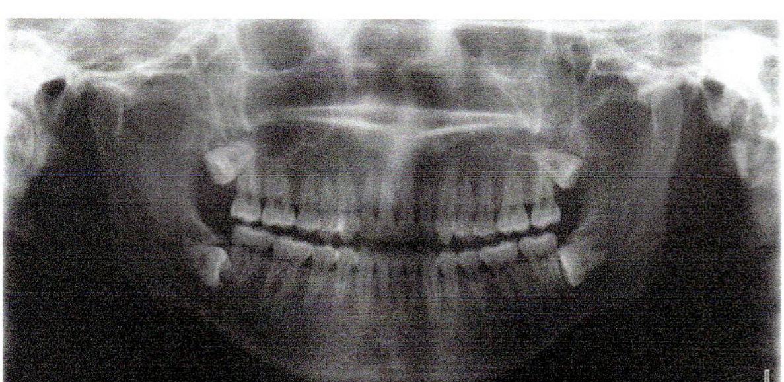

Fig. 5.1 Excellent quality panoramic radiograph including the TMJ regions

accommodate the maxillary and mandibular dental arches. The image layer represents a zone of maximal image sharpness, at the centre of which vertical and horizontal magnifications become equal. Structures outside the image layer become progressively more blurred the further they are from it, but their shape also becomes increasingly distorted. Structures bucco-labial to the image layer suffer from relatively less horizontal magnification than that in the vertical direction, while the reverse is the case for structures positioned palato-lingually. The detailed motion of panoramic equipment will vary between manufacturers, while patient anatomy will often deviate from the ideal model used in designing the equipment. Thus, a change in the equipment may change the appearance of the jaws including the TMJs. Furthermore, positioning of patients is critically important in determining the appearance of the panoramic image. In the context of the TMJ region, this means that absolute dimensions of the joint's bony components are unreliable and shape may be distorted [9, 10]. In particular, asymmetric positioning of the TMJs relative to the image layer, either due to poor operator technique or anatomical asymmetry, may introduce marked differences between the right and left sides that are not real (Fig. 5.2).

Panoramic radiography is not a reliable means of assessing the shape of the mandibular condyles [11–13]. In any case, Crow et al. reported that condylar shape alone is not an indicator of temporomandibular joint disorder or disease (TMD). They added that minor discrepancies may not be significant [14]. Consequently, it is important not to overestimate the veracity of diagnostic information obtained from panoramic images of the TMJ.

Panoramic radiographs are normally taken with the patient's anterior teeth in an edge-to-edge position, facilitated by a groove in the bite block. This should ensure that maxillary and mandibular teeth are in the focal plane. Of course, for some patients, this may not be possible, for example, in Class 3 skeletal relationships and/or Class III malocclusions or in the case of some partially or completely edentulous patients for whom positioning is less precise. For most patients, positioning the upper and lower anterior teeth in an edge-to-edge position requires some degree of mandibular protrusion. This will translate the condylar head anteriorly, to a degree dependent on the overjet and overbite, which may be helpful in reducing or removing superimposition of the temporal component of the joint (Fig. 5.3). If perfect imaging of the anterior mandibular teeth is not essential, it can be useful to ask the patient deliberately to protrude maximally, beyond the groove in the bite block, to achieve this.

5.2.1 Multifunction Panoramic Equipment

Many modern models of panoramic equipment incorporate more than a single function. Combined panoramic-cephalometric designs are common. Some panoramic systems have been combined with a simple form of linear tomography, while, more recently, hybrid panoramic/CBCT systems have become available. Selective field size selections, such as half (left or right side) or quadrant images (Fig. 5.4), paediatric settings and, in some cases, specific TMJ programmes are also sometimes included as standard or as options on modern panoramic equipment. These offer the advantage of a lower radiation dose [15, 16]. Some panoramic equipment also offers a choice of image layer shapes in an attempt to accommodate major variations in jaw anatomy.

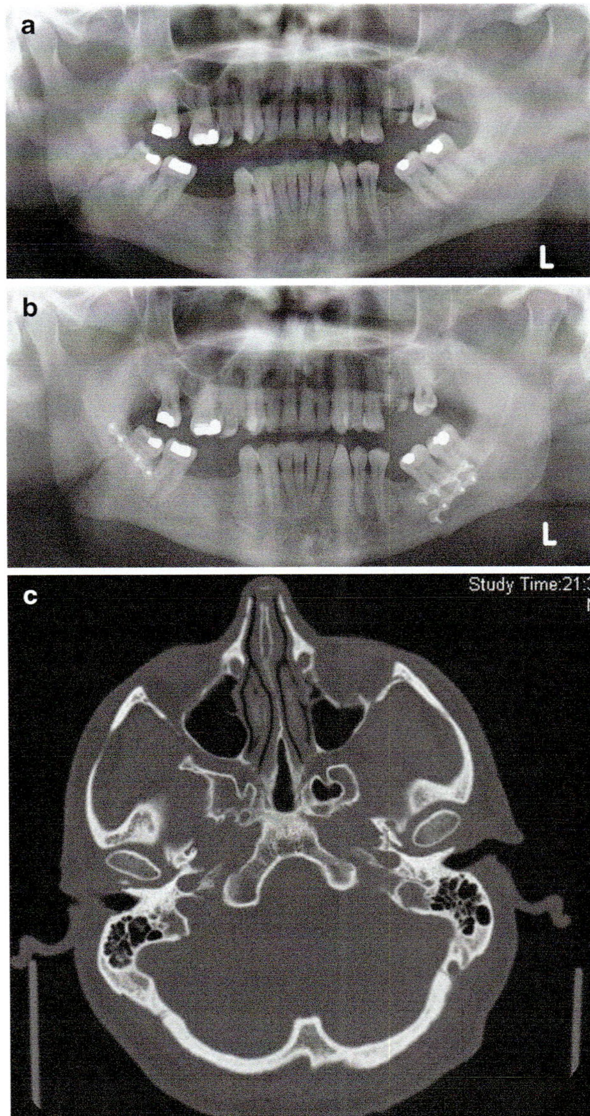

Fig. 5.2 Panoramic radiograph of a patient with mandibular fractures showing asymmetry of the condylar heads produced by positioning error. (**a**) Original image shows relative enlargement of the left condyle. (**b**) Radiograph taken after reduction and fixation of the fracture shows the left condyle at a more normal size. (**c**) Axial CT slice showing that the left condyle was of similar size to the right, perhaps even smaller in the medio-lateral direction

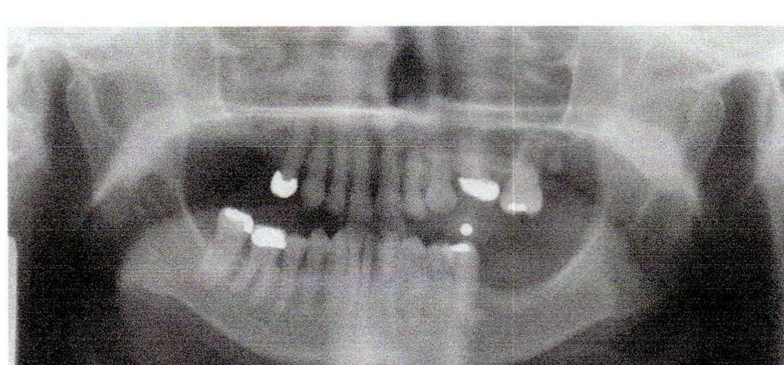

Fig. 5.3 Panoramic radiograph with protrusion leading to anterior condylar translation and consequent improved imaging of the condyles

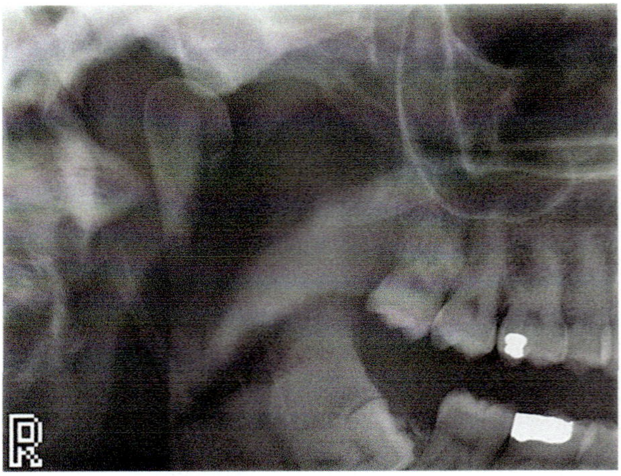

Fig. 5.4 Image of the right TMJ region, produced using a TMJ programme on a panoramic X-ray unit. Note the long styloid process and the anterior arch of the atlas vertebra just posterior to the condylar neck

5.3 Selection of Conventional Radiographs

Selection criteria (also known as "referral criteria" or "appropriateness criteria") have been described as "descriptions of clinical conditions derived from patient signs, symptoms and history that identify patients who are likely to benefit from a particular radiographic technique" [REF RP 136] [17]. Thus, imaging choices rely on the unique clinical history and examination of each patient and the clinician's provisional diagnosis. No imaging should be requested for any patient without conducting a history and clinical examination.

Today, the overwhelming majority of patients with TMJ symptoms can be managed with a very limited or no plain radiographic examination. At least transpharyngeal and transorbital radiographs are obsolete, while the same is generally true for the transcranial oblique lateral radiograph, although it is notable that a recent edition of an international standard textbook of radiographic positioning still includes it [5].

Involvement of the TMJ region in mandibular trauma is common. The prevalence of condylar fracture was 64.8% in patients with mandibular fractures, and the same study, using CT, found that glenoid fossa fracture was seen in 1.4% of patients with condylar fractures [18]. Panoramic radiography in conjunction with plain radiography, usually PA mandibular projections such as the reverse Towne's projection, is adequate for assessing *uncomplicated* mandibular trauma. It is, however, not appropriate in uncooperative or multiply injured patients [19]. There is evidence that CT picks up more fractures than panoramic radiography if the latter is used alone [20]. In cases of trauma involving the TMJ, cross-sectional imaging (CT or CBCT) may be appropriate. When there is disc or capsular injury to the TMJ or more severe condylar fractures (i.e. intracapsular), MR may be helpful to assess the soft tissues [19].

Lateral and postero-anterior (PA) cephalograms may be used to image patients with growth abnormalities related to or involving the TMJ, but their purpose is primarily as a means of imaging the jaws rather than to provide detailed images of the TMJs themselves.

In contemporary clinical practice, therefore, panoramic radiography is probably the only widely used plain radiographic technique, and even this is probably overused. Frequently, panoramic radiography is justified by dentists in terms of it providing an "overview" of the jaws and teeth or as a screening tool; the former is a diagnostically nebulous term, while the latter is widely discredited. As with all radiographic techniques, panoramic radiography should be used only when there are specific clinical indications. Various international guidelines in Europe, along with the Federal Drug Agency of the United States, expressly proscribe the use of panoramic radiography (and any other modality using radiation) as a tool for screening [17, 21]. Regrettably legal advice in many places in North America proposes that panoramic radiography be used for screening even when evidence exists to the contrary [22].

It is notable that for patients attending specialised TMD clinics, experienced clinicians may not use conventional radiography for the majority of patients. Most patients attending such clinics, or general dental practice, with symptoms related to the TMJs will have either myofascial pain or an internal derangement of the disc. In the former case, there are no radiological findings related to the bony components of the TMJ, so radiography will show nothing, while in the latter bony changes might be seen in some patients but are very unlikely to alter management. For experienced TMD clinicians, radiography is used in selected cases for which there is uncertainty about the provisional diagnosis and when there are symptoms which might be explicable as dental in origin but which are not localised or specific enough to be assessed using intraoral radiography. For inexperienced clinicians, panoramic radiography is probably being used as a "catch-all" for gross abnormalities or because of a perceived fear of missing something important.

Criteria for imaging of the TMJ have been described by several authors. For example, one author lists the criteria as: when osseous abnormality or infection is suspected, worsening symptoms despite conservative treatment or failed treatment, trauma, significant dysfunction, alteration in the range of motion, sensory or motor nerve abnormalities or significant changes in occlusion [4]. This wide range of clinical symptoms and signs is broad, and it is important to recognise that these criteria relate to imaging in general, not specifically conventional radiography. For example, where the clinician makes a confident provisional diagnosis of a non-reducing disc displacement, for which clinical history and examination can be accurate [23], referral directly for MR can be made without a radiograph.

Alteration of the range of jaw movement is a common finding in myofascial pain and internal derangement, but not all patients will benefit from a radiograph.

Specific clues were described to highlight where a panoramic radiograph (plus additional intraoral radiography if necessary) should be taken if a patient presents with trismus [24]:

- Inter-incisal opening less than 15 mm
- Progressively worsening trismus
- Absence of history of clicking
- Pain of non-myofascial origin (e.g. neuralgia)
- Swollen lymph glands
- Suspicious intraoral soft tissue lesion

Any one of these should trigger a radiographic examination.

Table 5.2 provides some clinical situations in which conventional radiography may, or may not, be indicated. Many of these will be discussed as conventional radiographic findings in TMJ disorders in Chap. 6.

Table 5.2 Potential indications for conventional radiography according to the provisional diagnosis made by the clinician based on clinical history and examination

Conditions included in the provisional clinical diagnosis	Conventional radiography normally indicated?	Comments
Facial pain for which there is insufficient confidence in a provisional diagnosis and when there are symptoms which might be explicable as dental in origin	Yes	Panoramic radiograph is a good starting point when provisional clinical diagnosis is uncertain and when there are symptoms which might be explicable as dental in origin. Intraoral dental radiographs may also be needed
Myofascial pain	No	No bony abnormality. Radiography will not alter management
Suspected disc derangement		
DD + R	No	Often no bony changes. Occasionally some degenerative changes are seen but do not alter management
DD − R	No	Radiographic findings will not alter management; MR is the appropriate imaging
Developmental abnormalities		Panoramic radiograph is a good starting point but will need supplementation by other radiographs or cross-sectional imaging
Condylar hypoplasia	Yes	
Condylar hyperplasia	Yes	
Coronoid hyperplasia	Yes	
Suspected and symptomatic degenerative joint diseases/arthritides		
Osteoarthrosis	Sometimes	Osteoarthrosis may show remodelling and deformity of the bony components of the TMJ, but the radiographic information may not affect management. Panoramic radiographs have limited diagnostic value
Rheumatoid arthritis	Yes	Panoramic radiograph is usually appropriate for symptomatic patients with rheumatoid or psoriatic arthritis
Psoriatic arthritis	Yes	
Ankylosing spondylitis	Yes	

Table 5.2 (continued)

Conditions included in the provisional clinical diagnosis	Conventional radiography normally indicated?	Comments
Trauma		Panoramic radiography with reverse Towne's projection is a good starting point but may need supplementation by cross-sectional imaging (CT or CBCT; MR)
Suspected mandibular fracture involving the condylar neck or head	Yes	
Suspected dislocation	Yes	Radiograph essential before attempting reduction
Suspected ankylosis	Yes	Panoramic radiograph is a good starting point, but if the findings confirm the possibility of bony ankylosis, this will need supplementation by cross-sectional imaging (CT or CBCT)
Suspected tumour	Yes	Panoramic radiograph is a good starting point but will need supplementation by cross-sectional imaging (CT or MR)
Others		Panoramic radiograph is a good starting point but may need supplementation by cross-sectional imaging (CT or MR)
Synovial chondromatosis	Yes	
Chondrocalcinosis	Yes	
Myositis ossificans	Yes	

DD + R disc displacement with reduction, *DD − R* disc displacement without reduction

References

1. Petersson A. What you can and cannot see in TMJ imaging—an overview related to the RDC/TMD diagnostic system. J Oral Rehabil. 2010;37:771–8. https://doi.org/10.1111/j.1365-2842.2010.02108.x.
2. Ahmad M, Hollender L, Anderson Q, Kartha K, Ohrbach R, Truelove EL, et al. Research diagnostic criteria for temporomandibular disorders (RDC/TMD): development of image analysis criteria and examiner reliability for image analysis. Oral Surg Oral Med Oral Pathol Oral Radiol Endod. 2009;107:844–60.
3. MacDonald D. Temporomandibular joint. In: Oral and maxillofacial radiology: a diagnostic approach. Ames: Wiley; 2011. p. 225–32.
4. Perschbacher S. Temporomandibular joint abnormalities. In: White SC, Pharoah MJ, editors. Oral radiology principles and interpretation. 7th ed. St Louis: Elsevier; 2014. p. 492–523.
5. Whitley AS, Jefferson G, Holmes K, Sloane C, Anderson C, Hoadley G. Clark's positioning in radiography. 13th ed. Boca Raton: CRC Press; 2015.
6. Boeddinghaus R, Whyte A. Trends in maxillofacial imaging. Clin Radiol. 2018;73:4–18. https://doi.org/10.1016/j.crad.2017.02.015.
7. Tamimi D, Jalali E, Hatcher D. Temporomandibular joint imaging. Radiol Clin North Am. 2018;56:157–75. https://doi.org/10.1016/j.rcl.2017.08.011.
8. Mallya SM, Lurie AG. Panoramic imaging. In: White SC, Pharoah MJ, editors. Oral radiology principles and interpretation. 7th ed. St Louis: Elsevier; 2014. p. 166–84.
9. Tűrp JC, Vach W, Harbich K, Alt KW, Strub JR. Determining mandibular condyle and ramus height with the help of an Orthopantomogram®—a valid method? J Oral Rehabil. 1996;23:395–400.

10. Van Elslande DC, Russett SJ, Major PW, Flores-Mir C. Mandibular asymmetry diagnosis with panoramic imaging. Am J Orthod Dentofac Orthop. 2008;134:183–92. https://doi.org/10.1016/j.ajodo.2007.07.021.
11. Mawani F, Lam EW, Heo G, McKee I, Raboud DW, Major PW. Condylar shape analysis using panoramic radiography units and conventional tomography. Oral Surg Oral Med Oral Pathol Oral Radiol Endod. 2005;99:341–8.
12. Schmitter M, Gabbert O, Ohlmann B, Hassel A, Wolff D, Rammelsberg P, et al. Assessment of the reliability and validity of panoramic imaging for assessment of mandibular condyle morphology using both MRI and clinical examination as the gold standard. Oral Surg Oral Med Oral Pathol Oral Radiol Endod. 2006;102:220–4.
13. Fallon SD, Fritz GW, Laskin DM. Panoramic imaging of the temporomandibular joint: an experimental study using cadaveric skulls. J Oral Maxillofac Surg. 2006;64:223–9.
14. Crow HC, Parks E, Campbell JH, Stucki DS, Daggy J. The utility of panoramic radiography in temporomandibular joint assessment. Dentomaxillofac Radiol. 2005;34:91–5.
15. Lecomber AR, Downes SL, Mokhtari M, Faulkner K. Optimisation of patient doses in programmable dental panoramic radiography. Dentomaxillofac Radiol. 2000;29:107–12.
16. Pakbaznejad Esmaeili E, Waltimo-Sirén J, Laatikainen T, Haukka J, Ekholm M. Application of segmented dental panoramic tomography among children: positive effect of continuing education in radiation protection. Dentomaxillofac Radiol. 2016;45:20160104. https://doi.org/10.1259/dmfr.20160104.
17. European Commission. Radiation protection 136. European guidelines on radiation protection in dental radiology. Luxembourg: Office for Official Publications of the European Communities; 2004. ISBN 92-894-5958-1. https://ec.europa.eu/energy/sites/ener/files/documents/136_0.pdf. Accessed 22 June 2018.
18. Ogura I, Sasaki Y, Kaneda T. Analysis of mandibular condylar and glenoid fossa fractures with computed tomography. Eur Radiol. 2014;24:902–6. https://doi.org/10.1007/s00330-013-3085-6.
19. iRefer guidelines: making the best use of clinical radiology. Version 8.0.1. London: Royal College of Radiologists. https://www.irefer.org.uk/. Accessed 22 June 2018.
20. Wilson IF, Lokeh A, Benjamin CI, Hilger PA, Hamlar DD, Ondrey FG, et al. Prospective comparison of panoramic tomography (zonography) and helical computed tomography in the diagnosis and operative management of mandibular fractures. Plast Reconstr Surg. 2001;107:1369–75.
21. American Dental Association and US Department of Health and Human Services. The selection of patients for dental radiographic examinations. Revision 2012. https://www.fda.gov/Radiation-EmittingProducts/RadiationEmittingProductsandProcedures/MedicalImaging/MedicalX-Rays/ucm116504.htm. Accessed 22 June 2018.
22. Kratz R, Walton JN, MacEntee MI, Nguyen CT, MacDonald DS. Panoramic radiographs made before complete removable dental prostheses fabrication: a retrospective study of clinical significance. J Prosthet Dent. 2017;118:26–30.
23. Schiffman E, Ohrbach R. Executive summary of the diagnostic criteria for Temporomandibular disorders for clinical and research applications. J Am Dent Assoc. 2016;147:438–45. https://doi.org/10.1016/j.adaj.2016.01.007.
24. Beddis HP, Davies SJ, Budenberg A, Horner K, Pemberton MN. Temporomandibular disorders, trismus and malignancy: development of a checklist to improve patient safety. Br Dent J. 2014;217:351–5. https://doi.org/10.1038/sj.bdj.2014.862.

Conventional Radiographic Findings in TMJ Disorders

6

David MacDonald and Keith Horner

6.1 Conventional Radiographic Anatomy

In Chap. 2, the normal anatomy of the TMJ was described in detail. On conventional radiographs it is important to recognise that only the bony components of the joint are seen. The intrinsic soft issue components of the TMJ, the fibrocartilage covering the surfaces of the condyle and articular fossa, the articular disc, the upper and lower joint spaces, the retrodiscal tissues and the fibrous capsule, are not visible radiographically. Similarly, the related muscles of mastication and ligaments are not seen. Recognition of this underlines how limited conventional radiography is in assessment of the TMJ.

As only panoramic radiographs and, perhaps, the PA facial bone (reverse Towne's) projection might be encountered in modern clinical practice, only the radiographic anatomy of these will be described. Figure 6.1a–d shows the TMJ and adjacent structures as seen on panoramic radiographs. Figure 6.2a, b shows the TMJ and adjacent structures as seen on a reverse Towne's projection.

6.1.1 The Mandibular Condyle

As described briefly in Sect. 5.1, the condyle has an ellipsoid shape. This is best appreciated when viewed from above (Fig. 6.3a). The condylar head is wider medio-laterally and narrower anteroposteriorly, with typical dimensions of about 20 mm

D. MacDonald
Division of Oral & Maxillofacial Radiology, Department of Oral, Biological and Medical Sciences, Faculty of Dentistry, University of British Columbia, Vancouver, BC, Canada

K. Horner (✉)
Division of Dentistry, School of Medical Sciences, Faculty of Biology, Medicine and Health, The University of Manchester, Manchester, UK
e-mail: keith.horner@manchester.ac.uk

I. Rozylo-Kalinowska, K. Orhan (eds.), *Imaging of the Temporomandibular Joint*, https://doi.org/10.1007/978-3-319-99468-0_6

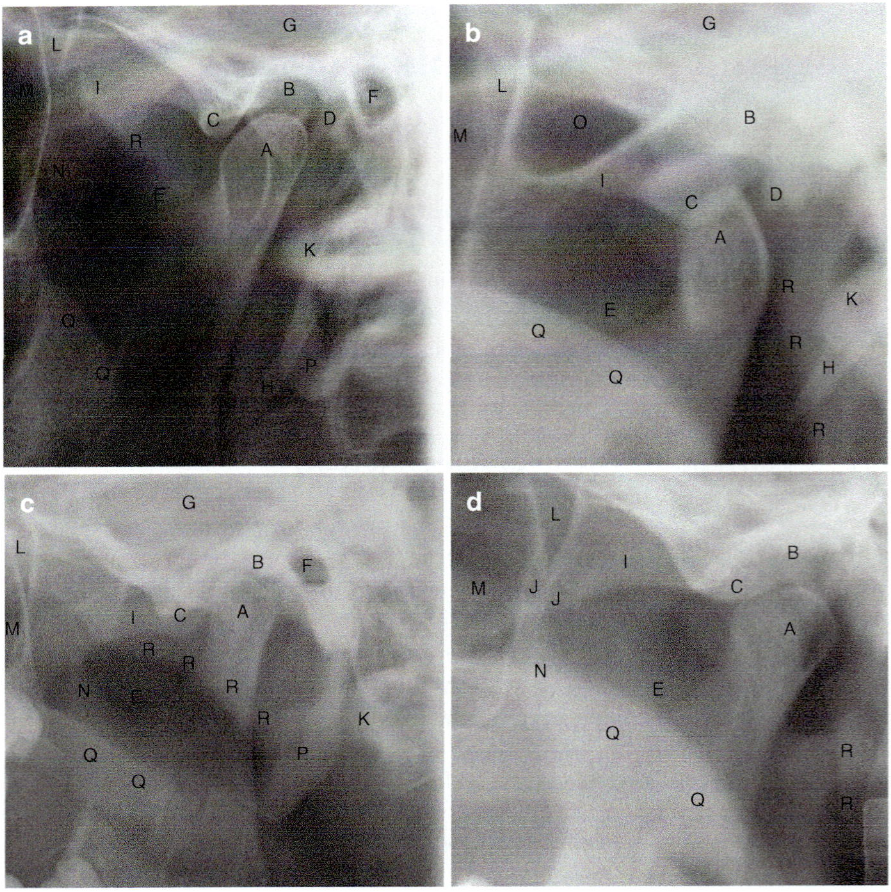

Fig. 6.1 TMJ region on sections of four panoramic radiographs (**a**–**d**), showing the main anatomical features. All show the left side. *A* condyle, *B* articular fossa, *C* articular eminence, *D* tympanic plate, *E* mandibular notch, *F* external auditory meatus, *G* middle cranial fossa, *H* styloid process, *I* zygomatic arch, *J* zygomatico-temporal suture, *K* anterior arch of atlas vertebra (C1), *L* pterygomaxillary fissure, *M* maxillary antrum, *N* coronoid process, *O* lateral extension of sphenoid sinus into lateral pterygoid plate (normal variant), *P* ear lobe, *Q* soft palate, *R* posterior wall of the nasopharynx

and 8–10 mm, respectively [1]. Viewed laterally, however, the condylar head has a more conical shape as it tapers down into a relatively narrow neck to join the ramus of the mandible (Fig. 6.3b to f photos of dry skull). The medio-lateral axis of the condyle is set at an angle of about 60–70° to the sagittal plane. A line through the axis, when extrapolated medially, meets its fellow close to the anterior aspect of the foramen magnum.

There is usually a distinct horizontal ridge on the anterior surface of the condyle, below which is a concavity called the pterygoid fovea (Fig. 6.3b, c). The fovea is the

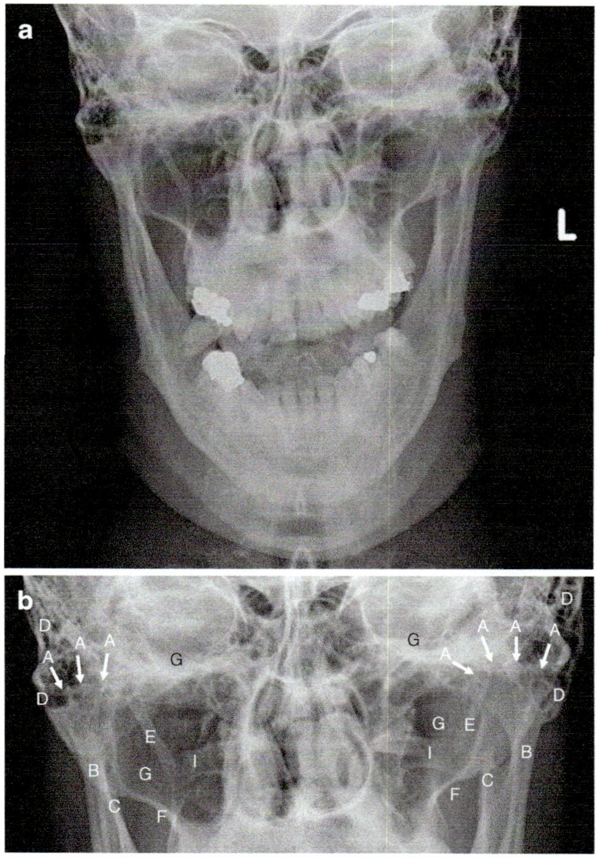

Fig. 6.2 (**a**) Reverse Towne's radiograph, with (**b**) magnified view of the TMJ regions, showing the main anatomical features. *A* condyle superior articulating surface (arrowed), *B* condylar neck, *C* coronoid process, *D* mastoid air cells, *E* styloid process (elongated on the right side), *F* zygomatic process of the maxilla, *G* maxillary antrum, *H* orbital floor, *I* lateral process of atlas vertebra

site of the attachment of the superior head of the lateral pterygoid muscle. As viewed from the lateral perspective, such as on panoramic radiographs, the anterior ridge above the fovea can give a "beaked" appearance to the condyle which could be misinterpreted as remodelling due to degenerative disease.

Condylar shape and size are variable in a normal population, and there may be asymmetry between condyles in an individual without it being classifiable as pathological. In addition, on plain radiographs, asymmetry may be seen for condyles of similar dimensions and shape if their long axes have different angulations to the coronal or sagittal plane, due to a different alignment with the X-ray beam (Fig. 6.4a–c). As described in Sect. 5.2, panoramic radiography may introduce asymmetry artefactually due to positioning faults or when a patient's morphology does not match the image layer shape and size (Fig. 5.2).

Bifid condyle is a uncommon anomaly of the TMJ, reported with a prevalence of 0.8% by Nikolova et al. [2]. As the name suggests, there is a notch or cleft, of variable depth, on the superior surface of the condylar head either in the anteroposterior

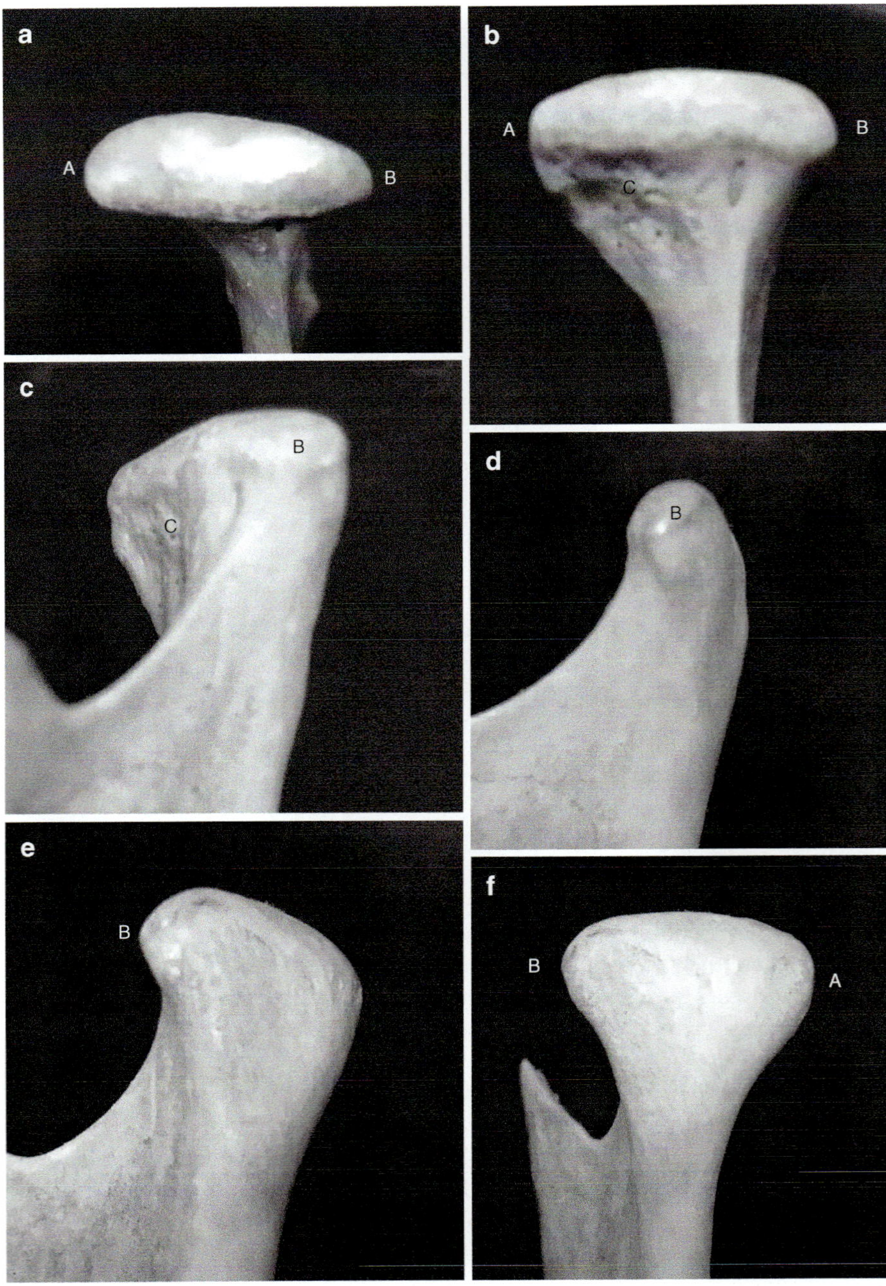

Fig. 6.3 Images of the mandibular condyle of the TMJ (dry skull). (**a**) Superior aspect, (**b**) anterior aspect, (**c**) anterolateral aspect, (**d**) lateral aspect, (**e**) posterolateral aspect, (**f**) posterior aspect. *A* medial pole, *B* lateral pole, *C* pterygoid fovea

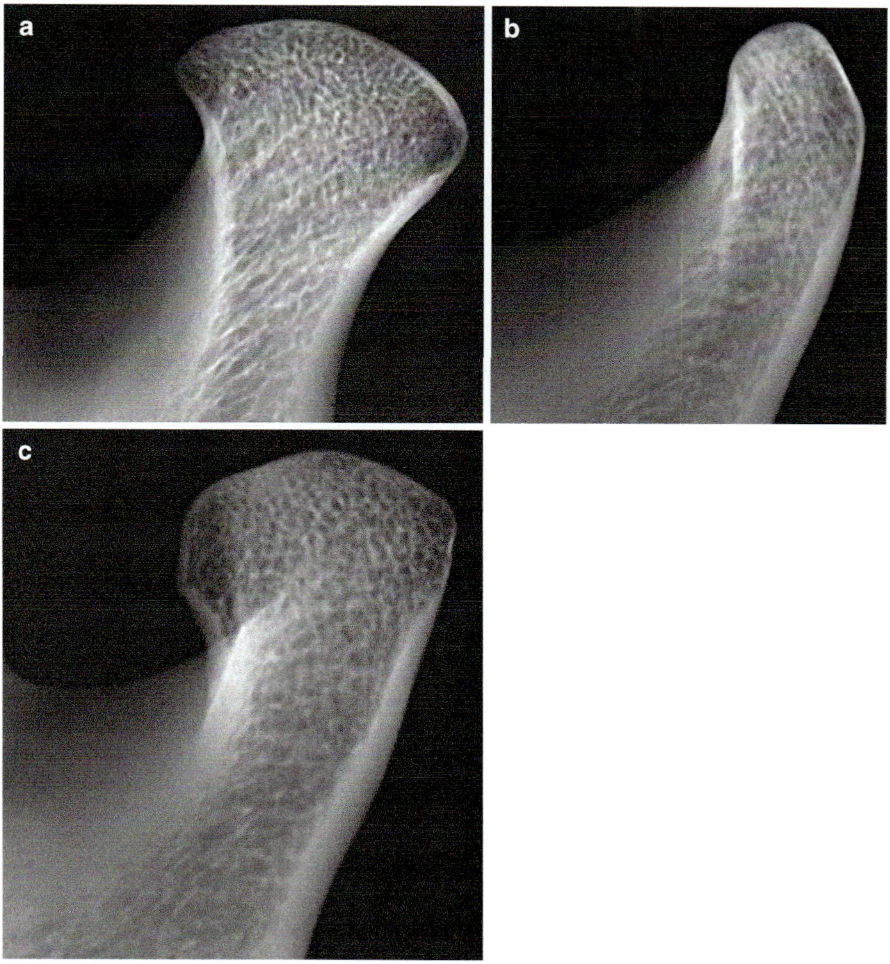

Fig. 6.4 Radiographs of the mandibular condyle of the TMJ, showing the change in the appearance of the condyle according to perspective. (**a**) Viewed from an anterior aspect, about 40° to a true lateral aspect. (**b**) Viewed from a true lateral aspect. (**c**) Viewed from a posterior aspect, about 40° to a true lateral aspect

or medio-lateral plane (Fig. 6.5). On panoramic radiography the parts of the condyle may be overlapped, although complete duplication of the condylar head has been described [4].

On panoramic radiographs, several structures can be superimposed on the condyle and condylar neck, although this is highly variable. Most common amongst these is superimposition of the temporal component of the joint, overlying the superior aspect of the condyle; as mentioned in Sect. 5.2, above, protrusion of the mandible might reduce this. The anterior arch of the atlas (first cervical vertebra) is quite commonly superimposed on the posterior aspect of the condylar neck (Fig. 6.1).

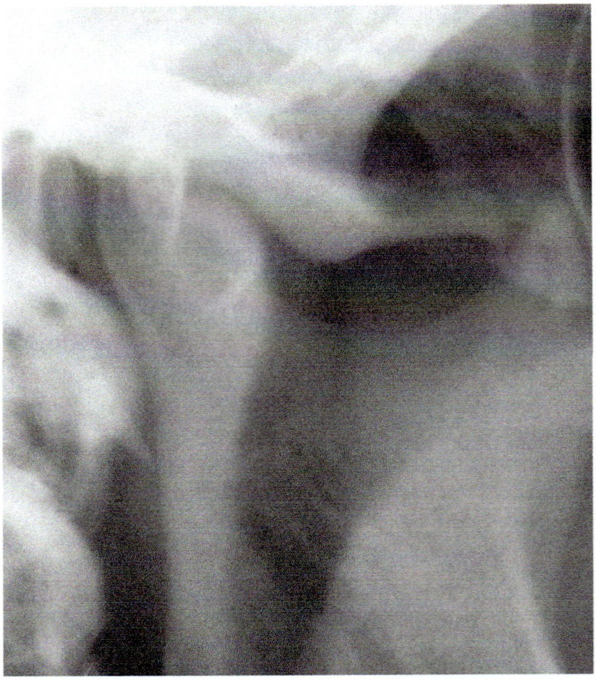

Fig. 6.5 Bifid right condyle on panoramic radiograph

The interface between the posterior nasopharyngeal soft tissues and airway frequently crosses over the condylar neck, producing a radiolucency where air overlies it (Fig. 6.1). Less frequently, air within the external ear/external auditory canal can be superimposed over the posterior aspect of the condyle.

6.1.2 The Temporal Component of the TMJ

This consists of the articular fossa (also known as the glenoid fossa), the articular eminence and, laterally, the articular tubercle (Fig. 6.6a, b). The morphology of the temporal component of the TMJ can vary in terms of size, medio-lateral width and anteroposterior length. The depth of the fossa and the steepness of the articular eminence also vary, reflecting normal individual variation. The TMJ develops over the first 4 or 5 years of life. Initially, there is a shallow articular fossa and lack of an articular eminence [1].

The temporal component of the TMJ can be pneumatised, to a variable degree, by air cells continuous with those of the mastoid process. Pneumatisation can extend into the articular eminence (Fig. 6.7). Miloglu et al. [3] reviewed the literature and found a wide age was affected, with a prevalence between 1% and 2.6%, although their study found 8% of subjects were affected, perhaps because they used cross-sectional imaging rather than panoramic radiographs. Orhan et al. [4] reported a prevalence of 3.4% in children and adolescents, based on viewing panoramic radiographs. Observers using the panoramic radiograph have only low to medium to low accuracy for diagnosis of pneumatisation of the articular eminence and TMJ fossa when compared with cross-sectional imaging [5].

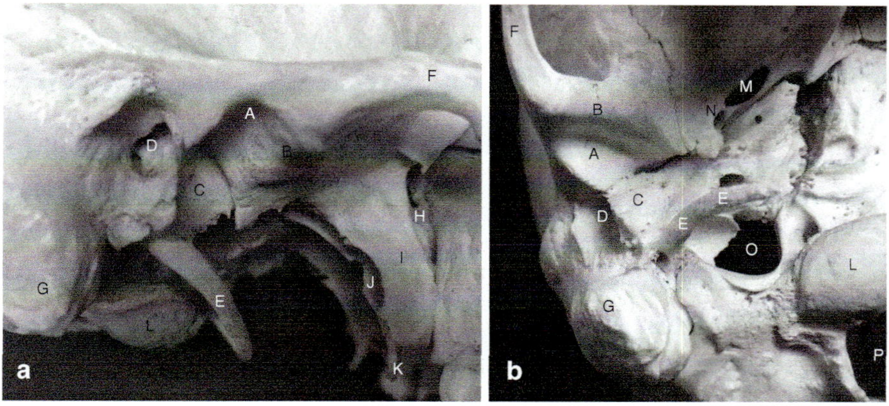

Fig. 6.6 Images of the temporal component of the TMJ (dry skull), (**a**) lateral view; (**b**) from below. *A* articular fossa, *B* articular eminence, *C* tympanic plate, *D* external auditory meatus, *E* styloid process, *F* zygomatic arch, *G* mastoid process, *H* pterygomaxillary fissure, *I* lateral pterygoid plate, *J* medial pterygoid plate, *K* pterygoid hamulus, *L* occipital condyle, *M* foramen ovale, *N* foramen spinosum, *O* jugular foramen, *P* foramen magnum

Fig. 6.7 Pneumatisation of the articular eminences on (**a**) panoramic radiograph, with (**b**) a close-up of the right TMJ region. The appearance in this case is of a multilocular radiolucency [Images courtesy of Prof. Kaan Orhan]

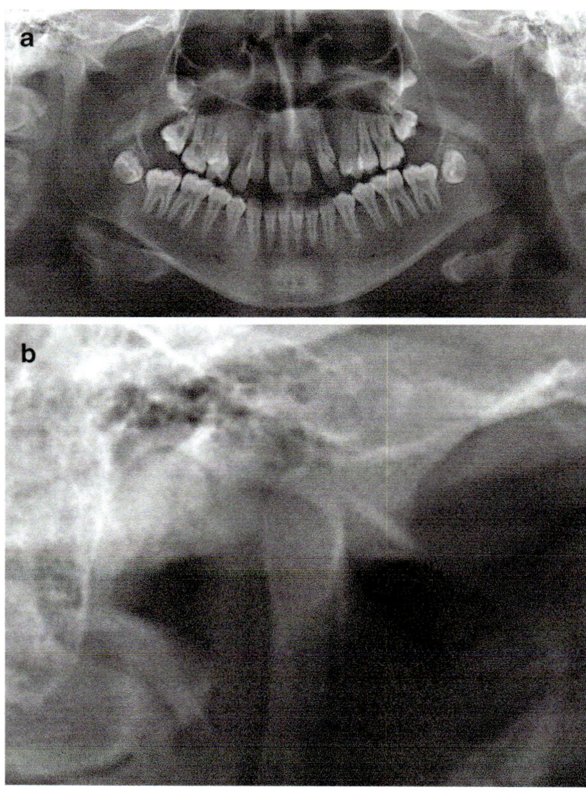

6.1.3 The "Joint Space"

A basic understanding of the anatomy of the TMJ means that to describe the gap seen on radiographs between the condylar head and the articular fossa as a "joint space" is wrong. This inter-bony gap contains the fibrocartilage layer over the bony part of the joint, the articular disc and the upper and lower joint spaces.

Before the advent of arthrography and MR, some significance was placed upon the dimensions of the gap between condylar head and articular fossa, often as seen on transcranial oblique lateral radiograph. Using that projection, the position of the condyle in the fossa and the joint space dimensions vary according to the patient position and radiographic technique [6, 7]. Furthermore, it should be noted that the caudal angulation of the X-ray beam for transcranial oblique lateral images means that it is the supero-lateral part of the "joint space" which is seen in profile.

On panoramic radiographs the patient's mandible is usually protruded. Thus, assessment of the condyle/articular fossa relationship is not possible. Similarly, patients are usually instructed to open their mouths as much as they can for reverse Towne's projection. Lateral and postero-anterior (PA) cephalograms superimpose the TMJs upon each other or on the base of the skull and give little information about the joints. In summary, currently used conventional radiographs do not provide useful information about joint space dimensions. Furthermore, the inter-bony space of the TMJ on conventional radiographs is of no obvious relevance to the management of patients with TMJ disorders. Although quantitative assessment of joint space dimensions is not of value in panoramic radiography, it is worth noting that limitation of movement of the condylar head may occur in temporomandibular disorders (TMDs). Asymmetry of anterior translation of the condyle, relative to the articular eminence, might be observed on panoramic radiographs when there is a unilateral problem but may be purely coincidental.

6.1.4 Related Bony Anatomical Structures

6.1.4.1 Styloid Process

The styloid process is a thin bony projection of the base of the skull postero-medial to the articular fossa. Its length is highly variable. The stylohyoid ligament, which attaches to the process, may undergo ossification to varying degrees (Figs. 6.1a, b and 6.8) which merely represents normal variation. Calcification of the stylohyoid complex occurs in one or more of four regions, each based on a centre of ossification. MacDonald-Jankowski [8] displayed the 12 most frequent patterns of calcification of the stylohyoid complex and revealed that they differed significantly in frequency between 2 major world communities, London and Hong Kong. The supposed association of an unusually long styloid process and ossification of the stylohyoid ligament with facial pain (Eagle's syndrome) means that patients' symptoms may be ascribed to the TMJ. Consequently, its recognition can be important.

6.1.4.2 External Ear

The external auditory meatus is posterior to the TMJ and may be included on the panoramic image as a round area of relative radiolucency (Fig. 6.1a, c).

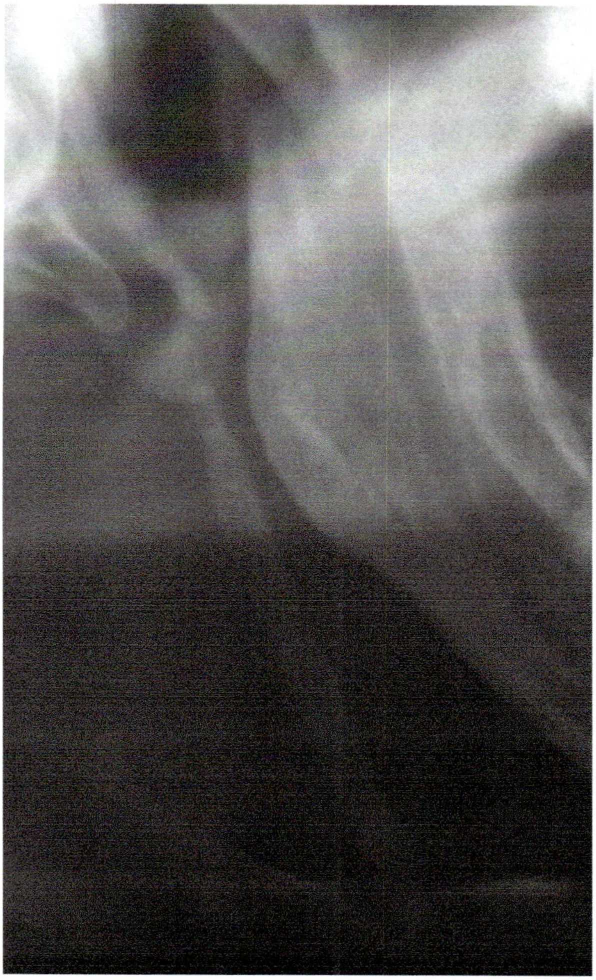

Fig. 6.8 Stylohyoid complex (a long styloid process and long segment of calcified stylohyoid ligament integrating the lesser horn of the hyoid, extending to the synovial joint at the junction between the greater horn and body of the hyoid), fractured condylar neck displaced forward by the pull of the lateral pterygoid muscle. The superimposition of the fractured ends appears as a radiopacity. The earlobe is superimposed upon the long styloid process. Acknowledgement: MacDonald. Wiley-Blackwell. 2011. P15

This is not important to the interpretation of the TMJ on conventional radiographs, but it is a useful landmark. The soft tissues of the external ear and the air spaces associated with them, however, may be superimposed on the TMJ (Fig. 6.1a–d).

6.2 Conventional Radiographic Findings in TMJ Disorders

There are numerous pathoses and developmental disorders which can affect the TMJ and associated structures. These will be considered in detail in other chapters. Here, content is limited to the radiological signs associated with many of these conditions that may be perceived on conventional radiographs. The indications for conventional radiography for some clinical situations are set out in Table 5.2.

6.2.1 Myalgia/Myofascial Pain

No radiological findings are relevant to the disorder.

6.2.2 Internal Derangement (Disc Displacement)

This common disorder is primarily soft tissue in origin, so usually there are no conventional radiological findings. Erosions and other remodelling changes consistent with OA may be seen in long-standing cases. MR is the imaging of choice, and some clinicians will not carry out radiography. Even if present, bony changes in cases of internal derangement are secondary to the main feature of the disorder, and it is hard to see their identification as having any relevance to management.

Some authors have suggested that a steep articular eminence is an aetiological factor in the development of internal disc derangement. The literature provides evidence both for and against this hypothesis [9–12].

6.2.3 Degenerative Joint Disease (Osteoarthrosis)

Remodelling of the bony components of the joint associated with loss of the articular cartilage and exposure of the bone leads to certain radiological signs:

- Shape change (flattening) of condylar head
- Sclerosis of the bone
- Erosion of bony surfaces
- Loose bodies in joint space
- Subsurface radiolucencies of condylar head (Ely's cysts)
- Narrowing of the gap between the bony articulating surfaces of the condyle and articular fossa

One, more or all of these radiological signs may occur in an affected joint. The final sign listed above is a key feature, but, for reasons described in Sect. 5.2, this space is not interpretable on panoramic radiographs but is appreciated on cross-sectional imaging. Some examples of radiological changes are shown in Fig. 6.9.

Using panoramic radiographs as the diagnostic imaging was associated with low sensitivity for flattening, erosions and osteophyte, but high specificities [13]. Winocur et al. [14] found that panoramic radiography had only 20% accuracy in cases with clinically diagnosed degenerative joint disease (DJD). They concluded that panoramic radiography should not be used routinely to assess DJD and that cross-sectional imaging should only be used if there was reason to expect that the findings might affect diagnosis and management.

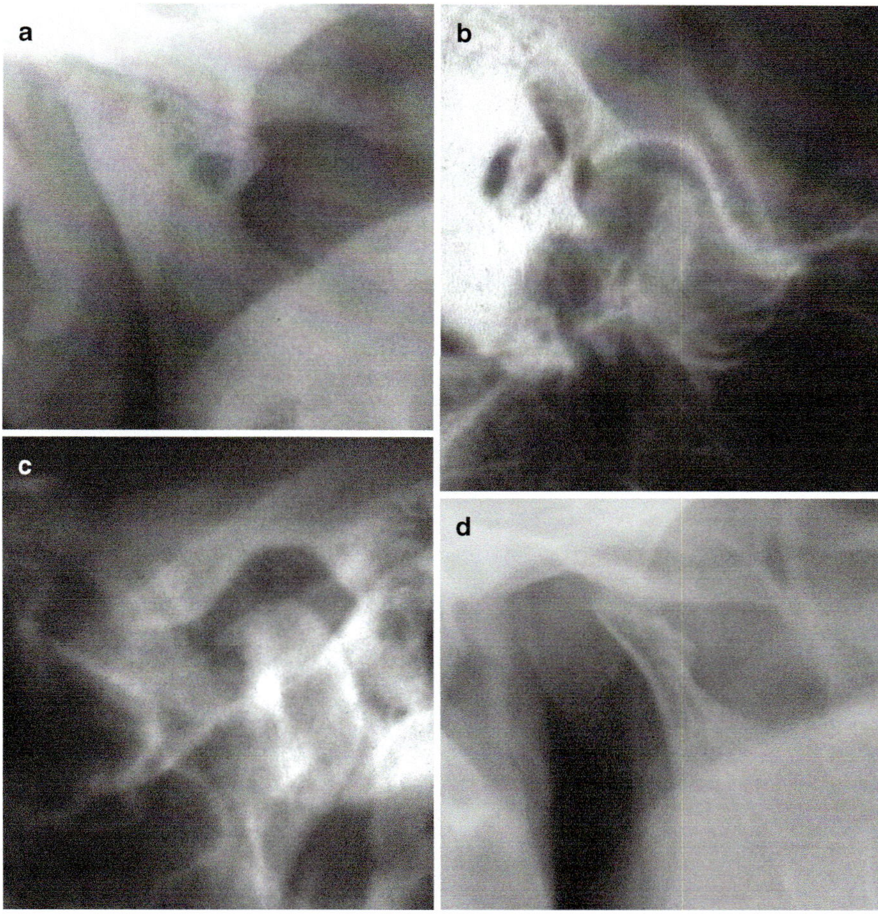

Fig. 6.9 Radiological findings in degenerative joint disease (osteoarthrosis). (**a**) Flattening, sclerosis and subsurface radiolucencies, with narrowing of the gap between the condyle and articular fossa surfaces. (**b**) A small erosion on the superior surface of the condylar head. (**c**) Prominent anterior "lipping" of the condylar head. (**d**) Irregular and sclerotic surface to the condyle with an overall shape change due to remodelling

6.2.4 Condylar Hypoplasia

Unilateral hypoplasia has a wide range of aetiologies, including congenital conditions such as hemifacial macrosomia (Fig. 6.10), infection, trauma and irradiation (Fig. 6.11). Bilateral hypoplasia is usually part of certain syndromes (Fig. 6.12). The radiological signs of hypoplasia may include:

- Facial asymmetry on cephalograms in unilateral cases
- Smaller condylar head
- Slender condylar neck

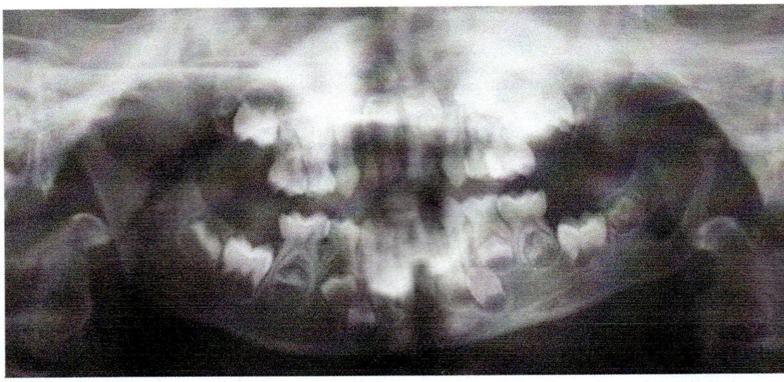

Fig. 6.10 Child patient with a congenital hypoplasia of the left side of the mandible, along with ear deformities, consistent with hemifacial microsomia. The condylar and coronoid processes are small and the ramus height very reduced in height. No normal articular eminence is evident

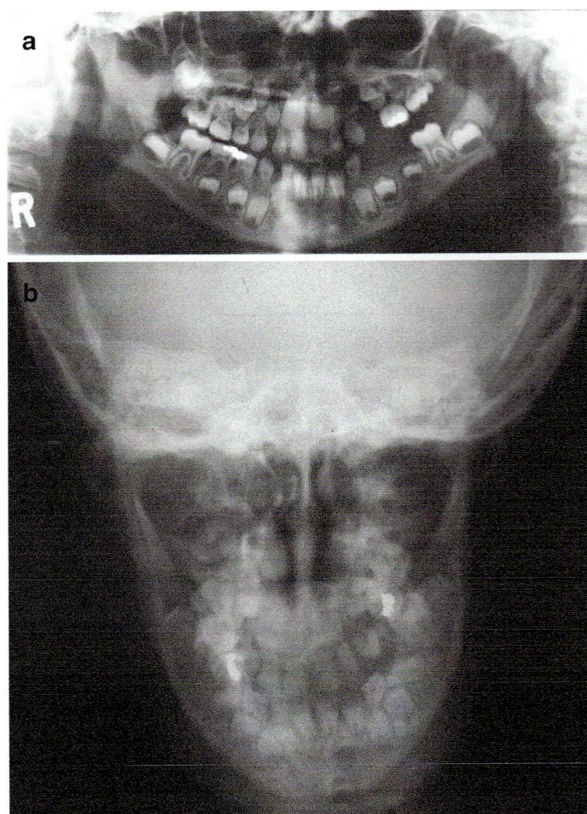

Fig. 6.11 Facial asymmetry with a hypoplastic left mandible in a child which started to develop following radiotherapy to the left orbit at age 2 to treat a malignant tumour. (**a**) The panoramic radiograph shows reduced height of the left ramus (angle to condyle distance). The condyle is slightly smaller on the left side. Note also the effects on dental development in the left maxilla, with arrested root development in the first molar and failure of development of the second molar. (**b**) The postero-anterior cephalogram shows the degree of asymmetry very well

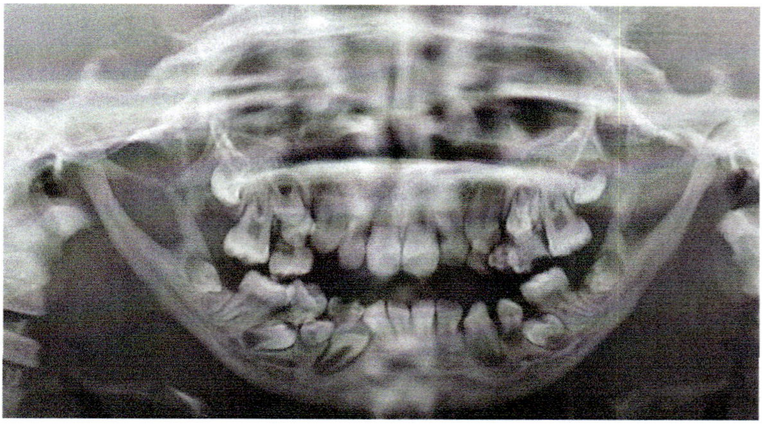

Fig. 6.12 Bilateral condylar hypoplasia as part of pyknodysostosis. There are no mandibular angles. The condylar and coronoid processes are thin and elongated, with small condylar heads

- Reduced height of the mandible (condyle to angle distance) on the affected side (unilateral cases) or bilaterally
- Concavity of the posterior border of the mandibular ramus
- Pronounced antegonial notch

Not all of these will occur in all cases.

It is important to recognise that mild skeletal asymmetry is a normal variation of anatomy. Panoramic radiographs, if properly taken, can confirm a clinical impression of asymmetry. This asymmetry may be a product of condylar hypoplasia or hyperplasia (see below). Due to errors in technique, which regrettably are not infrequent [15, 16], observed asymmetry on the panoramic radiograph for another reason should be confirmed by a clinical re-examination of the patient.

6.2.5 Condylar Hyperplasia

Usually a unilateral condition is seen typically in adolescents and young adults in which there is excessive or prolonged growth of the mandible [17].

The radiological signs of condylar hyperplasia may include:

- Facial asymmetry.
- Larger condylar head.
- Condylar head shape may be normal or sometimes abnormal.
- Increased height of the mandible on the affected side.

- Downward bowing of the lower border of the mandible on the affected side.
- Lateral bowing of the ramus on postero-anterior radiographs.

An example of condylar hyperplasia is shown in Fig. 6.13.

6.2.6 Coronoid Hyperplasia

Elongation of the coronoid process most often presents as progressive limitation of opening that may be ascribed to a TMJ disorder. It typically presents in young adult males, but paediatric cases can occur [18, 19]. It is often bilateral.

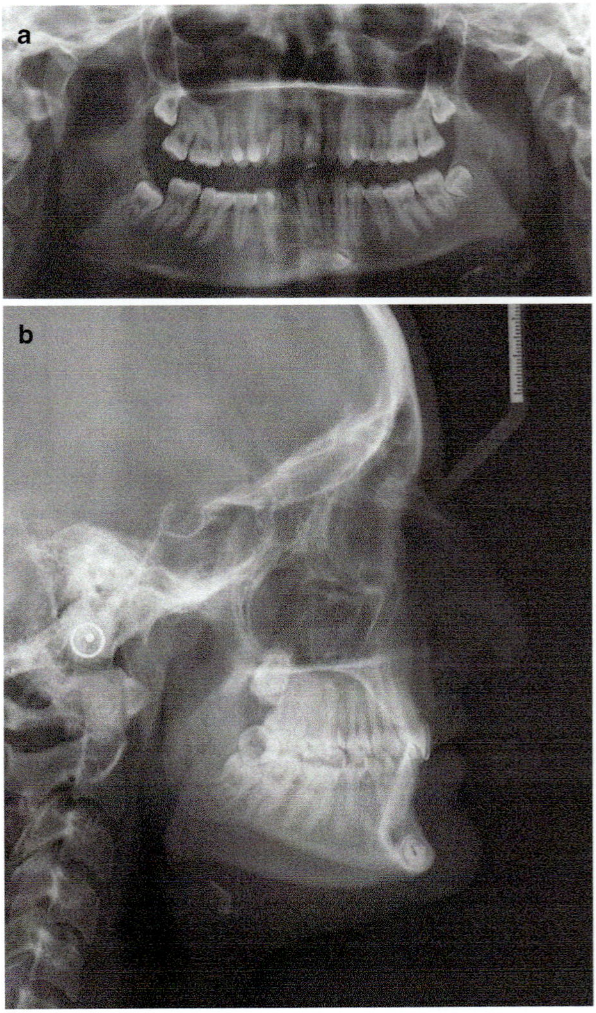

Fig. 6.13 Condylar hyperplasia affecting the right side on (**a**) a panoramic radiograph and (**b**) a lateral cephalogram. Note the greater height of the right ramus and the right body of mandible. The antegonial notch is less obvious than on the left side. The condylar neck is longer than that on the contralateral side. The size discrepancy shows very well on the cephalogram

The radiological signs of hyperplasia of the coronoid process of the mandible on plain radiographs are limited to:

- Elongation of the coronoid process at least 10 mm above the inferior edge of the zygomatic arch
- Variable change in shape or radiopacity of the coronoid process

It is not unusual, however, for the coronoid processes to be poorly seen on panoramic radiographs because of their thin width medio-laterally. A case of coronoid hyperplasia is shown in Fig. 6.14.

6.2.7 Rheumatoid Arthritis

This is a multi-joint condition and it is unusual for RA to present in the TMJ first. Consequently, the condition is likely to be suspected when a patient suffering from the condition presents with TMJ symptoms. It is often bilateral when affecting the TMJ.

The radiological signs of rheumatoid arthritis may include:

- Erosions, of both condylar head and the articular fossa, are the most prominent sign on conventional radiographs (Fig. 6.15).
- Shape change of the condylar head due to erosion: "sharpened pencil" appearance.
- Flattening of the articular eminence due to erosion.
- Developing anterior open bite on lateral cephalogram.
- Secondary changes of degenerative joint disease (see Sect. 6.2.3) in established cases.

Other systemic arthritides (e.g. psoriatic arthritis) have changes that are essentially the same.

6.2.8 Juvenile Idiopathic Arthritis

The radiological features of juvenile idiopathic arthritis (formerly known as juvenile rheumatoid arthritis) have close similarities with those of rheumatoid arthritis but due to the age of onset can result in significant impact on mandibular growth. This may result in micrognathia, anterior open bite and the classic "bird face" appearance [20]. Figure 6.16 shows a case of juvenile idiopathic arthritis with such changes.

Panoramic radiography has proven useful as the initial imaging of those child patients suspected of juvenile idiopathic arthritis. Abramowicz et al. [21] reported that the "abnormal condylar morphology and accentuated antegonial notching on panoramic radiography were found to be significantly correlated with synovitis" observed on MRI.

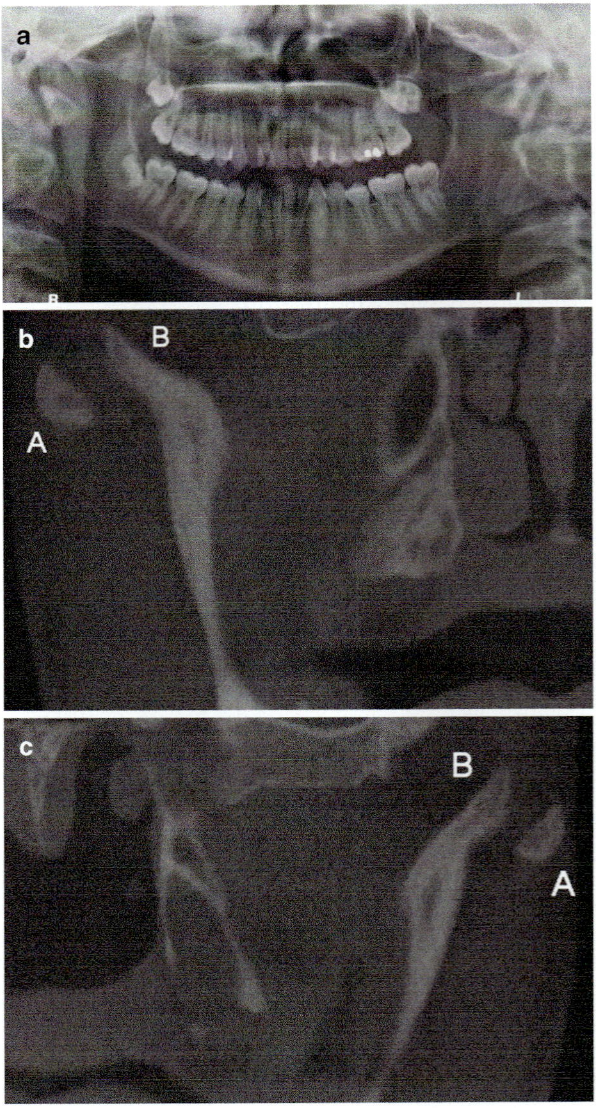

Fig. 6.14 Coronoid hyperplasia. (**a**) Panoramic radiograph of a 15 year-old male with marked limitation of opening of the mouth, initial diagnosed as a TMJ disorder. TMJs were normal on CBCT, but the coronoid processes on the (**b**) right and (**c**) left side were extremely elongated, extending above the level of the zygomatic arches. *A* the zygomatic arch, *B* the coronoid process. The coronoid processes were hitting the infratemporal surfaces of the zygomas on mouth opening

6.2.9 Trauma

The TMJ is frequently affected by facial trauma, and the first-line imaging may be conventional radiography, although cross-sectional imaging is increasingly used. Although subtle fractures of the condyle are frequently missed on conventional radiography, they are best displayed on an open-mouth reverse Towne's view [22]. Missed malunited fractures may present as a bifid condyle [22].

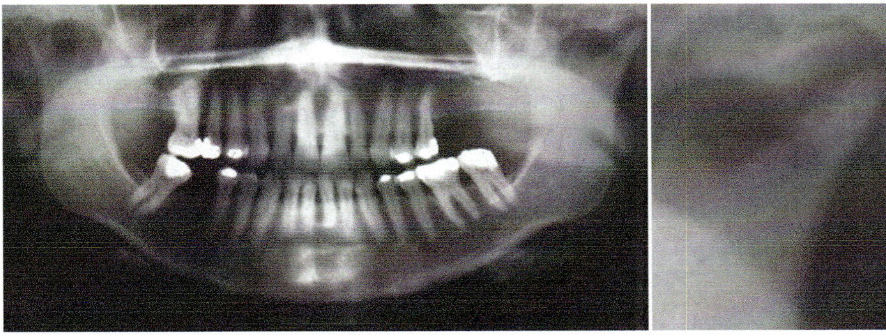

Fig. 6.15 Erosion of the left condyle in rheumatoid arthritis. Note the contralateral condyle appears normal

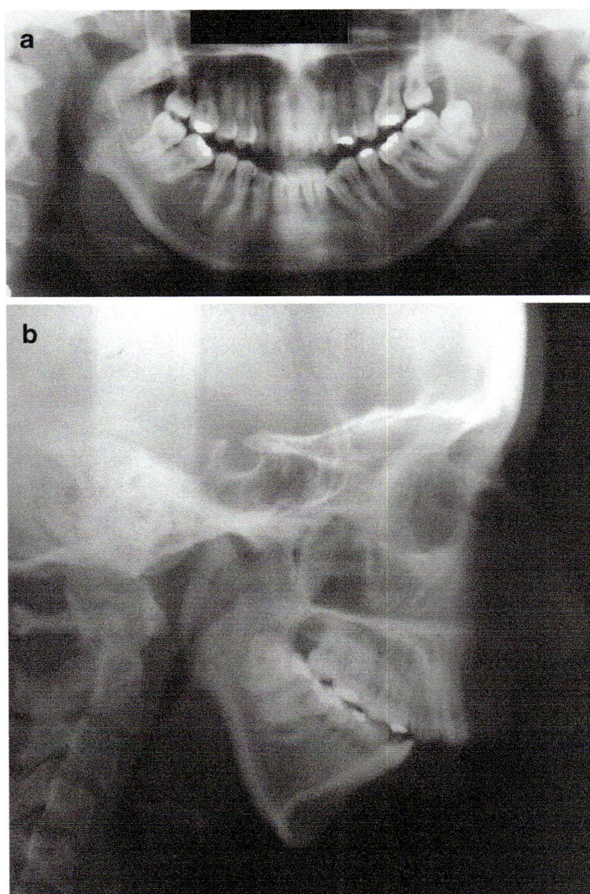

Fig. 6.16 Juvenile idiopathic arthritis. (**a**) Panoramic radiograph showing bilaterally very short condylar necks and accentuated antegonial notching. Note, however, the lack of detail of the condyles themselves. (**b**) Lateral cephalogram showing the short height of the mandibular rami and retrusive chin

6.2.9.1 Effusion

No radiological findings on conventional radiographs.

6.2.9.2 Dislocation

The diagnosis is primarily clinical, but the condyle, or condyles, may be seen to lie both anterior and superior to the articular eminence on panoramic radiographs (Fig. 6.16). Note, however, that the condyle can translate a long way forward in some individuals without it being dislocated.

6.2.9.3 Fracture

Fracture may be identified by one or more of the usual radiological signs:

- Radiolucent lines
- Step deformities of bony outlines
- Radiopaque bands where bone fragments overlap (Figs. 6.8 and 6.17)

The attachment of the lateral pterygoid muscle exerts an anterior and medial pull on the condyle, so fracture of the condylar neck is often accompanied by displacement of the condyle in an antero-medial direction (Fig. 6.18). This may be followed by an upward displacement of the ipsilateral ramus accompanied by a posterior open bite on the contralateral side. The latter sign might be seen on conventional radiographs, although it is most readily identified clinically.

6.2.10 Ankylosis

The radiological signs of ankylosis [23] may include:

- Deformity of the shape of the condyle and articular fossa, with loss of clear bony gap between them.

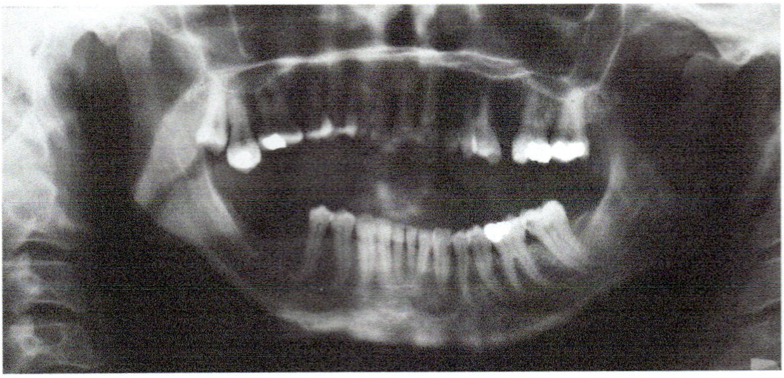

Fig. 6.17 Bilateral dislocation of the mandible. The condylar heads are anterior to the articular eminences but also have displaced superiorly, anterior to the articular eminences, particularly on the right side

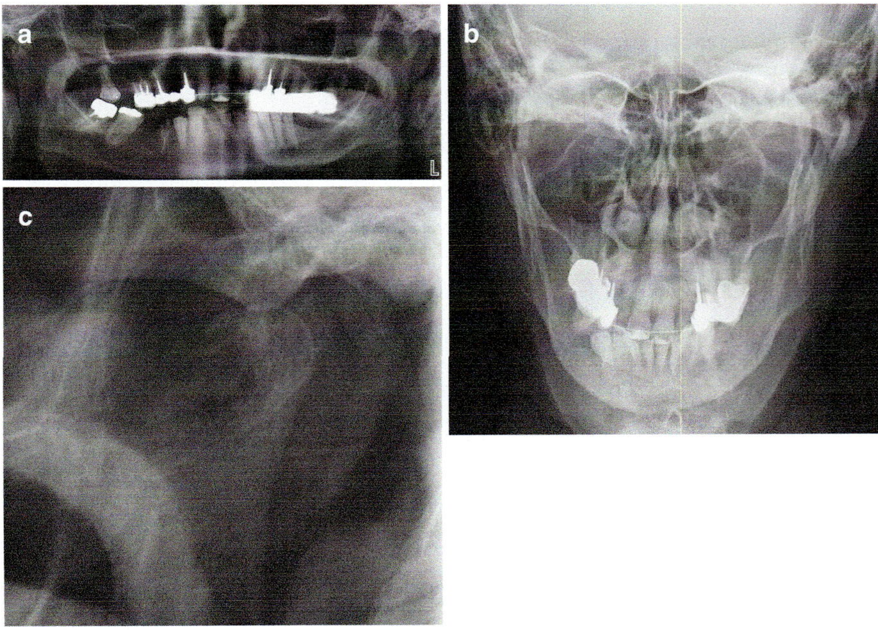

Fig. 6.18 Bilateral high condylar fracture on (**a**) panoramic and (**b**) reverse Towne's radiographs. The latter radiograph shows medial displacement of the condylar heads, while (**c**) shows a close-up of the left TMJ region on the panoramic radiograph, showing that the condylar fragment has also displaced anteriorly

- Sclerosis and enlargement of the joint bony components are commonly seen.
- Secondary changes include antegonial notching and elongation of the coronoid processes [24].

Figure 6.19 shows a case of ankylosis of the right TMJ. Differentiating between fibrous and bony ankylosis can be impossible without cross-sectional imaging.

6.2.11 Tumours

Osteochondroma is the most common benign tumour, appearing on conventional radiographs as an irregularly shaped enlargement of the condylar head, arising particularly from the anterior or antero-medial aspect of the condyle [25, 26]. Other benign tumours, including osteoma, may occur, but which will give a similar appearance. Figure 6.20 is a case of osteochondroma of the condyle.

Malignant tumours are rare, with metastatic tumours being the most likely. Extrinsic primary tumours may arise from adjacent structures such as the parotid gland. Primary tumours from the tissues of the TMJ itself are extremely rare. Radiological signs on plain radiographs will be very limited, principally to bone

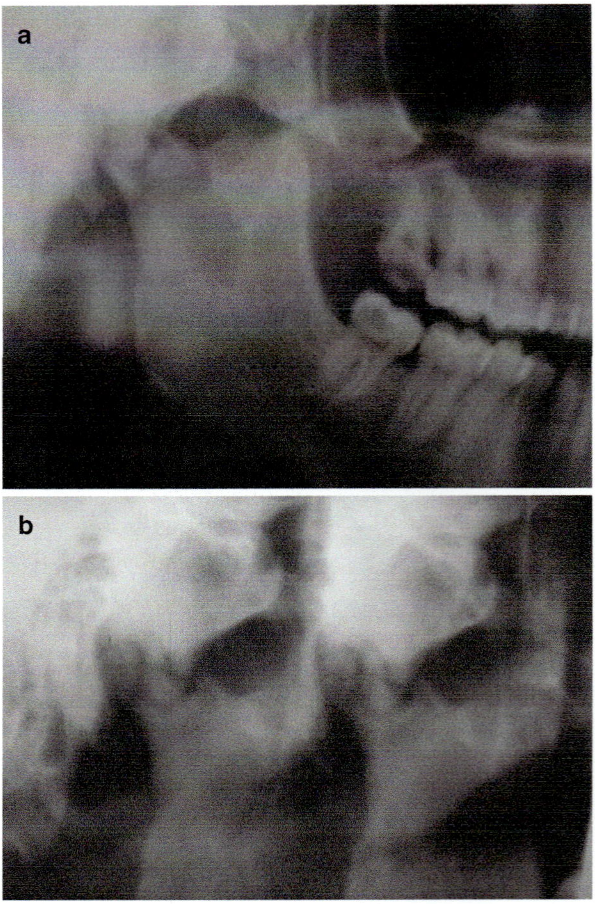

Fig. 6.19 (**a**) Part of a panoramic radiograph, showing deformity of normal anatomy of the right TMJ. There are bony irregularity and sclerosis, and it is impossible to see the condyle as a separate entity from the temporal bone. (**b**) Tomograms provide greater clarity of the anatomy, with the articular fossa and eminence shape more apparent, but any joint space is very narrow and not continuous [Images courtesy of Prof. Kaan Orhan]

destruction. This might be misinterpreted initially as attributable to other causes of erosion of the joint, such as rheumatoid arthritis or severe degenerative joint disease.

6.2.12 Others

6.2.12.1 Synovial (Osteo)chondromatosis

Ossification in the cartilaginous nodules which develop in the synovial membrane of joints in this condition can be seen on conventional radiographs (Fig. 6.21).

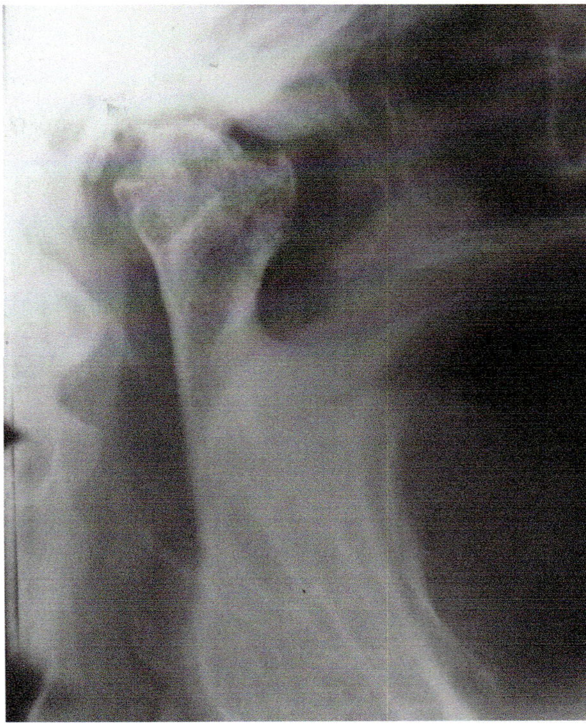

Fig. 6.20 Osteochondroma of the right condyle, producing an irregularly shaped enlargement. Transpharyngeal radiograph

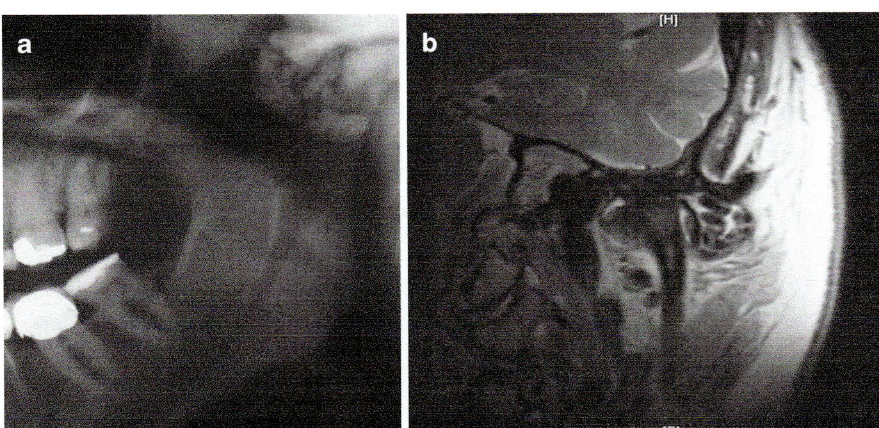

Fig. 6.21 Synovial osteochondromatosis of the left TMJ. (**a**) Panoramic radiograph of low quality received from a referring dentist showing a collection of multiple small radiopacities around the TMJ. (**b**) Coronal T1W MR cross-sectional image of the left TMJ region showing multiple hypointense nodules lateral to the condyle and medial to the condylar neck

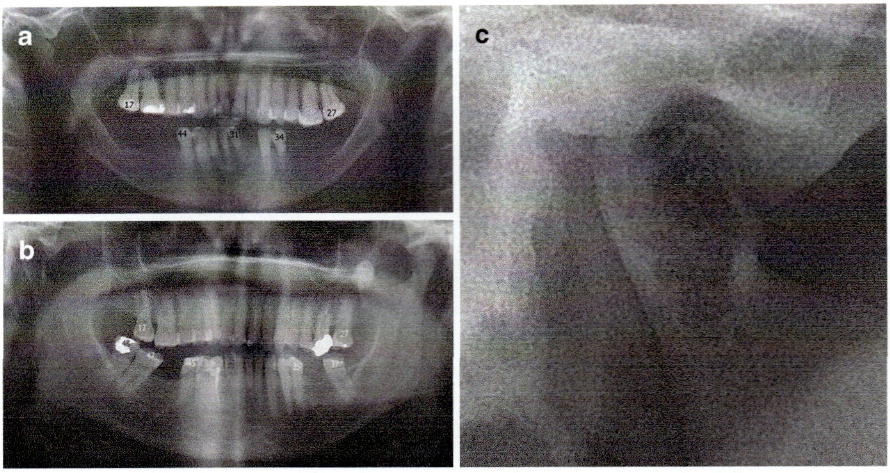

Fig. 6.22 Panoramic radiographs of two cases with scleroderma. (**a**) displays marked bilateral erosions of the ramus and antegonial notches areas. The right condylar head is larger and nearly of normal shape in comparison to the left condylar head. (**b**) The otherwise normal panoramic radiograph displays in (**c**) erosions of several parts of the right condylar head. Acknowledgement: Dr. Mervyn Gornitzky, Jewish General Hospital, Montreal, Canada

6.2.12.2 Systemic Sclerosis (Scleroderma)

The radiological signs of systemic sclerosis in the jaws include widening of periodontal ligaments and variable erosion of the bone. Erosions of the condyle were significantly more frequent in patients compared with controls in the large Canadian study [27]. Figure 6.22 shows three cases of this condition.

6.2.12.3 Neurofibromatosis

Patients with neurofibromatosis may have jaw abnormalities giving a striking appearance on panoramic radiographs [28]. Apart from localised enlargements of the mandibular canals due to neurofibromas, there may be other signs:

- Increase in bone density
- Enlarged mandibular foramen
- Lateral bowing of the mandibular ramus
- Increase in dimensions of the coronoid notch
- Decrease in the mandibular angle

Figure 6.23 shows a case of a patient with neurofibromatosis type I and mandibular changes.

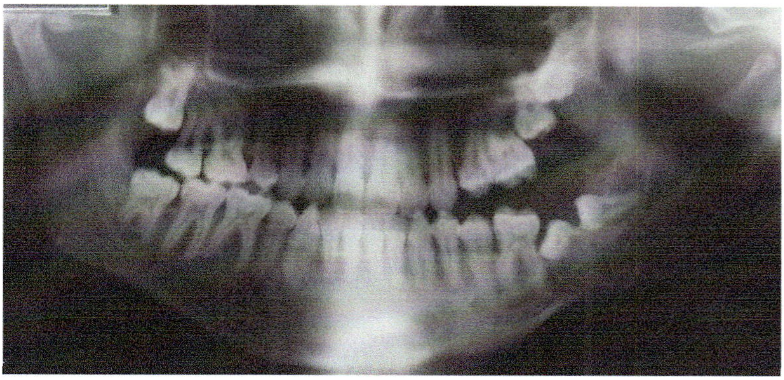

Fig. 6.23 A panoramic radiograph of a patient with neurofibromatosis type I. The left mandible is abnormally shaped, with an obtuse angle of the mandible and with elongated thin coronoid and condylar processes

References

1. Perschbacher S. Temporomandibular joint abnormalities. In: White SC, Pharoah MJ, editors. Oral radiology principles and interpretation. 7th ed. St Louis: Elsevier; 2014. p. 492–523.
2. Nikolova SY, Toneva DH, Lazarov NE. Incidence of a bifid mandibular condyle in dry mandibles. J Craniofac Surg. 2017;28:2168–73. https://doi.org/10.1097/SCS.0000000000003173.
3. Miloglu O, Yilmaz AB, Yildirim E, Akgul HM. Pneumatization of the articular eminence on cone beam computed tomography: prevalence, characteristics and a review of the literature. Dentomaxillofac Radiol. 2011;40:110–4. https://doi.org/10.1259/dmfr/75842018.
4. Orhan K, Oz U, Orhan AI, Ulker AE, Delilbasi C, Akcam O. Investigation of pneumatized articular eminence in orthodontic malocclusions. Orthod Craniofac Res. 2010;13:56–60. https://doi.org/10.1111/j.1601-6343.2009.01476.x.
5. de Rezende Barbosa GL, Nascimento Mdo C, Ladeira DB, Bomtorim VV, da Cruz AD, Almeida SM. Accuracy of digital panoramic radiography in the diagnosis of temporal bone pneumatization: a study in vivo using cone-beam-computed tomography. J Craniomaxillofac Surg. 2014;42:477–81. https://doi.org/10.1016/j.jcms.2013.06.005.
6. Gray RJ, Quayle AA, Horner K, Al-Gorashi AJ. The effects of positioning variations in transcranial radiographs of the temporomandibular joint: a laboratory study. Br J Oral Maxillofac Surg. 1991;29:241–9. Erratum in: Br J Oral Maxillofac Surg 1991;29:424
7. Knoernschild KL, Aquilino SA, Ruprecht A. Transcranial radiography and linear tomography: a comparative study. J Prosthet Dent. 1991;66:239–50.
8. MacDonald Jankowski DS. Calcification of the stylohyoid complex in Londoners and Hong Kong Chinese. Dentomaxillofac Radiol. 2001;30:35–9.
9. Ren YF, Isberg A, Westesson PL. Steepness of the articular eminence in the temporomandibular joint. Tomographic comparison between asymptomatic volunteers with normal disk position and patients with disk displacement. Oral Surg Oral Med Oral Pathol Oral Radiol Endod. 1995;80:258–66.

10. Sato S, Kawamura H, Motegi K, Takahashi K. Morphology of the mandibular fossa and the articular eminence in temporomandibular joints with anterior disk displacement. Int J Oral Maxillofac Surg. 1996;25(3):236–8.
11. Shahidi S, Vojdani M, Paknahad M. Correlation between articular eminence steepness measured with cone-beam computed tomography and clinical dysfunction index in patients with temporomandibular joint dysfunction. Oral Surg Oral Med Oral Pathol Oral Radiol. 2013;116:91–7. https://doi.org/10.1016/j.oooo.2013.04.001.
12. Paknahad M, Shahidi S, Akhlaghian M, Abolvardi M. Is mandibular fossa morphology and articular eminence inclination associated with temporomandibular dysfunction? J Dent (Shiraz). 2016 Jun;17(2):134–41.
13. Hintze H, Wiese M, Wenzel A. Comparison of three radiographic methods for detection of morphological temporomandibular joint changes: panoramic, scanographic and tomographic examination. Dentomaxillofac Radiol. 2009;38:134–40. https://doi.org/10.1259/dmfr/31066378.
14. Winocur E, Reiter S, Krichmer M, Kaffe I. Classifying degenerative joint disease by the RDC/TMD and by panoramic imaging: a retrospective analysis. J Oral Rehabil. 2010;37:171–7. https://doi.org/10.1111/j.1365-2842.2009.02035.x.
15. Rushton VE, Horner K, Worthington HV. The quality of panoramic radiographs in a sample of general dental practices. Br Dent J. 1999;186:630–3.
16. Kratz R, Nguyen CT, MacDonald DS, Walton JN. Dental students' interpretations of digital panoramic radiographs on completely edentate patients. J Dent Educ. 2018;82(3):313–21.
17. Rodrigues DB, Castro V. Condylar hyperplasia of the temporomandibular joint: types, treatment, and surgical implications. Oral Maxillofac Surg Clin North Am. 2015;27:155–67. https://doi.org/10.1016/j.coms.2014.09.011.
18. McLoughlin PM, Hopper C, Bowley NB. Hyperplasia of the mandibular coronoid process: an analysis of 31 cases and a review of the literature. J Oral Maxillofac Surg. 1995;53:250–5.
19. Jaskolka MS, Eppley BL, van Aalst JA. Mandibular coronoid hyperplasia in pediatric patients. J Craniofac Surg. 2007;18:849–54.
20. Twilt M, Schulten AJ, Nicolaas P, Dülger A, van Suijlekom-Smit LW. Facioskeletal changes in children with juvenile idiopathic arthritis. Ann Rheum Dis. 2006;65:823–5.
21. Abramowicz S, Simon LE, Susarla HK, Lee EY, Cheon JE, Kim S, Kaban LB. Are panoramic radiographs predictive of temporomandibular joint synovitis in children with juvenile idiopathic arthritis? J Oral Maxillofac Surg. 2014;72:1063–9.
22. Boeddinghaus R, Whyte A. Trends in maxillofacial imaging. Clin Radiol. 2018;73:4–18. https://doi.org/10.1016/j.crad.2017.02.015.
23. Wood RE, Harris AM, Nortjé CJ, Grotepass FW. The radiologic features of true ankylosis of the temporomandibular joint. An analysis of 25 cases. Dentomaxillofac Radiol. 1988;17:121–7.
24. Wang WH, Xu B, Zhang BJ, Lou HQ. Temporomandibular joint ankyloses contributing to coronoid process hyperplasia. Int J Oral Maxillofac Surg. 2016;45:1229–33.
25. Tamimi D, Jalali E, Hatcher D. Temporomandibular joint imaging. In: Tamimi D, editor. Oral and maxillofacial radiology, Radiologic clinics of North America, vol. 56; 2018. p. 157–75. https://doi.org/10.1016/j.rcl.2017.08.011.
26. Saito T, Utsunomiya T, Furutani M, Yamamoto H. Osteochondroma of the mandibular condyle: a case report and review of the literature. J Oral Sci. 2001;43:293–7.
27. Dagenais M, MacDonald D, Baron M, Hudson M, Tatibouet S, Steele R, et al. The Canadian Systemic Sclerosis Oral Health Study IV: oral radiographic manifestations in systemic sclerosis compared with the general population. Oral Surg Oral Med Oral Pathol Oral Radiol. 2015;120:104–11. https://doi.org/10.1016/j.oooo.2015.03.002.
28. Lee L, Yan YH, Pharoah MJ. Radiographic features of the mandible in neurofibromatosis: a report of 10 cases and review of the literature. Oral Surg Oral Med Oral Pathol Oral Radiol Endod. 1996;81:361–7.

7 Computed Tomography (CT)

Ingrid Różyło-Kalinowska

7.1 Basics of Computed Tomography Technique

Computed tomography (CT) is based on attenuation of X-ray beam passing through an examined object. The applied physical phenomenon is comparable to radiography, but the differences are the X-ray detectors making the obtained image tomographic (i.e. in slices), and not a sum up one. The first experiments with CT were carried out in the late 1960s and early 1970s, and the late Sir Godfrey Hounsfield is generally credited as the inventor of the imaging technique. CT has experienced huge progress since then, and numbers of examinations are constantly increasing worldwide.

A CT scanner facility contains a gantry, mobile table for patient positioning and technical workstation, while the obtained scans are transferred to a picture archiving and communication system (PACS) or less advanced on-site networks for analysis on imaging stations.

Inside the gantry there is one X-ray tube or, which more and more commonly nowadays, two X-rays tubes operating at different kilovoltage (dual-source CT), rotating around the mobile table supporting the examined patient. After passing through a patient's body, the attenuated X-rays are detected by parallel multiple rows of detectors (in older generations of CT scanners one row of detectors)—multi-slice computed tomography (MSCT). During the helical rotation of the X-ray tube(s) within the gantry, the table is constantly moving into it, thus bringing consecutive portions of the patient into the area of X-ray beam. The X-ray beam in CT is fan-shaped, which makes it different from cone beam in CBCT, but with more rows of detectors, the thickness of the fan-shaped beam in CT is getting wider.

I. Różyło-Kalinowska
Independent Unit of Propaedeutics of Dentomaxillofacial Radiology, Medical University of Lublin, Lublin, Poland
e-mail: rozylo.kalinowska@umlub.pl

I. Rozylo-Kalinowska, K. Orhan (eds.), *Imaging of the Temporomandibular Joint*, https://doi.org/10.1007/978-3-319-99468-0_7

Linear X-ray attenuation coefficient is calculated separately for each voxel, i.e. cuboid volumetric element which constitutes each scanned layer. Information about X-ray attenuation coefficients obtained during the whole scan is saved as raw data and then subjected to reconstruction processes resulting in visualization of slice images on computer screen. Further image processing is applied during image reconstruction and analysis. The initial slices are axial ones, i.e. perpendicular to long axis of patient's body/head. Then multiplanar reformatted reconstructions (MPR) are used to create coronal, sagittal, curved (e.g. panoramic curve), tangential (parallel to tangent to dental arch curve) and cross-sectional (perpendicular to tangent to dental arch curve)—along any chosen line. There are numerous pseudo-three-dimensional techniques. Shaded surface display (SSD) is based on display of surface pixels characterized by highest densities. Maximum intensity projection (MIP) is used to demonstrate contrast-enhanced blood vessels. Volume rendering (VR) is topographic imaging of those surfaces which have densities higher than a given threshold, e.g. to demonstrate blood vessels.

Linear attenuation coefficient of X-rays within individual images are transformed into the Hounsfield units (HU), which make it possible to estimate densities, and are arranged in the form of a Hounsfield scale. Zero density (0 HU) corresponds to water (distilled water at standard pressure). In the basic scale, air has density of −1000 HU while bone +1000. However, higher densities are also attained such as up to +3000 HU in cortical bone and + 30,000 HU in metallic foreign bodies. Different tissues and organs are characterized by different HU levels; thus density measurements are used in tissue differentiation and evaluation (Table 7.1). Human eye is not able to perceive differences between grey scale levels shown on screen corresponding to the whole Hounsfield scale; therefore the so-called windowing is applied. Windowing allows changing of window width (i.e. number of HU levels presented simultaneously on screen) and level. This way areas with HU higher than the upper threshold are shown as white, and areas with HU below the lower limit are shown as black. The monitor grey scale is applied to

Table 7.1 X-ray linear attenuation coefficient transformed to the Hounsfield units

Tissue or organ	Approximate HU values
Air	<−600
Fat	−60 to −120
Water	0
CSF	+15
Transudate	<+20
Exudate	>+20
Blood	+15 to +50
Thrombus	+50 to +75
Soft tissues	+30 to +80
Cancellous bone	>+300
Cortical bone	Up to +3000

demonstrate all HU levels between the set limits. Window level is the middle value of HU in a given window. CT image processing software makes it possible to change window width and level smoothly, but in general two basic windows are distinguished—soft tissue window and bone window. Soft tissue window is characterized by low level (HU corresponding to soft tissue densities) and small width—in order to demonstrate soft tissue with high detail rather than bone details. On the other hand, bone window has high level (HU of the bone) and is wide so as to visualize fine bone detail at the same time omitting most information on soft tissues. When CT densities are reported, hyperdense, isodense and hypodense areas are described. Examples of hyperdense structures include hard tissues of teeth, calcifications, dense foreign bodies, contrast-enhanced blood and freshly extravasated blood. Pathological areas can be described as hyperdense when compared with normal density of a studied organ or tissue, while isodense lesions have the same density as tissues in vicinity. Hypodense lesions are characterized by densities lower than surrounding tissues, and examples include cysts, inflammatory infiltrations and some tumours.

Before every CT examination, a scout scan is taken and range of scanning chosen. In many cases CT examination is performed in two phases—before and after contrast medium injection resulting in the so-called contrast enhancement of blood vessels and highly vascularized tissues or lesions. Most commonly contrast media are administered intravenously (into an antecubital vein) but can be injected also into a joint space. Contrast media applied in computed tomography are identical as those used in fluoroscopy (see Chapter 16). Adequate delay in the start of CT scanning must be set or bolus tracking applied triggering CT acquisition. Directly after the beginning of intravenous contrast media administration by means of an automatic injector, blood vessels are being filled (arterial phase). Next parenchyma is saturated, and then contrast medium flows into veins, from which it is finally secreted to urea. Velocity of contrast medium injection, contrast medium amount and concentration of iodine as well as delay in imaging from the beginning of contrast medium administration all influence the obtained image quality. These factors are individually set depending on purpose of imaging protocol and patient's characteristics. The aim of contrast media administration is to verify whether contrast enhancement occurs in comparison with baseline scans obtained before contrast media injection. Pre-contrast images demonstrate hyperdense areas such as calcifications or dense foreign bodies, while post-contrast scans reveal blood vessels and/or areas characterized by high vascularisation. Contrast-enhanced blood vessels are very well visible, and their high density is applied to reconstruct images in the form of the so-called angio-CT. Contrast enhancement is also useful in differentiation between vascularized and avascular lesions (tumour vs. cyst), better delineation of lesion margins and its internal structure.

7.2 Advantages and Disadvantages of CT

Advantages of CT include:

- Short scanning time
- Cross-sectional imaging
- High quality of multiplanar reconstructions
- High contrast resolution
- Objective density measurements using HU
- Assessment of contrast enhancement

Disadvantages of CT include:

- Average to high radiation exposure dose depending on the purpose of examination and number of phases acquired
- Image artefacts produced by metallic objects such as osteosynthesis plates, TMJ prostheses, dental implants, fixed orthodontic appliances, amalgam fillings and other dense objects such as dental fillings or foreign bodies. The use of the most up-to-date CT scanners allowing for spectral imaging resulting in synthesized monoenergetic images at predefined keV values may reduce artefacts at higher keV (kiloelectronovolts)
- Side effects of administered iodine contrast media

7.3 Contraindications for CT and Patient Preparation

Contraindications

- There are no absolute contraindications.
- Relative contraindications are mostly consequences of contrast media administration and do not occur when contrast enhancement is not applied.
- Also pregnancy is a relative contraindication since CT exams can be performed in life-threatening situations when scanning cannot be postponed until after childbirth.

Patient Preparation

- Informed consent must be obtained.
- Scheduled contrast-enhanced studies are performed on an empty stomach.
- Patient does not refrain from taking prescribed medications.

- Patients with thyroid pathology must have TSH blood level tested before CT with possible iodine contrast medium administration.
- Patients with kidney failure must have creatinine blood level tested before CT with possible iodine contrast medium administration.

7.4 Use of CT in Diagnostics of TMJ Lesions

The use of CT in diagnostics of TMJ lesions comprises:

- Congenital malformations such as condylar hypoplasia, condylar hyperplasia, bifid or trifid condyle
- Arthropathies such as rheumatoid arthritis, juvenile rheumatoid arthritis or psoriatic arthropathy to assess bone erosion
- Osteoarthritis [1]
- Condylar fractures [2]
- Bone and fibrous ankylosis to evaluate the presence of bony union as well as to evaluate treatment outcomes [3–5]
- Benign and malignant tumours to assess bone destruction, calcifications within joint space and tumour itself, soft-tissue tumour mass, contrast enhancement [6–8]
- Evaluation of condyle morphology in relation to sagittal split osteotomy [9]
- Virtual surgical planning (VSP) using computer-aided design/computer-aided manufacturing (CAD/CAM) of TMJ prosthesis [10, 11]

Recently four-dimensional CT was described as a novel imaging technique, which can be used to assess kinematic features of TMJ not visualized with other imaging modalities. During scanning 4D CT motion images are registered during mastication, and patient's condylar movement is evaluated. In this first study by Akashi et al. [12], the technique was successfully used to directly visualize the friction between the atrophic and flattened condylar surface and the articular eminence.

7.5 CT Anatomy of TMJ

CT anatomy of the TMJ is presented in Fig. 7.1 (axial slices, hard tissues) and Fig. 7.2 (axial slices soft tissues), Fig. 7.3 (coronal sections) and Fig. 7.4 (sagittal sections).

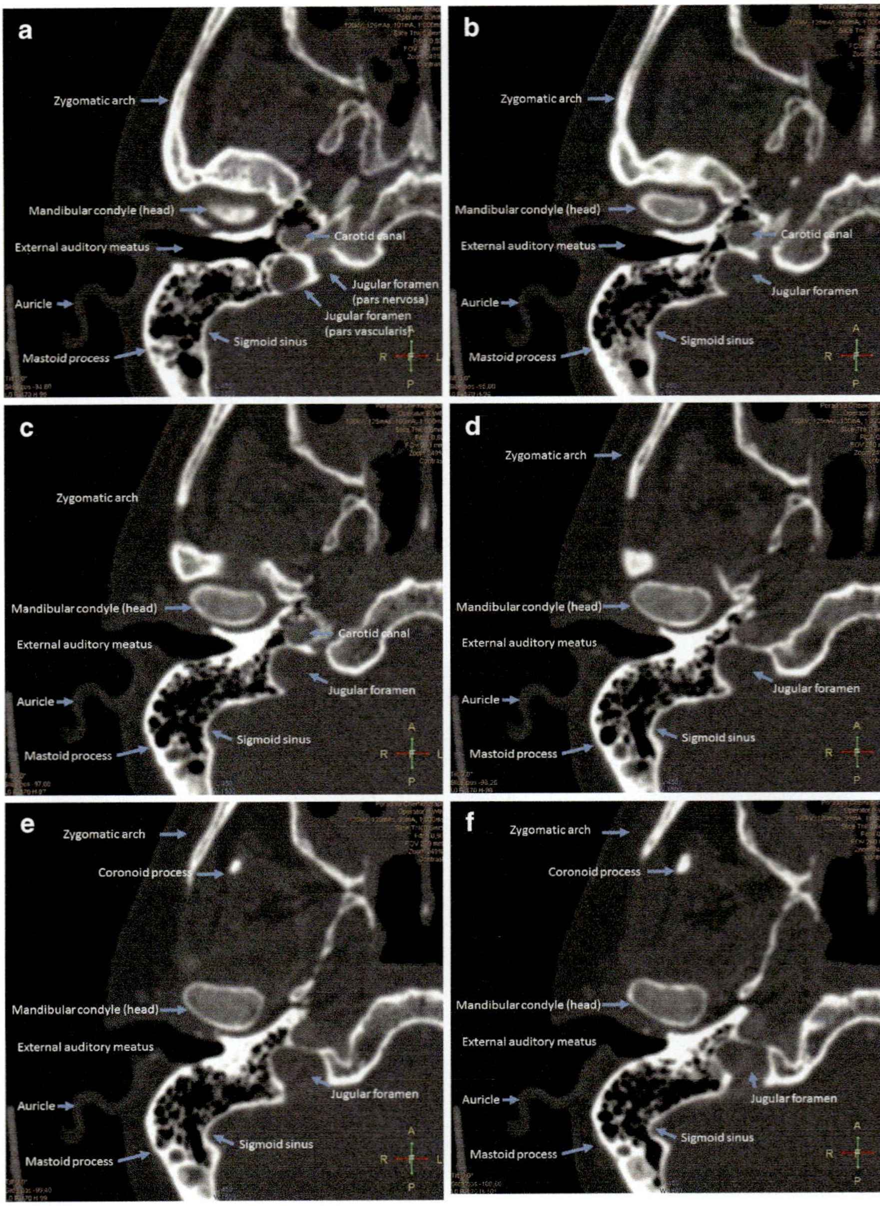

Fig. 7.1 (**a**–**h**) CT anatomy of the TMJ in axial slices, bone window

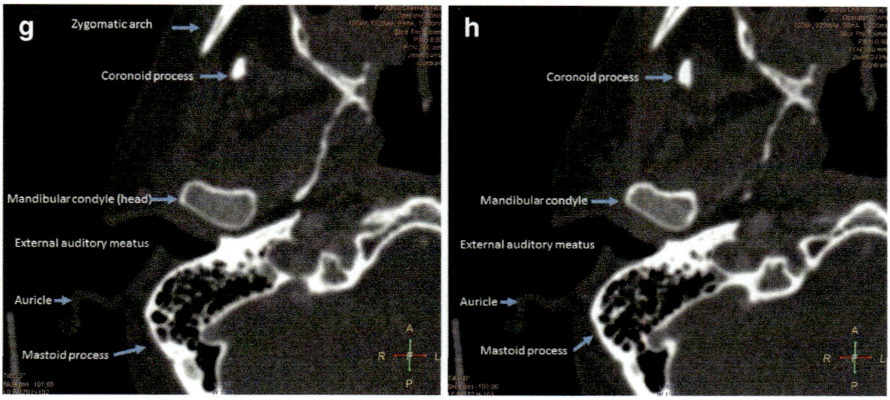

Fig. 7.1 (continued)

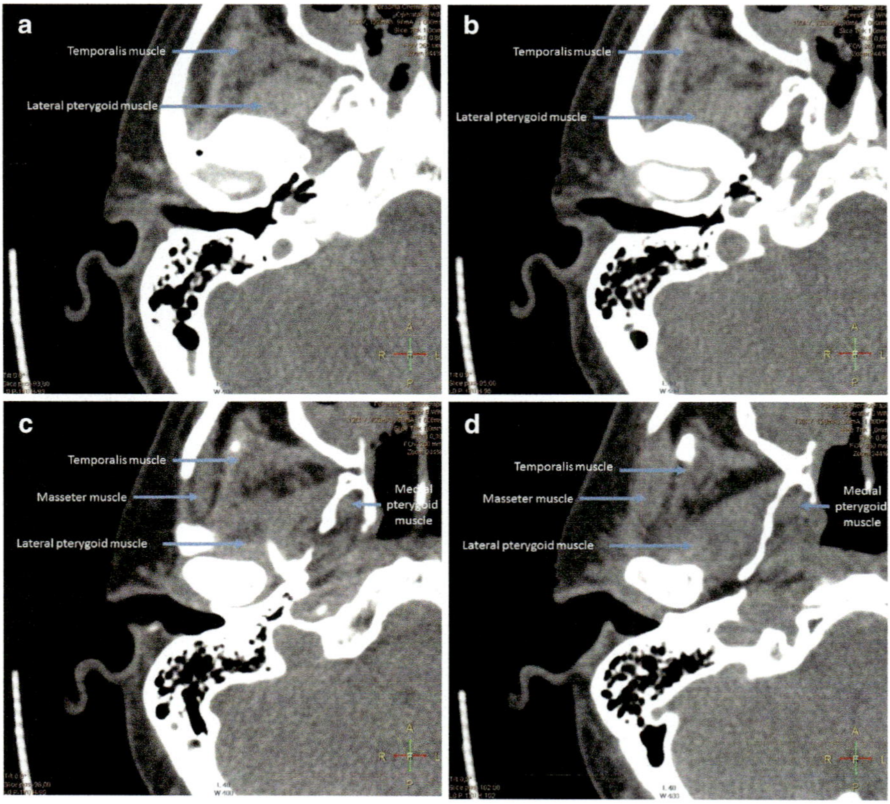

Fig. 7.2 (**a**–**e**) CT anatomy of the TMJ in axial slices, soft tissue window

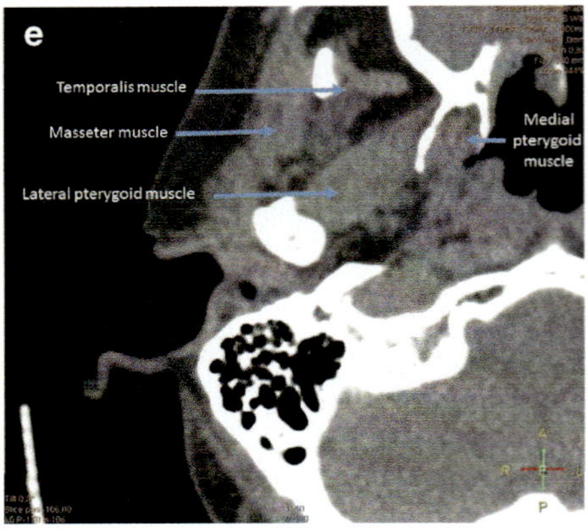

Fig. 7.2 (continued)

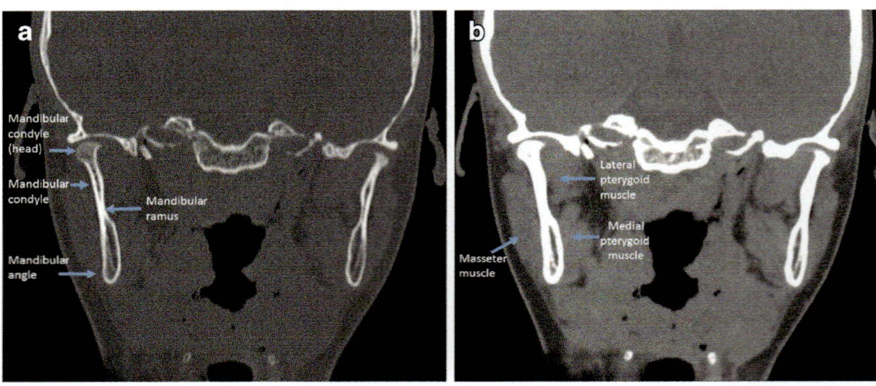

Fig. 7.3 CT anatomy of the TMJ in coronal images, (**a**) bone window, (**b**) soft tissue window

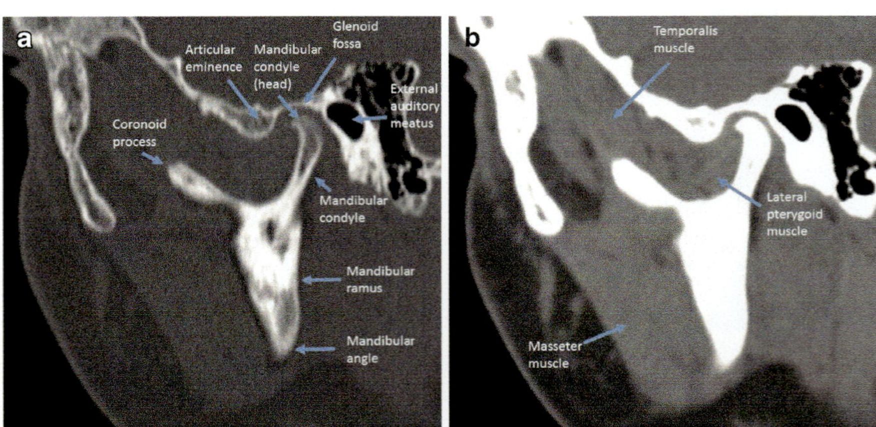

Fig. 7.4 CT anatomy of the TMJ in sagittal images, (**a**) bone window, (**b**) soft tissue window

References

1. Mani FM, Sivasubramanian SS. A study of temporomandibular joint osteoarthritis using computed tomographic imaging. Biom J. 2016;39(3):201–6.
2. Naeem A, Gemal H, Reed D. Imaging in traumatic mandibular fractures. Quant Imaging Med Surg. 2017;7(4):469–79.
3. Ranjit Kumar P, Naveen G, Raja Satish P, Srinivas Chakravarthy P, Krishna Prasad L. An unusual anterior dislocation of fractured mandibular condyle leading to pseudo-ankylosis in a 8 yr old child-A distinct case report. Int J Surg Case Rep. 2016;26:34–7.
4. Yuang X, Lu C, Dong M, He D, Yang C, Hu Y. Evaluation of the condyle remodelling after lateral arthroplasty in growing children with temporomandibular joint ankyloses. Sci Rep. 2017;7:9922.
5. Zhao J, He D, Yang C, Hu Y, Huang D, Ellis E 3rd. 3-D computed tomography measurement of mandibular growth after costochondral grafting in growing children with temporomandibular joint ankylosis and jaw deformity. Oral Surg Oral Med Oral Pathol Oral Radiol. 2017;124(4):333–8.
6. Guarda-Nardini L, Stellini E, Di Fiore A, Manfredini D. A rare case of misdiagnosed silent lung cancer with solitary metastasis to the temporomandibular joint condyle. J Oral Facial Pain Headache. 2017;31(2):180–5.
7. Hu Y, Kuang B, Chen Y, Shu J. Imaging features for diffuse-type tenosynovial giant cell tumor of the temporomandibular joint: A case report. Medicine (Baltimore). 2017;96(26):e7383. https://doi.org/10.1097/MD.0000000000007383.
8. Liu X, Huang Z, Zhu W, Liang P, Tao Q. Clinical and imaging findings of temporomandibular joint synovial chondromatosis: an analysis of 10 cases and literature review. J Oral Maxillofac Surg. 2016;74(11):2159–68.
9. Iguchi R, Yoshizawa K, Moroi A, Tsutsui T, Hotta A, Hiraide R, Takayama A, Tsunoda T, Saito Y, Sato M, Baba N, Ueki K. Comparison of temporomandibular joint and ramus morphology between class II and class III cases before and after bi-maxillary osteotomy. J Craniomaxillofac Surg. 2017;45(12):2002–9.
10. Lu C, He D, Yang C, Huang D, Ellis E 3rd. Computer-assisted surgical planning and simulation for unilateral condylar benign lesions causing facial asymmetry. Oral Surg Oral Med Oral Pathol Oral Radiol. 2017;123(4):453–8.
11. Tarsitano A, Battaglia S, Ramieri V, Cascone P, Ciocca L, Scotti R, Marchetti C. Short-term outcomes of mandibular reconstruction in oncological patients using a CAD-CAM prosthesis including a condyle supporting a fibular free flap. J Craniomaxillofac Surg. 2017;45(2):330–7.
12. Akashi M, Hasegawa T, Takahashi S, Komori T. Four-dimensional computed tomography evaluation of condylar movement in a patient with temporomandibular joint osteoarthritis. J Oral Maxillofac Surg. 2017;76(2):304–13. pii: S0278-2391(17)31282-X. https://doi.org/10.1016/j.joms.2017.10.012.

Cone Beam Computed Tomography (CBCT) in TMJ Imaging

8

Ingrid Różyło-Kalinowska

8.1 Basics of Cone Beam Computed Tomography

In cone beam computed tomography (CBCT), an X-ray beam in the form of a cone (hence the name) is used to obtain a sequence of several hundred X-rays during a 180- or 360-degree rotation of the tube around patient's head. Another name for this time of cross-sectional examination is digital volumetric tomography (DVT) or imaging (DVI), and this name is also justified as during the scan a certain volume is imaged in contrast to CT, where it is rather a distance from one level to another which is scanned in a patient. In CBCT field of view (FoV) must be chosen, and it varies between machines merchandised by different companies. In general FoVs can be divided into small, medium, and large depending on diameter and height of the scanned volume. In TMJ diagnostics medium and large FoVs usually are chosen. Small FoV can be virtually "stitched" to produce a larger volume, but it requires more than one X-ray acquisition; therefore in newer CBCT units, a selection of FoVs is available. Apart from dimensions, also FoV shape can be different—cylindrical, spherical, or jaw-shaped.

Majority of available CBCT units resemble panoramic machines with patient examined standing or sitting, and in fact in many devices, it is possible to obtain also a conventional 2D panoramic radiograph. Only a few CBCT devices are similar to CT with patient examined lying supine on a table. In general patient positioning is comparable to positioning for panoramic, but TMJ imaging requires careful selection and placement of FoV.

Image resolution depends on voxel size—the smaller a voxel is, the higher image resolution is obtained. Voxels in CBCT are isotropic, i.e., cubical with all margins equal in contrast to CT where voxels are anisotropic (of different heights depending

I. Różyło-Kalinowska
Independent Unit of Propaedeutics of Dentomaxillofacial Radiology,
Medical University of Lublin, Lublin, Poland
e-mail: rozylo.kalinowska@umlub.pl

I. Rozylo-Kalinowska, K. Orhan (eds.), *Imaging of the Temporomandibular Joint*, https://doi.org/10.1007/978-3-319-99468-0_8

on the purpose of examination). Voxel size in CBCT varies from 0.05 to 0.4 mm, and its choice is related to the aim of the imaging study.

Digital data obtained during image acquisition are reconstructed to produce axial, coronal, and sagittal images similar to MPRs in CT, as well as dedicated dental slices such as panoramic, cross-sectional, and tangential. Volume rendering (VR) and surface-shaded display (SSD) pseudo-three-dimensional images can be produced, as well.

8.2 Advantages and Disadvantages of CBCT

Advantages of CBCT include:

- High-resolution cross-sectional imaging of bone structures
- Relatively low patient exposure dose [1]
- High and growing availability of CBCT machines for dentists
- Relatively low cost of facilities, equipment, and examination itself when compared with CT
- Relatively high diagnostic accuracy for TMJ bone changes [2], comparable with CT [3]

Disadvantages of CBCT include:

- Lower image contrast than in CT.
- Higher image noise than in CT.
- Currently no precise estimation of Hounsfield units possible due to errors in estimation of densities.
- Still no reliable evaluation of soft tissues.
- Image artifacts generated by patient motion or metallic objects, e.g., osteosynthesis plate or TMJ prosthesis causing X-ray beam hardening (streak artifacts and/or cupping artifacts). However the latter are less pronounced in CBCT than in regular CT.
- Limited reliability for TMJ bone changes [2].

8.3 Contraindications for CBCT and Patient Preparation

No specific patient preparation is required for CBCT. However, evaluation of TMJs may require a standardized position of the jaws which is maintained owing to the use of a silicone index prepared by the referring dentist.

There are no absolute contraindications for CBCT, and pregnancy is a relative contraindication.

A limitation of CBCT application may be the lack of cooperation resulting in motion artifacts in small children or mentally disabled patients. Neonates and disabled patients not able to maintain vertical position of the head cannot be examined in machines in which patient positioning requires standing or sitting.

8.4 Indications for CBCT in TMJ Diagnostics

The use of CBCT in dentistry has been addressed by the European Academy of Dentomaxillofacial Radiology as "Basic Principles for Use of Dental Cone Beam CT—Consensus Guidelines of the European Academy of Dental and Maxillofacial Radiology" published in 2009 followed by the outcomes of the SEDENTEX-CT project published as "Cone Beam for Dental and Maxillofacial Radiology. Evidence Based Guidelines" as document no. 172.

So far the following applications of CBCT in TMJ diagnostics have been described:

- Evaluation of TMJ anatomy [4]
- Evaluation of condylar position in malocclusion [5]
- Developmental anomalies of TMJ, e.g., bifid condyle, condylar hyperplasia, coronoid hyperplasia [6]
- Osteoarthritis including assessment of osteophytes, erosion, flattening, subchondral sclerosis, and pseudocysts [7]
- Follow-up of progression or treatment of degenerative joint disease [8]
- Rheumatoid arthritis and juvenile idiopathic arthritis [9]
- Assessment of internal derangement, also in conjunction with MRI [10, 11]
- Relationship between the superior semicircular canal of the vestibulum and TMJ symptoms [12]
- Condylar fractures [13]
- TMJ ankylosis [14]
- TMJ cysts and tumors including synovial chondromatosis and metastasis [15–17]
- Changes in TMJ after mandibulotomy [18]
- Misdiagnosis of temporomandibular joint disorder in tumors [16]
- Measurement of styloid process length in patients with temporomandibular joint disorder (TMD) [19]
- Image-guided puncture [3, 17]

8.5 CBCT Radiological Anatomy of TMJ

Radiological anatomy of the TMJ in CBCT is presented in the Figs. 8.1, 8.2, and 8.3.

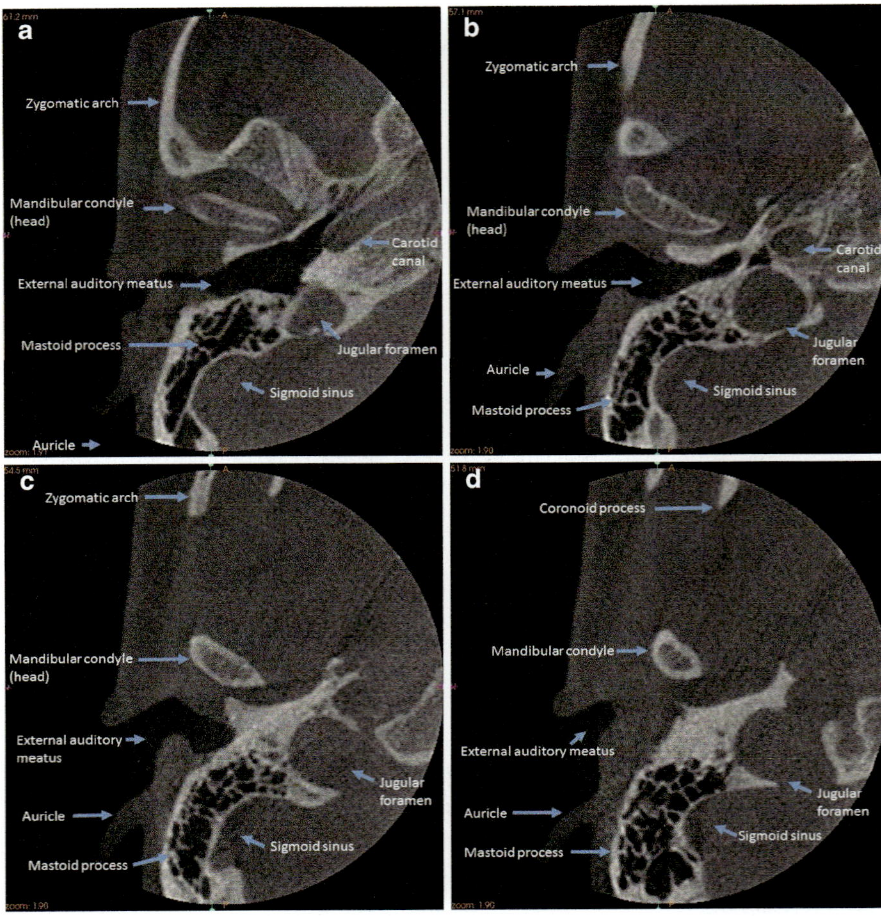

Fig. 8.1 (**a**–**d**) Radiological anatomy of the TMJ in CBCT—axial slices

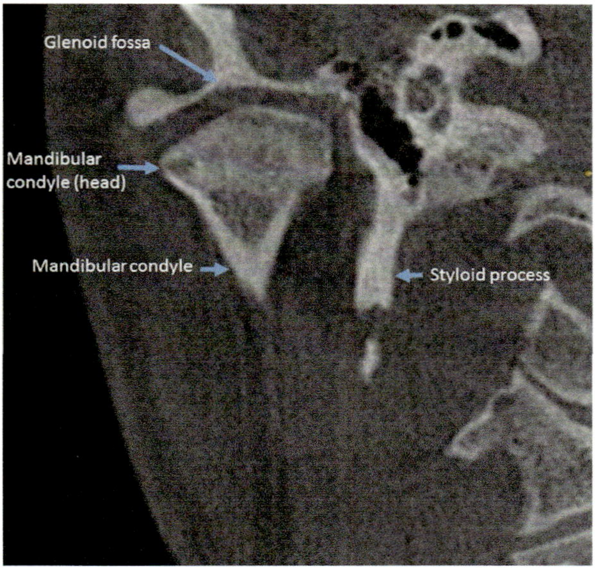

Fig. 8.2 Radiological anatomy of the TMJ in CBCT—image obtained along the long axis of the condyle

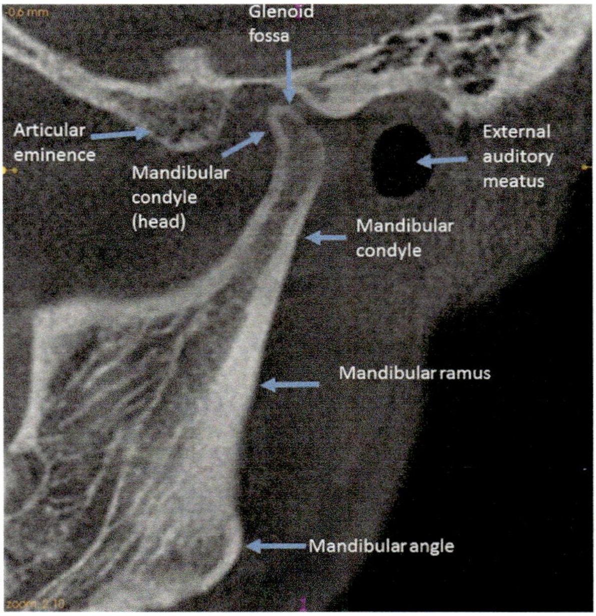

Fig. 8.3 Radiological anatomy of the TMJ in CBCT—image obtained along the short axis of the condyle (parasagittal)

References

1. Kadesjö N, Benchimol D, Falahat B, Näsström K, Shi XQ. Evaluation of the effective dose of cone beam computed tomography and multi-slice computed tomography for temporomandibular joint examinations at optimized exposure levels. Dentomaxillofac Radiol. 2015;2:20150041.
2. Ma RH, Yin S, Li G. The detection accuracy of cone beam CT for osseous defects of the temporomandibular joint: a systematic review and meta-analysis. Sci Rep. 2016;6:34714.
3. Honda K, Bjornland T. Image-guided puncture technique for the superior temporomandibular joint space: value of cone beam computed tomography (CBCT). Oral surg Oral Med Oral Pthol Oral Radiol Endod. 2006;102:281–6.
4. Caruso S, Storti E, Nota A, Ehsani S, Gatto R. Temporomandibular joint anatomy assessed by CBCT images. Biomed Res Int. 2017;2017:2916953.
5. Kaur A, Natt AS, Mehra SK, Maheshwari K, Singh G, Kaur A. Improved visualisation and assessment of condylar position in the glenoid fossa for different occlusions: A CBCT study. J Contemp Dent Pract. 2016;17(8):679–86.
6. Almasan OC, Hedesiu M, Baciut G, Baciut M, Bran S, Jacobs R. Nontraumatic bilateral bifid condyle and intermittent joint lock: a case report and literature review. J Oral Maxillofac Surg. 2011;69:e297–303. https://doi.org/10.1016/j.joms.2011.03.072. Accessed 25 Mar 2018.
7. Shi J, Lee S, Pan HC, Mohammad A, Lin A, Guo W, Chen E, Ahn A, Li J, Ting K, Kwak JH. Association of condylar bone quality with TMJ osteoarthritis. J Dent Res. 2017;96(8):888–94.
8. Hilgenberg-Sydney PB, Bonotto DV, Stechman-Neto J, Zwir LF, Pacheco-Pereira C, Canto GL, Porporatti AL. Diagnostic validity of CT to assess degenerative temporomandibular joint disease: a systematic review. Dentomaxillofac Radiol. 2018;47(5):20170389. https://doi.org/10.1259/dmfr.20170389. Accessed 23 Mar 2018.
9. El Assar de la Fuente S, Angenete O, Jellestad S, Tzaribachev N, Koos B, Rosendahl K. Juvenile idiopathic arthritis and the temporomandibular joint: A comprehensive review. J Craniomaxillofac Surg. 2016;44(5):597–607.
10. Alkhader M, Kuribayashi A, Ohbayashi N, Nakamura S, Kurabayashi T. Usefulness of cone beam computed tomography in temporomandibular joints with soft tissue pathology. Dentomaxillofac Radiol. 2010;39:343–8.
11. Al-Saleh MA, Punithakumar K, Lagravere M, Boulanger P, Jaremko JL, Major PW. Three-dimensional assessment of temporomandibular joint using MRI-CBCT image registration. PLoS One. 2017a;12(1):e0169555.
12. Kurt H, Orhan K, Aksoy S, Kursun S, Akbulut N, Bilecenoglu B. Evaluation of the superior semicircular canal morphology using cone beam computed tomography: a possible correlation for temporomandibular joint symptoms. Oral Surg Oral Med Oral Pathol Oral Radiol. 2014;117(3):e280–8. https://doi.org/10.1016/j.oooo.2014.01.011. Accessed 25 Mar 2018.
13. Tang Y, Wang X, Zhu Y, Sun H, Zhu M. A comparative evaluation of CBCT outcomes of two closed treatment methods in intracapsular condylar fractures. Oral Surg Oral Med Oral Pathol Oral Radiol. 2017;123(5):e141–7.
14. Liu L, Li J, Ji H, Zhang N, Wang Y, Zheng G, Wang H, Luo E. Cone-beam computed tomography evaluation of the maxillofacial features of patients with unilateral temporomandibular joint ankyloses undergoing condylar reconstruction with an autogenous coronoid process graft. PLoS One. 2017;12(3):e0173142.
15. Balasundaram A, Geist JR, Gordon SC, Klasser GD. Radiographic diagnosis of synovial chondromatosis of the temporomandibular joint: a case report. J Can Dent Assoc. 2009;75:711–4.
16. Emanuelsson J, Allen CM, Rydin K, Sjöström M. Osteoblastoma of the temporal articular tubercle misdiagnosed as a temporomandibular joint disorder. Int J Oral Maxillofac Surg. 2017;46(5):610–3.
17. Matsumoto K, Sato T, Iwanari S, Kameoka S, Oki H, Komiyama K, Honda K. The use of arthrography in the diagnosis of temporomandibular joint synovial chondromatosis.

Dentomaxillofac Radiol. 2013;42(1):15388284. https://doi.org/10.1259/dmfr/15388284. Accessed 25 Mar 2018.

18. Al-Saleh MA, Punithakumar K, Lagravere M, Boulanger P, Jaremko JL, Wolfaardt J, Major PW, Seikaly H. Three-dimensional morphological changes of the temporomandibular joint and functional effects after mandibulotomy. J Otolaryngol Head Neck Surg. 2017b;46(1):8.
19. Krohn S, Brockmeyer P, Kubein-Meesenburg D, Kirschneck C, Buergers R. Elongated styloid process in patients with temporomandibular disorders – is there a link? Ann Anat. 2018;217:118–24. https://doi.org/10.1016/j.aanat.2018.01.007. Accessed 23 Mar 2018.

Ultrasonography

9

Kaan Orhan and Ingrid Różyło-Kalinowska

9.1 Basics of Ultrasonography Physics and Technique

Ultrasonography (US) is performed using physical properties of ultrasound, i.e. acoustic waves with frequency above 20,000 Hz propagated within a patient's body. In clinical practice acoustic waves with frequency from 2 to 20 MHz are applied.

The source of ultrasound is a probe, also called a transducer, containing a piezoelectric device which on one hand emits acoustic wave and on the other is the receiver of acoustic signals which return from an examined object as mechanical oscillation of wave reflected off the object, known as echoes. Since patient tissues are not homogenous, ultrasound encounters different tissue interfaces and various internal structures leading to changes in the returning waves in comparison with the emitted ultrasound. Inside the examined object, reflection, deflection, scattering and absorption with release of thermal energy occur. Scattering and absorption result in attenuation of ultrasound wave, which decreases penetration depth of an acoustic wave. An ultrasound wave is reflected off a boundary between two tissues characterized by a different acoustic impedance, and this way returning echoes form images of tissue or organ interfaces. The part of acoustic wave picked up by piezoelectric elements in the transducer give rise to electric signal which is presented on screen in real time as a black and white two-dimensional image (B-mode). In this mode the so-called echogenicity is evaluated. An area which produces strong echoes is called hyperechoic, on the other hand, areas with no internal echoes are named anechoic. Hypoechoic lesions are characterized by echogenicity lower than structures in vicinity, while areas of the same or comparable echogenicity are called isoechoic.

K. Orhan
Department of Dentomaxillofacial Radiology, Ankara University, Faculty of Dentistry, Ankara, Turkey

I. Różyło-Kalinowska (✉)
Independent Unit of Propaedeutics of Dentomaxillofacial Radiology, Medical University of Lublin, Lublin, Poland

I. Rozylo-Kalinowska, K. Orhan (eds.), *Imaging of the Temporomandibular Joint*, https://doi.org/10.1007/978-3-319-99468-0_9

Post-acoustic shadowing occurs when ultrasound beam is completely reflected off the outer surface of a structure, e.g. condyle or a very dense lesion, such as calcification. When ultrasound beam travels through a very low-density lesion such as a cyst, the liquid content does not reflect ultrasound; thus a bigger portion of the beam reaches tissues located below the fluid collection, and more echoes are generated behind the lesion. This appearance is called post-acoustic enhancement.

Feasibility of an ultrasound unit depends on the applied probes. In diagnostics of TMJ, high-frequency linear probes (preferably over 12 MHz) with a relatively small "footprint" are used as they offer high resolution of image with a relatively low penetration depth which is sufficient in examinations of these superficially located joints. Intraoral probes are useful in imaging of masticatory muscles, instead of infrequent finger probes or finger-tip probes, an intraoperative "hockey stick" probe can be successfully applied.

Doppler ultrasound is based on the physical phenomenon called Doppler phenomenon which is change in frequency of a wave reflected off a moving object, and in case of medical imaging, movement of blood cells in blood vessels is registered. Blood cells flowing towards the probe reflect the acoustic wave increasing its frequency. On the contrary, when blood cells flow away from the probe, the frequency of wave coming back to the transducer decreases. In both situations difference between the frequency of wave emitted by probe and the frequency of returning wave is proportional to velocity of the moving object.

Doppler scanning ultrasound includes continuous wave examination (to study blood flow in big vessels without their identification), pulse wave Doppler (to measure velocity of blood flow), colour-coded Doppler (demonstrating direction of blood flow—inflowing towards the probe is shown as shades of red and outflowing as shades of blue), power-Doppler (enhancement of signal allowing demonstration of small blood vessels but without presentation of blood flow direction), Duplex Doppler (B-mode and spectral Doppler simultaneously applied) and Triplex Doppler (spectral and colour Doppler combined to allow localisation of blood vessel during blood flow measurement) [1].

US elastography offers a possibility of evaluation of stiffness of tissues on the basis of analysis of change of their shape when an external stimulus is applied such as exerted pressure or emission of an acoustic impulse propagated within tissues as the so-called shear wave. A coloured map represents areas with higher and lower stiffness in a qualitative manner. In some US machines, quantitative assessment is possible in the form of Young's modulus values given in kilopascals [2].

US scanning of TMJ is performed in a patient lying on a special examination bed or sitting upright. A water-soluble gel is generously administered on patient's skin within the region of interest in order to eliminate air bubbles from between the skin and the probe since ultrasound is strongly reflected by gases [3, 4]. The transducer is then placed parallel to the Frankfurt horizontal plane and at 60°–70° to the plane, parallel to the ramus of mandible, both in open and closed mouth position (Fig. 9.1a–d). However, it must be remembered that since US is a dynamic real-time examination, so during the study, the probe has to be moved gently over the studied area. Therefore the US images are never truly transverse or sagittal [5]. This obstacle can be overcome by using a 3-D US probe [6, 7]. During the examination multiple

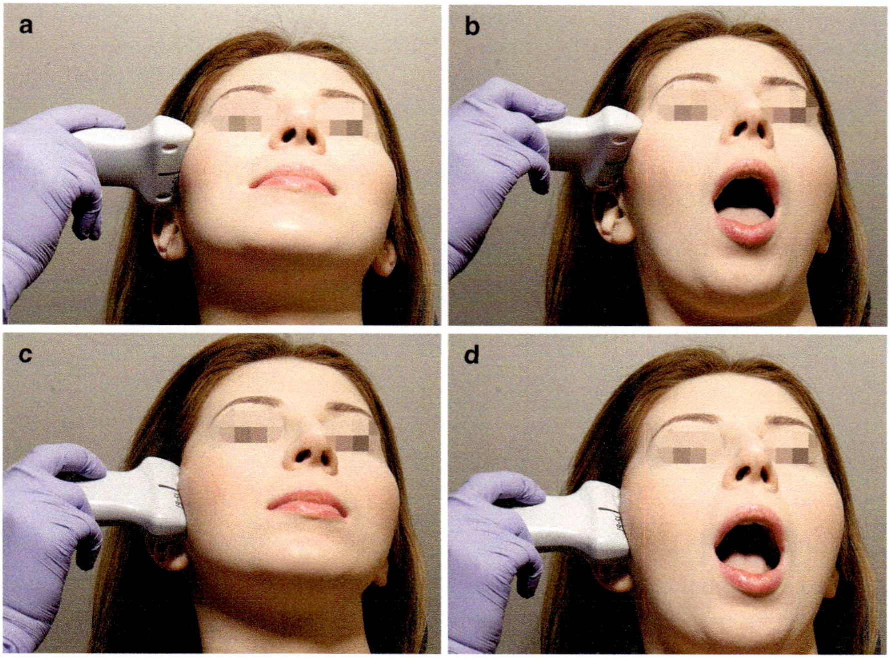

Fig. 9.1 Ultrasound examination of the right TMJ. The transducer is placed parallel to the Frankfurt horizontal plane in closed (**a**) and open (**b**) mouth position as well as at 60°–70° to the plane, parallel to the ramus of mandible, both in closed (**c**) and open (**d**) mouth position

images are captured, and condyle movement range can be registered, as well. Complementary US scanning of masticatory muscles may be performed.

9.2 Advantages and Disadvantages of Ultrasonography

Advantages of ultrasonography include availability, no harmful effects (even in pregnant females and children), high image resolution, real-time imaging and a relatively low cost when compared with other diagnostic imaging methods such as CT and MRI [4, 5, 8].

One of the disadvantages of US is high dependency on operator's skills and experience [9]. Another disadvantage of utmost importance in diagnostics of TMJ is that it is not possible to demonstrate structures located behind intact bone surface, as the beam is fully reflected off dense the outer cortex. Therefore only a part of TMJ is accessible for US—the articular capsule, the disc and cortex of laterosuperior aspect of the condyle are visible [10]. Another limitation of TMJ US imaging is osteoarthritis with reduction of joint space width and formation of bony spurs further decreasing area available for penetration with an ultrasound beam [3]. All this discourages some operators from using US in this joint at all, and MR is preferred for that purpose [11].

Reported sensitivity, specificity and accuracy values of ultrasound vary in broad ranges, e.g. according to Melis et al. [12], sensitivity of US in assessment of disc displacement falls between 13% and 100%, specificity from 62% to 100% and accuracy in the range of 51.8–100%. In a meta-analysis by Dong et al. [13] comprising 1096 subjects from 11 studies, for anterior disc displacement with reduction, the pooled sensitivity and specificity were 83% and 85%, respectively, while for the anterior disc displacement without reduction, the weighted sensitivity and specificity values were 72% and 90%, respectively.

9.3 Indications and Contraindications for Ultrasound

Within the head and neck, including area of the TMJ and masticatory muscles, US is used among others in diagnostic imaging of lymphadenopathy, salivary gland lesions, inflammations, cysts and tumours and masseter hypertrophy.

As far as TMJ is concerned, the following applications were described:

- Joint effusion [14, 15].
- Internal derangement [16] and disc displacement, mainly anterior with and without reduction [7, 10, 17–22]; no studies reported data on lateral or posterior disc displacement [23].
- Osteoarthrosis including condylar erosion [6, 9, 24, 25].
- Rheumatoid, psoriatic and juvenile idiopathic arthritis with TMJ involvement as well as polyarthritis [15, 19, 20, 26–29, 30, 31].
- Joint function basing on condylar translation range [32–37].
- Condylar movement using Duplex Doppler [1].
- Intrauterine TMJ dislocation [38].
- Guidance in fine needle aspiration cytology (FNAC).
- Guidance for TMJ arthrocentesis [39].
- Guidance in TMJ injections, e.g. with steroids.

There are neither contraindications for ultrasound scanning nor special patient preparation required. Use of a gel stand-off pad may be necessary in case of very superficially located lesions, but a thick layer of gel with limited pressure on the probe may be applied in its stead [8].

9.4 Normal Anatomy of TMJ in Ultrasound

Normal anatomy of TMJ in ultrasound is presented in Figs. 9.2, 9.3, 9.4, 9.5, 9.6 and 9.7.

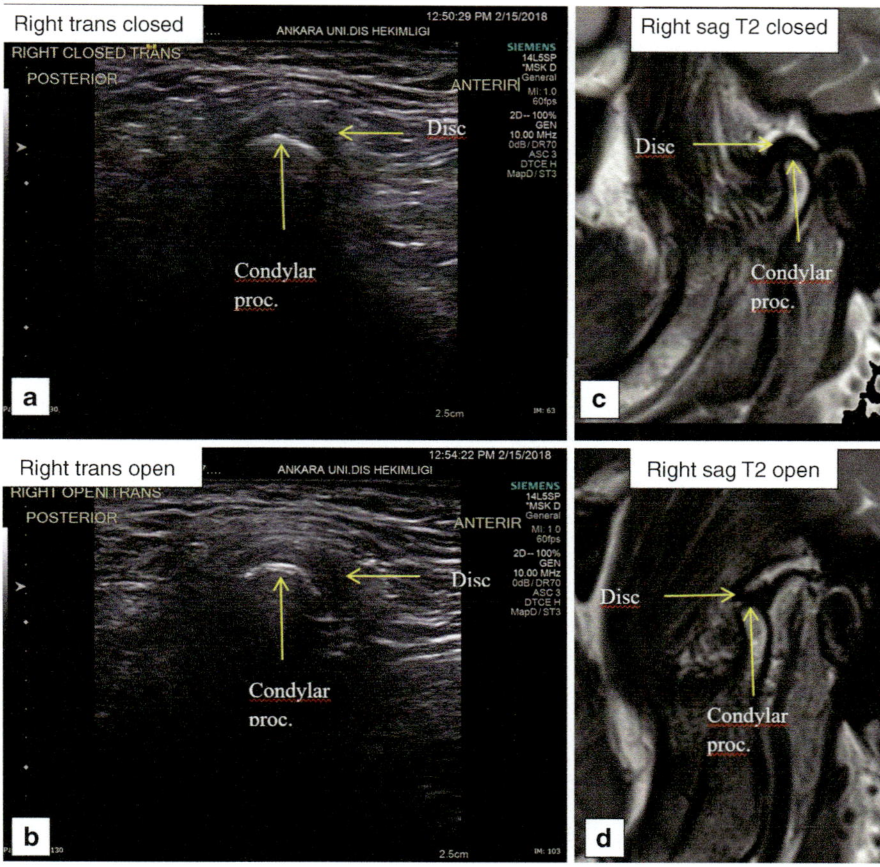

Fig. 9.2 (**a**) Closed mouth; (**b**) open mouth, US transducer placed transversally and MRI (sagittal plane); (**c**) closed mouth; (**d**) open mouth images showing right TMJ with normal disc position

9.5 Ultrasonography-Guided Invasive Procedures

9.5.1 Fine Needle Aspiration Biopsy

The golden standard for diagnosis of pathologies concerning the temporomandibular joint is histopathological evaluation. In literature, fine needle aspiration biopsy is a proven method for obtaining pathological specimen and continuing histopathological evaluation.

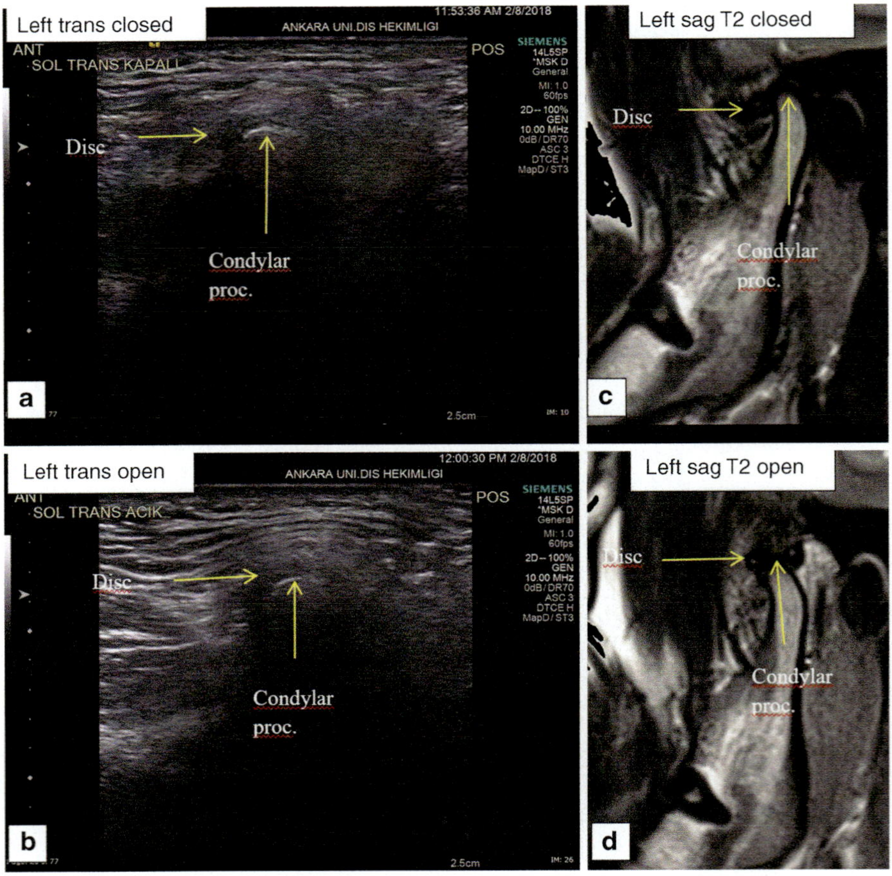

Fig. 9.3 (**a**) Closed mouth; (**b**) open mouth, US (transducer placed transversally) and MRI (sagittal plane); (**c**) closed mouth; (**d**) open mouth images showing left TMJ with disc displacement with reduction

Ultrasonography guidance while reaching the pathology is one of the primary methods that will ensure results that are more accurate. Features like easy access to this technology, ease of use for the radiologist, being a non-invasive procedure and easily tolerated by the patients have made this technology a routine while performing fine needle aspiration biopsy.

Ultrasonography-guided fine needle aspiration biopsy is a minor invasive procedure which can take place in an ambulatory setting; the patient can be discharged the same day and go back to daily routine.

9.5.2 Ultrasonography-Guided Fine Needle Aspiration Biopsy

Being an invasive procedure, fine needle aspiration biopsy should be planned under sterile conditions. Preparations should be made and checked before biopsy. As a

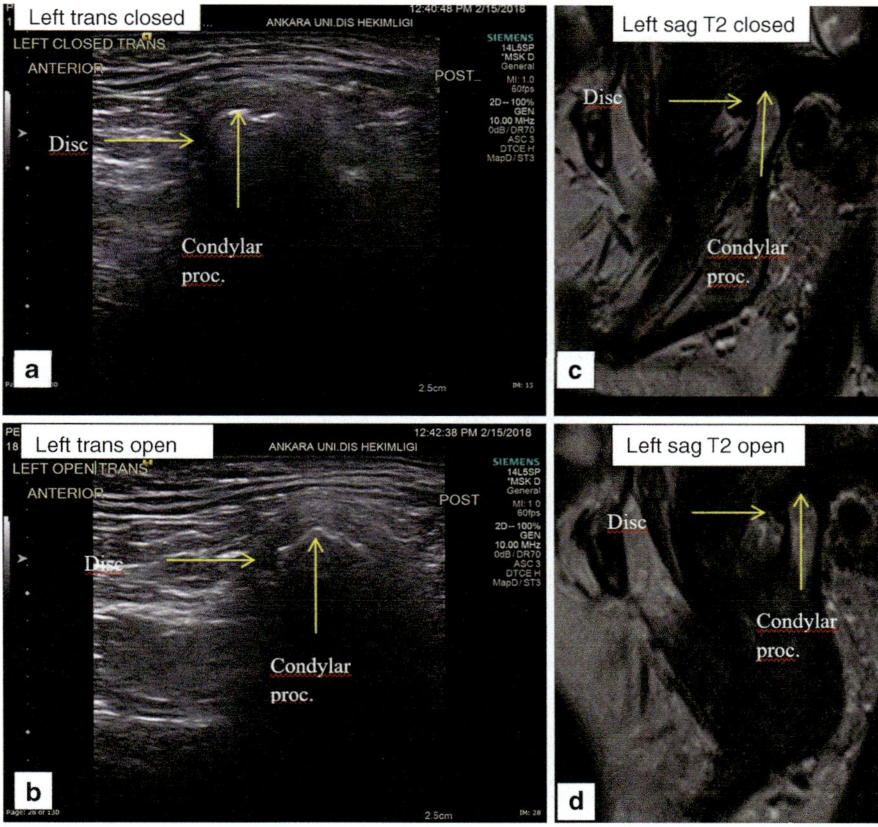

Fig. 9.4 (**a**) Closed mouth; (**b**) open mouth, US (transducer placed transversally) and MRI (sagittal plane); (**c**) closed mouth; (**d**) open mouth images showing left TMJ with disc displacement without reduction

minimal invasive method, ultrasonography-guided fine needle aspiration biopsy could be realized with only one operator, while two operators are commonly preferred. One operator performs the ultrasonography and guides the procedure, while the other performs biopsy.

Before passing on to the procedure, the anatomy of the region and pathology should be thoroughly examined with ultrasound by both the operators. This will give both the operators advantage before performing the biopsy. The area should then be wiped from the ultrasonography gel.

Sterile gloves should be worn, and the region should be cleaned with skin disinfectants to achieve antisepsis. A local anaesthetic solution containing 1:100.000 epinephrine should be carefully and slowly injected inside the temporomandibular joint capsule using a 27-gauge needle. This careful and slow application of local anaesthetic should prevent any discomfort during the procedure.

After local anaesthetic injection, the region must be palpated and 'manually sensed'. During palpation of the region, the patient should be instructed to slowly

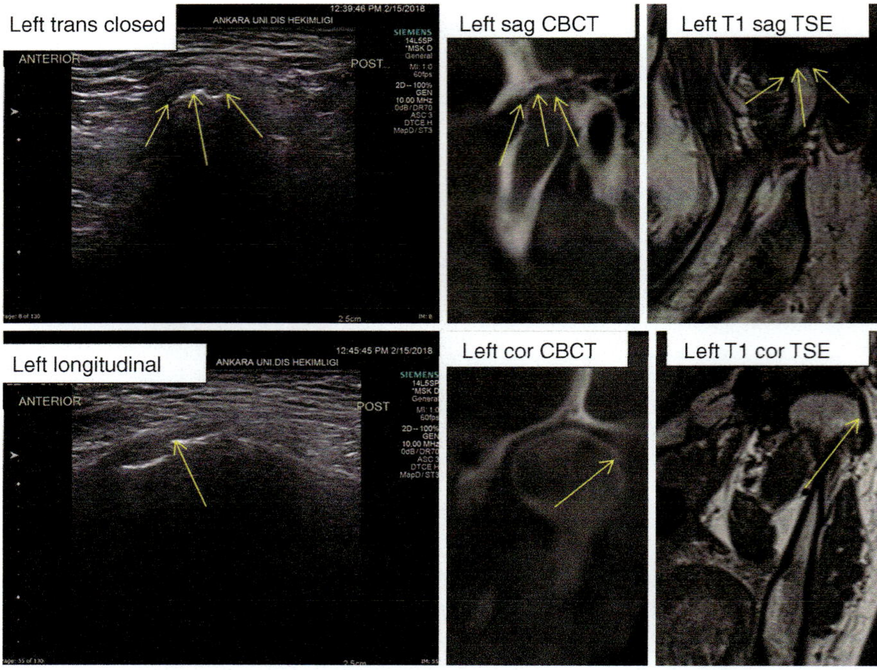

Fig. 9.5 Closed mouth US, CBCT and MRI of the same patient with degenerative bone changes of left TMJ

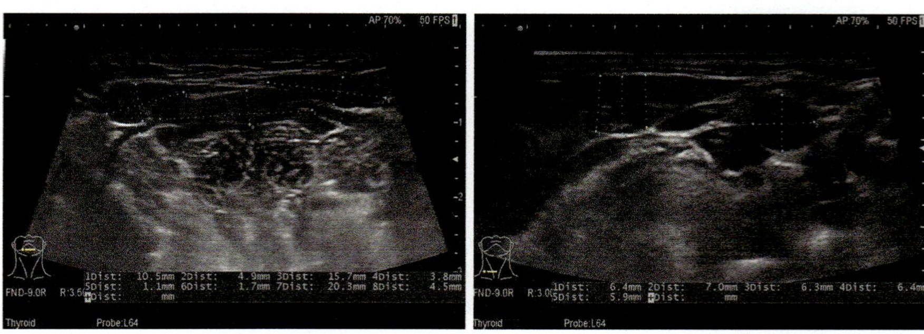

Fig. 9.6 USG showing the measurements for anterior belly of digastric, geniohyoid complex, mylohyoid thickness as well as sternocleidomastoid muscle

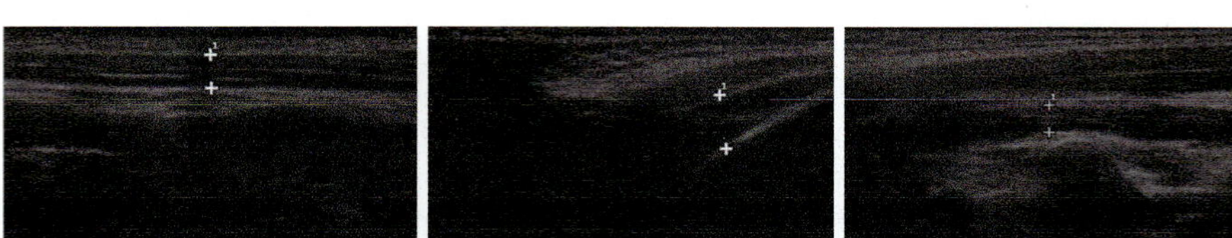

Fig. 9.7 USG showing the measurements for posterior belly of digastric muscle, mylohyoid thickness as well as sternocleidomastoid muscle

open and close the jaws. This motion will be helpful for detecting the zygomatic arch and mandibular condyle.

To identify the entrance point of the needle, a soft ruler and dermal pen can be used. The ruler should be directed from the outer cantus of the eye to the tip of the outer ear tragus. On this imaginary line, a mark should be made 10 mm away anteriorly from the tragus tip. Another mark should be made on a second imaginary line parallel to the first one just 2 mm below the first mark. This second mark will be entrance point of the needle. There will be approximately 25 mm from the skin mark to the temporomandibular joint.

A 23- or 27-gauge needle should be preferred. To increase the joint space, patient should be instructed to open the jaws widely. The radiologist should then position the ultrasonography probe anterior to the entrance point. This settlement will ensure a comfortable procedure for the operator performing the biopsy. After visualization of the temporomandibular joint structures and associative pathology, the needle should be inserted from the specified mark with the bevel facing the temporomandibular joint. After some advancement, the tip of the needle should be recognized through ultrasonography. The needle should be then advanced into the structures in a posterior and superior route, into the pathology (Fig. 9.8).

Coordination between the two operators is essential during this phase. The ultrasonography operator should help the other operator channel the needle in the correct direction. After access to the pathology, the needle should be advanced to the centre of the lesion. Under mild vacuum applied with the plunger biopsy, specimen should be obtained with light forward-backward movements of the needle. The needle should then be removed while mild vacuum continues, and the specimen should be spread on a lamella. The specimen should then be sent for histopathological evaluation.

Following biopsy, the area should be closed with a sticking plaster with slight pressure, to prevent haematoma formation. Intermittent cold-pack applications and anti-inflammatory medication will be useful during the postoperative period.

9.5.3 Core Biopsy

Core biopsy is an invasive method, in need of special equipment. While soft tissue core biopsy needles measure around 1 mm, hard tissue core biopsy needles may

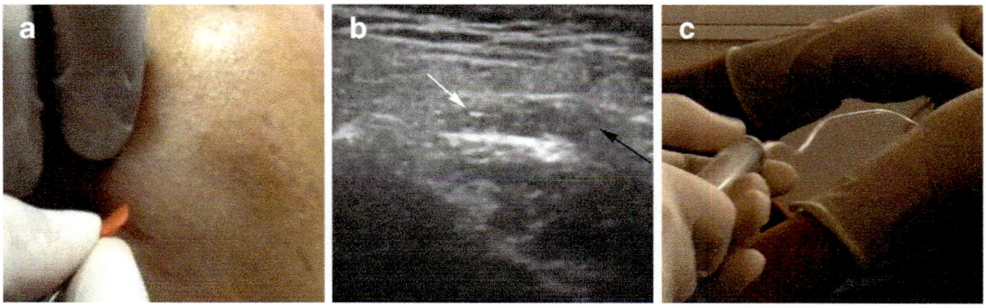

Fig. 9.8 Fine needle aspiration biopsy of TMJ mass, (**a**) the entrance of needle, (**b**) USG image showing needle (white arrow) and the mass (black arrow), (**c**) two hands technique

measure up to 2 mm diameter. The core biopsy needle, produced especially for this procedure, enters the lesion while its blade is closed; when it is triggered, the blade opens and closes in high speed, obtaining the specimen. The specimen with an approximate length of 1 cm is then extracted. This large tissue is very valuable for a correct histopathological diagnosis. Thus, the most important advantage of core biopsy is that chance of accurate histopathological diagnosis is higher and additional biopsy procedures are needed less. Nevertheless, haemorrhage may occur more frequently during this procedure.

9.5.4 Ultrasonography-Guided Core Biopsy

Preoperative preparation and technique are similar to those of fine needle aspiration biopsy. However postoperative complications such as pain and oedema will be more excessive since wider needles are used, the entrance port is larger and larger amount of tissue is incised.

Core biopsy under ultrasonography guidance will reduce the reliability of the procedure, lower the need for additional biopsies and shorten operation time while reducing patient comfort.

9.5.5 Intra-articular Sodium Hyaluronate Injection

Sodium hyaluronate is a material similar to the synovial fluid produced in the temporomandibular joint. It serves as a lubricant and absorber of traumas. It is commonly used to treat temporomandibular joint osteoarthritis. It is an agent effective in decreasing temporomandibular joint pain associated with intra-articular derangements unresponsive to conservative treatments.

9.5.6 Ultrasonography-Guided Sodium Hyaluronate Injection

Preoperative preparation and technique are similar to those of fine needle aspiration biopsy. The procedure should be planned under sterile conditions. Preparations should be made and checked before biopsy. As a minimal invasive method, ultrasonography-guided fine needle aspiration biopsy could be realized with only one operator, while two operators are commonly preferred.

Before passing on to the procedure, the anatomy of the region and pathology should be thoroughly examined with ultrasound by both the operators. This will give both the operators advantage before performing the procedure. The area should then be wiped from the ultrasonography gel.

Sterile gloves should be worn, and the region should be cleaned with skin disinfectants to achieve antisepsis. A local anaesthetic solution containing 1:100.000 epinephrine should be carefully and slowly injected inside the temporomandibular joint capsule using a 27-gauge needle. This careful and slow application of local anaesthetic should prevent any discomfort during the procedure.

After local anaesthetic injection, the region must be palpated and 'manually sensed'. During palpation of the region, the patient should be instructed to slowly open and close the jaws. This motion will be helpful for detecting the zygomatic arch and mandibular condyle.

To identify the entrance point of the needle, a soft ruler and dermal pen can be used. The ruler should be directed from the outer cantus of the eye to the tip of the outer ear tragus. On this imaginary line, a mark should be made 10 mm away anteriorly from the tragus tip. Another mark should be made on a second imaginary line parallel to the first one just 2 mm below the first mark. This second mark will be entrance point of the needle. There will be approximately 25 mm from the skin mark to the temporomandibular joint.

To increase the joint space, patient should be instructed to open the jaws widely. The radiologist should then position the ultrasonography probe anterior to the entrance point. This settlement will ensure a comfortable procedure for the operator performing the biopsy. After visualization of the temporomandibular joint structures and associative pathology, the needle should be inserted from the specified mark with the bevel facing the temporomandibular joint. After some advancement, the tip of the needle should be recognized through ultrasonography. The needle should be then advanced into the structures in a posterior and superior route, into the pathology. Sodium hyaluronate preparations are usually present in ready-to-use syringes. If such syringes are used, the presented needles should be used. If no needle is present, a 19-gauge needle can be used (Fig. 9.9).

Coordination between the two operators is essential during this phase. The ultrasonography operator should help the other operator channel the needle in the correct direction. After access to the upper temporomandibular joint space, the preparation should be slowly injected. A 1 ml volume is proved efficient for small joints such as the temporomandibular joint; repetitive applications can be made (Fig. 9.10).

Following injection, the area should be closed with a sticking plaster with slight pressure, to prevent haematoma formation. Intermittent cold-pack applications and anti-inflammatory medication will be useful during the postoperative period. Temporary pain or swelling of the affected joint may occur after injection.

9.5.7 Arthrocentesis

Arthrocentesis is an invasive procedure commonly preferred in conditions of internal derangements of the temporomandibular joint, opening intra-articular cohesions, painful clicking not responsive to conservative treatments and disc displacement without reduction. It is an ambulatory service, which can be applied in hospital or office settings, under general anaesthesia, sedation or local anaesthesia.

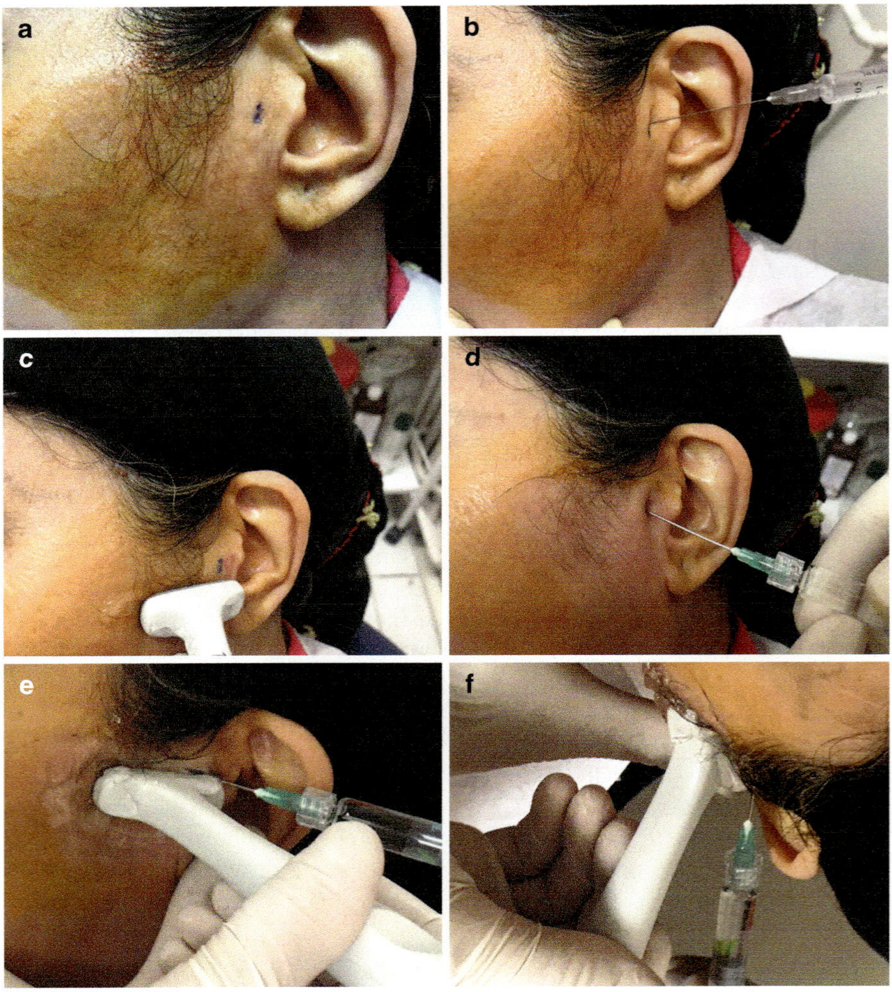

Fig. 9.9 Intra-articular sodium hyaluronate injection procedure, (**a**) identifying the entrance of the needle, (**b**) local anaesthesia application, (**c**) USGS examination before entrance, (**d**) the entrance of the needle, (**e**, **f**) US-guided intervention

The aim of this invasive procedure is to reduce inflammation by washing out demolished tissue products present in the articular joint. This washing out procedure can be performed with sterile solutions such as sodium chloride or lactated Ringer's solution. During the operation, two needles are used; while one needle is used to inject the preferred solution into the articular joint, the other needle serves as an exit port for the solution along with tissue demolition products. Afterwards, decrease in pain, increase in maximum mouth opening and long-term relief of symptoms are expected.

This procedure is commonly performed 'blind' using anatomic landmarks.

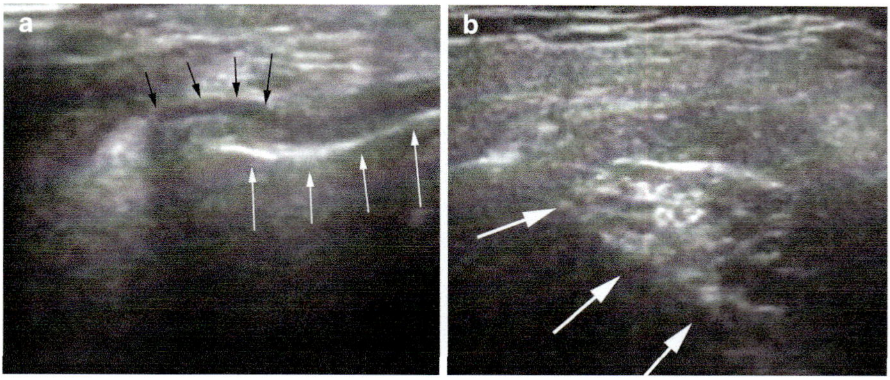

Fig. 9.10 (**a**) USG image before intra-articular sodium hyaluronate injection, black arrows show TMJ disc; white arrows show the needle. Note that the needle is entering lower compartment of the TMJ; (**b**) USG image shows the hyperechoic areas after injection

9.5.8 Ultrasonography-Guided Arthrocentesis

Ultrasonography-guided arthrocentesis essentially leans on the same principals with those of fine needle aspiration biopsy. The technique starts off with the radiologists and surgeons detailed ultrasonography evaluation of the related temporomandibular joint.

Sterile gloves should be worn, and the region should be cleaned with skin disinfectants to achieve antisepsis. A local anaesthetic solution containing 1:100.000 epinephrine should be carefully and slowly injected inside the temporomandibular joint capsule using a 27-gauge needle. This careful and slow application of local anaesthetic should prevent any discomfort during the procedure.

After local anaesthetic injection, the region must be palpated and 'manually sensed'. During palpation of the region, the patient should be instructed to slowly open and close the jaws. This motion will be helpful for detecting the zygomatic arch and mandibular condyle.

To identify the entrance point of the needle, a soft ruler and dermal pen can be used. The ruler should be directed from the outer cantus of the eye to the tip of the outer ear tragus. On this imaginary line, the first mark should be made 10 mm away anteriorly from the tragus tip and just 2 mm below on a second imaginary line parallel to the first one. This mark will be entrance point of the first needle. There will be approximately 25 mm from the skin mark to the temporomandibular joint. The second mark should be made 20 mm away anteriorly from the tragus tip and just 10 mm below on a second imaginary line parallel to the first one. This mark will be entrance point of the second needle.

Two 19-gauge needles should be preferred. To increase the joint space, patient should be instructed to open the jaws widely. The radiologist should then position the ultrasonography probe anterior to the entrance point. This settlement will ensure a comfortable procedure for the operator performing the biopsy. After visualization of the temporomandibular joint structures, the first needle should be inserted from the specified mark with the bevel facing the temporomandibular joint. After some advancement, the tip of the needle should be recognized through ultrasonography. The needles should be then advanced into the structures in a posterior and superior route, into the upper temporomandibular joint space.

Coordination between the two operators is essential during this phase. The ultrasonography operator should help the other operator channel the needle in the correct direction. After correct settlement of the needles, 300 ml of preferred solution should be slowly injected while exiting from the second needle. Thus the 'washing out' of the joint space is verified.

Following the procedure, the area should be closed with a sticking plaster with slight pressure, to prevent haematoma formation. Intermittent cold-pack applications and anti-inflammatory medication will be useful during the postoperative period.

9.5.9 Intramasseteric Botulinum Toxin Injections for Bruxism

The botulinum toxin (BT) is a neurotoxin produced by the *Clostridium botulinum* bacteria. When this toxin is injected into the muscles, it prevents neurotransmission, and the muscle fails to contract. It is commonly used in facial aesthetics to prevent wrinkles. In our healthcare area, it is commonly used to prevent bruxism, by affecting the masseter muscle. This procedure is a simple and fast ambulatory application. The effect of the BT is temporary; thus repetitive applications are required.

The masseter is a bulky muscle, and the needle must deliver the BT deeper into the muscle to achieve optimal effect. The muscle is covered with a dense fascial layer, so if the injections are made superficially under this layer, the optimal effect will not be achieved. The needle must penetrate this fascia and deliver the BT within the body of the muscle. While this procedure is commonly applied 'blinded', ultrasonography-guided applications ensure the BT is injected in the correct depth; it increases the effect of the BT and lowers the number of repetitions (Figs. 9.11 and 9.12).

9.5.10 Ultrasonography-Guided Intramasseteric Botulinum Toxin Injections

Usually with 20 units per side, the desired decrease on bruxism is acquired, although additional units may need to be administered to achieve the optimal effect. According to the achieved response to this initial treatment, the operator will be able to designate the needed dosage better with future treatments, and usually with 20 units per side, the desired decrease on bruxism is acquired; additional units may need to be administered to achieve the optimal effect.

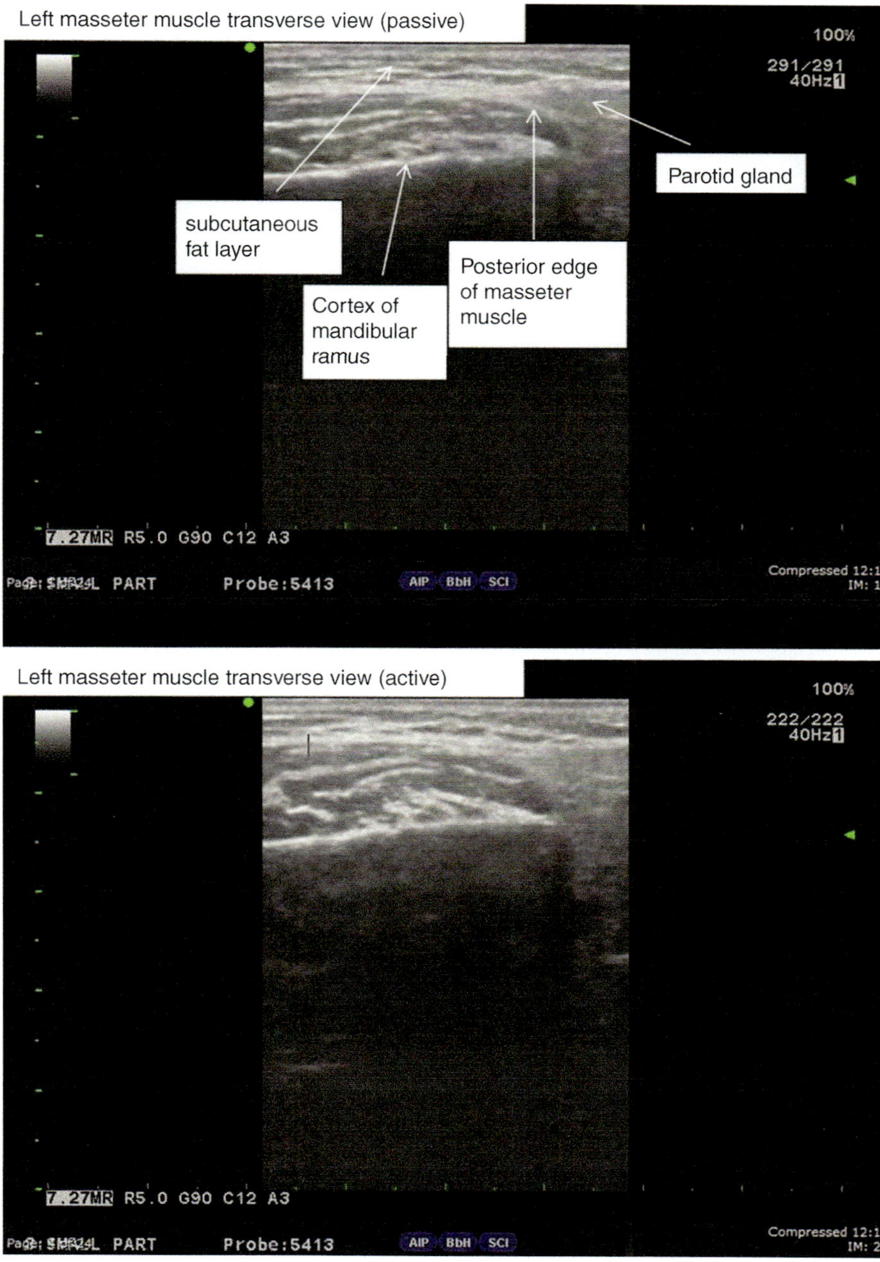

Fig. 9.11 Left masseter muscle transverse view passive and active USG images

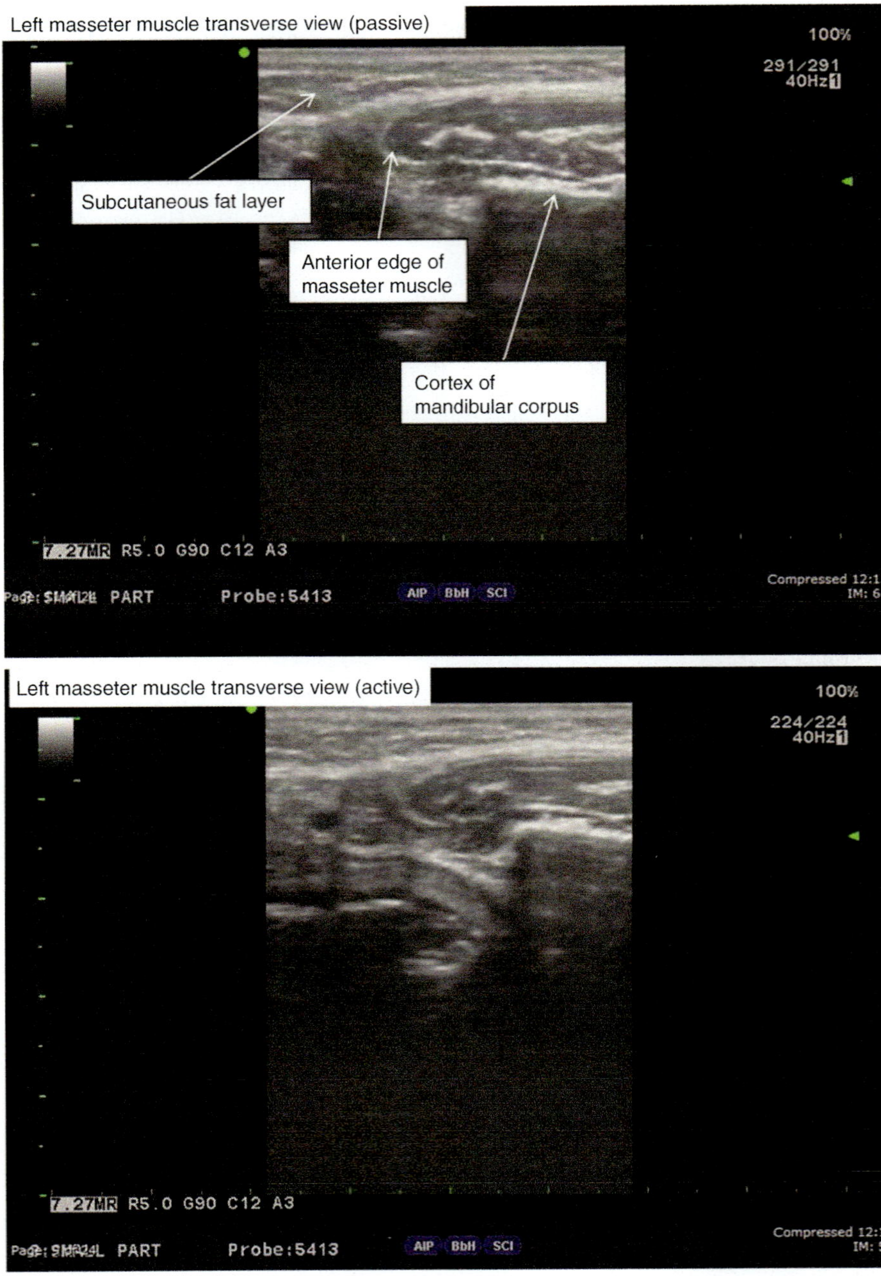

Fig. 9.12 Left masseter muscle transverse view passive and active USG images

Being an invasive procedure, intramasseteric botulinum toxin injections should be planned under sterile conditions. Preparations should be made and checked before biopsy.

Before passing on to the procedure, the anatomy of the region and the masseteric muscle should be thoroughly examined with ultrasound by both the operators. This will give both the operators advantage before performing the injections. The area should then be wiped from the ultrasonography gel.

The masseter muscle should be palpated, while the patient should be instructed to relax and bear down the jaw to determine the muscle. A line from the corner of the mouth up to the ear tragus should be traced with a dermal pen. Additionally, the anterior and posterior borders are designated and marked with a line. This defined area should not be crossed during injections. This way the risorius muscle and the zygomaticus major muscles will be protected. Protecting these muscles is important in protecting the patients smile (Figs. 9.13, 9.14, and 9.15).

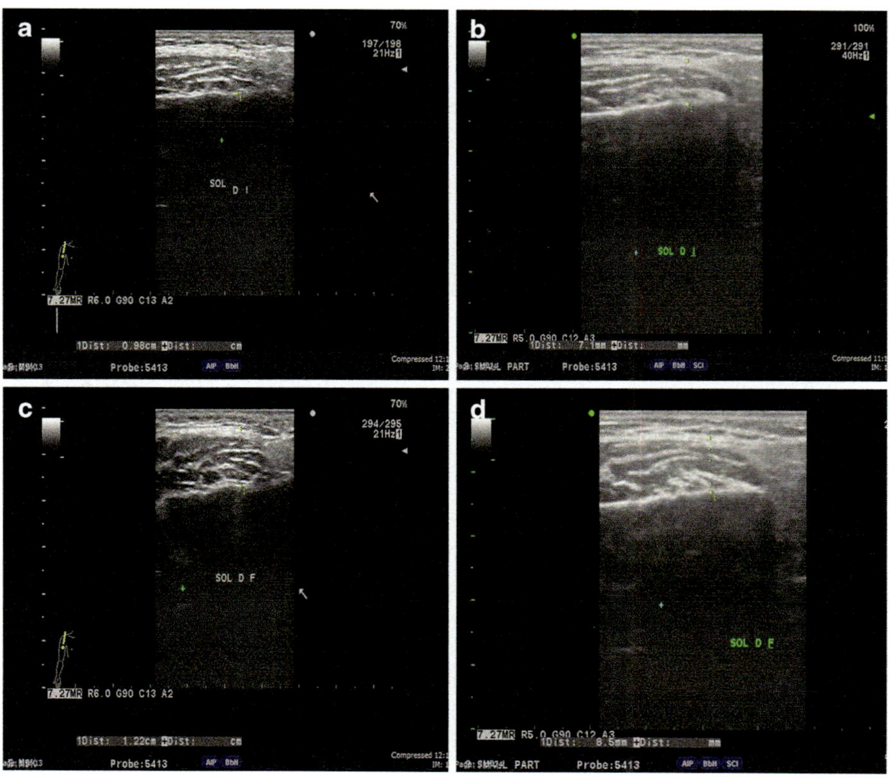

Fig. 9.13 USG images show (**a**) thickness of distal edge of left masseter muscle (passive before injection), (**b**) thickness of distal edge of left masseter muscle (passive 2 months after injection), (**c**) thickness of distal edge of left masseter muscle (active before injection), (**d**) thickness of distal edge of left masseter muscle (active 2 months after injection)

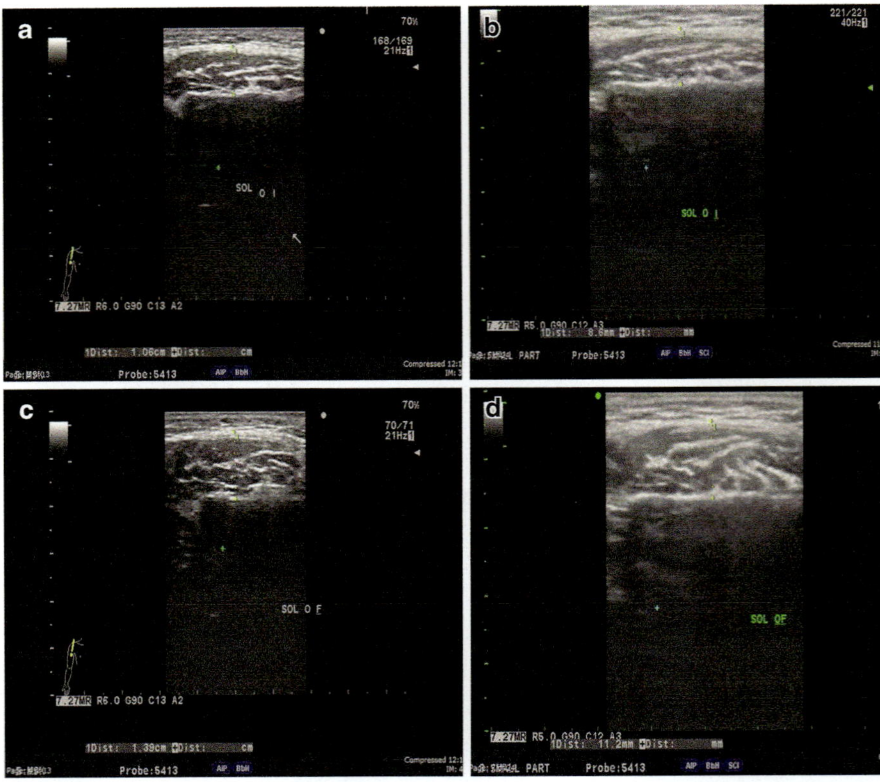

Fig. 9.14 USG images show (**a**) thickness of middle portion of left masseter muscle (passive 2 months after injection), (**b**) thickness of middle portion of left masseter muscle (passive before injection), (**c**) thickness of middle portion of left masseter muscle (active 2 months after injection), (**d**) thickness of middle portion of left masseter muscle (active before injection)

Sterile gloves should be worn, and the region should be cleaned with skin disinfectants to achieve antisepsis. The radiologist should then position the ultrasonography probe anterior to the anterior border. This settlement will ensure a comfortable procedure for the operator performing the injection. After visualization of the masseter muscle, the needle should be inserted, and after some advancement, the tip of the needle should be recognized through ultrasonography. The needle should be then advanced into the structures to advance into the deeper tissues of the masseter muscle. After appropriate depth is achieved, injection should be made. Usually 3–4 injection points will be sufficient (Fig. 9.16).

For the first 2–3 h after treatment, cold-pack application is recommended. The full effect may be noticed after 3–4 days or may even take longer. The results may last from 3 to 4 months on average but sometimes up to 6 months. After that, the patient will start to experience bruxism-related pain, and reapplication will be required (Fig. 9.17).

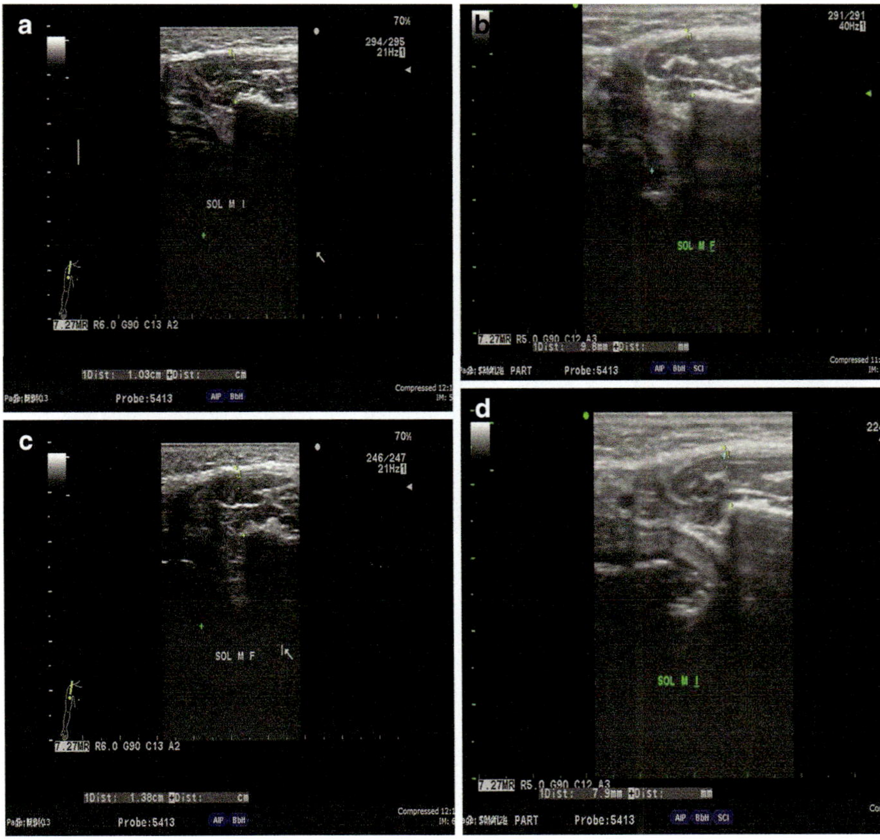

Fig. 9.15 USG images show (**a**) thickness of mesial edge of left masseter muscle (passive 2 months after injection), (**b**) thickness of mesial edge of left masseter muscle (passive before injection), (**c**) thickness of mesial edge of left masseter muscle (active 2 months after injection), (**d**) thickness of mesial edge of left masseter muscle (active before injection)

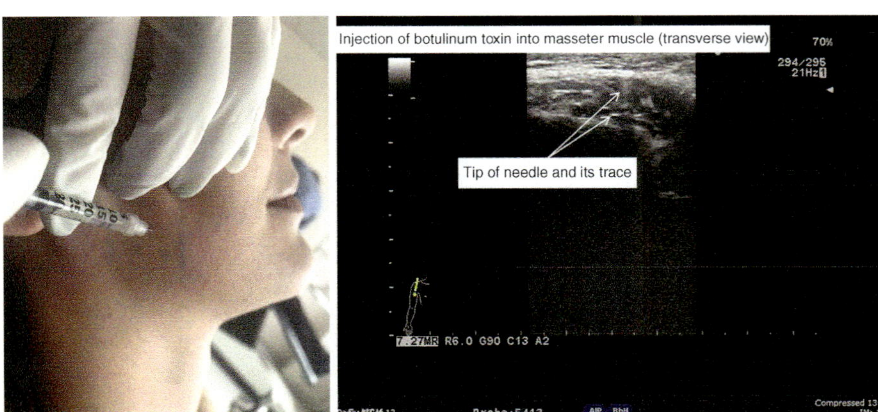

Fig. 9.16 Lateral photo showing the application and USG image after injection of botulinum toxin into masseter muscle (transverse view)

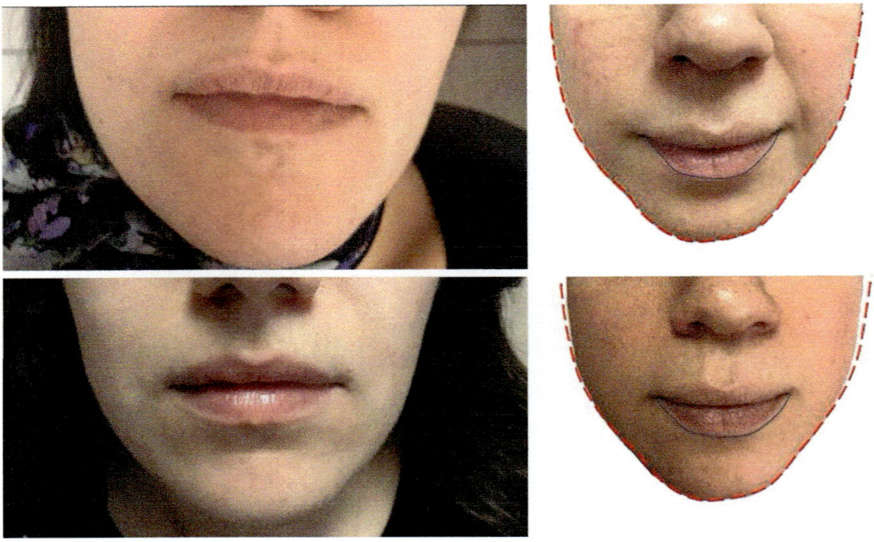

Fig. 9.17 Profile photos show pre- and postinjection of botulinum toxin with decreased masseter muscle hypertrophy

Acknowledgements The authors would like to thank to Associate Prof. Dr. Nilsun Bagis, Dr. Poyzan Bozkurt, Dr. Dilek Yılmaz, Dr. Katarzyna Portka and Dr. Leszek Szalewski for their contributions to the chapter.

References

1. Stagnitti A, Marini A, Impara L, Drudi FM, Lo Mele L, Odoardi GL. Duplex Doppler ultrasound study of the temporomandibular joint. J Ultrasound. 2012;15(2):111–4.
2. Yuan S, Magarik M, Lex AM, Fleischer AC. Clinical applications of sonoelastography. Expert Rev Med Devices. 2016;13(12):1107–17.
3. Katzberg RW. Is ultrasonography of the temporomandibular joint ready for prime time? Is there a "window" of opportunity? J Oral Maxillofac Surg. 2012;70(6):1310–4.
4. Whaites E, Drage N. Essentials of dental radiography and radiology. 5th ed. London: Churchill Livingstone; 2013.
5. Kundu H, Basavaraj P, Kote S, Singla A, Singh S. Assessment of TMJ disorders using ultrasonography as a diagnostic tool: a review. J Clin Diagn Res. 2013;7(12):3116–20.
6. Landes CA, Goral W, Mack MG, Sader R. 3-D sonography for diagnosis of osteoarthrosis and disk degeneration of the temporomandibular joint, compared with MRI. Ultrasound Med Biol. 2006;32(5):627–32.
7. Landes CA, Goral WA, Sader R, Mack MG. Three-dimensional versus two-dimensional sonography of the temporomandibular joint in comparison to MRI. Eur J Radiol. 2007;61(2):235–44.
8. Ahuja A, Evans R. Practical head and neck ultrasound. Cambridge: Cambridge University Press; 2013.
9. Manfredini D, Guarda-Nardini L. Ultrasonography of the temporomandibular joint: a literature review. Int J Oral Maxillofac Surg. 2009;38(12):1229–36. https://doi.org/10.1016/j.ijom.2009.07.014.

10. Manfredini D, Tognini F, Melchiorre D, Zampa V, Bosco M. Ultrasound assessment of increased capsular width as a predictor of temporomandibular joint effusions. Dentomaxillofac Radiol. 2003;32:359–64.
11. Weiss PF, Arabshani B, Johnson A, Bilaniuk LT, Zarnow D, Cahill AM, Feudtner C, Cron RQ. High prevalence of temporomandibular joint arthritis at disease onset in children with juvenile idiopathic arthritis, as detected by magnetic resonance imaging but not by ultrasound. Arthritis Rheum. 2008;58(4):1189–96. https://doi.org/10.1002/art.23401.
12. Melis M, Secci S, Ceneviz C. Use of US for diagnosis of temporomandibular joint disorders: a review. Am J Dent. 2007;20:73–8.
13. Dong XY, He S, Zhu L, Dong TY, Pan SS, Tang LJ, Zhu ZF. The diagnostic value of high-resolution ultrasonography for the detection of anterior disc displacement of the temporomandibular joint: a meta-analysis employing the HSROC statistical model. Int J Oral Maxillofac Surg. 2015;44:852–8.
14. Bas B, Yılmaz N, Gökce E, Akan H. Ultrasound assessment of increased capsular width in temporomandibular joint internal derangements: relationship with joint pain and magnetic resonance grading of joint effusion. Oral Surg Oral Med Oral Pathol Oral Radiol Endod. 2011;112(1):112–7.
15. Tognini F, Manfredini D, Mechiorre D, Zampa V, Bosco M. Ultrasonographic vs magnetic resonance imaging findings of temporomandibular joint effusion. Minerva Stomatol. 2003;52:365–72.
16. Uysal S, Kansu H, Akhan O, Kansu O. Comparison of ultrasonography with magnetic resonance imaging in the diagnosis of temporomandibular joint internal derangements: a preliminary investigation. Oral Surg Oral Med Oral Pathol Oral Radiol Endod. 2002;94(1):115–21.
17. Brandlmaier I, Rudisch A, Bodner G, Bertram S, Emshoff R. Temporomandibular joint internal derangement: detection with 12.5 MHz ultrasonography. J Oral Rehabil. 2003;30(8):796–801.
18. Emshoff R, Bertram S, Rudisch A, Gassner R. The diagnostic value of ultrasonography to determine the temporomandibular joint disc position. Oral Surg Oral Med Oral Pathol Oral Radiol Endod. 1997;84:688–96.
19. Emshoff R, Jank S, Bertram S, Rudisch A, Bodner G. Disk displacement of the temporomandibular joint: sonography versus MR imaging. AJR Am J Roentgenol. 2002;178(6):1557–62.
20. Emshoff R, Jank S, Rudisch A, Walch C, Bodner G. Error patterns and observer variations in the high-resolution ultrasonography imaging evaluation of the disk position of the temporomandibular joint. Oral Surg Oral Med Oral Pathol Oral Radiol Endod. 2002;93(3):369–75.
21. Kaya K, Dulgeroğlu D, Unsal Daelialioğlu S, Babadağ M, Tacal T, Barlak A. Diagnostic value of ultrasonography in the evaluation of the temporomandibular joint anterior disk displacement. J Cranio-Maxillofac Surg. 2010;38:391–5.
22. Tognini F, Manfredini D, Mechiorre D, Bosco M. Comparison of ultrasonography and magnetic resonance imaging in the evaluation of the temporomandibular joint disc displacement. J Oral Rehabil. 2005;32:248–53.
23. Li C, Su N, Yang X, Sh Z, Li L. Ultrasonography for detection of disc displacement of temporomandibular joint: a systematic review and meta-analysis. J Oral Maxillofac Surg. 2012;70(6):1300–9.
24. Emshoff R, Brandlmaier I, Bodner G, Rudisch A. Condylar erosion and disc displacement: detection with high-resolution ultrasonography. J Oral Maxillofac Surg. 2003;61(8):877–81.
25. Rudisch A, Emshoff R, Maurer H, Kovacs P, Bodner G. Pathologic-sonographic correlation in temporomandibular joint pathology. Eur Radiol. 2006;16(8):1750–6.
26. Assaf AT, Kahl-Nieke B, Feddersen J, Habermann CR. Is high-resolution ultrasonography suitable for the detection of temporomandibular joint involvement in children with juvenile idiopathic arthritis? Dentomaxillofac Radiol. 2013;42(3):20110379.
27. Hechler BL, Phero JA, Van Mater H, Matthews NS. Ultrasound versus magnetic resonance imaging of the temporomandibular joint in juvenile idiopathic arthritis: a systematic review. Int J Oral Maxillofac Surg. 2018;47(1):83–9.

28. Jank S, Zangerl A, Kloss FR, Laimer K, Missmann M, Schroeder D, Mur E. High resolution ultrasound investigation of the temporomandibular joint in patients with chronic polyarthritis. Int J Oral Maxillofac Surg. 2011;40(1):45–9.
29. Melchiorre D, Calderazzi A, Maddali Bongi S, Cristofani R, Bazzichi L, Eligi C, Maresca M, Ciompi M. A comparison of ultrasonography and magnetic resonance imaging in the evaluation of temporomandibular joint involvement in rheumatoid arthritis and psoriatic arthritis. Rheumatology. 2003;42:673–6.
30. Hayashi D, Roemer FW, Katur A, Felson DT, Yang SO, Alomran F, Guermazi A. Imaging of synovitis in osteoarthritis: current status and outlook. Semin Arthritis Rheum. 2011;41(2):116–30.
31. Katzberg RW, Conway WF, Ackerman SJ, Gonzales TS, Kheyfits V, Cronan MS. Pilot study to show the feasibility of high-resolution sagittal ultrasound imaging of the temporomandibular joint. J Oral Maxillofac Surg. 2017;75(6):1151–62.
32. Cakir-Ozkan N, Sarikaya B, Erkorkmaz U, Aktürk Y. Ultrasonographic evaluation of disc displacement of the temporomandibular joint compared with magnetic resonance imaging. J Oral Maxillofac Surg. 2010;68(5):1075–80.
33. Gateno J, Miloro M, Hendler BH, Horrow M. The use of ultrasound to determine the position of the mandibular condyle. J Oral Maxillofac Surg. 1993;51:1081–6.
34. Jank S, Emshoff R, Norer B, Missmann M, Nicasi A, Strobl H, Gassner R, Rudisch A, Bodner G. Diagnostic quality of dynamic high-resolution ultrasonography of the TMJ—a pilot study. Int J Oral Maxillofac Surg. 2005;34(2):132–7.
35. Jank S, Rudisch A, Bodner G, Brandlmaier I, Gerhard S, Emshoff R. High-resolution ultrasonography of the TMJ: helpful diagnostic approach for patients with TMJ disorders? J Craniomaxillofac Surg. 2001;29(6):366–71.
36. Landes CA, Sader R. Sonographic evaluation of the ranges of condylar translation and of temporomandibular joint space as well as first comparison with symptomatic joints. J Craniomaxillofac Surg. 2007;35:374–81.
37. Landes CA, Walendzik H, Klein C. Sonography of the temporomandibular joint from 60 examinations and comparison with MRI and axiography. J Craniomaxillofac Surg. 2000;28(6):352–61.
38. Çil AS, Bozkurt M, Bozkurt DK. Intrauterine temporomandibular joint dislocation: prenatal sonographic evaluation. Clin Med Res. 2014;12(1–2):58–60.
39. Dayisoylu EH, Cifci E, Uckan S. Ultrasound-guided arthrocentesis of the temporomandibular joint. Br J Oral Maxillofac Surg. 2013;51(7):667–8.

Magnetic Resonance Imaging of TMJ

10

Kaan Orhan and Seçil Aksoy

10.1 Principle of Magnetic Resonance Imaging (MRI)

Magnetic resonance imaging (MRI) is a noninvasive imaging modality which is based on the nuclear magnetic resonance (NMR). Isıdor Isaac Rabi discovered and observed the NMR process. Rabi is the first to use the "nuclear magnetic resonance (NMR)" term by publishing an article entitled "A New Method of Measuring Nuclear Magnetic Moment." In 1944 Rabi was awarded with the Nobel Prize in Physics. Paul Lauterbur and Peter Mansfield used NMR to produce images of the body [1].

In MRI, short radio-frequency (RF) pulse is used to produce the excellent soft tissue images instead of the other imaging techniques using ionizing radiation. MRI machine has three basic components. Magnet is the biggest and most important component of the MRI machine, generating strong magnetic field to realign the body's atoms. Strength of the magnetic field is defined by the units of Tesla (T). There are five types of magnets used in MRI system including permanent magnets, electromagnets (solenoid), resistive magnets, superconducting magnets, and hybrid magnets [2]. In 95% of the MRI machine, superconducting magnets are used to generate the strong and highly homogeneous magnetic field. Superconducting magnet consists of a main coil wound up with niobium-titanium (NbTi) wires that have no resistance to the flow of an electrical current and creates a magnetic field of up to 18 T. The gradient system which is used for slice selection and spatial encoding of the signal produce an additional magnetic field in the direction of the x, y, and z axes. Radio-frequency systems compromise RF transmitter and a highly sensitive receiver that produce the RF waves, excite the nuclei, select the slices, apply the gradients, and are used in signal

K. Orhan (✉)
Department of Dentomaxillofacial Radiology, Ankara University, Faculty of Dentistry, Ankara, Turkey

S. Aksoy
Department of Dentomaxillofacial Radiology, Near East University, Faculty of Dentistry, Mersin, Turkey

I. Rozylo-Kalinowska, K. Orhan (eds.), *Imaging of the Temporomandibular Joint*, https://doi.org/10.1007/978-3-319-99468-0_10

acquisition [3]. Externally applied magnetic field effects the specific magnetic nuclei, such as hydrogen (^{1}H), carbon (^{13}C), fluorine (^{19}F), sodium (^{23}Na), oxygen (^{17}O), nitrogen (^{15}N), and phosphor (^{31}P). These atoms are called NMR active atoms [2].

10.1.1 Protons

All the materials in the world are made from atoms. Atoms are composed of particles called protons, neutrons, and electrons. Atomic nucleus consists of the protons and neutrons are called nucleons together. Total number of the protons and neutrons give the atomic mass number. Electrons move around the nucleus in orbitals. The protons and neutrons are attracted to each other by a nuclear force that holds them together in the nucleus at a certain distance [1]. Proton and neutrons revolve around themselves; therefore nuclear magnetism consists of the movement of these particles, and this magnetism is used to produce MR images. The number of neutrons relative to the protons determines the stability of the nucleus. Proton and neutrons both act as a small magnet with the south and north poles, and in equilibrium situations, net magnetic moment of the atom is zero. Nuclear magnetism is only seen in atoms with odd atomic mass number [2, 4–7].

The magnetism generated by nucleon particles is very weak, so to get an image, billions of atoms are needed. For this reason, hydrogen isotope, which has only a proton and no neutron in its nucleus, is the most suitable atom for MRI because it is the most abundant atom in human body, especially in water and fat. The high concentration of hydrogen nuclei in the human body, coupled with its high "relative MR sensitivity," makes the nucleus most suitable for high-resolution MRI [2, 8].

The magnetic moment of the particles in the nucleus spinning around itself is parallel to the rotation axis. This magnetic moment, created by the protons, is directly related to the rotation of the protons around themselves, and this spinning motion is called the spin or angular momentum. Magnetic moment is defined by the vector system which shows the power and direction of the magnetic field. Hydrogen atom which behaves like a small magnet and planet earth has a south and north pole and a magnetic vector (Fig. 10.1). The spin vectors of protons within the normal tissue are randomly oriented in all directions [7, 9, 10].

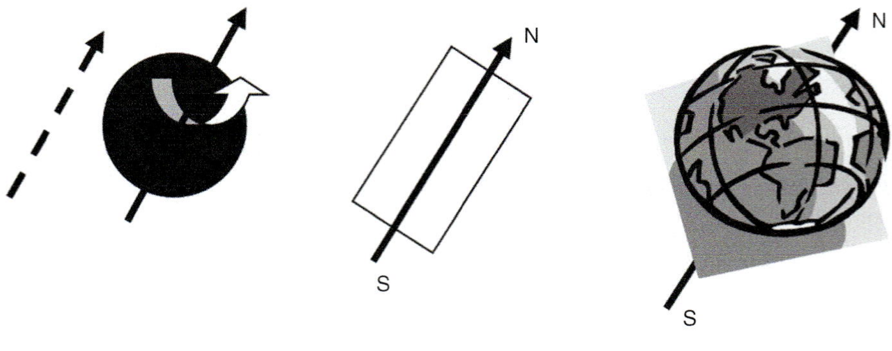

Fig. 10.1 Hydrogen atoms can be visualized as a small magnet or planet earth with a "north" and "south" pole

Once an external magnetic field (B_0) is applied, protons either align with (parallel/spin-up/low energy level) or against (anti parallel/spin-down/high energy level) it. However a slight excess of spins align parallel to the main magnetic field, causing net tissue magnetization. As the strength of the magnetic field increases, the number of parallel aligned atoms increases to [2–4, 7, 11].

10.1.2 Precession/Resonance

The magnetic vectors of protons do not align parallel or antiparallel exactly with the direction of the magnetic field (B_0). If an external magnetic field effects on a spinning protons and tries to change the orientation of the rotational axis, a second movement occurs, and protons begin to process at a rate known as the Larmor frequency around the lines of the applied magnetic field (Fig. 10.2); this process is called precession or oscillation [1–3, 7].

The frequency of the precession depends on the nature of the nucleus and on the strength of the external applied magnetic field. MRI scanners come in different field strength usually between 0.1 and 7 T with 1.5–3 T being the most common [7]. Larmor frequency (precession frequency or resonance frequency) is 63.86 MHz for the hydrogen atoms in a magnetic field of 1.5 T, and each magnetic nucleus has a special frequency in the same magnetic field [2, 5, 7]. Exposure of individual nuclei to RF pulse at the Larmor frequency causes nuclei in the lower energy state to reach into the higher energy state. Applications of the RF pulse cause the protons to change their magnetization alignment, and this newly formed magnetic vector is called transverse magnetization. Protons undergo a transition between the two energy states by the absorption of RF pulse, and after a while, they emitted the energy to return to their former position, which is called resonance [2, 3, 7].

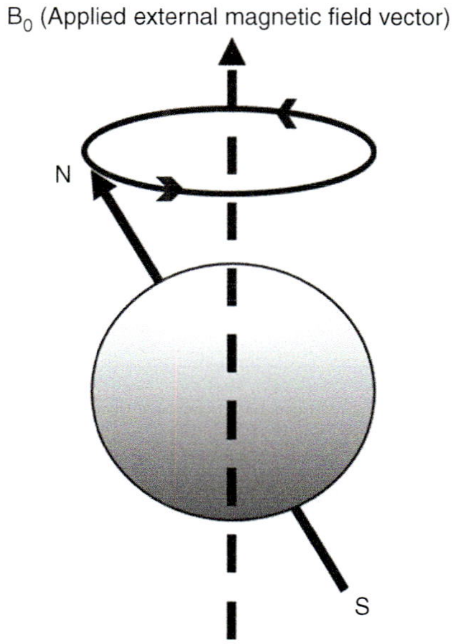

Fig. 10.2 Precession. Each spinning hydrogen nucleus precess around the direction of the external magnetic field, B_0, at the Larmor frequency

10.1.3 The Fundamentals of MRI

The transmission of the energy occurs in two ways within the tissue. These two independent processes reduce transverse magnetization and thus cause a return to the stable state present before excitation: spin-lattice interaction (longitudinal, thermal relaxation) and spin-spin interaction (transvers relaxation). These two processes cause T1 relaxation and T2 relaxation, respectively [3, 12]. The nuclei which precess around the direction of an applied magnetic field are out of phase initially. Application of the RF pulse causes the nuclei to precess in phase synchronously, and MR signal is formed, but it fades quickly, and nuclei become out of phase [6].

When a 90° RF pulse is applied to longitudinal magnetization, it tips down so that it creates transverse magnetization, an excited condition (Fig. 10.3).

RF pulse is usually applied in short pulses, each lasting microseconds, and when it is terminated, over a period of time, the nuclei return to its original longitudinal alignment (z axes), and energy is emitted from the tissue on relaxation [6, 11]. Absorption and vice versa emission of the energy induces an electric voltage or signal that can be detected by a receiver coil known as free induction decay (FID) [9, 11]. However, the MR signal quickly fades away due to the inhomogeneity in the magnetic field and microscopic local changes in the magnetic field (Fig. 10.4). The signal is lost in the milliseconds due to these reasons, and transverse relaxation which is caused by static magnetic field inhomogeneity and microscopic magnetic local differences is called T2* (T2 star) [9].

A 90° RF pulse application causes the net magnetization vector from the longitudinal plan into transverse plane which generates the detectable MR signal by a receiver coil positioned in this plane [2]. However if a uniform field of identical strength were generated throughout the body, RF pulse would excite all of the protons without a means of spatial localization, and signal would be detected from the whole body. To enable selected slice excitations, gradients should be used to produce deliberate variations in the main magnetic field. Thus, the Larmor frequencies of the protons outside the selected slice would change and would not be affected by

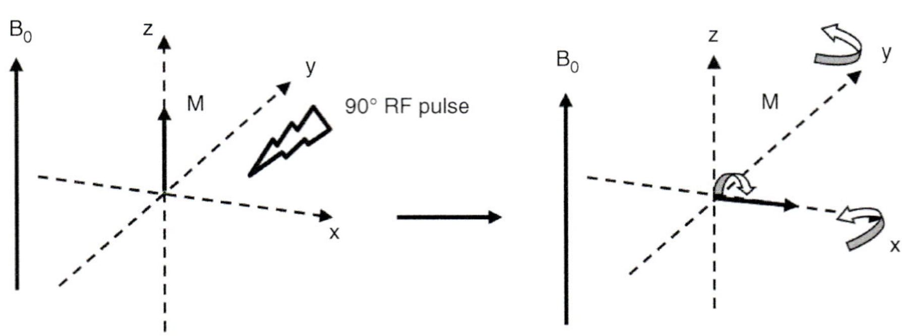

Fig. 10.3 In the presence of a magnetic field, net longitudinal magnetization occur in the z axis, and after a 90° RF pulse application, longitudinal magnetization tips down and rotate into transverse magnetization

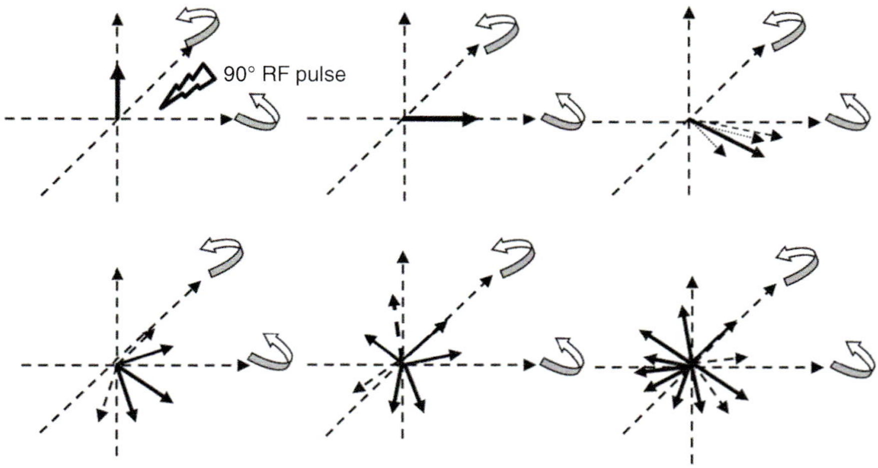

Fig. 10.4 Transverse magnetization is at maximum while the protons are in phase, due to the inter- and intramolecular interactions, protons begin to precess at different frequencies

the excitation pulse [3]. Gradient coils alter both the magnetic field magnitude and linear fashion so that a specific point along the axis of the gradient has a specific precessional frequency. This is known spatial encoding. Three sets of gradient coils are used in MR system one for each direction, and these are named according to the axis along which they act when they are switched on. Gradients accomplish the spatial localization in MRI, including slice selection, frequency encoding, and phase encoding. The location of the slice may be changed or moved along the slice selection gradient [2]. Slice thickness is determined by the amplitude of slice selection gradient and transmit bandwidth; shallow (weaker) gradient and broad transmit bandwidth generate thick slice, whereas steeper (strong) gradient and narrow transmit bandwidth generate thin slices [2, 3]. Frequency-encoding gradient that causes the precessional frequency of signal within the slice to be position along the axis of the gradient is changed in a linear fashion. Phase-encoding gradient is the spatial position of a signal along the short axis of the anatomy. The data are collected from all the gradients and stored into an array called k-space. K-space has two axes perpendicular to each other, while the horizontal axes represent the frequency information, vertical axes represent the phase information [2].

When the inhomogeneity of the magnet is reduced, the minimum there will only be transverse relaxation resulting from the microscopic local changes in the magnetic field that is called T2 or spin-echo relaxation. So perfectly homogeneous magnet is not possible; the influence of magnetic field inhomogeneity may be reduced by applying a 180° RF pulse. This method or sequence in which 180° RF pulses are used after 90° RF pulses is called the spin-echo (SE) sequence [3].

Determination of the amount of weighting depends on the acquisition parameters. Repetition time (TR) is the amount of the time from the application of an excitation pulse to the application of the next pulse and is therefore crucial for T1 contrast. T1 relaxation is the release of energy to the environment by which net magnetization vector recovers to its ground state in the direction of B_0 reaches thermodynamic equilibrium with its surroundings (the "lattice"). After the RF pulse has been applied, the signal will recover to 63% of its equilibrium value by this transfer of energy called T1 relaxation time [2, 6, 9, 11, 13]. Due to the different molecular structure in each tissue, it exhibits various T1 times. Application of shorter repetition times allows only partial recovery of tissue and the image contrast mainly affected by T1. The appearance of the tissue having a short T1 relaxation time such as fat on T1-weighted (T1W) image will appear as a bright because this tissue produces a stronger MR signal and has the highest level of magnetization at any particular time. On the other hand, a tissue with long T1 relaxation time such as cerebrospinal fluid produces weaker MR signals than tissue with short T1 and also appears dark because they do not regain their longitudinal magnetization on T1W images [2, 7, 13].

The time between the applications of the 90° RF pulse and MR signal sampling is called echo time (TE). The amount of the T2 relaxation is determined by TE. Short TE application results in the low T2 weighting, while long TE application results in the strong T2 weighting. Tissues with a long T2 relaxation time appear dark, whereas tissues with short T2 relaxation time such as cerebrospinal fluid appear bright on T2-weighted image [2, 7, 13].

10.1.4 Pixel/Voxel

Matrix of pixel or picture element is the smallest two-dimensional (2D) component of a digital image. Each pixel has 2D grid of row and columns determining the spatial resolution in-plane. This grid of pixels will hold signal intensity collected from the patient. A voxel is a rectangular cuboid volume element representing a value in the three-dimensional space, whose dimensions are set by the slice thickness, field of view (FOV), and matrix size by the scanning process [3, 14]. The voxel size represents the spatial resolution. The smaller the voxel, the greater the resolution.

10.1.5 Signal-to-Noise Ratio (SNR)

SNR is the quantitative value to the strength of the desired signal to its background reflections at a given point in time. The SNR in MRI depends on a slice thickness, receiver bandwidth, FOV, size of the (image) matrix, number of excitations (NEX), scan parameters (repetition time (TR), echo time (TE), flip angle), magnetic field strength, and selection of the transmit and receive coil (RF coil). SNR is proportional to the pixel size (FOV/matrix), slice thickness, number of excitations (NEX), and magnetic field strength, employing local coil, TR, and is inversely proportional to the receiver bandwidth, TE [3]. The higher the SNR in MR image, the more likely is the image quality. Noise is always present at the MRI, and even if the signal is high, the quality of the view will be low if the noise is high. The use of surface coil system can trade for increased image detail by using smaller voxels and influence both the statistical and the spatial distribution of noise [15].

10.1.6 Contrast-to-Noise Ratio (CNR)

CNR is the ability to differentiate two adjacent structures of high signal from areas of low signal such as gray and white matter, scaled to image noise [16]. The CNR increases with the T2-weighted images, contrast agents, chemical pre-saturation technique, and magnetization transfer contrast [2].

10.2 Image Acquisition in MRI (Common Sequences in MRI for TMJ)

The names of various sequences used by the MR manufacturers are listed in Table 10.1.

10.2.1 T1, T2, and Proton Density-Weighted Spin-Echo Images

The most commonly used sequence is spin echo. Because imaging appearance may vary depending on the acquisition parameters, T1, T2, and proton density (PD)-weighted images are obtained by changing the TR and TE (Table 10.2) [2, 4, 17].

T1W images tend to have short TR (typically 300–700 ms) and TE (20 ms) and best demonstrate the anatomy. Fat has high signal intensity and appears bright on T1W images, whereas the lower signal for more water content such as edema, tumor, infarction, inflammation, infection, and CSF will be dark. A contrast agent usually shortened the value of the T1 and brightened the image. Also subacute hemorrhage, melanin, protein-rich fluid, and slowly flowing blood have high signal intensity on T1W images [7] (Fig. 10.5).

Unlike the T1W images, T2W images are produced by using long TR (2000 ms) and TE (typically ≥60 ms). Since fluid has a long T2 relaxation time, edema, tumor, infarction, inflammation, infection, CSF, and subacute hemorrhage appear bright, while contrast agent, calcification, fat, protein-rich fluid, and flow void appear dark on T2W images. T2W images are appropriate and most frequently used for visualizing the pathologic conditions [7] (Fig. 10.6).

Proton density (PD)-weighted image tends to have long TR (to diminish the T1 effect) and short TE (to diminish the T2 effect) [17]. PDW images display the amount of the protons per unit tissue. Fat exhibits relatively high signal intensity but not as bright as in T1W image. Fluid presents intermediate signal on PDW images [3]. Also PDW images provide better contrast between gray and white matter rather than T2W. PDW imaging is particularly helpful to differentiate the CSF and pathology which have both high signals on T2W images [18] (Fig. 10.7).

Table 10.1 The list of the common names for MRI sequences abbreviations used by different manufacturers

	Common names for MRI sequences abbreviations used by different manufacturers								
	Philips	GE	Hitachi	Siemens	Fonar	Toshiba	Elscint	Shimadzu	Picker
Spin echo	SE	SE, MEMP, VEMP	SE	SE	SE	SE	SE	SE	SE
Turbo spin echo/fast spin echo	TSE	FSE	FSE	TSE	FSE	FSE	FSE	RISE	FSE
Single shot technique	Single shot TSE	SSFSE	Single shot FSE	HASTE		FASE			EXPRESS
Gradient echo	FFE	GRE, GRASS	GE	GRE	Field echo	Field echo	SHORT	Field echo	FAST
Coherent gradient echo	FFE	GRASS, FGR, FMPGR	Rephased, SARGE, GFEC	FISP	Field echo	Field echo	E/F SHORT	SSFP	FAST
Incoherent gradient echo (RF spoiled)	T1 FFE	SPGR	GE/GFE	FLASH	Field echo	Field echo	SHORT	STAGE T1W	RF spoiled FAST
Incoherent gradient echo (gradient spoiled)	T2 FFE	MPGR	GRE	FLASH	Field echo	Field echo	SHORT	STAGE	T1-FAST NOSE
Steady-state free precession	T2 FFE	SSFP, DE FGR	Time reversed SARGE	PSIF	Field echo		F/E SHORT	STERF	CE FAST
Balanced sequences/true FISP	Balanced FFE	FIESTA	BASG	True FISP		True SSFP		STERF	
True FISP/dual excitation		FIESTA-C		CISS					
Multi-echo data image combination	M-FFE	MERGE	ADAGE	MEDIC					
Inversion recovery	IR, IR-TSE	IR, MPIR, FASTIR	IR	IR, TIR	IR	IR	IR	IR	IR
Short T1 inversion recovery	STIR	STIR	STIR	STIR	STIR	STIR	STIR	STIR	STIR
Long tau inversion recovery	FLAIR	FLAIR	Fast FLAIR	Turbo dark fluid					
True inversion recovery	Real IR	T1 FLAIR	T1 FLAIR	True IR					
	Philips	GE	Hitachi	Siemens	Fonar	Toshiba	Elscint	Shimadzu	Picker

Table 10.2 Relative TR and TE differences in basic spin-echo sequences

	TR	TE
T1 weighted	Short	Short
T2 weighted	Long	Long
Proton density weighted	Long	Short

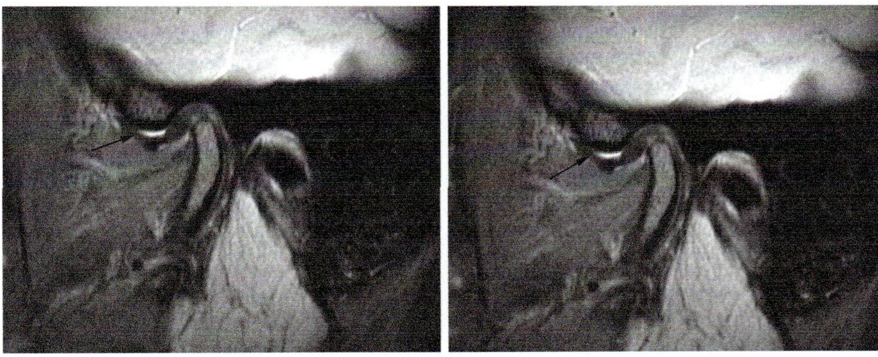

Fig. 10.5 T1-W sagittal MR image showing anatomical structures of TMJ clearly with superior joint compartment effusion (arrows)

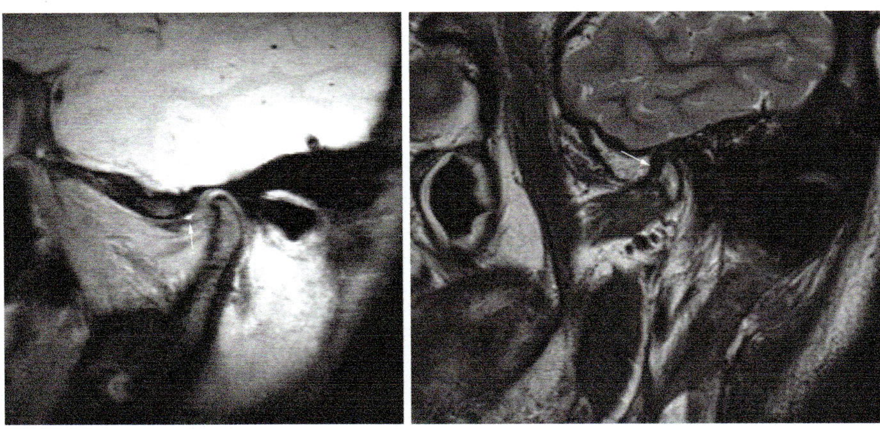

Fig. 10.6 MR image showing T1-W with effusion (white arrow) and T2-W sagittal images with degeneration of the condyle (black arrow)

10.2.2 Fast Spin Echo (FSE) and Turbo Spin-Echo Imaging (TSE)

Standard spin-echo sequences have relatively long acquisition times. Such an exemplary the acquisition time of a single T1W spin echo takes approximately 4 min; for T2W spin-echo image, this time increases 21 min with a 512 matrix size [17]. Conventional spin-echo sequences fill the k-space line by line until the entire space is filled per TR and scan time is very long. TR, number of excitations (NEX), and number of phase encodings affect the scan time and any changes in these parameter

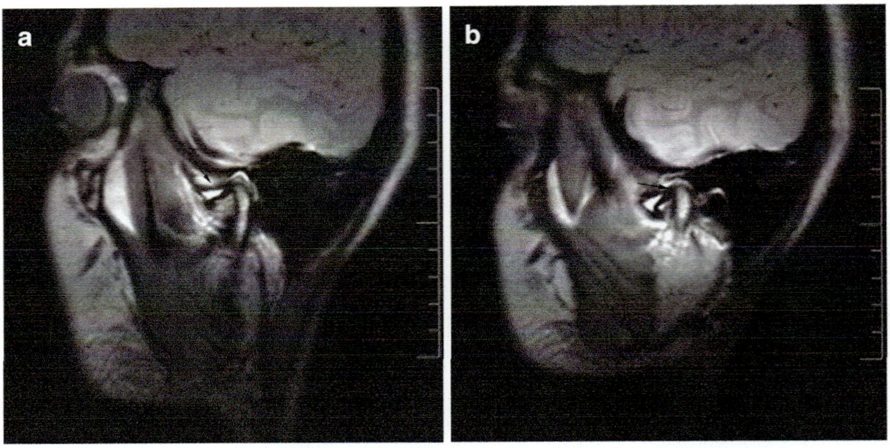

Fig. 10.7 (**a**) Proton-weighted sagittal MR images showing closed mouth and (**b**) open mouth position of a stuck disc (arrows)

image weighting, spatial resolution, and SNR in a negative way [2]. To decrease the acquisition time and reduce the motion artifact due to the long scan time, Hennig et al. developed the RARE (rapid acquisition with relaxation enhancement) sequence [19]. FSE sequence also called TSE depending on the manufacturers is characterized by multiple rapidly applied 180° rephrasing RF pulses after just one 90° excitation pulse and multiple echoes, to produce echo train. This number of the echoes is called echo train length (also known as the turbo factor). Instead of the one line in conventional spin-echo sequence, multiple lines are used to fill the k-space more rapidly in FSE sequences, and the scan time is decreased [2, 20]. Echo train length or turbo factor has an important role in image weighting. If the turbo factor is so high, scan time decrease, but image would be a mixture of weighting. To obtain a T1 and PDW fast spin-echo image, turbo factor has to be minimum, but in T2W image, larger turbo factor is needed [2] (Fig. 10.8).

10.2.3 Fat-Saturated TMJ Imaging

Since the majority of the body is composed of water and fat, these two parts constitute the major component of MR images. A relative difference in nuclear magnetic resonance frequency of the same water and fat's atomic nuclei depending on its molecular or molecular sites differences is known as chemical shift. If both water and lipid protons coexist in the same voxel, the signal from water and fat will be additive, and the out-of-phase transverse magnetization cancel each other out [3]. In clinical MR imaging, to prevent the signal loss, chemically selective RF pulses are applied to cause the signal from fat (or water) to be nulled (saturated), while the other signal is relatively unaffected before imaging [3, 5]. Fat suppression with chemically selective pulses is mainly used to suppress the signal coming from the

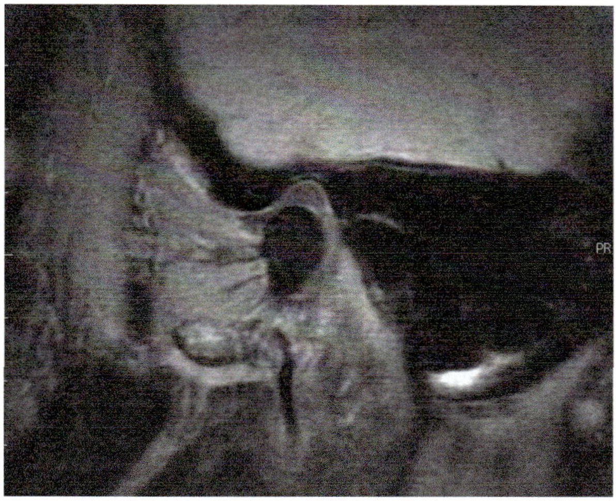

Fig. 10.8 T1-weighted turbo spin-echo images of TMJ disc and condyle clearly

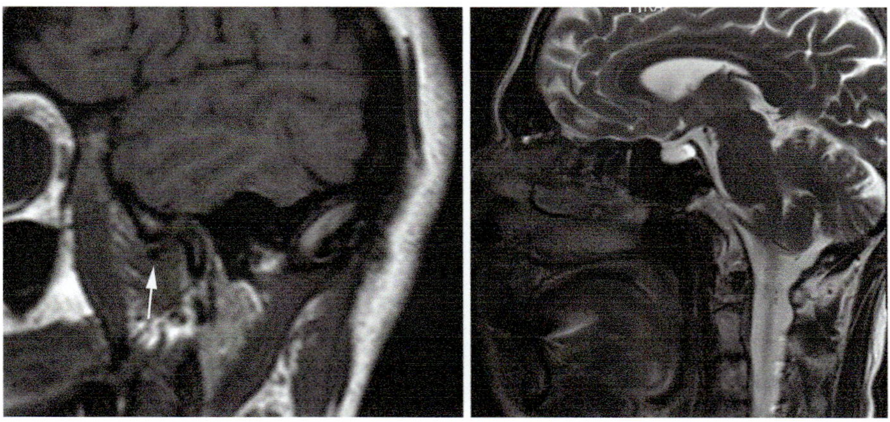

Fig. 10.9 T1- and T2-weighted STIR images. Note the disc displacement in the closed mouth position (arrow)

normal adipose tissue which causes the chemical shift artifact, to improve the visibility of the interested tissue, adrenal gland tumors, steatosis [21], fatty tumors (such as lipoma or liposarcoma), bone marrow edema, and extent of the pathologic lesion in the bone marrow [4].

As the fat saturation pulses are affected by the magnet inhomogeneity, highly uniform magnet is needed to obtain fat-saturated (FatSat) image. Inhomogeneity of the magnet results in partially saturated missing or incomplete fat [4]. A short frequency 90° fat sat pulse is applied; the fat protons magnetization deflected into the transverse plane before sequence imaging, and they produce no signal [20].

There are several techniques to achieve fat suppression including frequency-selective fat saturation (FS) and short-tau inversion recovery (STIR) (Fig. 10.9).

Dixon and spectral-attenuated inversionrecovery (SPAIR) techniques are the most commonly used two fat suppression methods [22]. Dixon technique is depending on the water/fat chemical shift differences. This technique is able to separate water and fat proton signals which are generated for in-phase and opposed-phase images, and then "fat-suppressed" water-only and "water-suppressed" fat-only images could be analytically calculated [22, 23] (Fig. 10.10).

10.2.4 Pseudo-Dynamic Imaging of TMJ

Pseudo-dynamic images is based on the static sequential step-by-step acquisitions which is obtained from the closed mouth to maximum open mouth position in various degree of the translation using bite block or mouth wedge [24, 25]. Pseudo-dynamic images can be played in cine loop to do a simulation of condylar movement [26]. Pseudo-dynamic image is not a real dynamic image; it is an artificial movement of the disc and condyle of the TMJ; physiological and pathological situations cannot directly visualize with this method [24, 25].

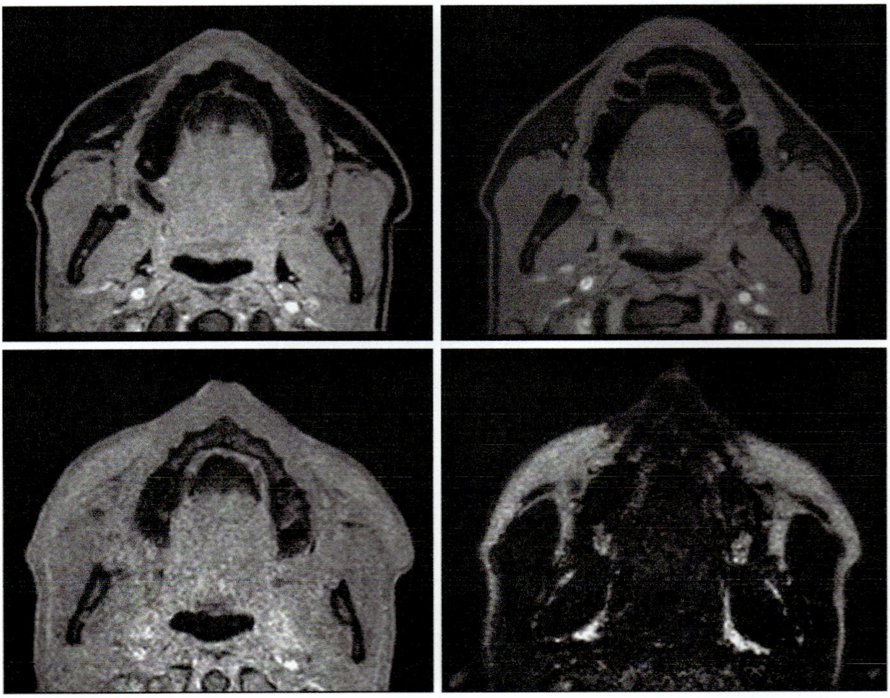

Fig. 10.10 Dixon-type sequences all produce four sets of images as shown below: water only, fat only, in phase, and out of phase. The fat-only images offer the potential for fat quantification. A minor disadvantage is an increase in minimum TR value (required to allow time for collection of the multiple echoes)

10.2.5 Dynamic Imaging of TMJ

10.2.5.1 Gradient Echo Imaging

Gradient echo (GRE) sequence, also known as gradient-recalled echo or fast field echo (FFE) sequences, uses gradient coils instead of a 180° refocusing RF pulse for producing an echo [3]. Frequency encoding is accomplished by applying gradients during data acquisition which are used to dephase (negative polarity) and rephase (positive polarity) transverse magnetization to create one or multiple echo signal [4]. In this sequence variable RF pulses (between 10° and 90°) also known as flip angle or tip angle are applied to create the transverse magnetization [20] (Fig. 10.11). After the α-degree RF pulse (characteristic flip angle), readout gradient is firstly applied with negative polarity and then reversed into positive polarity. This reversal of the gradients results in a regrowth of the signal and generates the echoes [5]. Since no 180° RF pulse is used, the main problem is the magnet inhomogeneities effect in this sequence. Depending on this technical characteristics, T2* dephasing with much shorter time than T2 occur in GRE [5, 20]. The most important advantage of the GRE sequence is short imaging time.

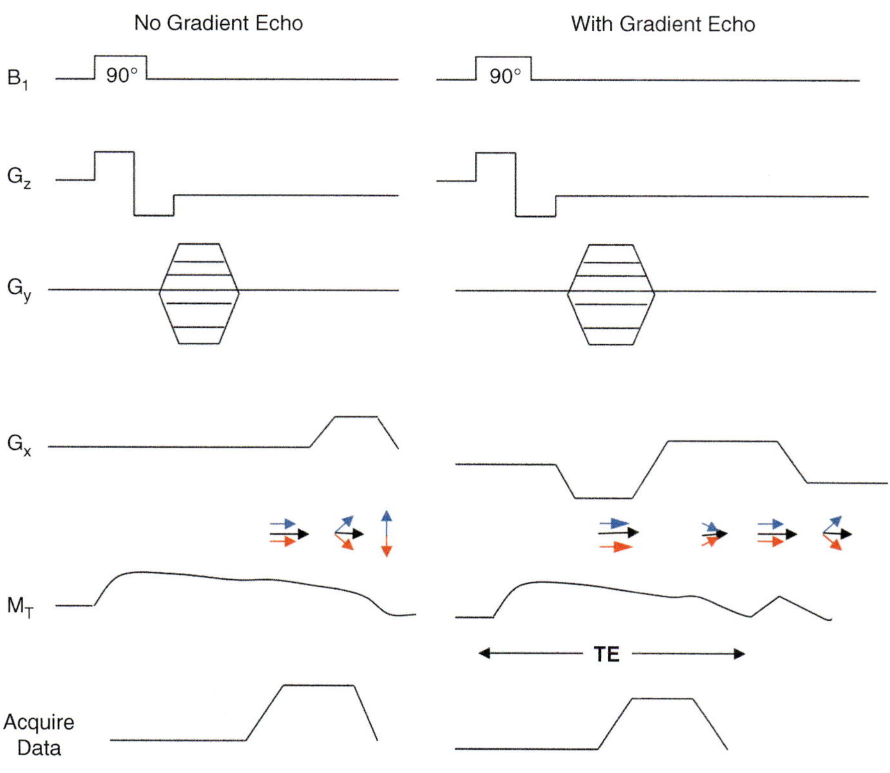

Fig. 10.11 Gradient echo pulse sequence formation diagram

T2* contrast affected by TE and T1 contrast is related with the flip angle and TR in this sequence. Larger flip angle and short TR introduces higher degree of T1 contrast, while lower flip angle and short TE accentuate T2* contrast [2, 3, 20]. Proton density contrast dominates when lower flip angle, longer TR, and shorter TE are used [2].

There are two broad categories of gradient echo sequences: incoherent gradient echo or gradient spoiled (spoiled residual transverse magnetization) and coherent gradient echo (refocused transverse magnetization). In the incoherent gradient echo sequence, the transverse magnetization is eliminated by a magnetic field gradient or a spoiler RF pulse.

A FFE sequence using a balanced gradient waveform. A balanced sequence starts out with a RF pulse of 90° or less and the spins in the steady state. Before the next TR in the slice phase and frequency encoding, gradients are balanced, so their net value is zero. Now the spins are prepared to accept the next RF pulse, and their corresponding signal can become part of the new transverse magnetization. Since the balanced gradients maintain the transverse and longitudinal magnetization, the result is that both T1 and T2 contrast are represented in the image. This pulse sequence produces images with increased signal from fluid, along with retaining T1-weighted tissue contrast. Because this form of sequence is extremely dependent on field homogeneity, it is essential to run a shimming prior to the acquisition. A fully balanced (refocused) sequence would yield higher signal, especially for tissues with long T2 relaxation times [20] (Figs. 10.12 and 10.13).

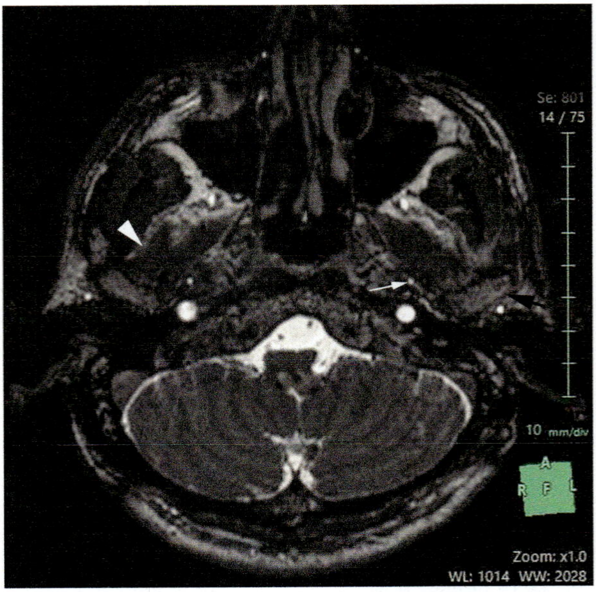

Fig. 10.12 An axial bFFE image of both TMJs showing increased signal from fluid (white arrow), along with retaining T1-weighted tissue contrast of the condyle (black arrow) and pterygoid muscle (arrow head)

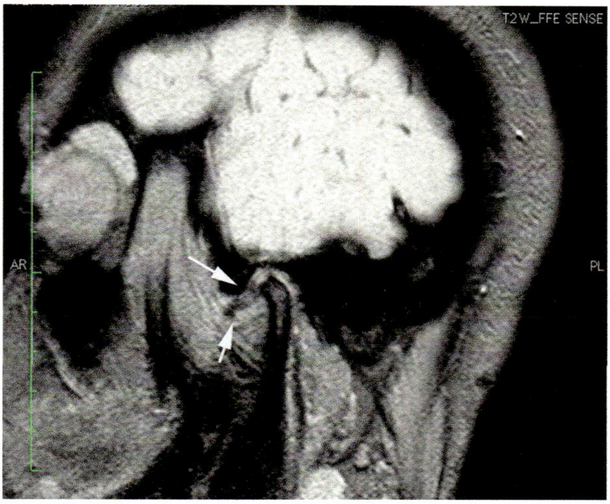

Fig. 10.13 A T2W-FFE image showing an anterior disc displacement without reduction case (arrows)

10.2.5.2 Echo Planar Imaging (EPI) Sequence

EPI allows ultrafast data acquisition (in 100–200 ms) and is performed by a series of gradient reversals in the readout direction [9]. EPI methods need strong and rapidly switched frequency-encoding gradients [3]. A gradient echo train is constituted by the application of the readout gradient continuously with positive and negative alternations [9]. If EPI sequence begins with the variable RF excitation pulse, it is called gradient echo EPI (GE–EPI), or if it begins with the 90° and 180° RF pulses, it is known as spin-echo EPI (SE–EPI). 180° refocusing pulse application needs for reducing artefacts caused by magnetic field inhomogeneities and chemical shift. SE–EPI has better image quality but longer scan time than GE–EPI [2].

10.2.5.3 Inversion Recovery (IR)

Inversion recovery pulse sequence is a variant of spin-echo sequence using the 180° inverting RF pulse to null or suppress the signal from certain tissues (e.g., fat or fluid). 180° RF pulse changes the direction of the nuclear magnetization from the positive z-direction into the negative z-direction. The regrowth of longitudinal magnetization starts to return the original orientation. After some relaxation occurrence process continue with the application of the 90° RF pulse. The time between the applications of the two RF pulses is called inversion time (TI) [3]. 90° RF pulse change the magnetization direction along negative y' axis or the positive y' axis depending on the inversion time used as an image contrast control [8]. Inversion recovery sequence provides heavily T1-weighted images which are primarily controlled by the TI value. A short TE application regarding to the T2 value decreases the T2 effect on IR sequence [20].

Two important clinical applications of the inversion recovery techniques are the short-tau inversion recovery (STIR) sequence and the fluid-attenuated inversion recovery (FLAIR) sequence [4].

Short-tau inversion recovery also known as short T1 inversion recovery sequence suppresses the tissue signal which has short T1 using a short IR [20]. Since the STIR sequence selectively suppresses the signal from fat, it provides excellent determination of the bone marrow edema [4] (Fig. 10.14).

FLAIR, a special inversion recovery technique, is used to null the signal from fluid (e.g., CSF, urine) using long inversion times. FLAIR sequence is very useful for evaluating the brain tissue [3, 4] (Fig. 10.15).

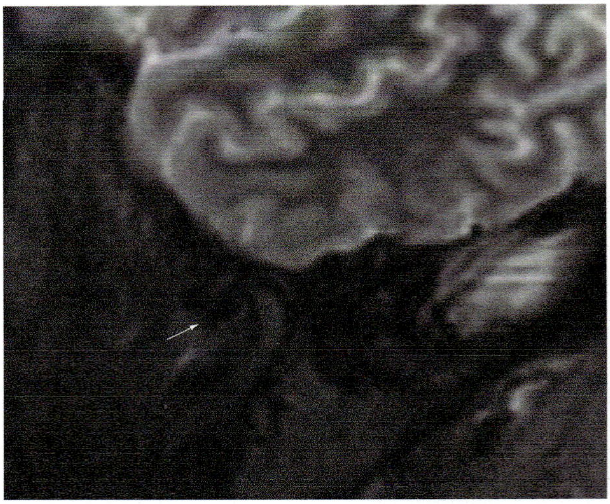

Fig. 10.14 Sagittal STIR image showing anterior disc displacement (arrow)

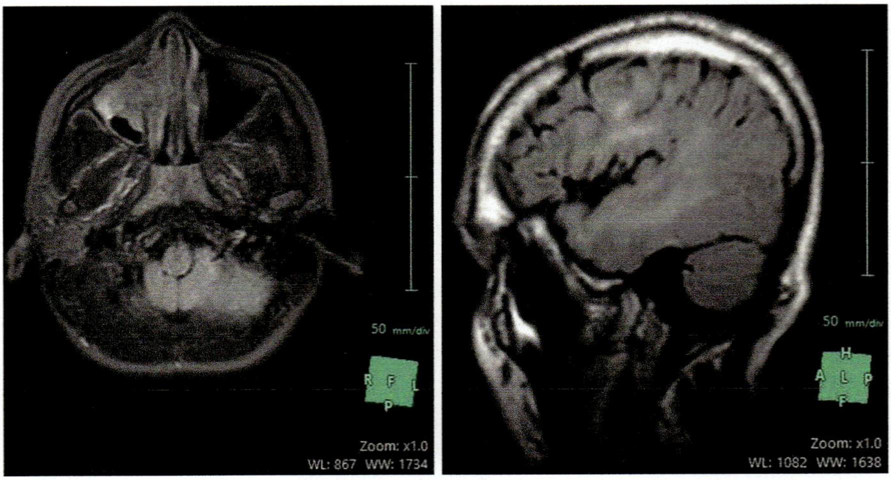

Fig. 10.15 Axial T1-W and sagittal T2W-FLAIR image showing TMJ structures. Note that the null is the signal from fluid

10.2.5.4 Half-Fourier Acquisition Single-Shot Turbo Spin-Echo (HASTE) Imaging

Half-fourier acquisition single-shot fast spin echo (HASTE) also known as single-shot fast spin echo (SSFSE) is a single-shot version of fast spin-echo which uses a single slice selective excitation and multiple refocusing RF pulses to reduce the number of phase-encoding steps with imaging times of 1 s or less [27]. Short acquisition time is an advantage to minimize the motion artifact and magnetic susceptibility [28]. Because a long time to repetition have to be selected to obtain an image in HASTE, sequence tissues with long TEs are well depicted, whereas tissues with short or medium TEs are not shown [3] (Fig. 10.16).

10.2.5.5 Steady-State Free Precession (SSFP)

SSFP is a highly effective unspoiled gradient echo sequence that accumulates signal from several echoes which are generated with repeatedly applied RF pulse. TR is usually kept as short as possible to minimize the acquisition time because SSFP sequences are very susceptible to artifacts caused by magnetic field inhomogeneities [4]. SSFP sequence image contrast is based on the ratio of T2/T1. Tissues which have high T2/T1 ratio appear bright, while tissues with a low T2/T1 appears dark on image. SSFP sequence is especially useful for evaluating the moving organs such as heart, vascular imaging [3], interventional MR imaging, and internal auditory canal in a short acquisition time with a high SNR [4].

GRASS (gradient-recalled acquisition in the steady state), FISP (fast imaging with steady-state precession), FIESTA (fast imaging employing steady-state

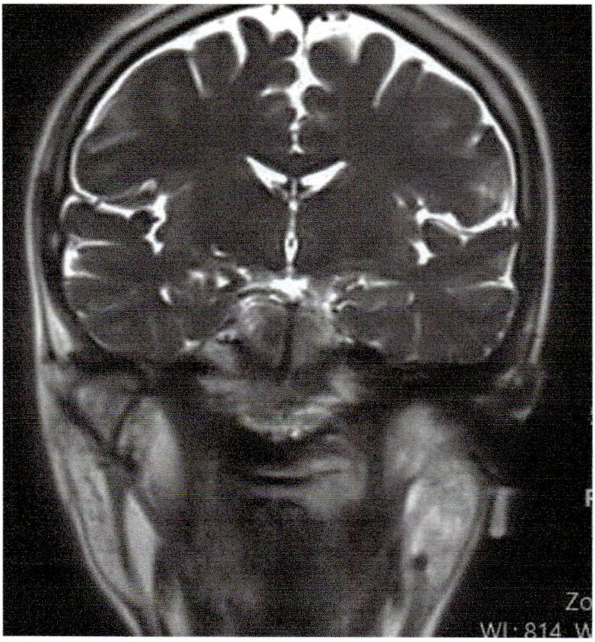

Fig. 10.16 Coronal T2W-HASTE image TMJ condyle on the right side

acquisition), balanced FFE (fast-field echo), and true FISP are the different names of the SSFP sequence depending on the manufacturers listed in Table 10.1.

Several studies used frequency-selective fat-saturated (FS) T2W sequence and found to be more sensitive than conventional T2W images in detecting marrow alterations and stated to be used instead of conventional T2W images [29–31], while the others used several sequences such as half-fourier acquisition single-shot turbo spin echo (HASTE) [32–34], fast low-angle shot (FLASH) [35, 36], and steady-state free precession (SSFP) (true fast imaging with steady-state precession (true FISP) [37], balanced fast field echo (bFFE), balanced turbo field echo (bTFE), and fast imaging employing steady-state acquisition sequence (FIESTA)24) especially for dynamic imaging of TMJ. Krohn et al. investigated the potential of real-time MR imaging (dynamic TMJ imaging) using 3T and concluded the advantage of 3T for this kind of imaging. Yen et al. developed an imaging protocol on a 3T system using the true FISP sequence that yielded an acceptable spatial and temporal resolution for dynamic MR imaging. In a recent study, used T2 mapping technique to evaluate TMJ disc ultrastructure. They concluded T2 relaxation time measurements could enable an ultrastructural analysis of the articular disc of the TMJ [38] (Fig. 10.17).

10.2.6 Advanced MRI Applications

10.2.6.1 Diffusion-Weighted Imaging (DWI)

Diffusion is the tendency of the molecules to move from a region where they are in high concentration to a region where they are in low concentration due to interactions with their surroundings. Two types of movement occur in tissues including coherent bulk flow and continuous movement in molecular space called as translational motion [9]. Diffusion is limited or restricted by various anatomical structures such as ligaments, membranes and macromolecules, as well as pathology. The net displacement of the molecules is named apparent diffusion coefficient (ADC) [2]. Diffusion constant in biological tissues may be measured by changing the b values (duration and interval of the gradients) with same imaging parameters [3]. If b value is zero, long TE and TR is resulted in T2W images; however, image weighting

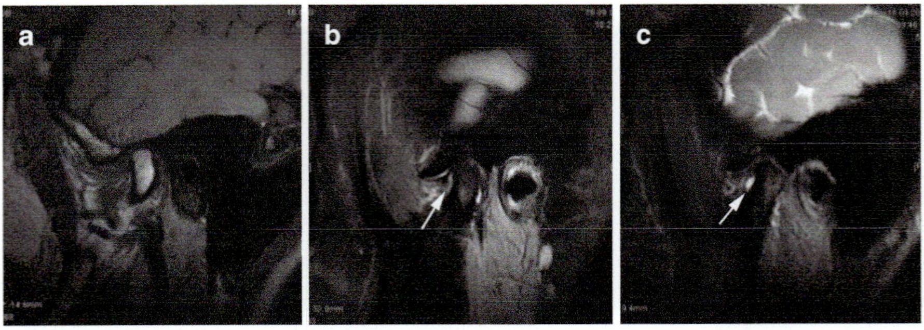

Fig. 10.17 (**a**) Conventional T2W image showing a normal bone marrow, (**b**) FS T2W, and 3D, (**c**) FIESTA-C sequences of the same patient demonstrated increased signal intensity with effusion in the inferior compartment of the joint and with the mandibular condyle bone marrow edema

changes into DWI when the b value (changing between the 500 and 1500 s/mm^2) increases [2]. ADC map is generated using the grayscale values which represent the mean ADCs of the corresponding voxels [3]. Pathologic tissues display high signal intensity on DWI and is characterized by lower ADC value than normal tissue due to the restriction of the diffusion when pathology is present [2].

DWI is very useful for evaluating the cholesteatoma, assessment of the malignant tumors, prediction and monitoring of treatment response, and differentiation of recurrent tumor from posttherapeutic changes in head and neck cancer [39] (Figs. 10.18 and 10.19).

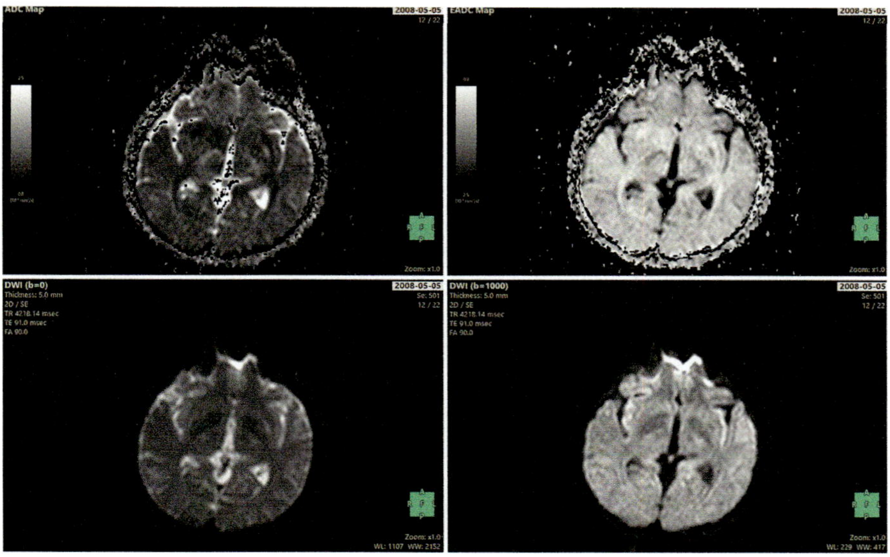

Fig. 10.18 DWI images showing ADC map, EADC map, b = 0, and b = 1000 images

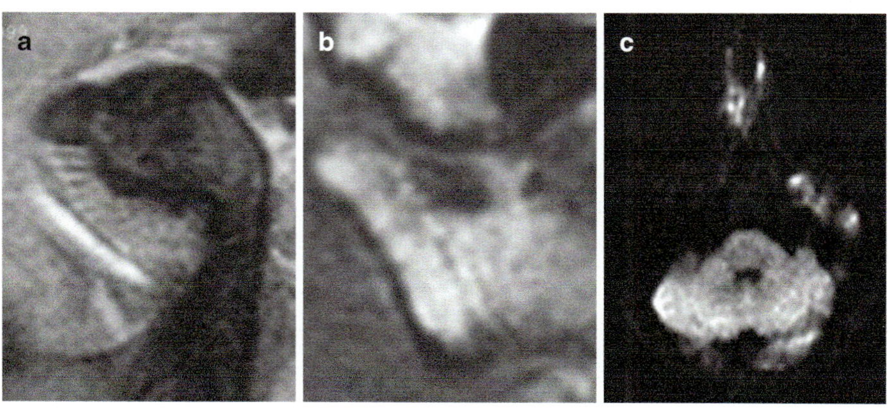

Fig. 10.19 (**a**) t1-W, (**b**) T2-W, and (**c**) diffusion-weighted images at b value1000 showing non-restricted diffusion in an osteochondroma case of the TMJ condyle

10.2.6.2 Perfusion-Weighted Imaging

Perfusion is a relative and/or absolute measurement of the parameters of regional blood flow, vascular supply to a tissue, and tissue activity [2]. Perfusion-weighted imaging is of great help to evaluate the microvascular blood flow in the brain, the myocardium, the lungs, the spleen, and the kidneys [2, 3]. This technique relies on the use of a tracer either a bolus injection of exogenous perfusion contrast agent such as gadolinium or endogenous saturating the protons in arterial blood with RF inversion or saturation pulses [2]. A paramagnetic contrast agent application results in a shortening of both longitudinal and transverse relaxation times, visceral with high perfusion appear as an increase in signal on T1-weighted images and a decrease on T2- or T2*-weighted images [2, 3]. (Figs. 10.20 and 10.21).

10.2.6.3 High-Speed Real-Time Radial FLASH MRI

Real-time MR imaging of moving spins focuses on the observation of dynamic processes such as tongue movement, cardiac imaging, and fetal imaging. This technique is based on acquisition of dynamic images in a short period of time. In order to achieve dynamic images, specific reconstruction algorithms should be used in order to constitute the MR images. FLASH sequence is one of them that can be used with regularized nonlinear inversion for achieving real-time phase-contrast imaging [40].

Fast low-angle shot (FLASH) is the most commonly used spoiled gradient-echo MRI sequence. FLASH uses radio-frequency excitation pulses with a low flip angle (less than 90°) and subsequent reading gradient reversal for producing a gradient echo signal. The small flip angle pulses create equilibrium of longitudinal magnetization. Transverse magnetization is eliminated by a strong gradient (spoiler gradient). T1-weighted and T2*-weighted contrast can be set with the FLASH sequence. In comparison to spin echo, FLASH is more sensitive to field inhomogeneities and susceptibility differences. On the other hand, it provides several advantages such as reduction in acquisition time due to short TR, lower specific absorption rate, and extra contrast due to imaging at in-phase and opposed-phase conditions [41, 42].

For FLASH imaging, due to transverse magnetization in steady state, there are three types of FLASH sequences such as spoiled, refocused FLASH, and balanced steady-state free precession (bSSFP). Spoiled FLASH employs RF spoiling or gradient spoiling to destroy the transverse magnetization. Gradient spoiling involves the application of the gradient pulses which results the dephasing of the residual magnetization [43]. For radial spoiled FLASH, the technique itself employs a fast low-angle shot sequence with proton density, T1 or T2/T1 contrast, and radial data encoding for motion robustness. High temporal resolution is achieved by an up to 20-fold undersampling of the radial data [41, 43, 44].

Radial views are acquired in a certain view order to fill the k-space. The simplest method fills the k-space in which the order plays a major role in dynamic imaging as the motion of the object. The distribution of radial views in k-space and different types of view order had been studied extensively [40]. The sequential reordering

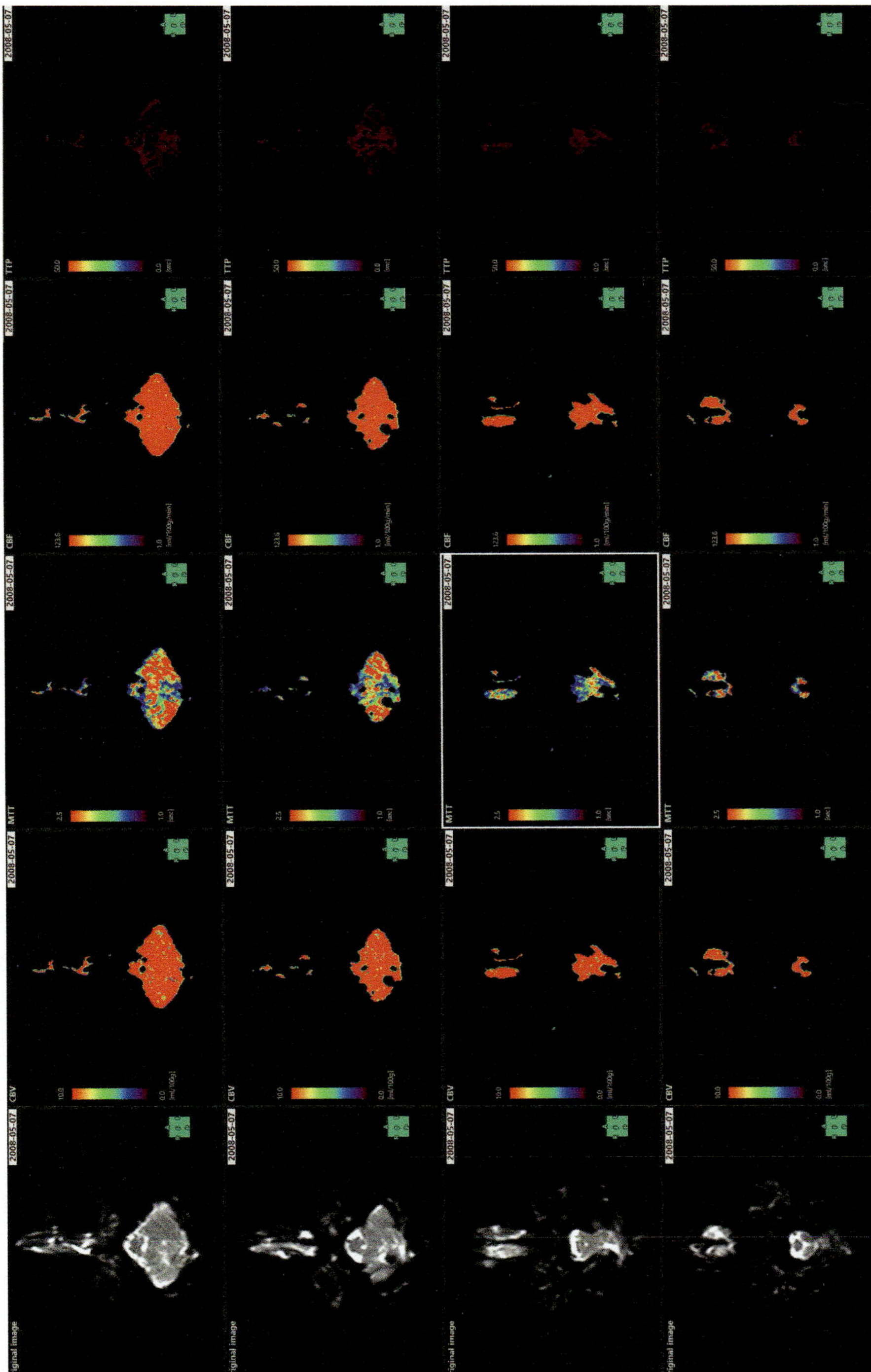

Fig. 10.20 MR perfusion study showing blood flow parameters

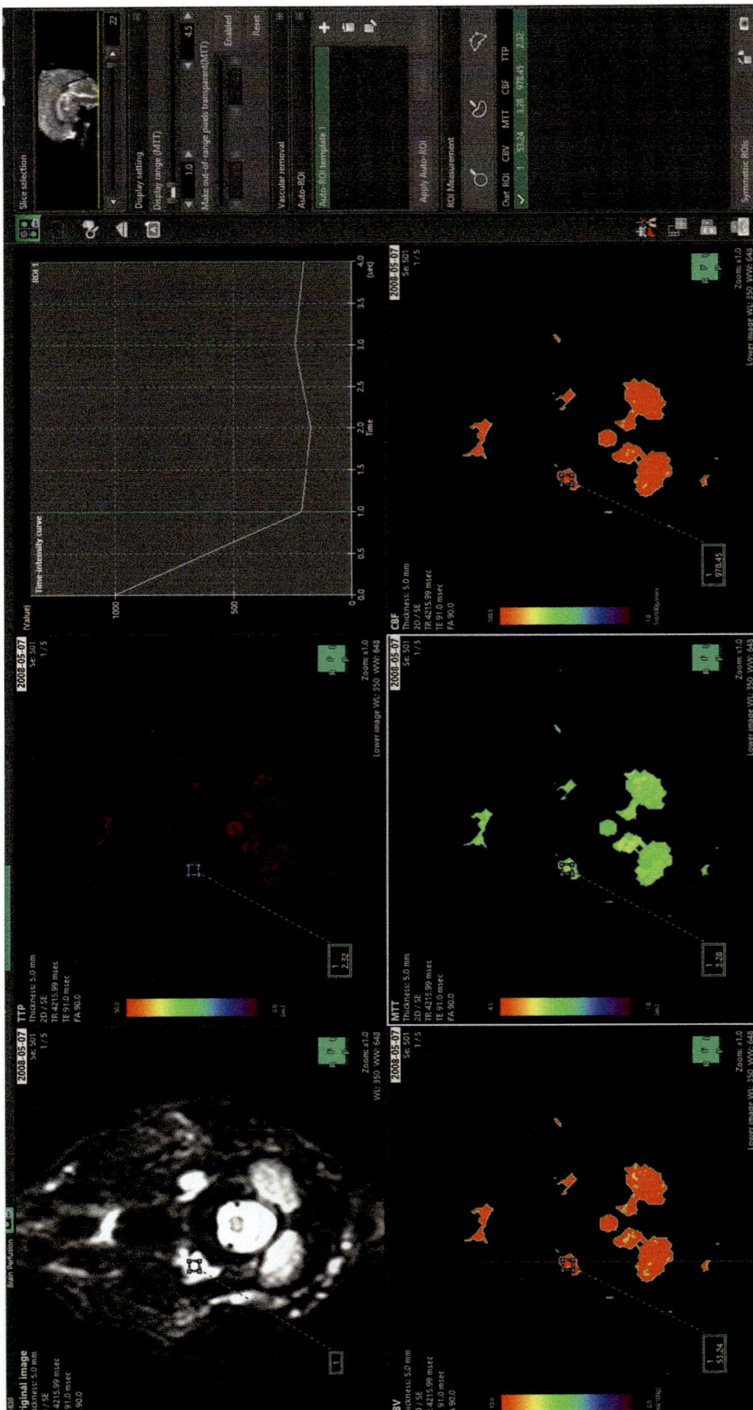

Fig. 10.21 MR perfusion study describes rate and level of blood flow (CBF) to tissues with time-intensity curve

scheme along with five radial turns was experimentally found to be optimal for dynamic imaging.

However, in this technique, the obstacle is the coil sensitivity esp. in parallel and real-time MRI due to short acquisition time. If the receive coil sensitivities are known, the image recovery an efficiently be solved using iterative methods. In practice, however, static sensitivities are obtained through extrapolation, and in a human subject during any type of movement (e.g., breathing or TMJ imaging) or when dynamically scanning, different planes and orientations (e.g., during real-time monitoring of minimally invasive procedures) can be effected dramatically. In such situations, extrapolating static sensitivities is not sufficient and thus should be corrected with various reconstruction algorithms [44, 45].

Increasing imaging speed is of utmost importance in in vivo MRI and can be simultaneously acquire several slices of an object, which allows for higher undersampling factors compared to single- or conventional multi-slice measurements by exploiting axial coil sensitivity information. Furthermore, these MRI benefits from an inherently increased SNR which contributes to an improved overall image quality. For real-time dynamic MRI changes during a physiologic process, there is need for undersampled data sets which can be solved with nonlinear inverse problem. Simultaneous multi- slice (SMS) MRI together with reconstruction techniques such as regularized nonlinear inversion (NLINV) formulates the image reconstruction as a nonlinear least-squares problem for dynamic imaging [46].

This approach has been tested for high spatial MRI, in particular MRI studies for articulation [47], brass playing [48] to swallowing [49, 50], etc. Although there are a couple of studies, so far no detail imaging was done for TMJ FLASH imaging. The easy way to recognize the FLASH images is to check for fluid-filled space around TMJ area (e.g., cerebrospinal fluid, synovial fluid in the joint). Fluids normally appear as dark on a FLASH image (Fig. 10.22). However, the application for TMJ is still not tested in detail for this imaging sequence and reconstruction.

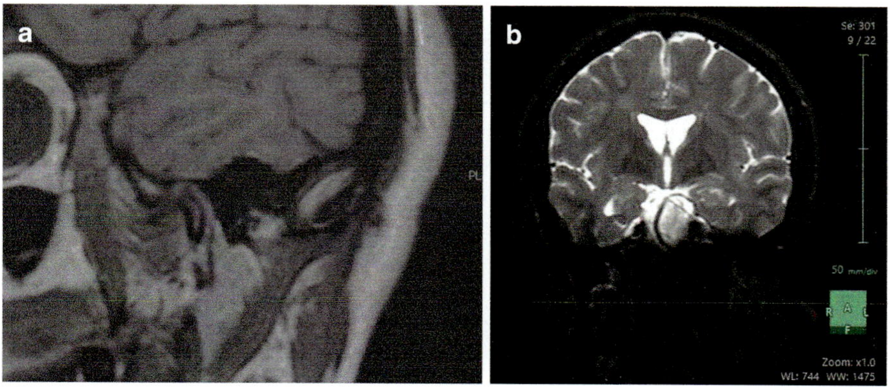

Fig. 10.22 (**a**) T1-W flash and (**b**) T2-W FLASH sequences. Note that the easy way to detect FLASH images is to check for fluid the filled space which fluids normally appear as dark

10.3 Contrast Media and Contrast Enhancement

Image contrast in medical MR imaging is due to differences in signal intensity (SI) between the two tissues [3]. Since the earliest stages of development of this imaging modality, contrast enhancement media have been used for magnetic resonance imaging. The contrast agent used in computerized tomography and magnetic resonance imaging is working with completely different mechanism. The contrast agent used in computerized tomography accumulates in the tissue and visualized with the ability to absorb X-ray photons. On the other hand, the contrast agent used in magnetic resonance imaging indirectly functions with changes in the local magnetic environment [51]. The contrast agent used in this imaging is pharmaceutical preparations applied in MR imaging to further enhance natural contrast and also to obtain dynamic (pharmacokinetic) information. To achieve these goals, the contrast agents used for MRI must have certain physicochemical properties as well as a suitable pharmacokinetic profile.

The MR contrast medical changes its contrast properties of biological tissues in two basic ways.

- Directly by changing the proton density of a tissue or
- Indirectly, by altering the local magnetic field and the resonance properties of a tissue and thus the T1 and/or T2 values [3]

The use of contrast media enhances the sensitivity and specificity of the MRI sequences by chancing the intrinsic properties of tissue depending on the tissue vascularity, capillary permeability, and extracellular fluid volume following oral or intravenous administration [52, 53]. There are several different contrast agents available for MR imaging. Some of the contrast materials used in magnetic resonance imaging are gadolinium-based, while others include gadolinium-free materials. Gadolinium (Gd)-based chelates entering clinical use in 1998 represent the basis of intravenous contrast-enhanced MR imaging [54]. This Gd chelates are highly water soluble and contain Gd ion. Gadolinium is an earth metal which has special paramagnetic properties, making it useful as a contrast agent for MRI scans. The paramagnetic properties of this contrast agents result from the numerous unpaired electrons that exist within its inner shells. These unpaired electrons can interact with adjacent resonating protons and cause the protons to relax more rapidly. This result in a shortening of both longitudinal and transverse relaxation with consequent reduction in the T1 and T2 values of the tissue in which it accumulates [52, 53]. This is depicted as an increase in T1-weighted image and a decrease in T2-weighted image signal. In practice, the signal increase detected on T1-weighted imaging is better appreciated than any corresponding signal decrease in T2-weighted imaging and makes T1-weighted imaging the method of choice for intravenous contrast studies [55]. Fat suppression is often used to suppress the high signal from fat and obtain a reliable acquisition of contrast material-enhanced images [52].

Gadolinium-based contrast agents (GBCAs) are used to enhance the image approved by the Food and Drug Administration (FDA) including Ablavar (gadofosveset trisodium), Dotarem (gadoterate meglumine), Eovist (gadoxetate disodium), Gadavist (gadobutrol), Magnevist (gadopentetate dimeglumine), MultiHance (gadobenate dimeglumine), Omniscan (gadodiamide), OptiMARK (gadoversetamide), and ProHance (gadoteridol).

The standard dose of extracellular contrast material administration shortens T1, which leads to an increase in signal intensity in vessels and tissues due to tissue perfusion or disruption of the capillary barrier (brain, spinal cord, eyes, testes). The extracellular contrast medium is administered intravenously as a bolus or drip infusion at a dose of 0.1–0.3 mmol/kg body weight. In MR angiography, higher doses were administered consecutively up to 0.5 mmol/kg body weight [3]. The major elimination pathway of these agents is through glomerular filtration and renal excretion. Half-life is usually 90 min, but it takes 24 h for complete elimination of the agents. Contrast agents used in MR imaging have several advantages over those used in CT. CT agents are direct agents; they contain an atom (iodine, barium) that attenuates or scatters the incident X-ray beam, differently from the surrounding tissue. This scattering permits direct visualization of the agent itself regardless of its location. Most MRI contrast agents are indirect agents and never directly visualized in the image, affecting the relaxation times of water protons in nearby tissues. The incidence of side effects due to MRI agents is very low, as the concentration and dosage of MRI contrast medium is significantly lower compared to CT [9].

Gadolinium contrast agents are considered to be safer than the nonionic iodinated contrast material. Gadolinium contrasting substances are less reactive than iodized substances, and most of them are minor and self-limiting [56]. European Society of Magnetic Resonance in Medicine and Biology (ESMRMB) classified adverse reaction to gadolinium-based contrast agent (Gd-CA) into the four groups [57]. The vast majority of these reactions are mild, including coldness at the injection site, nausea with or without vomiting, headache, warmth or pain at the injection site, paresthesias, dizziness, and itching. Reactions resembling an "allergic" response are very unusual and vary. A rash hives, or urticaria are the most frequent of this group, and very rarely there may be bronchospasm. Severe, life-threatening anaphylactoid or nonallergic anaphylactic reactions are exceedingly rare. Fatal reactions to gadolinium chelate agents occur but are extremely rare. Gadolinium chelates administered to patients with acute renal failure or severe chronic kidney disease can result in a syndrome of nephrogenic systemic fibrosis (NSF) [57].

Contrast media application is resulted in some adverse reaction in very rare cases, and frequency of the anaphylaxis or allergic-like reactions is less than 0.5% of patients [58, 59]. Late side effect reactions occur between 1 h and 7 days after administration of intravascular iodinated contrast media [60]. The most commonly identified symptoms in acute minor reactions include flushing, nausea, arm pain, pruritus, vomiting, headache, and mild urticaria [61]. Most of the reactions are self-limited, and up to the three-quarters resolve within the first 3 days and others in 7 days. Serious late reactions have been reported that require treatment at the hospital, permanent disability, or even death; however, it is very rare [60].

Nephrogenic systemic fibrosis (NSF) is a potentially debilitating disease. The exact pathogenesis of nephrogenic systemic fibrosis is uncertain, but the disease has been associated with the use of gadolinium-based contrast agents in patients with predominantly acute renal failure or end-stage renal disease [62]. The time between the initial NSF-eliciting gadodiamide exposure and the appearance of the first symptom is commonly referred to as the symptom-free, or asymptomatic period may extend from 0 to 53 days with an average of 2 weeks [63]. In most of the NSF patient, skin involvement is the initial symptom that begins with the swelling in the distal parts of the extremities [64]. Whereas some of the NSF patients have symptoms such as leg pain and swelling, pneumonitis, and diarrhea appearing more acutely within less than 24 h, the others may have more chronic symptoms like contractures that firstly appear up to 2 months. Skin thickening may be aggressive and in relationship with persistent pain and loss of elasticity in the skin and muscle. In some patients NSF may progress to physical disability, whereas some of them need to use wheelchair. In some patients, skin thickening results in contractures with the inhibition of flexion and extension in the joints [63]. The severity of the disease is directly proportional to the amount of the drug or contrast agent, but there is an exposure limit required for the patient to show the symptoms. Disease can occur even at lower doses if the agent is given over a specific dose or if the patient is susceptible to the agent. In order to prevent this disease, in MRI, it is important to choose the substance that releases least gadolinium in the body and to ensure that the agent has high stability and relaxation [65].

10.4 Image Artifacts

Artifacts are one of the most important handicap of MR images. An artifact is defined as a distortion in MRI signal intensity with no identifiable anatomical source in the imaging field.

Artifacts can be categorized in many ways; the first group is a consequence of motion of patient tissue during the measurement. The second group is produced primarily as a result of the particular measurement technique and/or specific measurement parameters. The last group is independent of the patient or measurement technique; it occurs because of the malfunction of the MR, external source, or the scanner during shooting [9].

Routine MR imaging usually involves two types of motion artifacts:

- With respiratory, peristalsis, or from the beating heart
- Pulsatile blood flow or cerebrospinal fluid (flow artifacts) [3]

Patient motion during the acquisition of a magnetic resonance image can cause blurring and ghosting artifacts in the image [66]. These movement artifacts also appear to be an antagonistic problem in other examination methods; however, the duration of the examination in MRI is longer than the other imaging techniques, which causes the artifacts to become apparent. In addition, because the routine examinations are carried out with the multi-slice technique, the motion within the examination period reflects many interactions in our examination plan. Basically, the artifact is caused by the encoding of the signal from the tissue into the wrong voxels during the frequency-coding and phase-coding gradients or by multiple coding of the same voxel. Cardiac, respiratory movements, vascular pulsations, CSF pulsations, periodic or intestinal peristalsis, and swallowing like physiological movements of the patient lead to significant artifacts in the image. The most commonly used method to remove artifacts that are caused by periodic movements today is the "physiological gate" technique (cardiac gating, breathing gating). This means that the signal is recorded only in one phase of these physiological periodic movements [1].

10.4.1 Aliasing Artifacts

Wrap or aliasing produces an image where anatomy that exists outside the FOV is folded onto the top of anatomy inside the FOV [2]. This artifact is often seen on the phase-coding or frequency-coding axis or both axes when the region under examination is smaller than the patient volume or when working with a small FOV [1]. Aliasing artifact can be reduced or eliminated by increasing the FOV, changing the gradient axes relative to the patient, and displaying only the central portion of the actual FOV, use of surface coils, or inner volume imaging techniques [67].

10.4.2 Chemical Shift Artifact

The chemical shift phenomenon refers to the signal intensity alterations seen in MR imaging that result from the inherent differences in the resonant frequencies of precessing protons [68]. Hydrogen is our target in MR images. This makes the water our target. But the oil also contains hydrogen and carbon to generate the signal. They also generate a lot of signal. We often see chemical shift artifacts as dark and shiny lines at the water and oil boundary.

10.4.3 Out-of-Phase Artifact

This is also called chemical misregistration. This artifact is caused when the precession of fat and water are out of phase. When hydrogen protons in fat and water are in phase within a pixel, the signal is produced in these tissues. When fat and water hydrogen protons are out of phase within a pixel, no signal is produced. This will be represented as a dark signal boarder around organs [2].

10.4.4 Zipper Artifact

Zipper artifacts are common in conventional MR imaging and originate from contamination of the nuclear MR imaging signal by spurious radio-frequency (RF) noise, a result of either a compromised faraday cage or faulty equipment within the scanning room [69]. A conventional zipper artifact appears as one line or a series of alternating black and white lines, giving the artifact its name. Because a zipper artifact results from a set of contaminant RFs, it fills one or more lines in the image at a given location along the frequency-encoding axis [69, 70]. In parallel MR imaging, zipper artifacts appear along the frequency-encoding axis. The RF noise also leads to reconstruction errors in the form of a subtle ghost that can overlap with areas beyond the zipper artifact. If not severe, a zipper artifact may not prevent interpretation of conventional MR images, which may cause the origin of the artifact to be ignored.

Depending on the source, RF noise and the subsequent zipper artifact may disappear and reappear at different times during the examination. First, a zipper may be visible in the image itself. Reconstruction programs recognize zippers as anatomy that should be present in the sensitivity map. Second, in addition to being seen on images, a zipper may appear during calibration scanning, which leads to a faulty sensitivity map. Both cases may lead to problems in reconstruction. In the second case, differences between calibration and imaging protocols, such as bandwidth and pulse sequence timing, change the position and appearance of zipper artifacts [69].

10.4.5 Magnetic Susceptibility Artifact

Magnetic susceptibility artifacts are the result of microscopic gradients of the magnetic field strength at the interfaces of regions of different magnetic susceptibility. Paramagnetic materials such as platinum, titanium, and gadolinium have positive susceptibility and augment the external field. Diamagnetic substances (water, most biological substances) have negative susceptibility and slightly weaken the external field. Ferromagnetic materials (iron, cobalt, nickel) have strong nonlinear positive susceptibility. There are two main effects of magnetic susceptibility [71]. First, ferromagnetic materials can lead to a strong distortion of the B_0 field and the linearity of the frequency encoding gradient close to the object. This frequency shift results in geometric distortion of the image. Second, susceptibility gradients result in different precession frequencies of adjacent protons, resulting in stronger dephasing of spins. The net results are bright and dark areas with spatial distortion of surrounding anatomy. Lightweight reduction of artifact may also be achieved using wide broadband width techniques that enhance gradient strength [70].

10.4.6 Herringbone Artifact

A crisscross or herringbone artifact is due to a data processing or reconstruction error. It is characterized by an obliquely oriented stripe that is seen throughout the image. These artifacts can usually be eliminated by reconstructing the image again [3].

10.4.7 Truncation

This artifact is also known as “ringing artifact” or “Gibbs phenomenon.” It is usually seen along the phase-encoding axis and in 128 phase-encoding step numbers (such as matrix 128 × 256). This artifact occurs in Fourier transformation, and it is not possible to perform signal sampling for the required time for the image. This artifact is often lost when using 256 phase-coding step numbers. Therefore, to avoid this artifact, the number of phase-coding steps can be increased, or the frequency-coding gradient axes can be shifted by phase coding [1, 70].

10.4.8 Shading Artifact

The signal intensity of each voxel is directly related to the radio frequency in that region. When the transmitter or receiver coil generates an unequal radio-frequency field, the signal intensity will not be equal. This artificial object is intimate in all views of the spinal column obtained with a surface bobbin because the radiofrequency field is significantly reduced from the bobbin; this significant reduction causes a gradual loss of image brightness. This type of artifact is eliminated by breaking the loop and thereby preventing the induction of eddy currents [72].

10.4.9 Partial Volume

Partial volume artifact occurs when a voxel signal represents an average of different tissues, which results in a loss of resolution. To avoid this artifact, thinner slices should be chosen, but this can lead to a poor SNR [70].

10.4.10 Artifacts Due to Metal

Artifacts caused by dental restorations, such as dental crowns, dental fillings, and orthodontic appliances, are common problems in MRI and CT scans of the head and neck. The presence of ferromagnetic metals in some dental materials causes magnetic field homogeneity, where metal-based materials form their own magnetic fields and dramatically alter the frequency of pressing the protons in adjacent tissues. The tissues adjacent to the ferromagnetic components are influenced by the induced magnetic field of the metal, so either a different frequency precipitates or fails, thus not producing a useful signal [73].

Surgical implants: The knowledge about the amount and distribution of artifacts through different implant materials in various image modalities and settings might help support the decision for choice of implant material in the clinical setting, accounting for the image modality needed for future diagnostic or monitoring purposes. Within the limits of the current in vitro study, zirconium implants are the most suitable for MRI, and only minimal artifacts are exhibited, especially in the T1W series, without a significant reduction in image quality. Corresponding titanium and titanium zirconium alloy implants exhibit large artifacts on both T1W and T2W images, leading to a reduction in diagnostic image quality near the implant [74].

Orthodontic devices (e.g., fixed or removable orthodontic and maxillofacial orthopedic devices) constitute the major portion of metal artifacts among other metallic dental objects such as metal crowns and titanium implants with regard to the extent of artifact in MRI. Various orthodontic brackets are available in market in terms of texture including stainless steel (SS), ceramic, ceramic with SS slots, plastic, and titanium brackets [75]. Not all the brackets should be removed before the MR imaging, and particular decision should be made individually considering the area of interest to be studied and type of brackets worn. It has been shown that 3M orthodontic brackets, in combination with NiTi wires in particular, cause smaller signal-free zones. In general, it is known that 3M and Dentaurum orthodontic brackets with NiTi wires generate less artifacts than SS braids with the same brackets. When nickel-free orthodontic brands are compared to nickel-containing brands, the effect on the size of the signal-free zones is not significant [76] (Fig. 10.23).

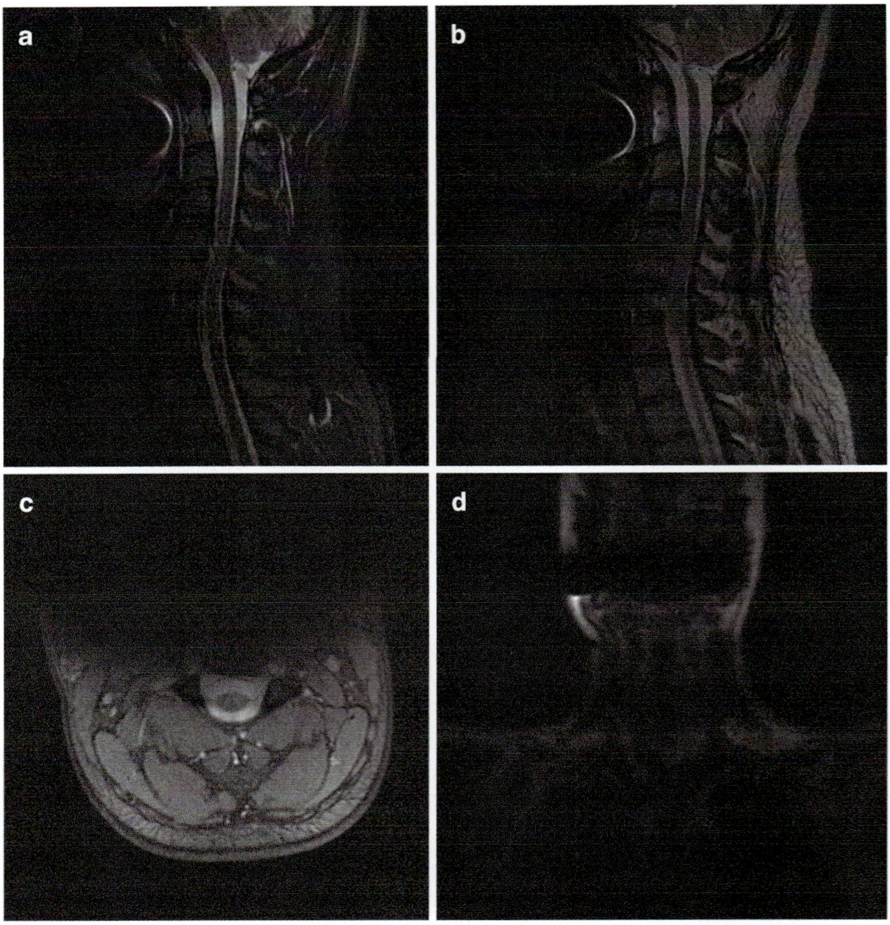

Fig. 10.23 (**a**) STIR, (**b**) T2-W, (**c**) MERGE, (**d**) coronal T1-W image showing artifact due to orthodontic bracelets' and wires

10.5 Contraindications for the Procedure

10.5.1 Metallic Implants and Vascular Clips

If a clip is made of non-ferromagnetic material and there is no concern with MR-associated heating, a patient may undergo MR immediately after implantation [77]. If the clip is made of titanium or titanium alloy, MR imaging can be done. However, if the clip is declared to be ferromagnetic or otherwise incompatible with MR, the examination must be canceled [78].

10.5.2 Foreign Bodies

If there is any doubt about the presence or location of foreign bodies, an X-ray should be taken before the MRI. The same holds true for bullets or grenade fragments. Shifting of metal foreign bodies under the influence of the magnetic field could damage vital structures such as vessels or nerves [79]. The most widely used types in clinical practice have been tested at magnetic fields of 1.5 T and 3 T and were found to be safe for MRI [78].

10.5.3 Coronary and Peripheral Artery Stents

Most coronary artery and peripheral vascular stents are made of stainless steel or nitinol. Some stents may contains variable amounts of platinum, cobalt alloy, gold, tantalum, MP35N, or other materials. That means most coronary and peripheral vascular stents are non-ferromagnetic or weakly ferromagnetic [80]. Extensive studies have led to the conclusion that MR scanning of patients after stent implantation can be performed without risk at any time at 3 T or less. However, stents generally cause artifacts that impair evaluation of the stent itself [77].

10.5.4 Prosthetic Heart Valves and Annuloplasty Rings

Although prosthetic heart valves and annuloplasty rings are made from a variety of materials, numerous studies have demonstrated that MRI examinations are safe. Even mechanical heart valves that are composed of a variety of metals are not contraindicated for MR imaging at 3 T or less any time after implantation. Depending on the amount of metal contained, there are some minor interactions with the magnetic field, but the resulting forces are much less compared to those of the beating heart and pulsatile blood flow. Sternal wires are usually made of stainless steel or alloy and are not a contraindication to MRI [78].

10.5.5 Inferior Vena Cava Filters

Many inferior vena cava filters are made of nonferromagnetic materials, whereas some others are composed of weakly ferromagnetic materials. Devices such as inferior vena cava filters are attached with hooks. As is typical for healing processes throughout the body, it is generally believed that inferior vena cava filters become incorporated securely into the vessel wall, primarily due to tissue ingrowth, within 4–6 weeks after implantation [81]. Therefore, it is unlikely that such implants would become moved or dislodged as a result of exposure to static magnetic fields of MR systems operating at up to 1.5 T [78]. Studies of MR examination of both animals and humans with implanted inferior vena cava filters have thus far not reported complications or symptomatic filter displacement [81].

10.5.6 Permanent Cardiac Pacemakers and Implantable Cardioverter Defibrillators

It has been estimated that a patient with a pacemaker or implanted defibrillator has a 50–75% likelihood of having a clinical indication for MR imaging over the lifetime of their device. These devices contain metal with variable ferromagnetic qualities, as well as complex electrical systems [77]. The real danger for pacemaker patients undergoing MRI examination is competitive rhythm in the case of asynchronously pacing generators and spontaneous, sometimes tachyarrhythmic heart rhythms. It is neither inhibition of the pacemaker nor heating of the lead tip that poses a real risk. Patients with magnet function off can safely be examined, if scanning is restricted to the refractory period of the pacemaker. Patients with non-programmable magnet function can be examined only if spontaneous beats are absent. Patients with asynchronous pacing and tachyarrhythmias should be handled in a special way, either by careful monitoring with a defibrillator at hand or by programming the output parameters to below threshold. Pacemakers with programmable magnet function should preferably be implanted, for the benefit of patients who may later require MRI examination [82].

10.5.7 Permanent Contraceptive Devices

Contraceptive devices have been tested for MR imaging safety, including intrauterine devices (IUDs) and contraceptive diaphragms. IUDs may be made entirely of nonmetallic materials, such as plastic, or a combination of nonmetallic and metallic materials. Typically, copper is the metal used in IUDs [83]. Therefore, heating and displacement might be the consequence of MRI. However, the results of various studies indicate that these devices are safe when patients are examined using magnets of 1.5 T or less. It is a general recommendation to inform the patient that displacement of the device might have occurred following the procedure, with consequently inappropriate anti-contraceptive effects. Therefore, the correct position of the device should be checked by ultrasound after the intervention [78]. The metallic component of an IUD may cause artifacts; however, such artifacts are relatively minor because of the low magnetic susceptibility of copper and relatively small size of the IUD [83].

10.5.8 Cochlear Implants

Cochlear implants are mechanical devices used for patients with severe sensory-neural hearing loss, which has an inner magnet [84]. These systems consist of complex electric and metal components. Various systems are in use, and the implantation numbers are increasing. This makes the compatibility of cochlear implants with MRI an increasingly relevant topic. Numerous devices have been tested for MRI safety. In general it is most important to know precisely which implant is present and the intended MRI procedure. Force and torque induced by the magnetic field of the MRI represent a hazard for the implant. Thus, cochlear implants represent a relative contraindication to MRI, and only after careful evaluation of the individual risk can an MRI possibly be performed [78].

10.5.9 Other Potential Contraindications

10.5.9.1 Tattoos and Cosmetics

Both tattoos and cosmetics may contain particles of iron oxides or other metals that, by interacting with the magnetic field, can cause sensations of heat, burns, swelling, or local irritation during an MRI examination [85]. If possible cosmetics should be removed before scanning. The same holds true for piercing material. If removal is not possible, an icepack/cold compress may be used. In a review of the literature, Shellock and Crues conclude that neither tattoos nor cosmetics are a contraindication for MRI, provided that appropriate precautions are taken [86].

10.5.9.2 Claustrophobia

Claustrophobic reactions happen in 1–15% of all patients who undergo an MR examination and consequently cannot be imaged or require sedation. The extent of claustrophobia is very variable and depends on the type of scanner, position in the scanner, gender, and age. When a patient reports that he or she is suffering from claustrophobia, it has to be taken seriously; besides the possible option of sedating the patient, the incidence of claustrophobia can be reduced by a factor of three by using recently developed scanners with a conical-shaped short magnet bore and reduced acoustic noise [78]. Oral benzodiazepines, prism glasses, communication devices, having a relative or friend present in the room, and music are other long-established options to reduce claustrophobic responses to MR examinations [87].

10.5.9.3 Pregnancy and Postpartum

Diagnostic imaging might be required during pregnancy for several reasons. MR procedures have been used to evaluate obstetric, placental, and fetal abnormalities in pregnant patients for more than 18 years [86]. The existing safety issues are related to possible adverse biological effects by the magnetic fields. MRI may be used in pregnant women if other non-ionizing forms of diagnostic imaging are inadequate or if the examination provides important information that would otherwise require exposure to ionizing radiation (e.g., fluoroscopy, computed tomography). If the diagnostic information outweighs concerns about potential negative effects clinically, the MRI examination can be performed with oral and written informed consent provided [78].

10.5.10 MRI and Contrast Agent

10.5.10.1 Paramagnetic Contrast Media During Pregnancy and Breast-Feeding

Although gadolinium containing contrast media cross the placental barrier, no published data of teratogenic or mutagenic effects on the fetus related to the administration of gadopentetate dimeglumine, gadoteridol, gadobenate, dimeglumine, or gadoversetamide in pregnant women exist [78].

Paramagnetic contrast media are filtered and eliminated by the kidneys; however, the mammary gland can also contribute to their excretion to a small extent, and so breast milk may contain an extremely small amount of contrast medium. With the data demonstrating the safety of intravenous and oral gadolinium-containing contrast agents in infants and the low amounts of gadolinium found to be excreted in human breast milk, it is timely to reconsider the justification for a 24 h precautionary suspension of breast-feeding following gadolinium containing contrast agent administration. The need for a 24-h suspension must be weighed against the distress to mother and infant resulting from the disruption in breast-feeding [88].

10.5.10.2 Renal Insufficiency

Nephrogenic systemic fibrosis (NSF) is a sclerosing disorder found in patients with impaired renal function after MRI examinations with gadolinium-based contrast agents (GBCA); symptoms usually develop up to 4 weeks after exposure. GBCA are renally eliminated, and so all patients with impaired renal function are at risk of retaining GBCA after exposure [89].

10.6 MRI in Diagnostics of TMJ

Magnetic resonance imaging (MRI) is claimed to be the method of choice for diagnosing TMJ involving soft tissue pathologies. MRI has been used to obtain information regarding especially articular disc position within the TMJ in patients. It provides a direct form of soft tissue visualization with excellent spatial and contrast resolution on sagittal and coronal MR images of the TMJ. The intra-articular disc composed of fibrous connective tissue and is located between the condyle and mandibular fossa. The disc divides the joint cavity into two comportments, called the lower and upper joint spaces, which are located below and above the disc, respectively. MRI can also provide essential information about position, morphology, and signal intensity characteristics of the TMJ structures (Figs. 10.24, 10.25, and 10.26).

10.6.1 MR Imaging of the TMJ Anatomy

In TMJ imaging although inflammation and fluid has low signal on T1W images, T2W images well depict both fluid and inflammatory changes with high signal intensity due to the increase in mobile protons resulting in a longer T2. The soft tissues of the bilaminar zone and lateral pterygoid attachments show moderate signal on T2W images but still lower than the T1W images. The signal returning from the yellow marrow is much lower than on T1W images due to the short T2 relaxation times of fat [90].

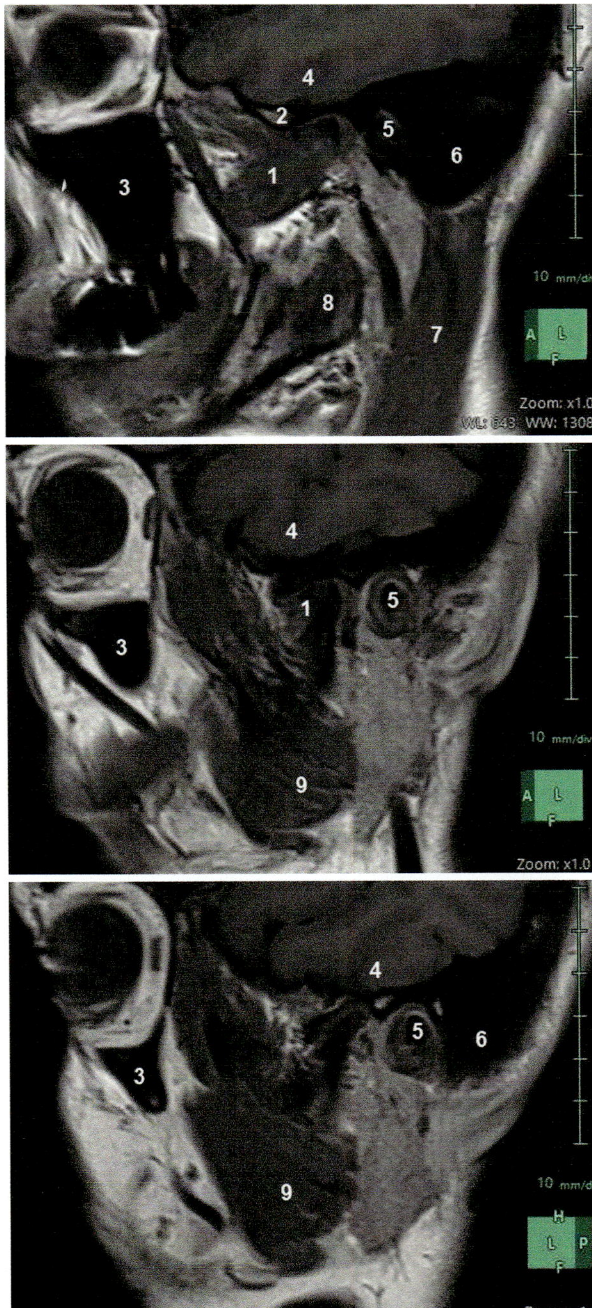

Fig. 10.24 Sagittal MR images showing anatomical landmarks. (1.) Lateral pterygoid muscle, (2.) articular eminence, (3.) maxillary sinus, (4.) temporal lobe of brain, (5.) external acoustic canal, (6.) mastoid air cells, (7.) sternocleidomastoid muscle, (8.) medial pterygoid muscle, (9.) masseter muscle

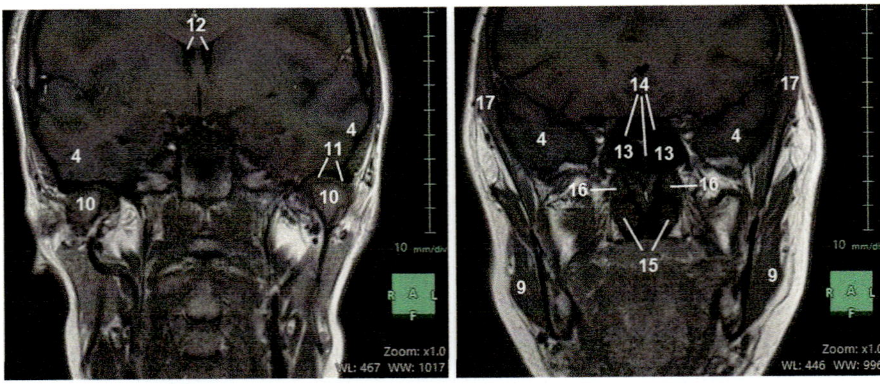

Fig. 10.25 Coronal MR images showing anatomical landmarks. 10. Condyle, (11.) disc, (12.) lateral ventricles, (13.) sphenoid sinus, (14.) sphenoid sinus septum, (15.) concha nasalis inferior, (16.) concha nasalis medius, (17.) temporal muscle

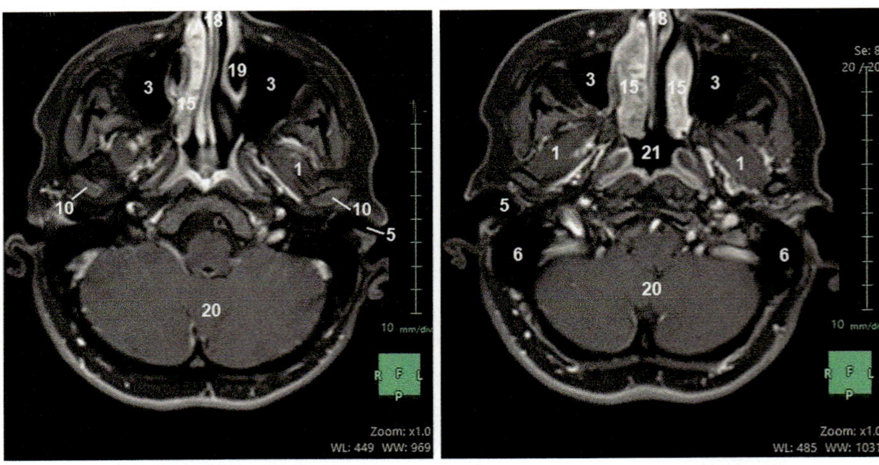

Fig. 10.26 Axial MR images showing anatomical landmarks. (18.) Nasal septum, (19.) nasolacrimal canal, (20.) cerebellum, (21.) nasopharynx

The yellow marrow within the condyle, zygomatic process, and articular eminence has a high signal due to its higher lipid content. The areas with intermediate signal are soft tissues in the bilaminar zone and lateral pterygoid attachments [90]. Temporomandibular joint (TMJ) disc presents low signal on T1W images [7, 90, 91]. Posterior disc attachment presents high signal relative to low signal in the posterior band of the fibrous disc [91].

In TMJ evaluation parasagittal and paracoronal T1W and PDW images in the closed mouth position best demonstrate the gross joint anatomy rather than T2W images [26, 92, 93]. TMJ disc still has low signal intensity unlike lateral pterygoid fat pat that shows high signal intensity (appears as bright) on PDW sequence [91]. While muscle exhibits intermediate signal intensity, fluid tends toward slightly higher or equal signal compared to muscle and cortical bone of the mandibular condyle produce low signal intensity on PDW images [94]. Also posterior disc attachments present high signal intensity in contrast to the posterior band's lower signal [91, 95].

MR allows the imaging of the TMJ structures especially evaluating the disc position in both sagittal and coronal planes and the disc movement in open and closed mouth positions [96]. The articular disc is normally biconcave in shape and has three different parts including anterior (with intermediate thickness), intermediate (the thinnest part), and posterior band (the thickest part). Normally the posterior band of the articular disc lies at the superior or 12 o'clock position relative to the condyle when the jaw is in closed position. Centrally thinner intermediate zone of the articular disc lies between the condylar head and articular tubercle in open mouth position [91, 97–99], and medial part is thicker than the lateral part [7]. Usually low signal intensity of the avascular fibrous disc is well determined between the relatively high signals from the surrounding soft tissues lateral pterygoid muscle fat pat. Similarly cortex of the condyle has no signal; however, it is well demonstrated between the relatively high signal intensity of the cartilaginous and synovial tissue superiorly and bright signal of yellow marrow in the cancellous part of the condylar head inferiorly. In the coronal oblique plane, the disc has an arc-shaped configurations and is perfectly centered on the condyle and attached to the condylar poles [91] (Figs. 10.27 and 10.28).

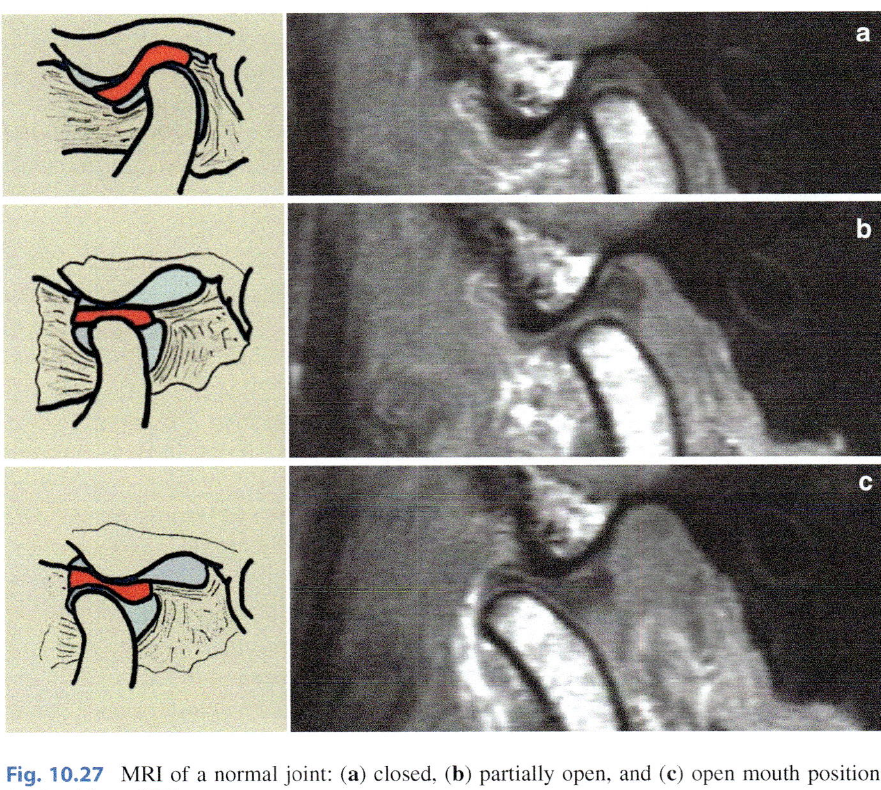

Fig. 10.27 MRI of a normal joint: (**a**) closed, (**b**) partially open, and (**c**) open mouth positions (derived from [97])

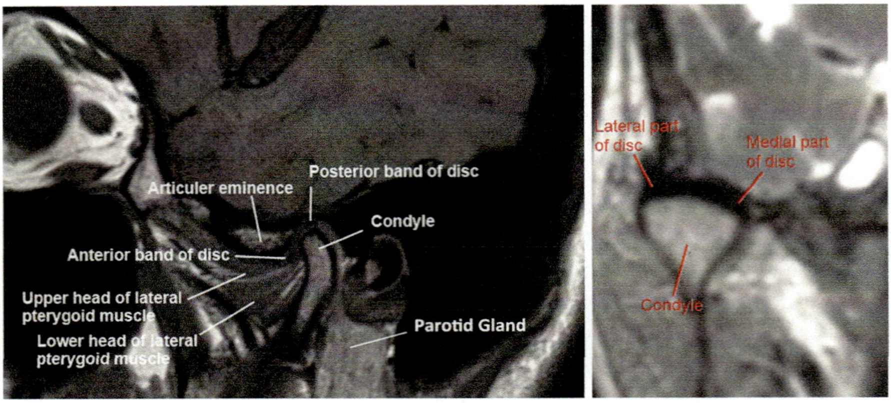

Fig. 10.28 Sagittal and coronal MR images showing the anatomical landmarks of TMJ

10.6.2 Disc Displacements

Temporomandibular disorders (TMD) are the most common nonodontogenic pain in the dentomaxillofacial region. Its prevalence is ranging between 16 and 68% and very variable depending on the study population, age, and gender [100]. However when evaluating the prevalence of joint pathology, the differences between objective diagnosis and subjective patient-reported pain are a challenging problem in terms of making a definitive diagnosis [97]. Disc displacements nearly affect up to one-third of asymptomatic volunteers in at least one TMJ [99, 101]. It is important to demonstrate the normal disc since some of the patients having TMD symptoms have normal disc [90]. In general, the most common breakdown in the masticatory system is the muscles, TMJs, and the dentition with developmental disorders. Among these groups, the disc displacements are the most encountered disorder type for TMJ.

Displacement or misalignment of the disc occurs when the disc is displaced from its normal position in relation to the head of the mandibular condyle in open and closed mouth position. Articular disc is most often displaced anteriorly. The type of the displacement may range partial or complete, uni- or multidirectional, and with or without reduction [7].

Partial anterior disc displacement (PADD): The disc is anteriorly misaligned in the lateral or medial part of the joint. The disc displaced in the medial or lateral slices but normally positioned in the other sagittal slices, which was not displaced laterally or medially in the coronal slices. If the disc is recaptured by the condyle and the disc condyle relationship appears normal when the jaw is opened, it was considered PADD [97, 98, 102] (Fig. 10.29).

Anterior disc displacement with reduction (ADDwR). In all sagittal sections, the posterior band of the disc is anterior position relative to the condylar head when the mouth is closed. While opening the mouth, the disc is recaptured by the condyle and returns to its normal position. In the maximum opening of the mouth disc–condyle relationship appears normally [97, 98, 102] (Fig. 10.30).

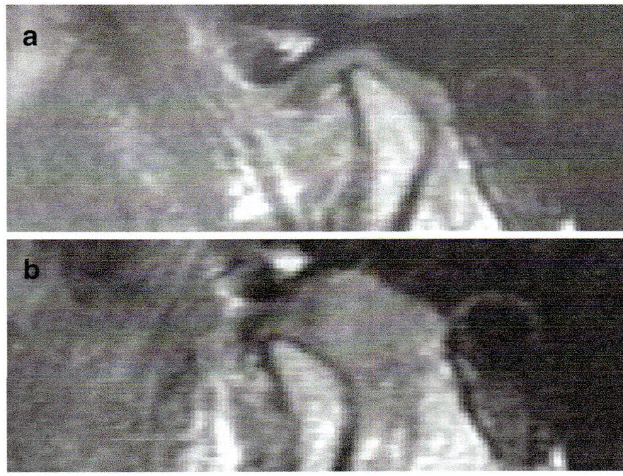

Fig. 10.29 T1-W image of partial anterior disc displacement (**a**) closed and (**b**) open mouth positions (derived from [97])

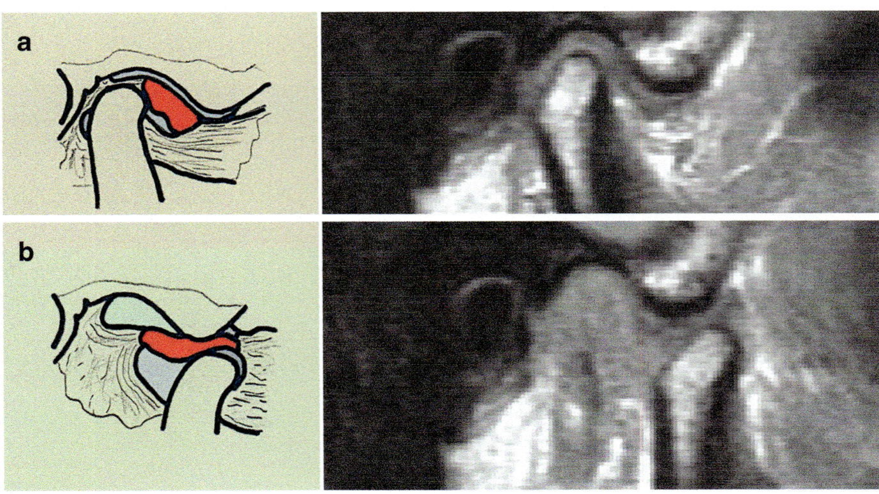

Fig. 10.30 MRI of ADDwR: (**a**) closed and (**b**) open mouths positions (derived from [97])

Anterior disc displacement without reduction (ADDwoR): In the closed mouth positions, the posterior band of the disc is anterior to the superior aspect of the condylar head in all sagittal sections and does not reduce during the mouth opening. When the jaw is opened, the disc is compressed anteriorly, regardless of whether its morphology is modified [97, 98, 102] (Fig. 10.31).

Sideways disc displacement (medial disc displacement/lateral disc displacement) (MDD/LDD without an anterior component): Sideways displacements of the disc are well depicted in the coronal plane. The disc crosses over one of the sagittal planes tangential to one of the condylar poles without an anterior component [91, 97, 98, 102] (Fig. 10.32).

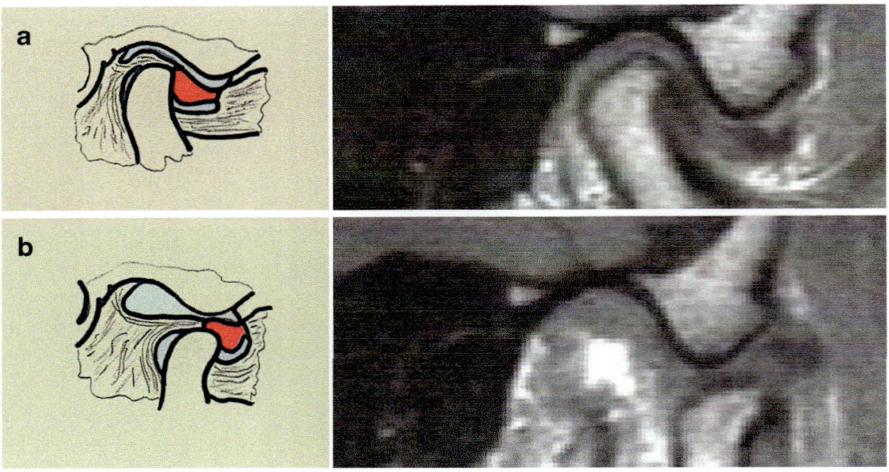

Fig. 10.31 MRI of ADDwoR: (**a**) closed and (**b**) open mouth positions (derived from [97])

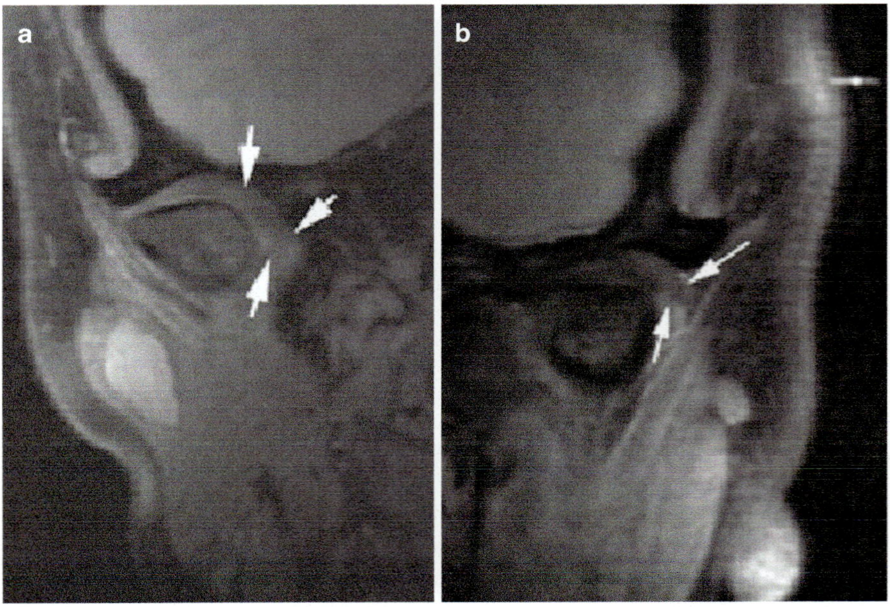

Fig. 10.32 MRI of (**a**) medial and (**b**) lateral disc displacement (derived from [97])

Stuck disc (STD) or disc adhesion: Although stuck disc is not a type disc displacement, they may occur together. A STD is defined as the disc remains in the same plane in relation to the mandibular fossa or articular tubercle during jaw movements [97, 98, 102] (Fig. 10.7).

Disc morphology may be classified into six categories: biconcave (a disc with clearly identifiable posterior and anterior bands and a tapered intermediate zone), biplanar (a disc with equal thickness in all three parts), biconvex (a humped disc), enlargement in the posterior band (a disc in which the posterior band is thicker and longer anteroposteriorly), Y shaped, and folded (irregular) [97]. Some researchers classified the disc morphology into the five categories according to disc shape: biconcave (both upper and lower surfaces are concave), biplanar (the disc is of even thickness), hemiconvex (upper surface is concave, while the lower is convex), biconvex (both upper and lower surfaces are convex), and folded (the disc is folded at the center) [102–104] (Fig. 10.33).

10.6.3 Bony Changes

Correlation between the MR imaging features and clinical symptoms of the TMD (such as pain) is still controversial. MR evidence of the joint effusion, condyle marrow suggesting edema, or osteonecrosis may be possible cause of the pain in TMJ.

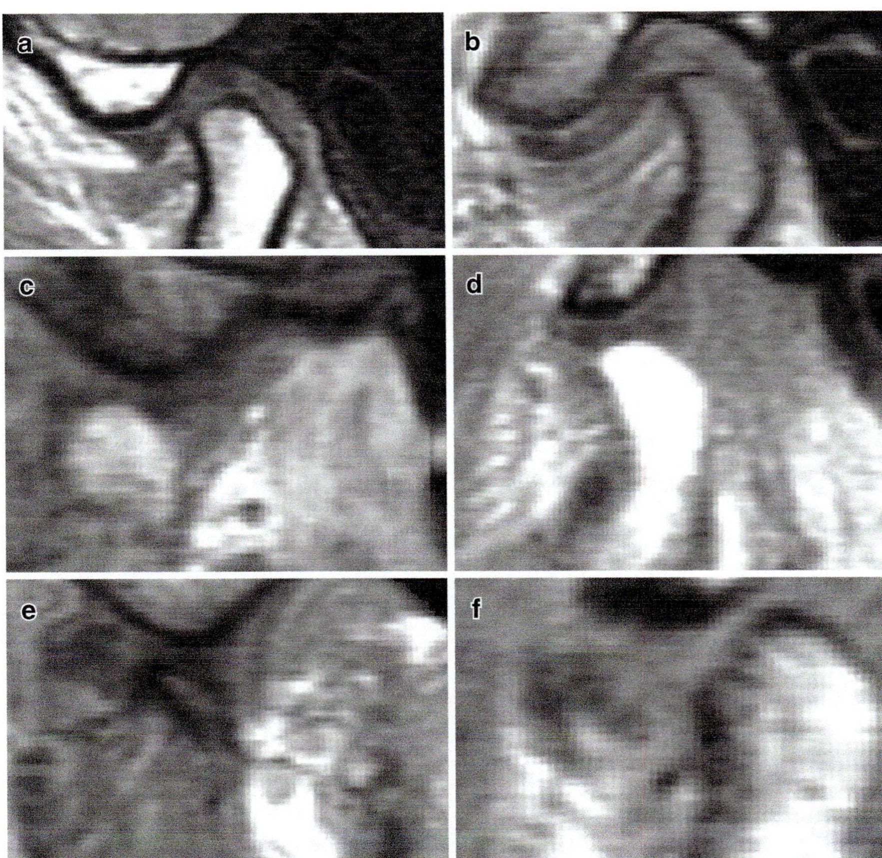

Fig. 10.33 MRI showing (**a**) biconcave disc, (**b**) biplane disc, (**c**) biconvex disc, (**d**) enlarged posterior band of the disc, (**e**) Y-shaped disc, and (**f**) folded disc (derived from [97])

For now, MRI is the only noninvasive imaging modality to evaluate the bone marrow in vivo. In MR images signal intensity is directly related to the relative content of fat, water, and cells in the marrow [30]. The normal bone marrow is hyperintense on T1W images and hypointense on T2W images. Reversal of these characteristics, decrease in signal intensity on T1W images, and bright signal on T2W images may be related with the medullary edema [92].

Bone marrow alterations may be categorized into three groups including normal bone marrow (homogeneous bright signal on proton density (PD) and homogeneous intermediate signal on T2-weighted images), marrow edema (decreased signal on PD and increased signal on T2-weighted images; edema pattern), and osteonecrosis (with decreased signal on PD and on T2-weighted images; sclerosis pattern or combination of edema pattern and sclerosis pattern; "combined" pattern) [105, 106]. Bone marrow edema may be a precursor condition for osteonecrotic development in temporomandibular disorder (TMD) patients [106–108] (Fig. 10.34).

Joint effusion which demonstrates the increased intra-articular fluid is classified into four groups including no fluid (no bright T2 signals from joint compartments), minimal fluid (dots or lines of bright T2 signals along articular surfaces), moderate fluid (more than the amount of bright T2 signals defined as minimal fluid and less than the amount defined as marked fluid), and marked fluid (equal to this amount of bright T2 signals or more) [105] (Figs. 10.5 and 10.6).

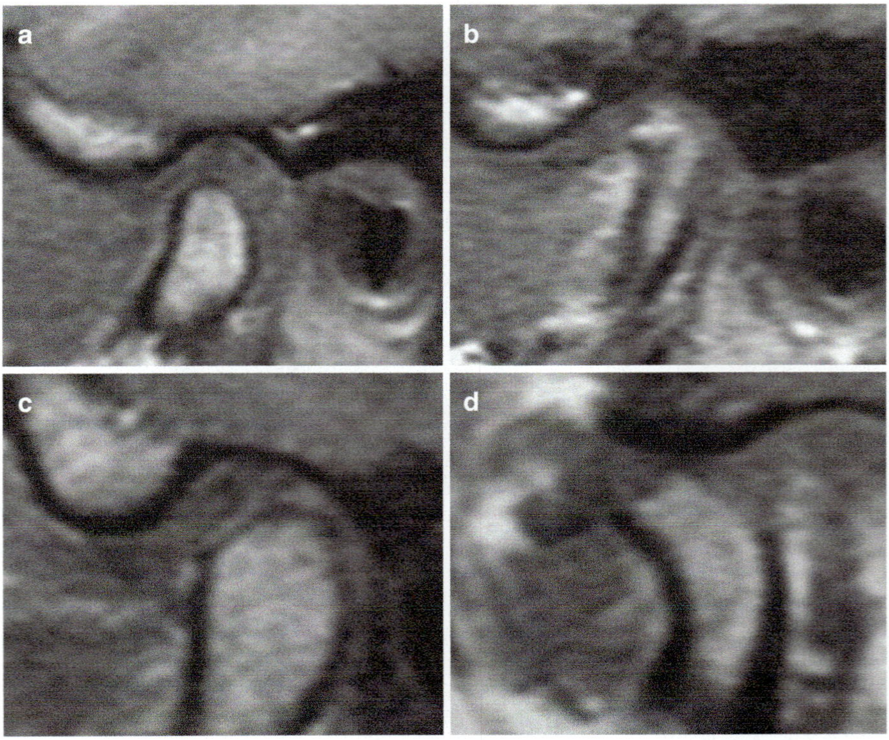

Fig. 10.34 Oblique sagittal T1-weighted MRI shows (**a**) normal condyle, (**b**) iso to high signal in condyle marrow consistent with bone marrow edema, (**c**) flattening of TMJ condyle, (**d**) mild osteoarthritis

There are many lesions both benign and malignant that can lead to bony destruction (see pathology) (Fig. 10.35). Apart from these lesions, several radiographic signs of the osteoarthritis are defined as osteophytes, subchondral sclerosis, generalized sclerosis, and cortical bone erosions [94]. Osteoarthritis

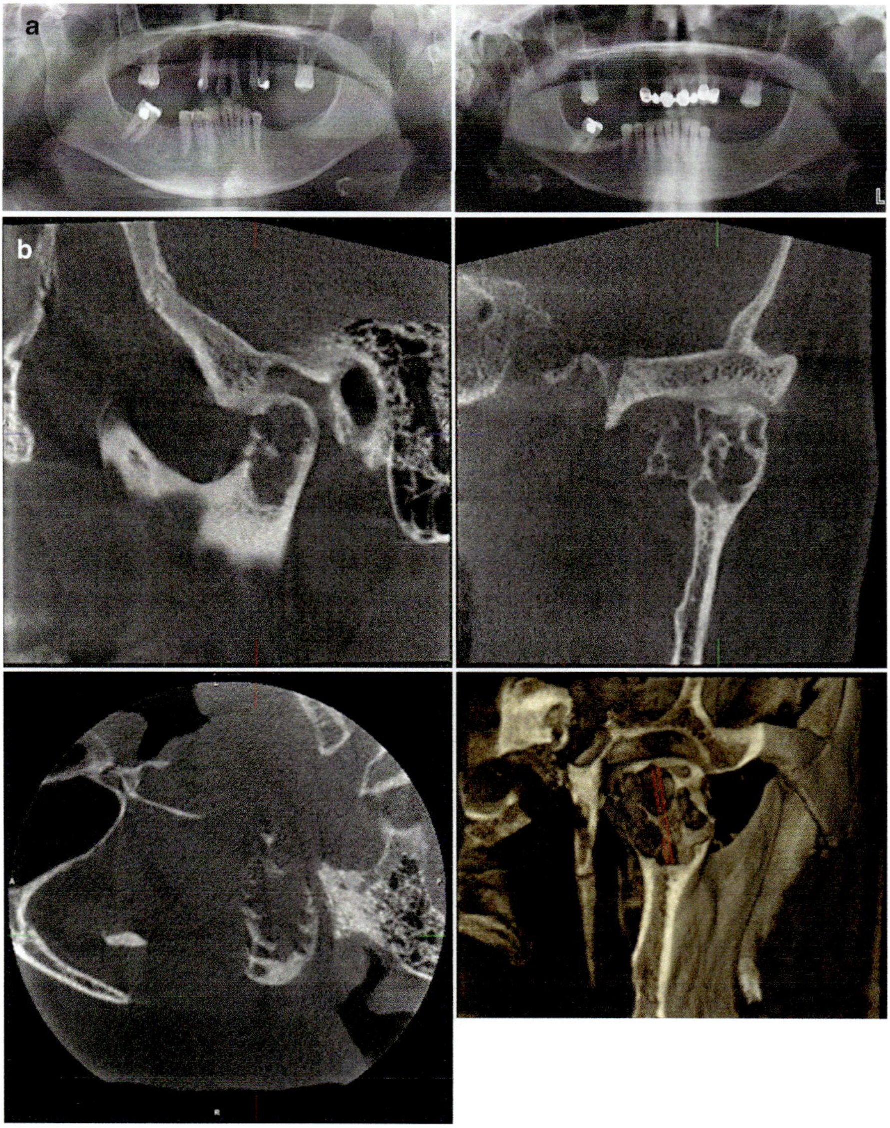

Fig. 10.35 A case of pigmented villonodular synovitis (PVNS) in a 62-year-old female patient, (**a**) panoramic radiographs in 2011 and 2017 with destruction of condyle, (**b**) CBCT images showing destruction with 3D reconstructions, (**c**) T1-W coronal image showing low signal, and (**d**) intermediate to high signal intensity in T2-W coronal image, (**e**) sagittal T1-W image enlarging mass extending around TMJ capsule, (**f**) DWI (b = 1000) showing the diffusion restriction area for the mass, (**g**) USG of the PVNS showing well vascularized hypo/isoechoic mass

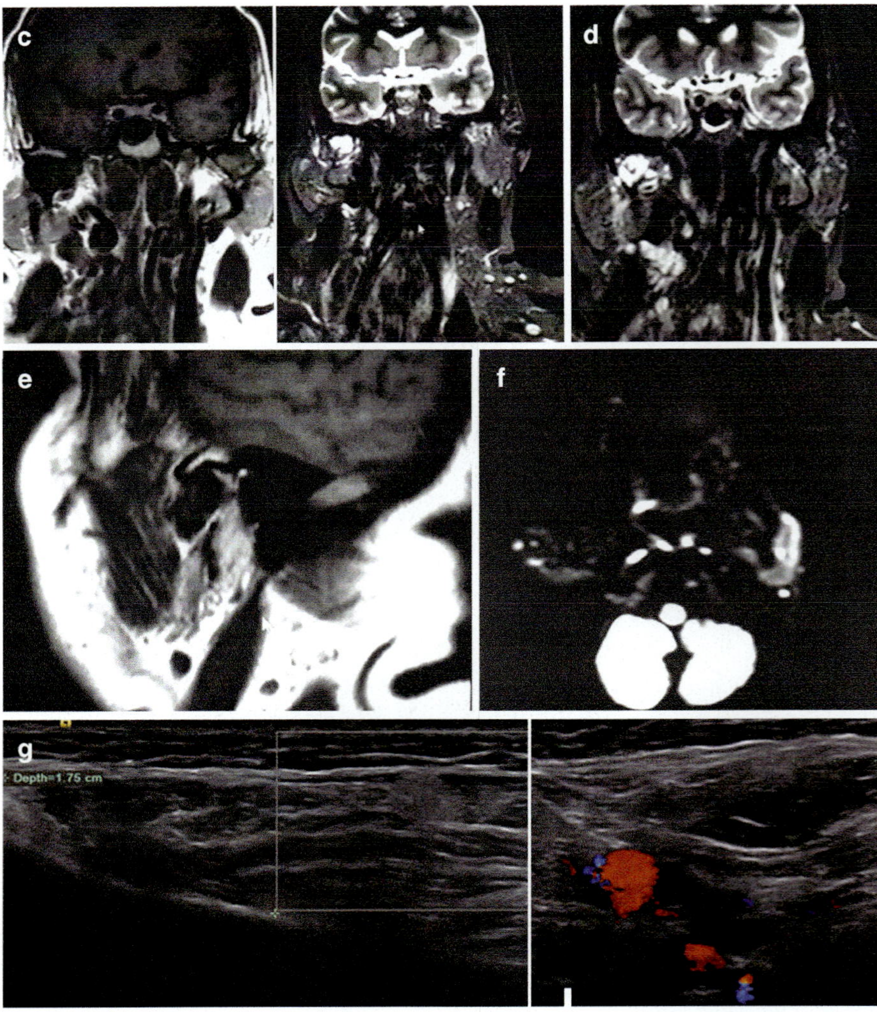

Fig. 10.35 (continued)

appears as a focal alteration (decrease) in signals on T1 and T2W images. Also focal increased signal on T2W images may show subchondral cyst [105]. Sclerosis represents low signal on both T1 and T2W images [109] (Fig. 10.36). More over, MRI is the modality of choice for confirming the diagnosis such as empty sella which shows same signal intensity with cerebrospinal fluid (Fig. 10.37).

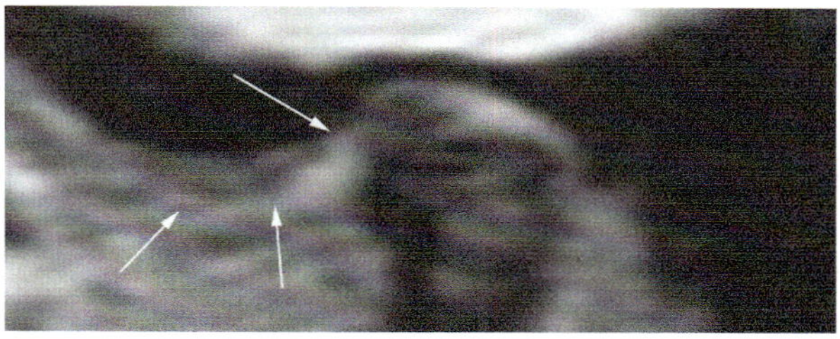

Fig. 10.36 T2-W image showing high signal intensity of bone marrow and resorption of the condyle with perforation of the disc (arrows)

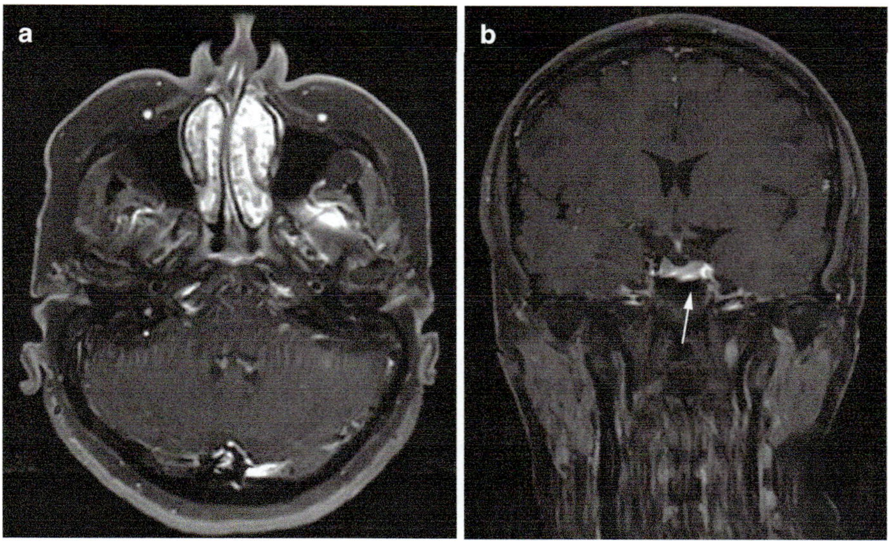

Fig. 10.37 (**a**) Axial, (**b**) coronal T1-W contrast-enhanced MR images showing a case of empty sella showing iso/high-intense signal intensity with CSF leak in the middle part of the sella (arrow)

Acknowledgments The authors would like to thank to Dr. Arzu Alan for providing PVNS images, and Dr. Melis Mısırlı for contribution of the chapter.

References

1. Konez O. Manyetik rezonans görüntüleme temel bilgiler. İstanbul: Nobel Offset Matbaa; 1995.
2. Westbrook C, Roth CK, Talbot J, editors. MRI in practice. 4th ed. West Sussex: Wiley; 2011.
3. Weishaupt D, Köchli VD, Marincek B. How does MRI work? 2nd ed. Berlin: Springer; 2006.

4. Bitar R, Leung G, Perng R, Tadros S, Moody AR, Sarrazin J, McGregor C, Christakis M, Symons S, Nelson A, Roberts TP. MR pulse sequences: what every radiologist wants to know but is afraid to ask. Radiographics. 2006;26(2):513–37.
5. Gibby WA. Basic principles of magnetic resonance imaging. Neurosurg Clin N Am. 2005;16:1–64.
6. Jacobson HG. Fundamentals of magnetic resonance imaging. Council on Scientific Affairs. JAMA. 1987;258:3417–23.
7. White CS, Pharoah JM, editors. Oral radiology principles and interpretation. 7th ed. St.Louis: Mosby; 2014.
8. Landini L, Positano L, Satanrelli MF, editors. Advanced image processing in magnetic resonance imaging. Boca Raton: Taylor and Francis Group; 2005.
9. Brown MA, Semelka RC. MRI basıc principles and application. 3rd ed. New York: Wiley; 2003.
10. Diren BH. *Manyetik Rezonans Görüntüleme temel bilgiler*. Ankara: Mine Offset Matbaa; 1994.
11. Grover VP, Tognarelli JM, Crossey MM, Cox IJ, Taylor-Robinson SD, McPhail MJ. Magnetic resonance imaging: principles and techniques: lessons for clinicians. J Clin Exp Hepatol. 2015;5(3):246–55.
12. Collins CM. Electromagnetics in magnetic resonance imaging: physical principles, related applications, and ongoing developments. 1st ed. San Rafael: Morgan & Claypool Publishers; 2016.
13. Pooley RA. AAPM/RSNA physics tutorial for residents: fundamental physics of MR imaging. Radiographics. 2005;25(4):1087–99.
14. Runge MV, Nitz WR, Schmeets SH. The physics of clinical MR taught through images. 2nd ed. New York: Thieme; 2007.
15. Dietrich O, Raya JG, Reeder SB, Reiser MF, Schoenberg SO. Measurement of signal-to-noise ratios in MR images: influence of multichannel coils, parallel imaging, and reconstruction filters. J Magn Reson Imaging. 2007;26(2):375–85.
16. Scherzinger AL, Hendee WR. Basic principles of magnetic resonance imaging-an update. West J Med. 1985;143(6):782–92.
17. Jung BA, Weigel M. Spin echo magnetic resonance imaging. J Magn Reson Imaging. 2013;37(4):805–17.
18. Mangrum W, Christianson K, Duncan SM, Hoang P, Song AW, Merkle E. Duke review of MRI principles: case review series. 1st ed. Philadelphia: Elsevier; 2012.
19. Hennig J, Nauerth A, Friedburg H. RARE imaging: a fast imaging method for clinical MR. Magn Reson Med. 1986;3(6):823–33.
20. Calle D, Navarro T. Basic pulse sequences in magnetic resonance imaging. Methods Mol Biol. 2018;1718:21–37.
21. Delfaut EM, Beltran J, Johnson G, Rousseau J, Marchandise X, Cotten A. Fat suppression in MR imaging: techniques and pitfalls. Radiographics. 1999;19(2):373–82.
22. Brandão S, Seixas D, Ayres-Basto M, Castro S, Neto J, Martins C, Ferreira JC, Parada F. Comparing T1-weighted and T2-weighted three-point Dixon technique with conventional T1-weighted fat-saturation and short-tau inversion recovery (STIR) techniques for the study of the lumbar spine in a short-bore MRI machine. Clin Radiol. 2013;68(11):e617–23.
23. Ma J. Dixon techniques for water and fat imaging. J Magn Reson Imaging. 2008;28(3):543–58.
24. Behr M, Held P, Leibrock A, Fellner C, Handel G. Diagnostic potential of pseudo-dynamic MRI (CINE mode) for evaluation of internal derangement of the TMJ. Eur J Radiol. 1996;23(3):212–5.
25. Lin WC, Lo CP, Chiang IC, Hsu CC, Hsu WL, Liu DW, Juan YH, Liu GC. The use of pseudo-dynamic magnetic resonance imaging for evaluating the relationship between temporomandibular joint anterior disc displacement and joint pain. Int J Oral Maxillofac Surg. 2012;41(12):1501–4.
26. Styles C, Whyte A. MRI in the assessment of internal derangement and pain within the temporomandibular joint: a pictorial essay. Br J Oral Maxillofac Surg. 2002;40(3):220–8.

27. Semelka RC, Kelekis NL, Thomasson D, Brown MA, Laub GA. HASTE MR imaging: description of technique and preliminary results in the abdomen. J Magn Reson Imaging. 1996;6(4):698–9.
28. Henzler T, Dietrich O, Krissak R, Wichmann T, Lanz T, Reiser MF, Schoenberg SO, Fink C. Half-Fourier-acquisition single-shot turbo spin-echo (HASTE) MRI of the lung at 3 tesla using parallel imaging with 32-receiver channel technology. J Magn Reson Imaging. 2009;30(3):541–6.
29. Morimoto Y, Tanaka T, Masumi SI, Tominaga K, Shibuya T, Kito S, et al. Significance of frequency-selective fat saturation T2-weighted MR images for the detection of bone marrow edema in the mandibular condyle. Cranio. 2004;22:115–23.
30. Orhan K, Delilbasi C, Paksoy C. Magnetic resonance imaging evaluation of mandibular condyle bone marrow and temporomandibular joint disc signal intensity in anaemia patients. Dentomaxillofac Radiol. 2009;38(5):247–54.
31. Tanaka T, Morimoto Y, Masumi S, Tominaga K, Ohba T. Utility of frequency-selective fat saturation T2-weighted MR images for the detection of joint effusion in the temporomandibular joint. Dentomaxillofac Radiol. 2002;31:305–12.
32. Barchetti F, Stagnitti A, Glorioso M, Al Ansari N, Barchetti G, Pranno N, et al. Static and dynamic MR imaging in the evaluation of temporomandibular disorders. Eur Rev Med Pharmacol Sci. 2014;18:2983–7.
33. Cassetta M, Barchetti F, Pranno N, Marini M. Comparing proton density and turbo spin echo T2 weighted static sequences with dynamic half-Fourier single-shot TSE pulse sequence at 3.0 T in diagnosis of temporomandibular joint disorders: a prospective study. Dentomaxillofac Radiol. 2014;43:1–7.
34. Wang EY, Mulholland TP, Pramanik BK, Nusbaum AO, Babb J, Pavone AG, et al. Dynamic sagittal half-Fourier acquired single-shot turbo spin-echo MR imaging of the temporomandibular joint: initial experience and comparison with sagittal oblique proton-attenuation images. Am J Neuroradiol. 2007;28:1126–32.
35. Conway WF, Hayes CW, Campbell RL. Dynamic magnetic resonance imaging of the temporomandibular joint using FLASH sequences. J Oral Maxillofac Surg. 1988;46:930–8.
36. Held P, Moritz M, Fellner C, Behr M, Gmeinwieser J. Magnetic resonance of the disk of the temporomandibular joint. MR imaging protocol. Clin Imaging. 1996;20:204–11.
37. Shimazaki Y, Saito K, Matsukawa S, Onizawa R, Kotake F, Nishio R, et al. Image quality using dynamic MR imaging of the temporomandibular joint with true-FISP sequence. Magn Reson Med Sci. 2007;6:15–20.
38. Schmid-Schwap M, Bristela M, Pittschieler E, Skolka A, Szomolanyi P, Weber M, et al. Biochemical analysis of the articular disc of the temporomandibular joint with magnetic resonance T2 mapping: a feasibility study. Clin Oral Investig. 2014;18:1865–71.
39. Widmann G, Henninger B, Kremser C, Jaschke W. MRI sequences in head & neck radiology—state of the art. Rofo. 2017;189(5):413–22.
40. Zhang S. Real-time magnetic resonance imaging [PhD thesis]. Goettingen: Georg-August-University; 2009.
41. Joseph AA. Real-time MRI of moving spins using undersampled radial FLASH [PhD thesis]. Bayerischen Julius-Maximilians-Universität Würzburg; 2013.
42. Wang X. Real-time MRI and model-based reconstruction techniques for parameter mapping of spin-lattice relaxation [PhD thesis]. Goettingen: Georg-August-University; 2016.
43. Roeloffs V, Voit D, Frahm J. Spoiling without additional gradients: radial FLASH MRI with randomized radiofrequency phases. Magn Reson Med. 2016;75:2094–9.
44. Uecker M, Thorsten H, Block KT, Frahm J. Image reconstruction by regularized nonlinear inversion—joint estimation of coil sensitivities and image content. Magn Reson Med. 2008;60:674–82.
45. Schaetz A, Voit D, Frahm J, Uecker M. Accelerated computing in magnetic resonance imaging – real-time imaging using non-linear inverse reconstruction. Comput Math Methods Med. 2017;2017:3527269.
46. Uecker M, Zhang S, Voit D, Merboldt KL, Frahm J. Real-time MRI: recent advances using radial FLASH. Imaging Med. 2012;4(4):1–22.

47. Niebergall A, Zhang S, Kunay E, Keydana G, Job M, Uecker M, et al. Real-time MRI of speaking at a resolution of 33 ms: Undersampled radial FLASH with 258 nonlinear inverse reconstruction. Magn Reson Med. 2013;69:477–85.
48. Iltis PW, Frahm J, Voit D, Joseph AA, Schoonderwaldt E, Altenmüller E. High speed real-time MRI of fast tongue movements in elite horn players. Quant Imaging Med Surg. 2015;5: 374–81.
49. Olthoff A, Carstens PO, Zhang S, von Fintel E, Friede T, Lotz J, et al. Evaluation of dysphagia by novel real-time magnetic resonance imaging. Neurology. 2016;264(87):1–7.
50. Zhang S, Joseph AA, Gross L, Ghadimi M, Frahm J, Beham A. Diagnosis of gastroesophageal reflux disease using real-time magnetic resonance imaging. Sci Rep. 2015;5:12112. https://doi.org/10.1038/srep12112.
51. Kuriashkin IV, Losonsky JM. Contrast enhancement in magnetic resonance imaging using intravenous paramagnetic contrast media: a review. Vet Radiol Ultrasound. 2000;41(1):4–7.
52. Hodgson JR. The basic science of MRI. Orthop Trauma. 2011;25(2):119–30.
53. Ibrahim MA, Dublin AB. Magnetic resonance imaging (MRI), gadolinium. StatPearls [Internet]. Treasure Island: StatPearls Publishing; 2018.
54. Czeyda-Pommersheim F, Martin DR, Costello JR, Kalb B. Contrast agents for MR imaging. Magn Reson Imaging Clin N Am. 2017;25(4):705–11.
55. Currie S, Hoggard N, Craven IJ, Hadjivassiliou M, Wilkinson ID. Understanding MRI: basic MR physics for physicians. Postgrad Med J. 2013;89(1050):209–23.
56. Runge VM. Safety of approved MR contrast media for intravenous injection. J Magn Reson Imaging. 2000;12(2):205–13.
57. European Society of Magnetic Resonance in Medicine and Biology (ESMRMB) recommendation on adverse reactions to gadolinium based contrast agents (Gd-CA). 2008.
58. Dillman JR, Ellis JH, Cohan RH, Strouse PJ, Jan SC. Frequency and severity of acute allergic-like reactions to gadolinium-containing i.v. contrast media in children and adults. AJR Am J Roentgenol. 2007;189(6):1533–8.
59. Li A, Wong CS, Wong MK, Lee CM, Au Yeung MC. Acute adverse reactions to magnetic resonance contrast media—gadolinium chelates. Br J Radiol. 2006;79(941):368–71.
60. Thomsen HS, Webb JAW, editors. Contrast media. 2nd ed. Berlin: Springer; 2009. p. 123–8.
61. Hayat MA. Cancer imaging: instrumentation and applications. 1st ed. Amsterdam: Academic Press; 2007.
62. Cheong BY, Muthupillai R. Nephrogenic systemic fibrosis: a concise review for cardiologists. Tex Heart Inst J. 2010;37(5):508–15.
63. Marckmann P. An epidemic outbreak of nephrogenic systemic fibrosis in a Danish hospital. Eur J Radiol. 2008;66(2):187–90.
64. Cowper SE, Rabach M, Girardi M. Clinical and histological findings in nephrogenic systemic fibrosis. Eur J Radiol. 2008;66(2):191–9.
65. Thomsen HS, Marckmann P, Logager VB. Nephrogenic systemic fibrosis (NSF): a late adverse reaction to some of the gadolinium based contrast agents. Cancer Imaging. 2007;7:130–7.
66. Atkinson D, Hill DL, Stoyle PN, Summers PE, Clare S, Bowtell R, Keevil SF. Automatic compensation of motion artifacts in MRI. Magn Reson Med. 1999;41(1):163–70.
67. Pusey E, Yoon C, Anselmo ML, Lufkin RB. Aliasing artifacts in MR imaging. Comput Med Imaging Graph. 1988;12(4):219–24.
68. Hood MN, Ho VB, Smirniotopoulos JG, Szumowski J. Chemical shift: the artifact and clinical tool revisited. Radiographics. 1999;19(2):357–71.
69. Yanasak NE, Kelly MJ. MR imaging artifacts and parallel imaging techniques with calibration scanning: a new twist on old problems. Radiographics. 2014;34(2):532–48.
70. Stadler A, Schima W, Ba-Ssalamah A, Kettenbach J, Eisenhuber E. Artifacts in body MR imaging: their appearance and how to eliminate them. Eur Radiol. 2007;17(5):1242–55.
71. Arena L, Morehouse HT, Safir J. MR imaging artifacts that simulate disease: how to recognize and eliminate them. Radiographics. 1995;15(6):1373–94.
72. Taber KH, Herrick RC, Weathers SW, Kumar AJ, Schomer DF, Hayman LA. Pitfalls and artifacts encountered in clinical MR imaging of the spine. Radiographics. 1998;18(6): 1499–521.

73. Klinke T, Daboul A, Maron J, Gredes T, Puls R, Jaghsi A, Biffar R. Artifacts in magnetic resonance imaging and computed tomography caused by dental materials. PLoS One. 2012;7(2):e31766.
74. Smeets R, Schöllchen M, Gauer T, Aarabi G, Assaf AT, Rendenbach C, Beck-Broichsitter B, Semmusch J, Sedlacik J, Heiland M, Fiehler J, Siemonsen S. Artefacts in multimodal imaging of titanium, zirconium and binary titanium-zirconium alloy dental implants: an in vitro study. Dentomaxillofac Radiol. 2017;46(2):20160267.
75. Poorsattar-Bejeh Mir A, Rahmati-Kamel M. Should the orthodontic brackets always be removed prior to magnetic resonance imaging (MRI)? J Oral Biol Craniofac Res. 2016;6(2):142–52.
76. Dalili Kajan Z, Khademi J, Alizadeh A, Babaei Hemmaty Y, Atrkar Roushan Z. A comparative study of metal artifacts from common metal orthodontic brackets in magnetic resonance imaging. Imaging Sci Dent. 2015;45(3):159–68.
77. Levine GN, Gomes AS, Arai AE, Bluemke DA, Flamm SD, Kanal E, Manning WJ, Martin ET, Smith JM, Wilke N, Shellock FS, American Heart Association Committee on Diagnostic and Interventional Cardiac Catheterization; American Heart Association Council on Clinical Cardiology; American Heart Association Council on Cardiovascular Radiology and Intervention. Safety of magnetic resonance imaging in patients with cardiovascular devices: an American Heart Association scientific statement from the Committee on Diagnostic and Interventional Cardiac Catheterization, Council on Clinical Cardiology, and the Council on Cardiovascular Radiology and Intervention: endorsed by the American College of Cardiology Foundation, the North American Society for Cardiac Imaging, and the Society for Cardiovascular Magnetic Resonance. Circulation. 2007;116(24):2878–91.
78. Dill T. Contraindications to magnetic resonance imaging: non-invasive imaging. Heart. 2008;94(7):943–8.
79. Campbell EA, Wilbert CD. Foreign body, imaging. SourceStat pearls [Internet]. Treasure Island: StatPearls Publishing; 2018.
80. Shellock FG, Crues JV. MRI: biologic effects, safety and patient management. 1st ed. Los Angeles: Biomedical Research Publishing Group; 2014.
81. Liebman CE, Messersmith RN, Levin DN, Lu CT. MR imaging of inferior vena caval filters: safety and artifacts. AJR Am J Roentgenol. 1988;150(5):1174–6.
82. Irnich W, Irnich B, Bartsch C, Stertmann WA, Gufler H, Weiler G. Do we need pacemakers resistant to magnetic resonance imaging? Europace. 2005;7(4):353–65.
83. Shellock FG. New metallic implant used for permanent contraception in women: evaluation of MR safety. AJR Am J Roentgenol. 2002;178(6):1513–6.
84. Öztürk E, Doruk C, Orhan KS, Çelik M, Polat B, Güldiken Y. A rare complication of Cochlear implantation after magnetic resonance imaging: reversion of the magnet. J Craniofac Surg. 2017;28(4):e372–4.
85. Tope WD, Shellock FG. Magnetic resonance imaging and permanent cosmetics (tattoos): survey of complications and adverse events. J Magn Reson Imaging. 2002;15(2):180–4.
86. Shellock FG, Crues JV. MR procedures: biologic effects, safety, and patient care. Radiology. 2004;232(3):635–52.
87. Dewey M, Schink T, Dewey CF. Claustrophobia during magnetic resonance imaging: cohort study in over 55,000 patients. J Magn Reson Imaging. 2007;26(5):1322–7.
88. Hylton NM. Suspension of breast-feeding following gadopentetate dimeglumine administration. Radiology. 2000;216(2):325–6.
89. Cowper SE. Nephrogenic systemic fibrosis: an overview. J Am Coll Radiol. 2008;5(1):23–8.
90. Harms SE, Wilk RM, Wolford LM, Chiles DG, Milam SB. The temporomandibular joint: magnetic resonance imaging using surface coils. Radiology. 1985;157(1):133–6.
91. Katzberg RW. Temporomandibular joint imaging. Radiology. 1989;170(2):297–307.
92. Alonso MBCC, Gamba TO, Lopes SLP, Cruz AD, Freitas DQ, Haiter-Neto F. Magnetic resonance imaging of the temporomandibular joint acquired using different parameters. J Morphol Sci. 2014;31(2):103–9.
93. Yang ZJ, Song DH, Dong LL, Li B, Tong DD, Li Q, Zhang FH. Magnetic resonance imaging of temporomandibular joint: morphometric study of asymptomatic volunteers. J Craniofac Surg. 2015;26(2):425–9.

94. Matthews NS. Dislocation of the Temporomandibular joint. 1st ed. New York: Springer; 2018.
95. Bag AK, Gaddikeri S, Singhal A, Hardin S, Tran BD, Medina JA, Curé JK. Imaging of the temporomandibular joint: an update. World J Radiol. 2014;6(8):567–82.
96. Brooks SL, Brand JW, Gibbs SJ, Hollender L, Lurie AG, Omnell KA, Westesson PL, White SC. Imaging of the temporomandibular joint: a position paper of the American Academy of Oral and Maxillofacial Radiology. Oral Surg Oral Med Oral Pathol Oral Radiol Endod. 1997;83(5):609–18.
97. Arslan A, Orhan K, Paksoy SC, Ucok O, Ozbek M, Dural S, Kanli A. MRI evaluation of the classification, frequency and disk morphology of temporomandibular joint disk displacement: a multicenter retrospective study in a Turkish population. Oral Radiol. 2009;25:14–21.
98. Foucart JM, Carpentier P, Pajoni D, Marguelles-Bonnet R, Pharaboz C. MR of 732 TMJs: anterior, rotational, partial and sideways disc displacements. Eur J Radiol. 1998;28(1):86–94.
99. Tasaki MM, Westesson PL, Isberg AM, Ren YF, Tallents RH. Classification and prevalence of temporomandibular joint disk displacement in patients and symptom-free volunteers. Am J Orthod Dentofac Orthop. 1996;109(3):249–62.
100. Sena MF, Mesquita KS, Santos FR, Silva FW, Serrano KV. Prevalence of temporomandibular dysfunction in children and adolescents. Rev Paul Pediatr. 2013;31(4):538–45.
101. Katzberg RW, Westesson PL, Tallents RH, Drake CM. Anatomic disorders of the temporomandibular joint disc in asymptomatic subjects. J Oral Maxillofac Surg. 1996;54(2):147–53. discussion 153–5.
102. Orhan K, Nishiyama H, Tadashi S, Murakami S, Furukawa S. Comparison of altered signal intensity, position, and morphology of the TMJ disc in MR images corrected for variations in surface coil sensitivity. Oral Surg Oral Med Oral Pathol Oral Radiol Endod. 2006;101(4):515–22.
103. Murakami S, Takahashi A, Nishiyama H, Fujishita M, Fuchihata H. Magnetic resonance evaluation of the temporomandibular joint disc position and configuration. Dentomaxillofac Radiol. 1993;22(4):205–7.
104. Taşkaya-Yilmaz N, Oğütcen-Toller M. Magnetic resonance imaging evaluation of temporomandibular joint disc deformities in relation to type of disc displacement. J Oral Maxillofac Surg. 2001;59(8):860–6.
105. Larheim TA, Katzberg RW, Westesson PL, Tallents RH, Moss ME. MR evidence of temporomandibular joint fluid and condyle marrow alterations: occurrence in asymptomatic volunteers and symptomatic patients. Int J Oral Maxillofac Surg. 2001;30(2):113–7.
106. Larheim TA, Westesson PL, Hicks DG, Eriksson L, Brown DA. Osteonecrosis of the temporomandibular joint: correlation of magnetic resonance imaging and histology. J Oral Maxillofac Surg. 1999;57(8):888–99.
107. Sano T, Westesson PL, Larheim TA, Rubin SJ, Tallents RH. Osteoarthritis and abnormal bone marrow of the mandibular condyle. Oral Surg Oral Med Oral Pathol Oral Radiol Endod. 1999;87(2):243–52.
108. Sano T. Recent developments in understanding temporomandibular joint disorders. Part 1: bone marrow abnormalities of the mandibular condyle. Dentomaxillofac Radiol. 2000;29(1):7–10.
109. Lieberman JM, Gardner CL, Motta AO, Schwartz RD. Prevalence of bone marrow signal abnormalities observed in the temporo-mandibular joint using magnetic resonance imaging. J Oral Maxillofac Surg. 1996;54:434–9.

Incidental Findings in TMJ Imaging

11

Kaan Orhan, Seçil Aksoy, Ismail Hakan Avsever,
and Kaan Gündüz

11.1 Incidental Findings in TMJ Imaging

MRI has been usually used to obtain information from the soft tissue of the TMJ especially for evaluating the articular disc and its pathology. Even if small field of view (FOV) and surface coils are used in TMJ MR imaging, it should be expected that some incidental findings may appear outside the primary area of interest. These incidental findings are common in TMJ MRIs. Orhan et al. [1] evaluated the incidental findings in TMJ MRI and found 117 incidental findings in 15% of the patients.

11.1.1 Epidermoid Cyst

Most commonly known as a sebaceous cyst but also known as epidermoid inclusion cyst or epidermal cyst is a slow-growing benign cyst which arises from the epidermis and develops out of the ectodermal tissue. Histologically the lining of

K. Orhan (✉)
Department of Dentomaxillofacial Radiology, Ankara University, Faculty of Dentistry, Ankara, Turkey

S. Aksoy
Department of Dentomaxillofacial Radiology, Near East University, Faculty of Dentistry, Mersin, Turkey

I. H. Avsever
Health Sciences University, Faculty of Gulhane Dentistry, Department of Dentomaxillofacial Radiology, Ankara, Turkey

K. Gündüz
Ondokuz Mayıs University, Faculty of Dentistry, Department of Dentomaxillofacial Radiology, Samsun, Turkey

I. Rozylo-Kalinowska, K. Orhan (eds.), *Imaging of the Temporomandibular Joint*, https://doi.org/10.1007/978-3-319-99468-0_11

the cyst contains only epithelium [2]. Panoramic radiographs are not able to show these cysts even if they are located on the dentomaxillofacial region. Epidermoid cyst usually appears as a hypoattenuated well-circumscribed cystic mass with near cerebrospinal fluid (CSF) density on computed tomography (CT) images and does not enhance after the administration of the contrast material [3]. This non-tender and dome-shaped cyst has low signal intensity on T1-W images while high signal intensity in T2-W images with focal low signal intensity debris [4]. Cyst signal intensity in MRI is varying broadly according to the composition of the cyst, but most of the intracranial epidermoid cysts have low signal intensity on T1-W images and high or equal signal on T2-W images when compared the cerebral cortex [5]. While DWI demonstrates high signal intensity, ADC maps have iso- or slightly hyperintense relative to the brain tissue [6]. Seven percent of epidermoid cyst is seen in head and neck region, whereas in oral cavity they account for only 1.6% [7].

11.1.2 Arachnoid Cyst

Arachnoid cysts are CFS-filled sacs that appear in the arachnoid membrane which is lining the brain (intracranial) and spinal cord (spinal). These cysts have low signal intensity on T1-W images, and high signal intensity on T2-W images resembles to the CSF [8]. Arachnoid cysts are usually asymptomatic and found incidentally on CT or MR images. It was determined as a CSF-like density mass in CT scans with a 0–20 Hounsfield unit (HU) attenuation values. They can cause the remodeling of the bony wall in calvaria, may compress the adjacent brain tissue, and do not enhance after the contrast material [9, 10]. It is important to differentiate the arachnoid and epidermoid cysts; both have the same signal intensity in conventional MR sequences; DWI is used in this situation, showing characteristic high signal for ECs compared with low signal for arachnoid cysts with very high diffusivity [6, 10] (Figs. 11.1 and 11.2).

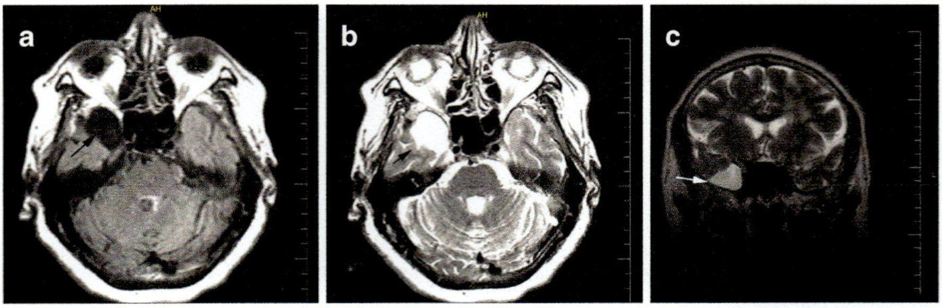

Fig. 11.1 A lesion of CSF intensity appearance displaces the temporal lobe posteriorly (arrow). T1 and T2-W images shows no enhancement. Features are characteristic of an arachnoid cyst (arrows)

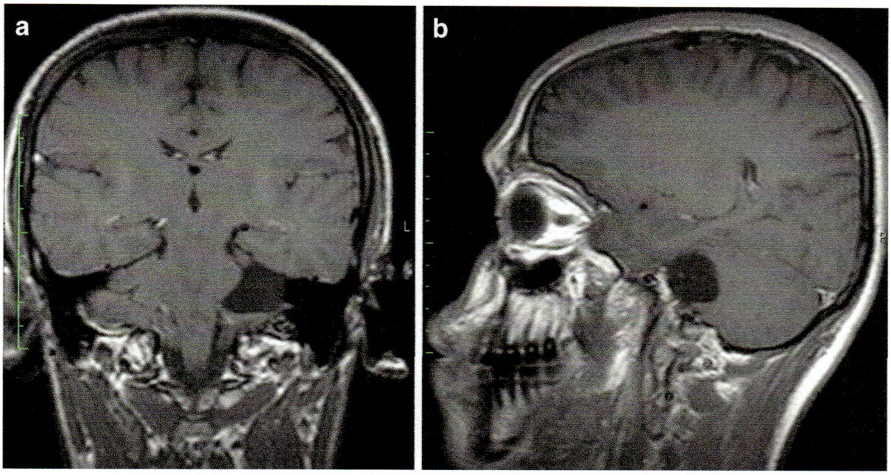

Fig. 11.2 A typical arachnoid cyst. (**a**) Low signal intensity on T1-W images, (**b**) high signal intensity on T2-W images

11.1.3 Thornwald Cyst

Thornwald cyst (also spelled as a Thornwaldt cyst or Tornwaldt cyst) is a common incidental benign lesions located in the superficial surface of the superior constrictor muscle and lined by the respiratory epithelium [11]. Obstruction of the pharyngeal bursa that communicates the roof of the nasopharynx and notochord causes the development of the Thornwald cyst [12] and does not involve the adjacent bony structures. This cyst appears as a hyperintense area on both T1- and T2-W images due to the high proteinaceous content concentration [12, 13]. If the cyst contains less protein, it will appear as hypo- or isointense on T1-W and hyperintense on T2-W images. After the gadolinium injection, the cyst content will not enhance [12]. Most of the patients are asymptomatic and found incidentally on images or while performing nasal endoscopic examination. CT images show low-attenuation soft tissue mass in the high posterior midline nasopharynx, and image characteristics are similar to CSF [12, 13] (Fig. 11.3).

11.1.4 Nasopharyngeal/Squamous Cell Carcinoma

Nasopharyngeal carcinoma (NPC) is a primary malignancy of the nasopharynx originating from the epithelial cells in lateral wall of the nasopharynx especially around the fossa of Rosenmuller and the Eustachian cushion [14–16]. Nasopharyngeal carcinoma is classified as squamous cell carcinoma and nonkeratinizing carcinoma (subdivided this type to differentiated nonkeratinizing carcinoma and undifferentiated carcinoma

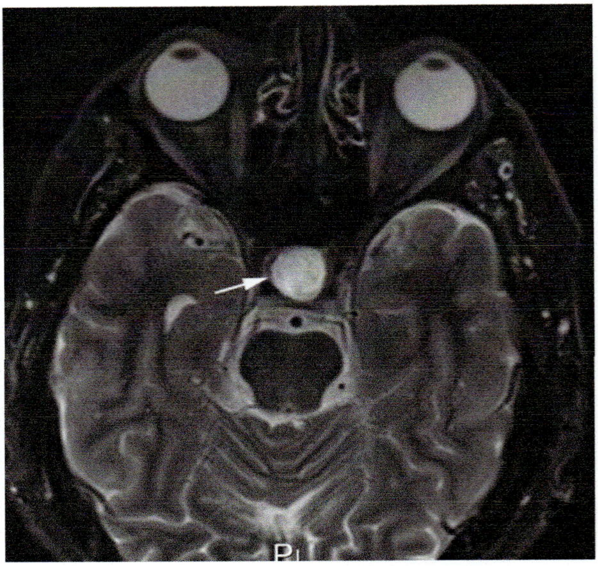

Fig. 11.3 A typical Thornwald cyst appearing on MR images as hyperintense area due to the high proteinaceous content

subtypes) by the World Health Organization (WHO) [17]. Etiological factors of this malignancy include the Epstein-Barr virus (EBV) (especially in children), genetic susceptibility and environmental carcinogens, and consumption of food (in particular salted fish) containing carcinogenic volatile nitrosamines [14]. MRI is sensitive than CT to perineural spread and for demonstrating early the bone marrow changes of infiltration (see normal bone marrow signal of the clivus), although not all bone marrow changes represent tumor extension. Signal characteristics on T1-W typically isointense to muscle, on T2-W image isointense to somewhat hyperintense to muscle fat saturation is helpful. Postcontrast sequences should be fat-saturated; prominent heterogeneous enhancement is typical. Perineural extension should be taken into consideration [18]. On CT images it is difficult to differentiate the small nasopharyngeal carcinomas from the muscles in consequent of resemblance density of the tumor with muscles [10].

11.1.5 Pleomorphic Adenoma

Pleomorphic adenomas (also known as benign mixed tumor) are the most common salivary gland tumors (accounts for approximately 60–70% of all benign tumors of the salivary glands), which mostly affect the superficial lobe of the parotid gland [19]. Pleomorphic adenoma is originating from the ductal epithelium of both salivary glands containing epithelial and mesenchymal components. The CT appearance of pleomorphic adenoma is well-defined mass that has parallel density to the muscle and shows mild to moderate contrast enhancement [10, 19]. This tumor represents various signal intensities in different MRI sequences such as relatively hypointense on T1-W images, isointense on proton density-weighted images, and hyperintense on T2-W images [20]. Pleomorphic adenomas have hypoechoic appearance compared with the normal parenchyma of the salivary gland on ultrasound (US). Also this tumor most commonly has lobulated shape, well-defined borders, heterogeneous echotexture, distal acoustic enhancement, and grade 0 or 1 vascularity. Peripheral vascularity is common in more than half of this tumor [21]. Ultrasound elastography shows generally heterogeneous stiff appearance, but this feature is not specific for the pleomorphic adenoma and may be seen also in a significant portion of the malignant tumor [22]. Klintworth et al. [23] defined specific elastographic findings for parotid gland tumors, and they reported that "dens core" sign (with a central zone of very stiff tissue with softer tissue in the vicinity) is specifically related with pleomorphic adenoma (Fig. 11.4).

11.1.6 Warthin's Tumor

Warthin's tumor, also known as a papillary cystadenoma lymphomatosum, adenolymphoma, lymphomatous adenoma, is the second most common benign neoplasm of the salivary gland and is arising from the ductal component of them [20]. More males than females suffer from this tumor, and it is found bilaterally in 10% of patients [18]. Warthin's tumor has low signal intensity on T1-W images compared with the high signal intensity of the parotid gland. On T2-W images tumor is heterogeneous and variable in signal intensity [10]. On CT scans, tumor density is equivalent to soft tissue or cystic density [20]. This tumor has hypoechoic appearance on US like the pleomorphic adenoma comparing with the normal parenchyma. Characteristic sonographic features of the Warthin's tumor include generally oval shape, well-defined borders, distal acoustic enhancement, heterogeneous echotexture, and grade 2 or 3 vascularity with central or mixed perfusion. Also more than half of the tumors have cystic areas [21]. Klintworth et al. [23] reported that "half-half" sign (with a stiff area located in the superficial half of a lesion while the deeper part has a softer appearance) is specifically related with Warthin's tumor.

11.1.7 Oncocytoma

Oncocytoma is a rare benign tumor arising from large, eosinophilic, granular, polygonal epithelial cells. This tumor usually occurs in the eighth decade of life with a slightly female predominance [24]. This tumor has variable tissue signal on different MR sequences such as relatively hypointense on T1-W images, intermediate on fat-saturated T2-W, and postcontrast T1-W images [10]. CT scans demonstrate the homogeneous well-circumscribed tumoral mass showing moderate enhancement after the contrast material administration [25]. This tumor has no specific imaging features and represents well-defined, hypoechoic solid mass with posterior enhancement on US [26].

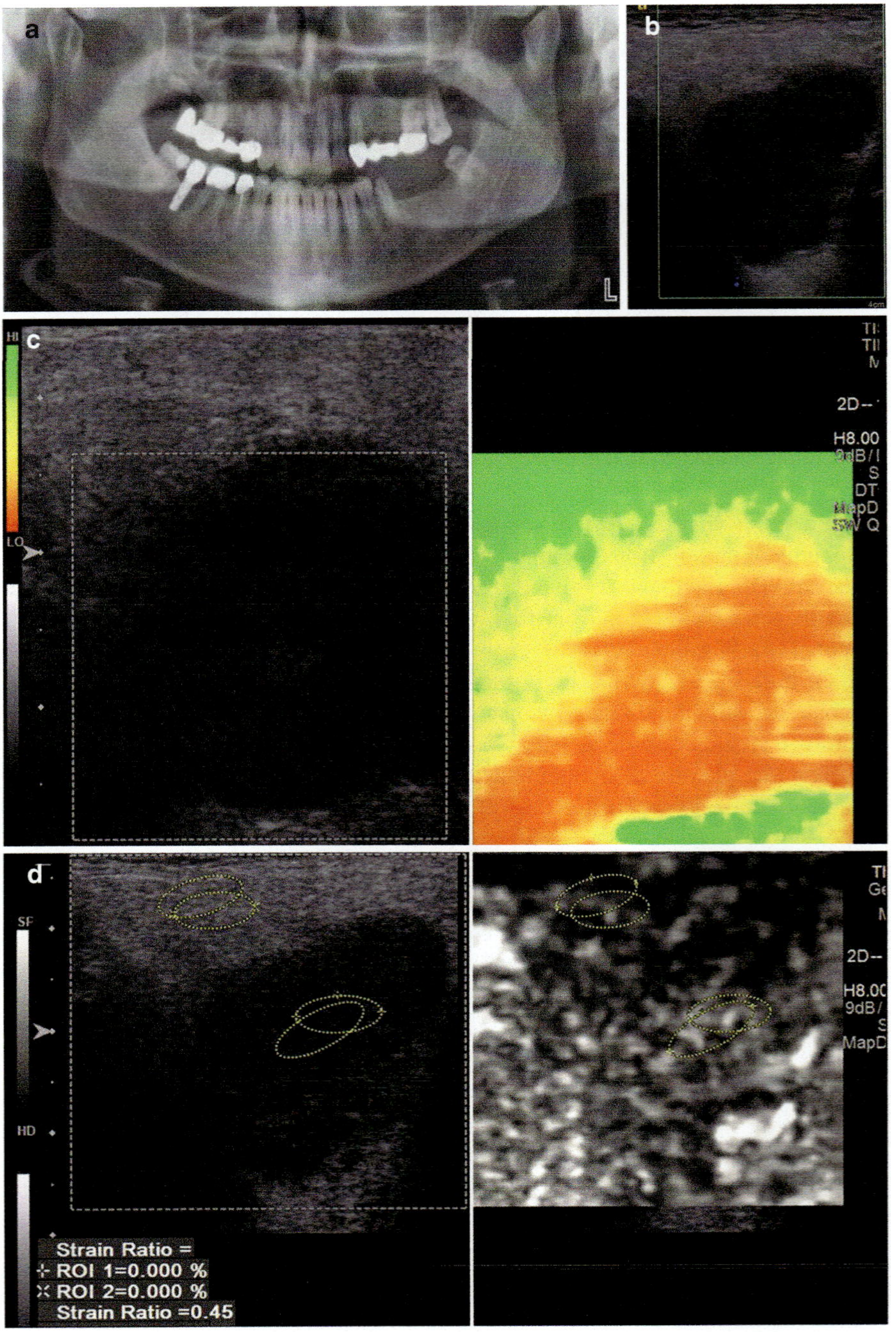

Fig. 11.4 (**a**) Panoramic radiography of a 45-year-old male patient who presented with pain, swelling, and limited mouth opening in right TMJ. The panoramic radiography showing flattening of both TMJs, (**b**) USG of the right parotid region revealed a huge mass in the parotid gland with hypoechoic nature, (**c**) sonoelastography of the lesion revealed an intermedia but predominantly soft lesion, (**d**) strain ration of the lesion, later diagnosed as pleomorphic adenoma of the parotid gland

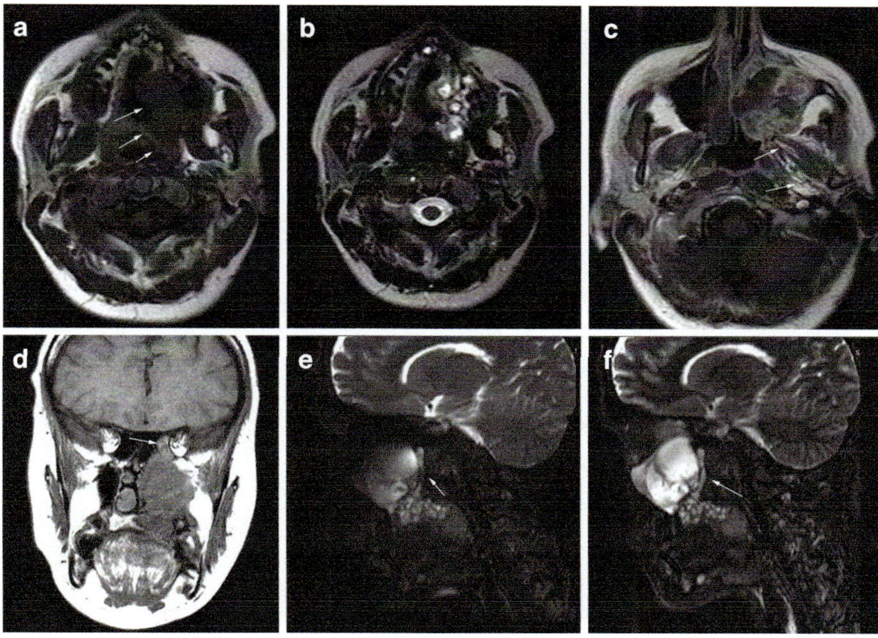

Fig. 11.5 A 28-year-old female patient with adenoid cystic carcinoma, (**a**) T1-W image isointense to hypointense compared to muscles (arrow), (**b**) T2-W image high signal intensity with different signal intensity areas, (**c**) T1 C+ Mr. showing the spread of the tumor into the masticator space through TMJ area, (**d**) coronal T1-W image showing the extend and spread of the lesion into cranial fossa, (**e**) T2-W images showing perineural spread using fossa pterygopalatine (arrow), (**f**) STIR images also showing clearly perineural spread (arrow)

11.1.8 Adenoid Cystic Carcinoma

Adenoid cystic carcinoma (ACC) is a malignant tumor of secretory glands and most commonly located in major and minor salivary glands. ACC accounts for 23% of malignant salivary gland tumors, but most of the tumors occur in the minor salivary gland [20]. Most common localization of the ACC is hard palate [27]. Perineural invasion of ACC is more common and allows the tumors to spread the parapharyngeal space or intracranial tissues that can be determined with MRI or CT [19]. CT scans demonstrate the ACC isodense to muscle [10]. This tumor has no specific imaging features and represents hypoechoic cystic mass on US images. Postcontrast MRI demonstrates the nerve enhancement and enlargement in perineural invasion [20]. This tumor has intermediate signal intensity on T1-W images and slightly high signal intensity on T2-W images [28] (Fig. 11.5).

11.1.9 Lymphomas of Major Salivary Glands

Lymphomas generally occur with the neoplastic proliferation of the lymphoid cells in lymph nodes. However lymphomas arise not only from the lymph nodes but also

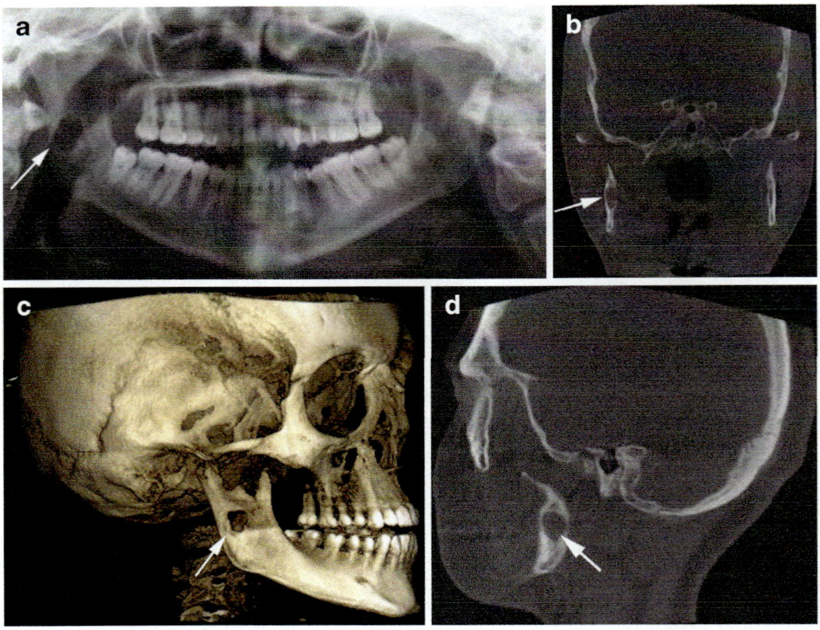

Fig. 11.6 (**a**) Panoramic radiography of 24-year-old female patient who presented with pain and limited mouth opening around TMJ, showing a solitary radiolucent lesion in the ramus of the mandible, (**b**) coronal CBCT image showing the thinning of the cortex of the mandible from the lingual region, (**c, d**) 3D and sagittal representation of the lesion. The lesion was diagnosed as histopathologically a rare plasmacytoma case

from the extranodal areas such as salivary gland, Waldeyer ring, gastrointestinal system, bone and tonsils, etc. [20]. Among them, the most common site of extranodal localization is parotid and submandibular gland [29]. Primary location of the neoplastic proliferation of the lymphoid cells in the salivary gland is rare with an incidence of 1.7–7.7% of all major salivary gland tumors. This tumor affects predominantly females [24]. This tumor is isodense compared with the muscle and has well-circumscribed margins on CT scans. But extranodal extensions have less well-defined borders and necrosis areas. On MRI lymphomas are hypointense on T1-W images and hypo- to hyperintense on T2-W images [30]. US features of the non-Hodgkin's lymphoma include hypoechoic lymphomatous node with peripheral and hilar vascularity [31] (Figs. 11.6, 11.7, and 11.8).

11.1.10 Astrocytoma

Astrocytomas are malignant tumors of the brain and spinal cord that originate from immortalized astrocytes which are a particular kind of glial cells, star-shaped cells in the cerebrum and spinal cord. These tumors are classified into the four World Health Organization (WHO) categories: Grade I includes pilocytic astrocytoma and subependymal giant cell astrocytoma; Grade II includes pleomorphic

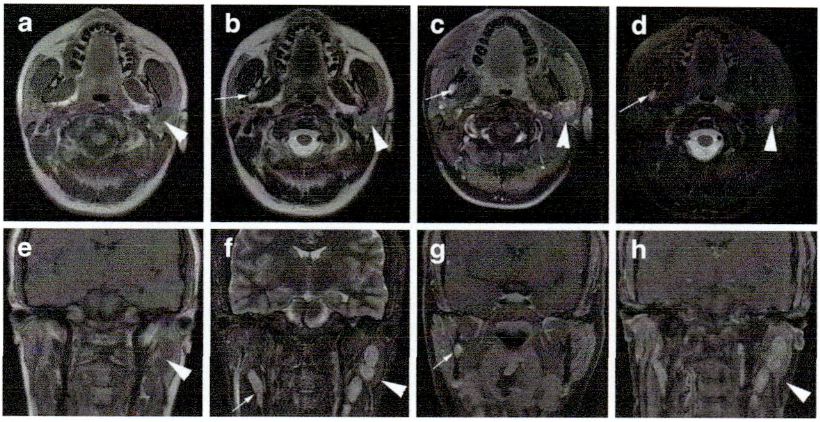

Fig. 11.7 (**a–d**) MR images of the same plasmacytoma case who incidentally diagnosed as non-Hodgkin's lymphoma in the left parotid gland. Axial T1 image showing the lesion isointense to muscle. This lobulated lesion does involve the tail of the parotid gland. The mass shows high T2 signal, enhancement, and diffusion restriction (arrow head) and the right site arrow showing the plasmacytoma in the right ramus of the mandible. (**e–h**) The lesion is enhancing, multi-lobulated mass arising largely posteroinferior to the right parotid gland but involving the parotid tail consistent with multiple enlarged lymph nodes (arrow head); the corresponding site plasmacytoma in the mandible can also be seen on coronal T1-weighted images (arrow)

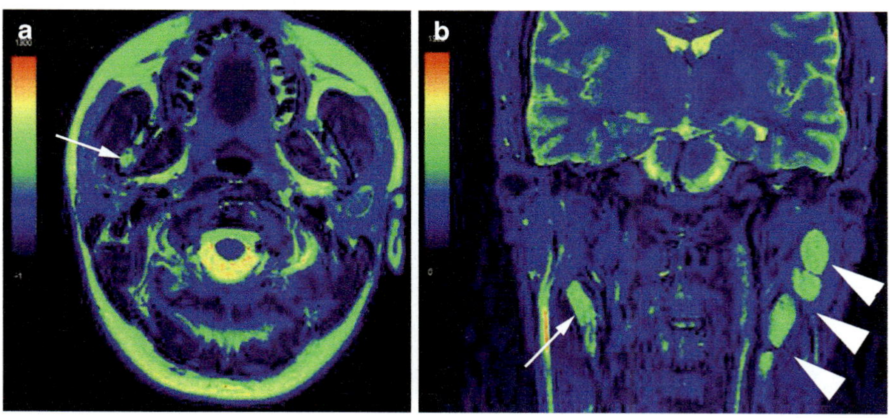

Fig. 11.8 (**a, b**) MR perfusion images; axial and coronal color ADC map shows the lesions as enhancing lesion with high ADC and a solid lesion (arrow) with intermediate ADC

xanthoastrocytoma, oligodendroglioma, and diffuse astrocytoma; Grade III includes anaplastic astrocytoma, anaplastic oligodendroglioma, and anaplastic pleomorphic xanthoastrocytoma; and Grade IV includes glioblastoma and diffuse midline glioma [32]. Spinal cord astrocytomas peak at third and fifth decades of life with a slightly male predominance. MRI is useful to demonstrate spinal cord edema, drop metastasis, and leptomeningeal spread [33]. Low-grade astrocytomas are determined as ill-defined areas of decreased attenuation involving the white matter on CT scans [34]. Low-grade astrocytomas are best seen on MRI with multimodality images.

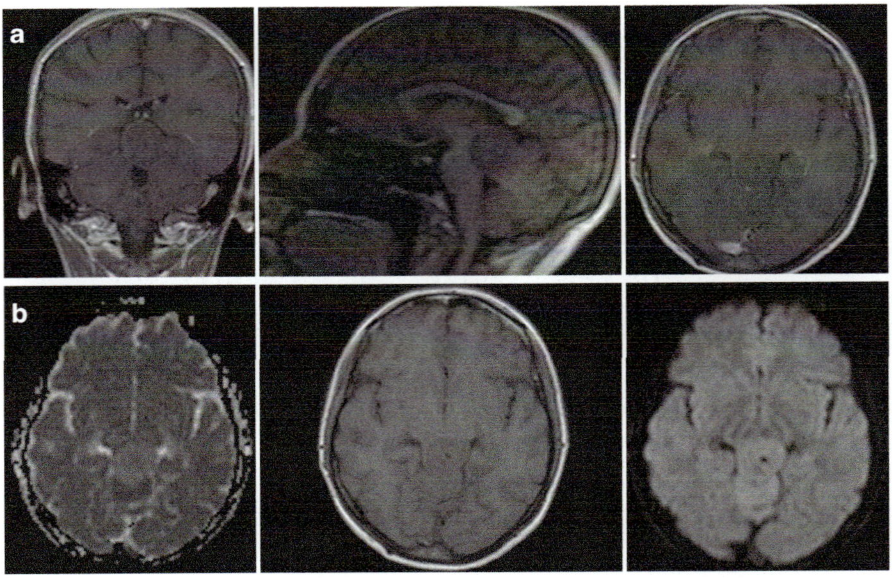

Fig. 11.9 An 18-year-old female patient with low-grade astrocytoma referred for temporal and TMJ pain. (**a**) T1-W image shows a lesion isointense to hypointense compared to white matter. (**b**) DWI has facilitated diffusion, with lower ADC values (arrows) with microcystic change which is a unique behavior for the infiltrative astrocytoma

T1-W image is isointense to hypointense compared to white matter and causes expansion of the adjacent cortex. T2/FLAIR is usually mass-like hyperintense signal. The "microcystic changes" along the lines of spread of the infiltrative astrocytoma are a unique behavior for the infiltrative astrocytoma. DWI/ADC typically has expedited diffusion, with lower ADC values suggesting a higher-grade tumor. Contrast is usually no enhancement, but small ill-defined areas of enhancement are not rare; however, when enhancement is seen, it should be considered as a warning sign for progression to a higher grade (Fig. 11.9).

11.1.11 Meningioma

Meningiomas are usually slow-growing tumors that develop from the meninges that surround the brain and spinal cord. This tumor is classified into three WHO categories: Grade I includes meningioma, Grade II includes atypical meningioma, and Grade III includes anaplastic (malignant) meningioma [32]. From these types approximately 80% of the cases occur in Grade I (benign) [24]. Incidental detection of asymptomatic meningiomas is getting higher with the advanced imaging modalities. Some of the conditions may be related with the growing tumor such as gender, hyperintensity on T2-W images, tumor size at the initial diagnosis, and tumor with no calcification [35]. On unenhanced CT, the tumor appears as hyperdense or isodense mass compared with the adjacent brain tissue and shows homogeneous enhancement after contrast material administration [19]. Spinal meningioma shows

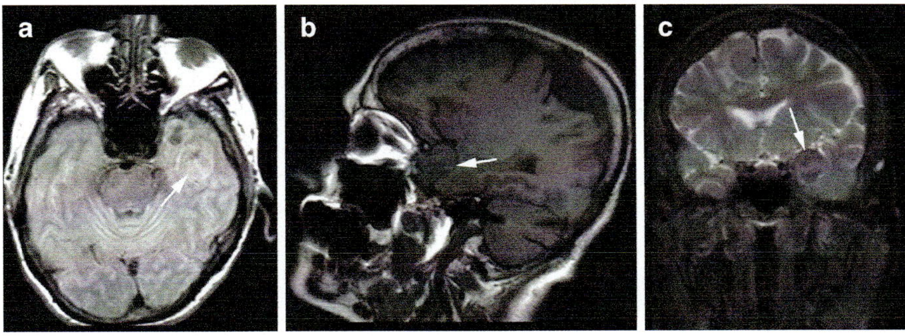

Fig. 11.10 (**a**) PD TSE TRA image showing isointense image in the left temporal region, (**b**) T1-W image showing same isointense image, (**c**) T2-W image showing heterogenous iso- to high-intensity meningioma

isointensity relative to the spinal cord parenchyma on T1- and T2-W images [33]. Diffusion-weighted images may be useful for differentiating Grade I tumor from Grade II/III [36] (Fig. 11.10).

11.1.12 Hemangiopericytoma

Hemangiopericytoma is a kind of soft tissue sarcoma that arises from the Zimmerman's pericytes surrounding the blood vessels in various parts of the body [37] but predominantly located in the lower extremities, pelvis, or retroperitoneum [38]. Hemangiopericytomas have no gender predilection with a mean presentation in sixth and seventh decades of life [37]. Only 15% and 25% of the hemangioma-pericytomas occur in the head and neck region [39]. On CT scans, hemangiopericytomas reveal round homogeneous masses with a sharp outline and often displace the adjacent structures [40, 41]. On T1-W images tumor shows intermediate signal intensity relative to the gray matter; after the gadolinium administration, it enhances heterogeneously [24]. Contrast T1-W images shows intense enhancement and heterogeneous signal intensity. There may be a dural tail sign in Grade II tumors. On T2-W images the lesion is isointense to gray matter multiple flow voids on MRI. DWI shows an intermediate restricted diffusion.

11.1.13 Osteoma

It is still unclear if osteomas are benign tumors or hamartomas. Osteomas originate from the cartilage and embryonal periosteum that are usually nodular or pedunculated polyp attached to the bone with a narrow stalk. It occurs almost exclusively in the head and neck region, particularly in the posterior mandible and also in paranasal sinuses especially in frontal sinuses and are most often encountered after 40 years of age [20]. Multiple osteomas which develop in the head and neck region and multiple epidermoid cysts of the skin and polyposis of the colon and rectum are the part of the Gardner syndrome [19, 20]. Histologically osteomas are divided into (1) ivory or compact osteoma, (2) spongious or trabecular osteoma, and (3) combination of the first two types [20, 42]. On MR T1-W and T2-W images, the ivory osteoma appears as a hypointense area and may be misinterpreted as air within the paranasal sinuses or nasal fossae [42]. While the CT appearance of the compact osteoma is very dense calcified, well-defined lesions, trabecular osteoma's density is changing depending on the fibrous component of the lesion [19, 42].

11.1.14 Cholesteatoma

Cholesteatoma is a destructive and expanding well-demarcated noncancerous cystic lesion consisting of keratinizing squamous epithelium in the middle ear and/or mastoid process [43, 44]. Cyst cavity is filled with the keratinous debris [45]. Cholesteatomas may be classified as either congenital or acquired types. Congenital cholesteatomas are derived from persistent embryologic remnants in the form of epithelial foci in the middle ear [44]. The pathogenesis of acquired cholesteatoma is explained on the invagination of the tympanic membrane, basal cell hyperplasia, epithelial in-growth through perforation, and squamous metaplasia of middle ear epithelium [43]. CT scans demonstrate the expansile nonenhancing hypodense lesions with neighboring smooth bony erosion [18]. Generally cholesteatomas have nonspecific signal intensity on basic MRI sequences, but non-echo planar diffusion-weighted imaging is more specific to diagnose these lesions and differentiate the primer and recurrent cholesteatoma. Cholesteatomas have high signal relative to the brain tissue on DWI [46, 47].

For cholesteatomatous tissue on MRI shows an intermediate to hypointense signal on T1-W images and appears hyperintense on the corresponding T2-W images. This hyperintensity is, however, significantly less as compared to that seen in inflammatory lesions [48]. Diffusion-weighted MRI is particularly sensitive to cholesteatoma tissue especially in diagnosis of intracranial and extracranial epidermoid cysts as middle ear cholesteatomas have similar histopathological characteristics to epidermoid cysts; this MR sequence should be used for evaluations such pathologies. Non-echo planar DWI for cholesteatoma diagnosis can be performed on 1.5 T or 3 T scanners indifferently. High sensitivity and negative predictive value and relatively lower specificity and positive predictive value are achieved by a single non-echo planar DWI protocol [49] (Fig. 11.11).

11.1.15 Fibrosarcoma

Fibrosarcoma is a malignant spindle cell tumor of fibrous connective tissue with herringbone architecture or interlacing fascicular pattern without expression of other connective tissue cell markers [50–53]. Fibrosarcomas have no sex predilection with a mean age in fourth decade [20]. Clinical diagnosis of the soft tissue sarcoma in the head and neck region is often a challenging problem due to growing in a considerable size without any symptoms, and even if the symptoms is present,

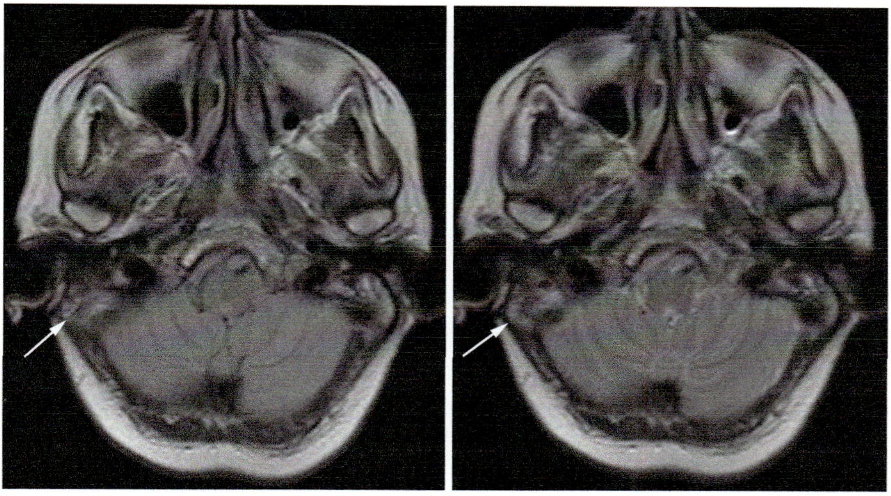

Fig. 11.11 Temporal bone, acquired cholesteatoma. T1-weighted axial MRI shows a soft tissue mass in the region of the right tegmen tympani (arrows)

it may be frequently overlooked as dental problem such as TMD [51, 52, 54]. On CT scans fibrosarcomas are determined as an isodense attenuating soft tissue masses. On T1-W images fibrosarcomas have low signal intensity and on T2-W images show both low and high signal intensity (heterogeneous) together in comparison with adjacent muscle [55].

11.1.16 Otomastoiditis

Otomastoiditis that can be classified into two distinct entities: acute and chronic otomastoiditis is an inflammatory disease of the middle air and mastoid air cells. While acute otomastoiditis may be related with the leukemia, mononucleosis, sarcoma of the temporal bone, and Kawasaki disease, chronic otomastoiditis is thought to be primarily due to Eustachian tube dysfunction [56–58]. Acute otomastoiditis presents opacification of the mastoid air cells [57, 58]. CT scans demonstrate the mastoid air cells filled with the soft tissue mass instead of the air [59]. MRI can be used for evaluating the otomastoiditis, however, with solely MRI it is difficult to diagnose the infection related to mastoid region. MRI characteristic of acute otomastoiditis are nonspecific debris within the middle ear and mastoid, possibly with several fluid levels which can be seen bright signal areas on T2-weighted images. For chronic otomastoiditis with cholesteatoma, MR signal characteristics are nonspecific; ordinarily, both T1 and T2 relaxation times are relatively long [57, 58]. Signal characteristics are mostly low signal on T1-W and high signal on T2-W images. DWI/ADC diffusion restriction may be present; mucosal contrast enhancement is present in the majority of the cases on T1-W contrast images (Fig. 11.12).

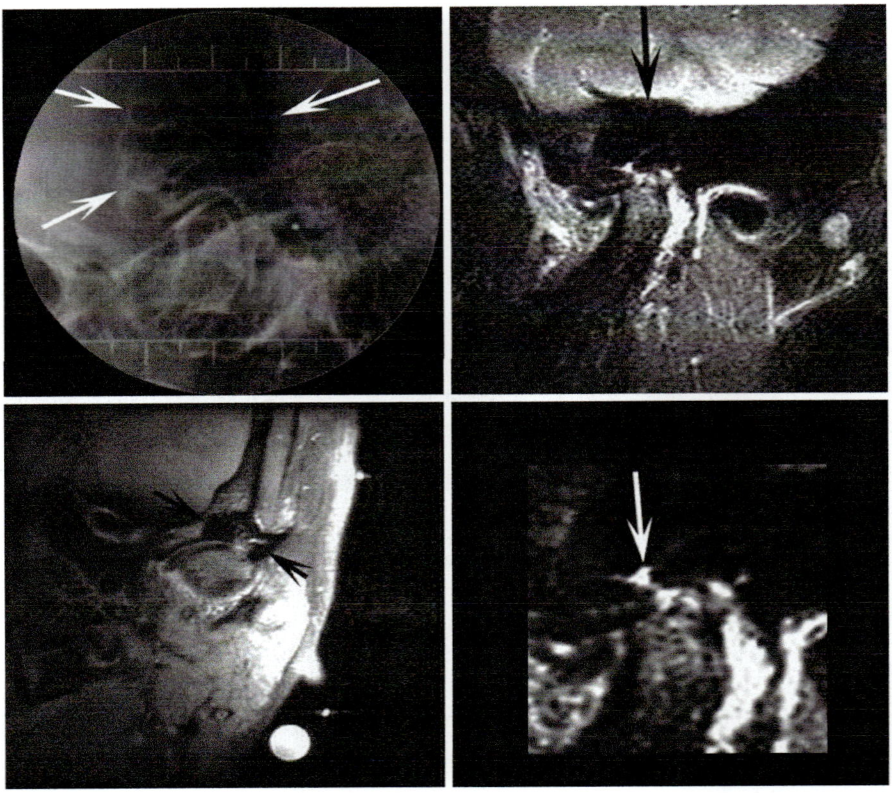

Fig. 11.12 MR images showing a well-pneumatized articular eminence and otomastoiditis at left articular eminence (arrows), coronal T1-W hypointense, while sagittal T2-W image showing bright signals above the TMJ condyle (arrows) (derived from [57])

11.1.17 Empty Sella

An empty sella is used to describe the extension of the subarachnoid space cerebrospinal fluid toward the intrasellar region through a defect in the diaphragma sella resulting in displacement of pituitary gland against the sellar wall with or without enlargement of the sella turcica [60]. Empty sella is divided into two types based on the reason: primary and secondary. Primary empty sella appears without any pathological changes in the pituitary gland, while secondary empty sella is caused by some pathologic conditions such as pituitary adenoma (radiation, drug or surgical therapy), postpartum pituitary necrosis, or lymphocytic hypophysitis [61]. Primary empty sella is asymptomatic and may be found incidentally, but secondary empty sella may be related to endocrine dysfunction, cerebrospinal fluid rhinorrhea, and visual abnormality. On CT scans an empty sella appears as a CSF or water-filled cavity density instead of normal pituitary gland tissue [62]. MRI is the modality of choice for confirming the diagnosis. On T1-W and T2-W images, empty sella shows the same signal intensity with cerebrospinal fluid [63]. Both MR images demonstrate

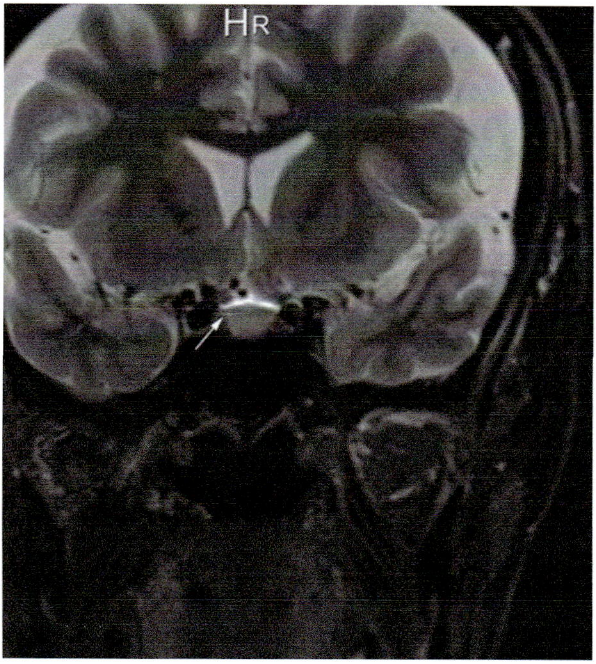

Fig. 11.13 Coronal T1-W contrast-enhanced MR images showing a case of empty sella showing iso-/high intense signal intensity with CSF leak in the middle part of the sella (arrows)

the sella to be filled with CSF, and the infundibulum can be seen to traverse the space, thereby excluding a cystic mass. This is known as the infundibulum sign (Fig. 11.13).

11.1.18 Internal Carotid Artery (ICA) Dissection

ICA dissection, like arterial dissection elsewhere, is a separation of the layers artery wall as a result of trauma and defects. As the blood enters the wall of the artery, thrombus form occurs which can lead to stroke, pseudoaneurysm, vessel occlusion, and stroke [64]. On CT, ICA dissections is eccentric lumen surrounded by the crescent shaped mural thickening which is hypodense relative to muscle [65, 66]. Fat-saturated T1-W images are useful to identify this pathology [67]. MR images mostly shows a high signal crescent sign within the wall of the vessel which can be best seen T1 fat saturation or T2 and abnormal vessel contour on MR angiography (Fig. 11.14).

11.1.19 Venous Angioma (VA)

Venous angiomas (VA) are vascular malformations in which veins are the predominant vascular constituent. Because venous angiomas are infrequently symptomatic, their clinical significance remains unclear. When symptomatic, they are associated mainly with seizures or bleeding or headache or scatter pain around the area. Although cerebral angiography is the definitive study of choice, it is no longer

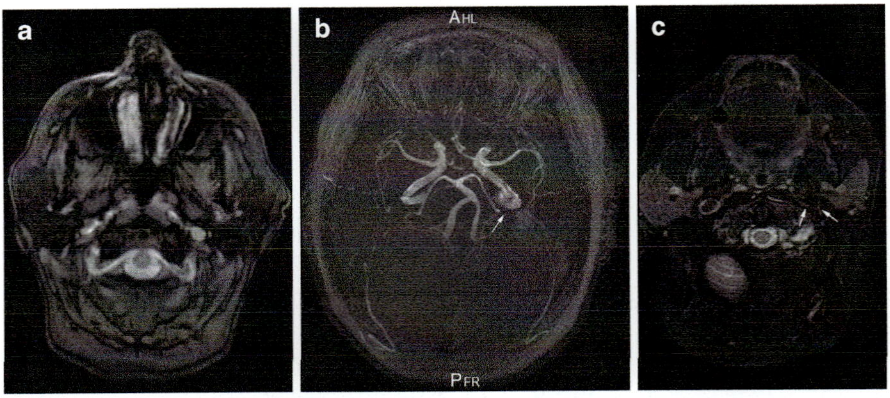

Fig. 11.14 (**a**) T1-W axial, (**b**) axial 3D TOF, (**c**) STIR images showing ICA on the left side (arrows)

judged necessary with uncomplicated vascular malformations. Cerebral developmental venous anomalies are usually incidentally detected and can be easily diagnosed as a linear or curvilinear focus of enhancement with contrast-enhanced CT images, and early CT findings of the VA include round, 1–2 cm focus enhancement [68]. Contrast-enhanced computed tomography (CT), which is no doubt responsible for the recent increase in the number of reported cases of VAS, is yielding to the far superior imaging ability of magnetic resonance (MR) as it becomes routinely available. MR imaging is thus becoming the primary study of choice. The most characteristic feature is an enlarged draining vein, followed by increased signal on T2-weighted images and decreased signal on T1-weighted images in adjacent parenchyma. T2 imaging is more successful in showing the lesions than T1 imaging. Best options are to find it as a gradient-echo or blood oxygen level-dependent sequence on MRI (Fig. 11.15).

11.1.20 Schwannoma

Temporal bone is also related to neuronal pathologies. One of them is a vestibular/acoustic schwannoma that derives from glial-neurilemmal junction of nerve sheath, mostly vestibular division of the CN VIII. It is visible in the internal auditory meatus or cerebellopontine/pontine angle [69]. On CT scans schwannomas are usually oval or spindle in shape and have well-defined borders [70]. On contrast-enhanced CT, a schwannoma displays mottle central lucency with peripheral intensification. CT images demonstrate the tumor and neighboring bony structure relation and the erosion and destruction of the bone clearly [71]. Besides typical symptoms such as tinnitus and sensorineural hearing loss, patients also complain on headache, vertigo, facial pain, and weakness; even big lesions may often be incidental and asymptomatic findings. Large tumors may develop mass effect with cerebellar and brainstem symptoms, e.g., hydrocephalus and cranial nerve dysfunction other than CNVIII. The

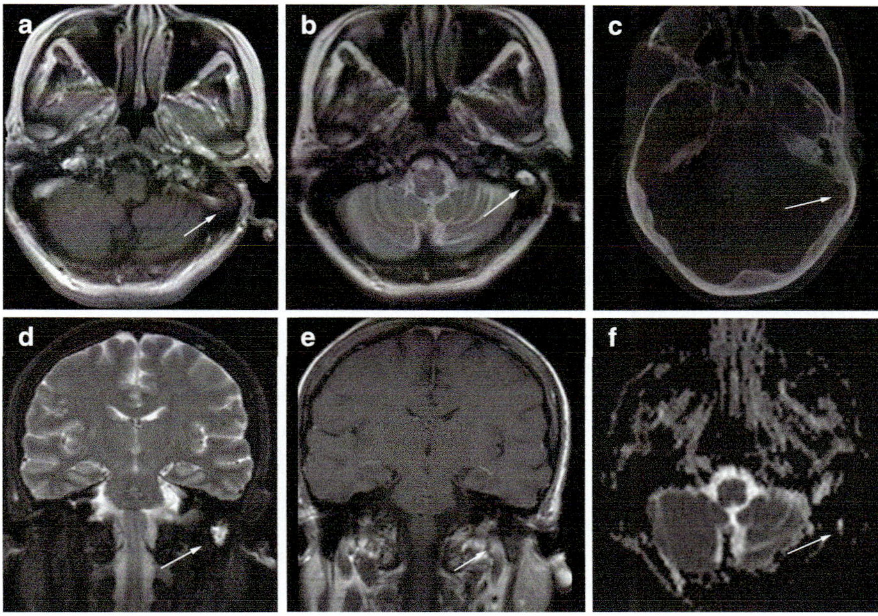

Fig. 11.15 A 62-year-old female patient referred with scattered pain around TMJ, (**a**) T1-W axial hypointense signal changes in the sigmoid sinus, (**b**) T2-W image shows the high signal intensity area, (**c**) axial CBCT showing an enlarged sigmoid sinus region, (**d**) coronal T2-W hyperintense, (**e**) coronal T1-W shows hypointense lesion, (**f**) DWI images diffusion restricted area which is consistent with venous angioma

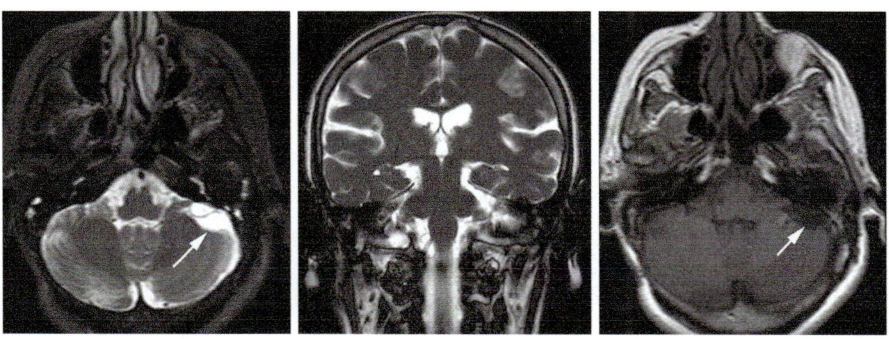

Fig. 11.16 A 38-year-old male patient with scattered pain around TMJ showing hypo- or isointense in T1- or heterogeneously hyperintense to adjacent brain in T2-weighted which is consistent with acoustic schwannoma

signal of the tumor is slightly hypo- or isointense in T1- or heterogeneously hyperintense to adjacent brain in T2-weighted images. Cystic areas show signal typical for fluid. In both modalities, most tumors show intense contrast enhancement with or without cystic degeneration and hemorrhagic areas (Fig. 11.16).

11.2 Incidental Calcifications in Maxillofacial Area

11.2.1 Tonsilloliths

Tonsillar calcifications also known as "tonsilloliths" are white-yellowish-calcified deposits which are commonly located in tonsillar crypts. Mesolella et al. [72] reported that calcified masses occur with a variation of sizes ranging from a few millimeters to several centimeters. Small-sized calculi are common and asymptomatic, but the giant-sized tonsilloliths are rare [73, 74]. Symptoms include dysphagia, recurrent sore throat, foreign body sensation, and halitosis [74]. The mechanisms of formation are still controversial. It is believed that they occurred due to repeated inflammation of the tonsillar crypts with recurrent tonsillitis. Repeated episodes of inflammation may cause cryptal fibrosis. Bacterial and epithelial debris accumulates within these crypts, and calcification occurs subsequent to the deposition of inorganic salts which derived from saliva [73, 75]. In addition, it is reported that tonsilloliths are primarily consisted of calcium hydroxyapatite/calcium carbonate and some other minerals such as magnesium, sodium, silica, potassium, copper, aluminum, iron, and ammonia radicals [72, 74, 76]. The most common cause of tonsillitis is viral infection including enteroviruses, particularly coxsackie virus, respiratory viruses (e.g., adenovirus, rhinovirus, influenza virus, coronavirus, parainfluenza virus, and respiratory syncytial virus), and viruses of the Herpesviridae family like Epstein-Barr virus (EBV), cytomegalovirus (CMV), and herpes simplex virus (HSV), while the most common bacterial pathogen is Group A β-hemolytic streptococcus in pediatric population [77].

Panoramic radiograph images can incidentally identify tonsilloliths as well as CBCT images [74]. Centurion et al. [78] suggested that CBCT images are more suitable to differentiate tonsilloliths than panoramic images. They are mostly seen as single or multiple, bilateral or unilateral, round, oval, dot-shaped, or irregular radiopacities around tonsillar area in CBCT scans. The study, which was conducted by Oda et al. [79], was reported that the prevalence of tonsilloliths was 46.1% in 482 CBCT scans. On MR images, it appears as hypo- to isointense to surrounding muscles on T1-W and hyperintense to surrounding muscles on T2-W images (Fig. 11.17).

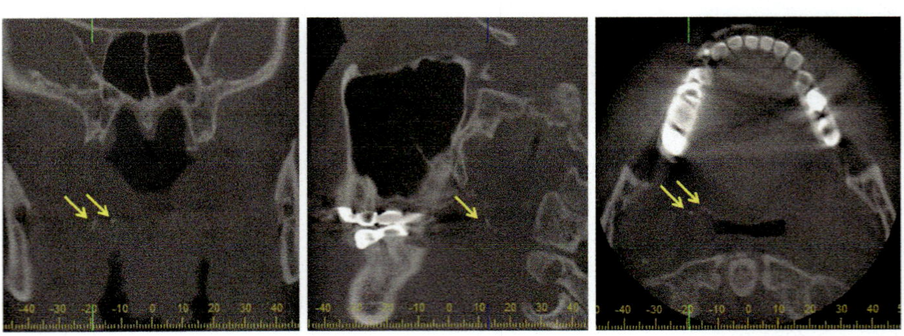

Fig. 11.17 Coronal, sagittal, and axial views of a CBCT image show multiple, irregular-shaped calcified masses in tonsillar region (arrows)

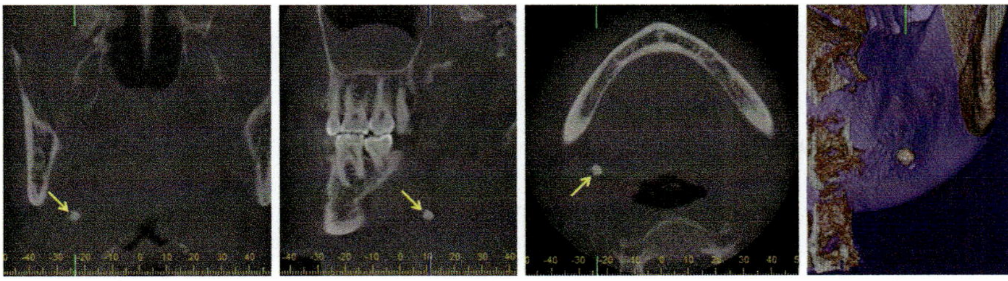

Fig. 11.18 Coronal, sagittal, axial, and 3D reconstructed views of a unilateral sialolith (arrows)

11.2.2 Sialolith

Salivary stones also known as "sialoliths" are described as an aggregation calcified deposits found within the salivary glands or ducts. It consists of hydroxyapatite, calcium and phosphate salts, desquamated epithelial cells, bacterial debris, and foreign bodies [20, 80]. They frequently occur in submandibular gland or its ducts (80–90%); calcified masses in the parotid and sublingual are, respectively, seen in 10–20% and 1–7% [20, 80]. They can also occur in minor salivary glands, primarily in the upper lip and buccal mucosa. According to literature, incidences of sialoliths are low, between 0.2% and 1.01% [81, 82].

The radiographic features are dependent on their internal structure. Homogeneously radiopaque deposits are easily seen in conventional radiographic techniques, but some of them have multiple layers of calcification. Low mineral content sialoliths are frequently seen in CBCT scans even they were asymptomatic [20]. No matter whether they are well calcified or not, salivary deposits are an incidental finding in TMJ CBCT images. If a sialolith is located in the ducts of salivary glands, then it is usually well defined, smooth, cylindric, round, or ovoid. On the contrary, if it tends to occur in the hilum of salivary gland, then it is larger and irregular-shaped [20, 83, 84] (Fig. 11.18).

11.2.3 Antrolith/Rhinolith

Antroliths are calcified masses which occurred in the paranasal sinuses [85]. If these calcified bodies occur in nasal cavity, then they are called as rhinolith [86]. These calcified bodies occur as a result of mineral salt deposition around a nidus within the nasal cavity. This core may be endogenous or exogenous. Endogenous sources could be originated from dental structures, blood, mucus, and bone fragments. Exogenous sources are the foreign bodies such as coin, bead, or weed introduced into the sinus cavities [20, 87]. Antroliths occur within the maxillary sinus above the floor of the antrum; rhinoliths are found in nasal cavity [87]. Antroliths and rhinoliths can appear as incidental findings on CBCT. They are frequently asymptomatic unless they are larger [88, 89]. According to literature, incidences of antroliths are between 0.12% and 3% [90, 91] (Fig. 11.19).

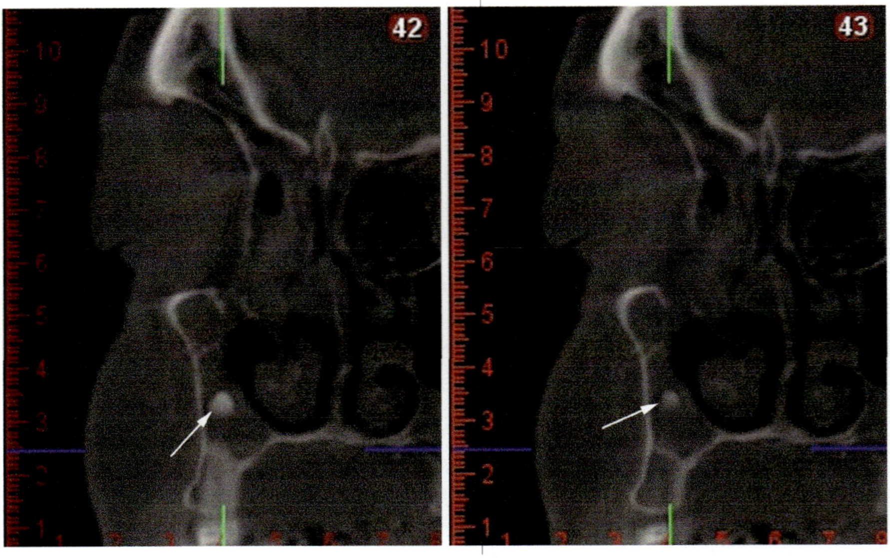

Fig. 11.19 Coronal views showing a calcified antrolith in the right maxillary sinus (arrows)

11.2.4 Fungal Infection (Aspergilloma)

Fungal infection of the sinuses is the inflammation of the lining mucosa of the paranasal sinuses due to fungal infection such as aspergillosis, mucormycosis, candidiasis, histoplasmosis, cryptococcosis, coccidioidomycosis, North American blastomycosis, rhinosporidiosis, and myospherulosis [58]. Fungal infection of the sinuses is classified as invasive and noninvasive due to the presence or absence of hyphae within the mucosal and other tissues of the paranasal sinuses [92] and divided into five subgroups. Aspergillosis is the most common fungal pathogen of the sinuses and usually affects the immunocompromised patients [93]. At noncontrast CT scans, aspergilloma is characterized by a hyperdense mass with occasional calcifications. This hyperattenuating lesion is usually surrounded by a hypodense mucosal thickening [94]. MR features can change due to the stage of the disease, mostly the lesions hypointensity on T1-WI and T2-WI. On T1-W image the lesion is hypointense because of the inflamed mucosal thickness and on T2-W usually appears as hyperintense peripheral inflamed mucosal thickness, and low T2 signal or signal void is due to high concentration of various metals such as iron, magnesium, and manganese concentrated by fungal organisms (Fig. 11.20).

11.2.5 Osteoma Cutis

Osteoma cutis is a rare soft tissue ossification in the skin or subcutaneous tissues. It is characterized a focal development of bone formation within the dermis. It may be primary but mostly secondary. Kishi et al. [95] reported a study which was based on

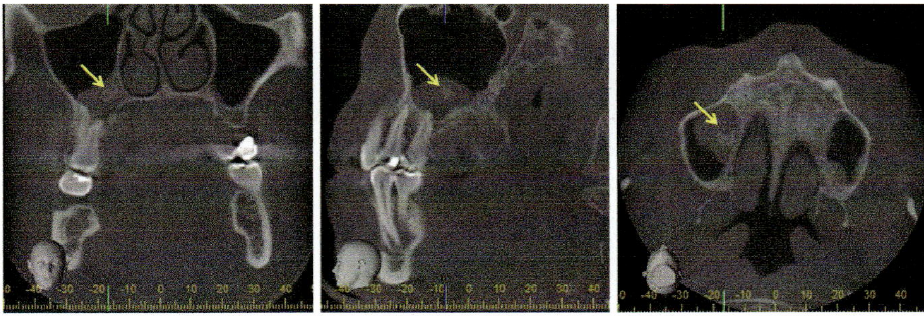

Fig. 11.20 An irregular calcified mass in the right maxillary sinus which was consisted with aspergillosis of the maxillary sinus (arrows)

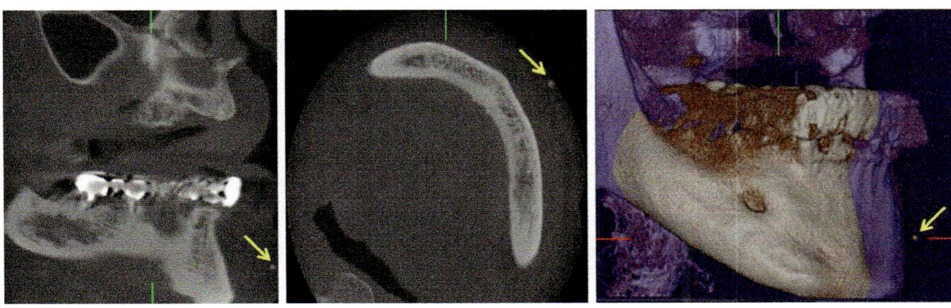

Fig. 11.21 Sagittal, axial, and 3D views of the CBCT scan show a calcified mass in soft tissue, asymptomatic incidental osteoma cutis case

examination of occlusal films, and they found that osteoma cutis can be detected during dental radiographic examinations and calculated their incidence to be 2.2%. But Shigehara et al. [96] reported their incidence was 28%. The most common involved regions include the face, scalp, fingers, cheeks, and lips. Majority of the cases are asymptomatic, and they may detect radiographically as an incidental finding. Radiographically, they appear as smoothly outlined radiopaque formations due to their homogeneous internal structure [20, 97]. But mostly they are superimposed to the tooth root or dense bone. Imaging by using an intraoral film may be possible only when it is located between cheeks and alveolar process. Or a posteroanterior skull view should be performed while the cheeks blown outward [20]. They are easily visualized by CBCT only when they are carefully examined (Fig. 11.21).

11.2.6 Calcified Lymph Nodes

Calcified lymph nodes are one of the calcification of structures in head and neck region. They are often an asymptomatic condition diagnosed accidentally during radiographic examination. Lymph node calcifications can occur in patients with chronic inflammatory diseases or tuberculosis. It can occur also in the patients who have been treated for lymphoma [98]. They may be able to detect on palpation. Due to underlying serious conditions, diagnosing and monitoring is crucially important. The most commonly involved nodes are the submandibular and superficial and deep cervical nodes. Radiographically, they present below the inferior border of the mandible and near the mandibular angle, and they usually appear well-defined, lobulated irregularly shaped opacities. The irregular shape is described as "cauliflower-like" [20]. Edwards et al. [90] reported that the incidence of calcified lymph nodes was rare, nearly 0.12%.

11.2.7 Cysticercosis

Cysticercosis is a parasitic tissue infection caused by larval cysts of *Taenia solium*. This affects the central nervous system, muscle, eyes, and skin. Infection is found most often in rural, developing countries where hygiene is poor. Cysticercosis can lead to neurologic and ocular complications, and rarely death. From the first located in the tissues, till death of the larvae, they are not visible in radiographic images. After their death calcification starts in subcutaneous and muscular sites [20]. Muscular cysticercosis appears as "grains of rice" and dot-shaped or well-defined ellipsoidal calcifications and is found incidentally in radiographic images [99].

Life cycle of the *Taenia solium* is completed in two different hosts including pork and human first as a larva (in the intermediate host) which develops from egg and then as an adult tapeworm (in the definitive host). Infection of *Taenia solium* can result in two distinct conditions in the human host: taeniasis and cysticercosis [100, 101]. Taeniasis and cysticercosis are highly endemic in developing countries in Latin America, most parts of Asia (including China and the Indian subcontinent), Eastern Europe, and most of Africa. Whereas infection with the adult tapeworm causes intestinal taeniasis, fecal-oral contamination of the larval *Taenia solium* results in cysticercosis [102]. Cysticercosis in human may affect the brain, muscle, skin, liver, lung, subcutaneous tissue, and heart as well as in the oral and perioral tissues especially in the masticatory muscles where the majority die and become densely calcified [20]. Both T1- and T2-W images show hypointensive area with a null signal due to parasite itself. The nidus due to central location of the parasite can be seen in STIR images (Fig. 11.16). Extraoral conventional imaging modalities such as panoramic or cephalometric images are enough to visualize calcifications. CBCT evaluations easily reveal these calcifications. Calcified masses may be found in the region of masseter and suprahyoid muscles, tongue, buccal mucosa, or lips [20, 103] (Fig. 11.22).

11.2.8 Phlebolith

Phleboliths are the deposition of calcium salts which occurred in organized intravascular thrombi by the venous congestion or stagnation. It is always prediction of presence of hemangioma, because they are mostly found in veins, venulae, or the sinusoidal vessels of hemangiomas [20, 104]. Phleboliths are usually multiple; their shape is round or oval, up to 6 mm in diameter with a smooth periphery. Internal structure commonly has laminated appearance as a bull's eye view [20]. They may

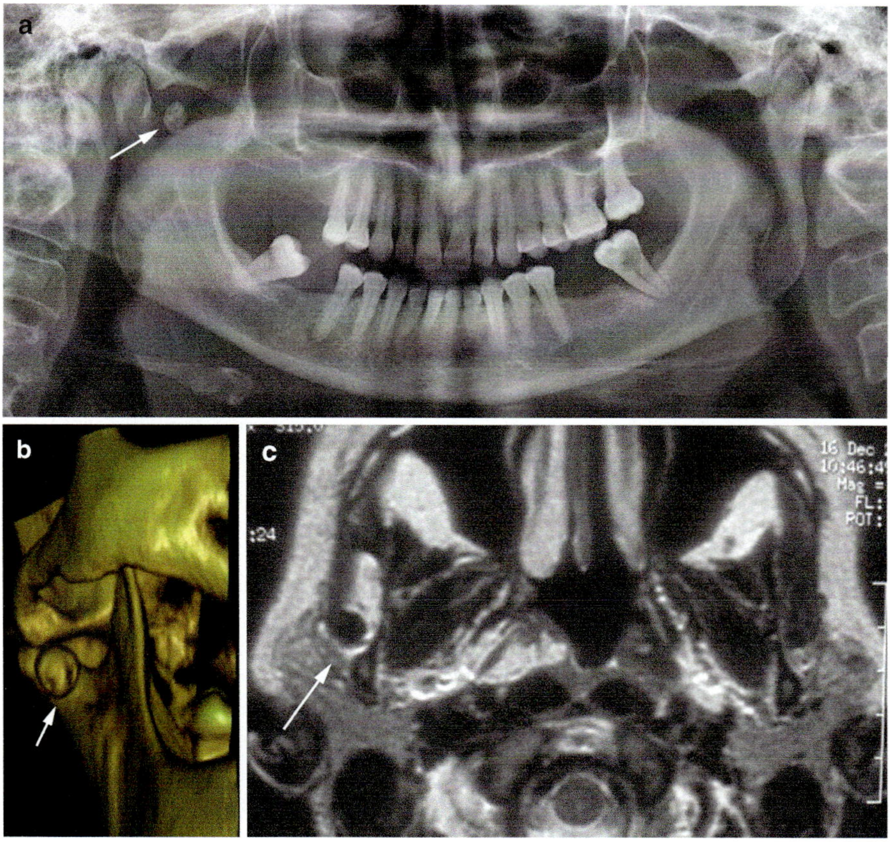

Fig. 11.22 (**a**) Panoramic image showing calcification around TMJ with limitation of mouth opening symptom, (**b**) 3D CBCT showing the exact location of the calcification, (**c**) T1-W MR image showing a signal void area on the master muscle, consistent with maxillofacial cysticercosis

detect by conventional radiographic techniques as well as MR, USG, CT, and CBCT [104]. Differential diagnosis should be made with sialoliths [20].

11.2.9 Myositis Ossificans

Myositis ossificans is a benign process characterized by arising bone or bone-like tissue within muscles, tendons, or ligaments. There are two types: localized traumatic or progressive. Localized myositis ossificans can occur as a result of acute or chronic trauma. It may occur not only when applied an intramuscular injection but only heavy muscular strain by sport [20, 104]. Progressive myositis ossificans is a rare hereditary disease which arises as a result of spontaneous mutation. The mostly involved muscles of maxillofacial area are masseter and sternocleidomastoideus. The less common muscles are medial and lateral pterygoid, buccinator, and temporalis [20].

Progressive form also known as fibrodysplasia ossificans progressiva is a rare autosomal dominant genetic disorder and most commonly affects male without any external injury of the muscle [20]. Myositis ossificans circumscripta occur as a result of some traumatic injury to muscle such as acute and chronic trauma, heavy muscular strain, infections, burns, neuromuscular disorders, hemophilia, tetanus, and drug abuse [105]. Masseter and sternocleidomastoid muscles are most commonly affected in the head and neck region [20]. Also it may be localized in other masticatory muscles [106, 107]. MRI appearances depend on the age of the lesion. Early lesions can be misleading before the maturation, however soft tissue may appear with edema. T1-W images show ill-defined isointense images; T2-W shows mostly edema as high signal. The signal intensity may change depending on the localization of the lesion in which central part mostly seen with heterogeneous signal intensity T1-W contrast enhancement is often present. Standard radiographs do not disclose any anomaly in the early stages of myositis ossificans. Typically, they are distant from adjacent bony structures [108]. CT scan examination is more sensitive than radiography for detecting ossification and may also show a central fatty metaplastic area [109].

11.2.10 Intracranial Calcifications

Intracranial calcifications can be physiological or pathological. They often occur due to mineral or metal deposition in the blood vessels, glands, cortices, or other structures within the brain [110]. The most common sites include the pineal gland, habenula, choroid plexus, basal ganglia, falx, tentorium, petroclinoid ligaments, and sagittal sinus [111]. According to the literature, intracranial calcifications were common and occur at any age and of any ethnicity [81]. Kwak et al. [112] reported that intracranial calcifications have male predilection. According to literature reports, incidence rates of intracranial calcifications vary from 0.42% [81] to 71% [113]. The great differences between incidence rates may be due to many reasons such as sample size, the size of the FOV, radiologic imaging devices, and their different abilities in detecting pathologies.

Since the CBCT gained widespread popularity in dentistry, sensors can easily display larger anatomical fields including intracranial area. Calcified deposits within intracranial region can incidentally detected in most CBCT scans. Medical CTs or CBCT is more effective displaying modalities rather than two-dimensional conventional techniques. It is also reported by Sedghizadeh et al. [110] that CBCT scans have some limitations compared with CT such as low soft tissue contrast and high noise. CT allows for better identification of anatomical structures or pathologies than CBCT (Fig. 11.23).

11.2.11 Stylohyoid Ligament Calcification

The stylohyoid chain consists of two bony structures and a fibrous cord known as the stylohyoid ligament [114, 115]. Because of congenital factors, trauma, and age-related factors, this fibrous cord starts to be ossified. Due to its close relationship

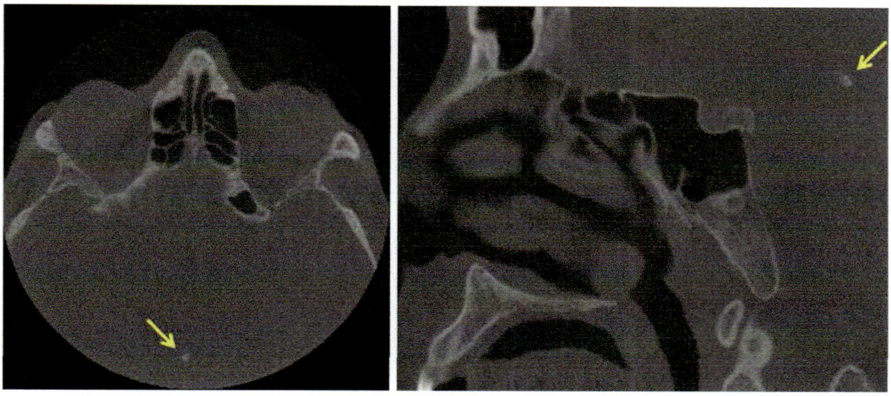

Fig. 11.23 A pineal gland calcification is incidentally found in CBCT examination (arrows)

with some important anatomical structures, ossification or elongation of this complex may lead some symptoms such as dysphagia and head-neck pain. Ossification of the stylohyoid ligament is a common condition which is found as an incidental finding in routine dental radiographic examination [114]. According to literature, incidence rates of stylohyoid ligament ossifications are between 2% and 30% [115]. Panoramic radiographs are routinely used in dentistry, and it allows to identify calcified stylohyoid ligament especially in asymptomatic patients. It extends forward from the mastoid region and crosses and superimposed to the ramus toward the hyoid bone. It appears as long, tapering, thin, interrupted by a jointlike junction or a straight structure [20]. Although panoramic radiography has frequently been used to show elongation or ossification of stylohyoid ligament, it also has some disadvantages such as superposition. Hence, CT and CBCT should be used for appropriate evaluation of this structure [115] (Fig. 11.24).

11.2.12 Arterial Calcifications

Arterial calcifications are a common consequence of aging and are more frequent in patients with some systemic diseases such as diabetes, dyslipidemia, genetic diseases, and diseases involving disturbances of calcium metabolism. They are a result of the deposition of calcium salts in the cells of the media or intima of the arterial wall [116]. Arterial calcifications have two different forms which identified radiographically and histologically: Mönckeberg's medial calcinosis and calcified atherosclerotic plaque [20]. Calcifications of tunica media of medium-sized arteries are described as Mönckeberg's medial calcinosis. The etiology is not well understood, but it is believed that glucose intolerance, age, sex, osteoporosis, or chronic renal failure is related. Medial calcinosis does not obstruct the lumina of the arteries, so tissue or organ ischemia is not seen [117]. Hence, it is mostly asymptomatic. Only it is clearly seen in three-dimensional imaging modalities and plain radiography techniques as an incidental finding. Radiographically, calcified vessels of Mönckeberg appear as a parallel pair of thin, radiopaque lines which were described

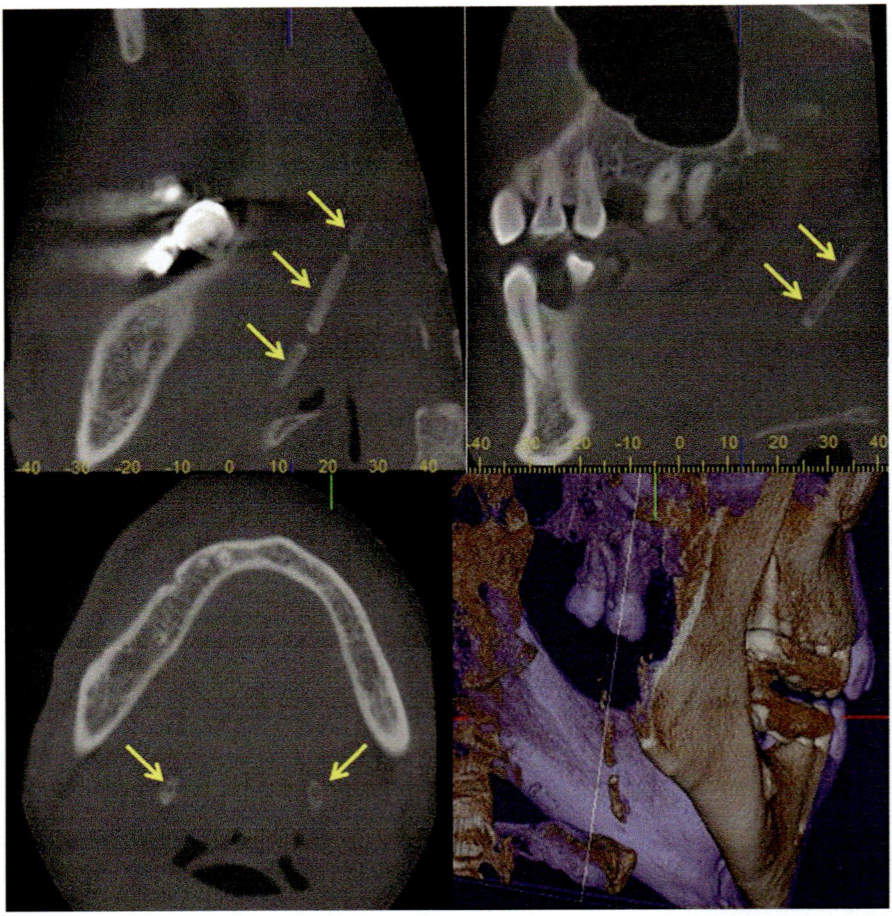

Fig. 11.24 Sagittal, axial, and 3D reconstructed views of elongated stylohyoid ligament (arrows)

as "tram tracks," "pipestem," or "tramline." In cross section, involved vessels can view a circular or ringlike pattern [20, 118].

One another arterial calcification is known as atherosclerosis. It is characterized by deposition of calcium in the atheromatous plaques within the intima of arteries. It causes narrowing the lumen of the affected vessels. The most common location for an atherosclerotic plaque lesion is at the carotid bifurcation; therefore, it may be visible in the panoramic radiograph. It may be seen as a heterogeneous radiopacity at the level of the intervertebral space between C3 and C4. They are usually multiple, unilateral or bilateral, irregular, and sharply defined from the surrounding soft tissues [20]. These plaques have an aspect mostly circular when small and mostly linear or thin rectangular when enlarged. They are usually located posterior to the angle of mandible, approximately at the inferior margin of third cervical vertebra near the hyoid bone [119].

Panoramic radiographs, which are used routinely in dental practice, can often show the presence of carotid atheroma. But authors suggested that angiography was

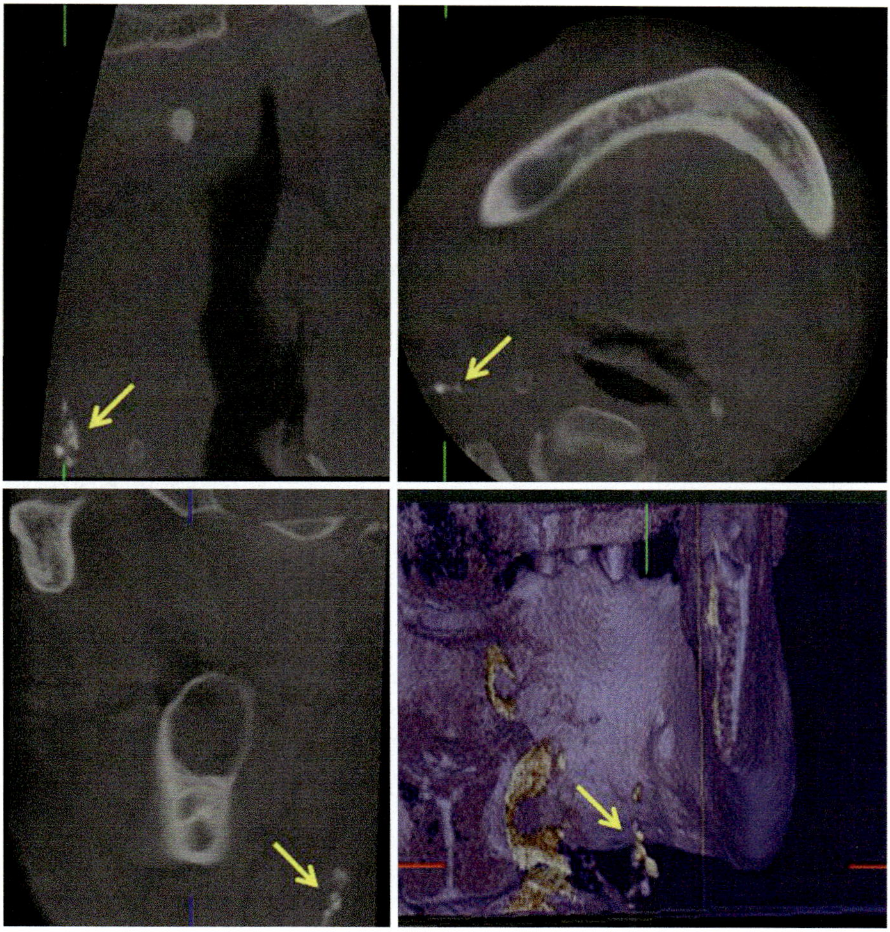

Fig. 11.25 Calcified atherosclerotic plaques are easily visualized in the CBCT scans. Notice that they are multiple-, unilateral-, and irregular-shaped calcified masses (arrows)

considered as a gold standard. Because of its possible complications, color Doppler imaging, also called laser Doppler fluxometry or duplex scan, has been increasingly used to diagnose atheroma because it is a fast, accurate, and painless method of diagnosis [119]. Besides, it is also well known that CBCT or CT reveals precious benefits to detect arterial calcifications [120] (Fig. 11.25).

11.3 Paranasal Sinus Findings in TMJ Imaging

The paranasal sinuses are four-paired air-filled spaces which surround the nasal cavity. They consist of maxillary, frontal, and sphenoid sinuses and ethmoid cells. Their infectious diseases can mimic of an odontogenic infection, and practitioners should be careful diagnosing pathologies and familiar with variations [20].

Since the first invention of three-dimensional imaging modalities, paranasal sinus evaluations were made by using conventional imaging techniques. As everybody knows, two-dimensional plain radiographic techniques have some limitations such as superimpositions, magnifications, distortions, and low-image quality. Because of these limitations, some pathologies, calcifications, and anatomical variations may be missed [121]. Especially in dentistry, panoramic radiography is routinely used by practitioners to evaluate dentomaxillofacial region. Panoramic radiography allows clinicians to evaluate not only normal anatomy, pathologies, and variations but also TMJ and paranasal sinuses. Evaluation of paranasal sinuses is quite difficult in panoramic images because of superimpositions. To overcome these limitations, CBCT use in dentistry spreads. Due to higher diagnostic sensitivity and specificity levels of CBCT, it became the first imaging tool option by clinicians. It became possible to make further analysis of the findings which could not have detected by conventional imaging modalities [81, 121].

As mentioned in previous chapters, "Any findings on a radiographic image which are not related to the research areas of interest" could be a description of "incidental findings." Paranasal sinus findings are one of these incidental findings. And correct identification of pathologies or variations will reduce further diagnostic assessments [81].

11.3.1 Maxillary and Sphenoid Sinusitis

Sinusitis is a condition in which the lining of the paranasal sinuses is inflamed due to an allergen, bacteria, or virus resulting in symptoms. Sinusitis is named depending on the involved sinus and is classified into the three (acute, subacute and chronic) categories based upon symptom duration [20]. Acute sinusitis describes the short-term (less than 4 weeks) infection or inflammation of the mucosa. Subacute sinusitis is defined as symptoms of 4–12-week duration. If the inflammation persists more than 12 weeks, it is considered chronic [122, 123]. Signal characteristics depend on the affected regions of the sinuses. In acute stages, on T1-W image due to mucosal thickening, the lesion is isointense to soft tissue, but the fluid shows hypointense areas. On T2-W images both mucosal thickening and fluid can show variable hyperintensity. On contrast-enhanced images, the T1-W images show enhancement only along with the inflamed mucosa (Fig. 11.26).

11.3.2 Sinus Opacifications

Sinus opacifications are common finding of paranasal sinuses. Radiopaque appearance of paranasal sinuses occurs in some cases such as mucosal thickening, air-fluid level, mucocele, mucous retention cyst, and total or partial opacifications.

Sinus mucosal thickening also known as mucositis is a common radiographic finding. All paranasal sinuses composed of respiratory epithelium and considered as normal if they are about 0.8–1 mm [20, 82]. Besides, some reports have considered mucosal thickening as ≥ 2 or ≥ 3 mm [82, 124, 125].

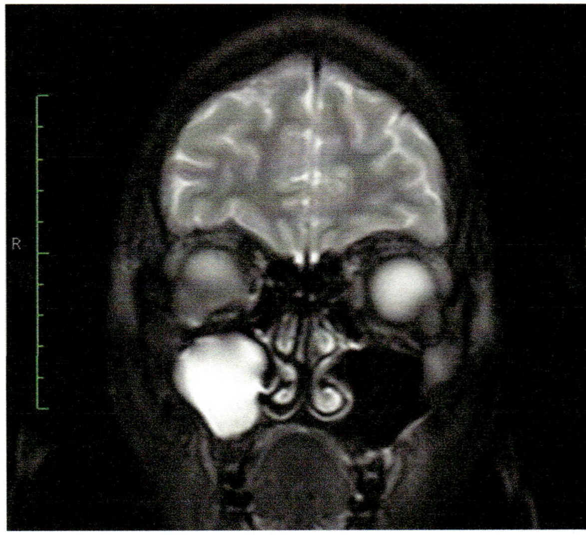

Fig. 11.26 T2-W FSE FS coronal image showing maxillary sinusitis with excessive pain symptom of the patient

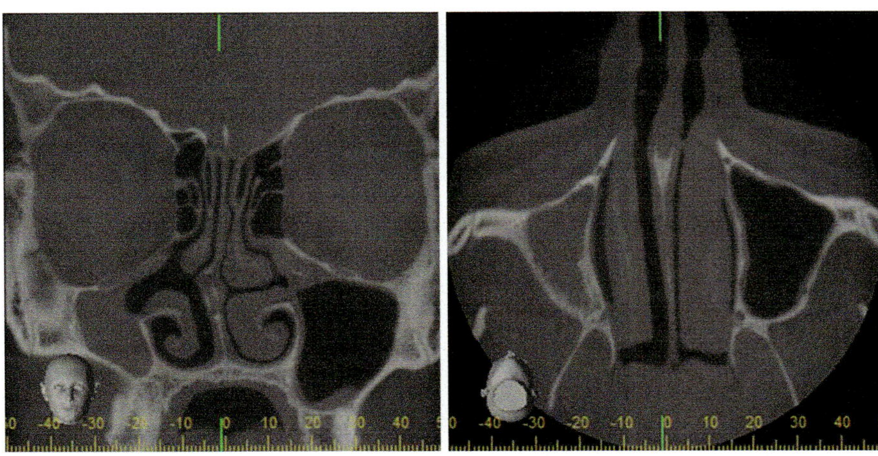

Fig. 11.27 Coronal and axial views of total opacification of right maxillary sinus

Lana et al. [125] reported that mucosal thickening was the most commonly detected lesion. They found mucosal thickening in 313 patients (62.6%). Avsever et al. [121] reported that incidence was 27.35%.

Normally, sinus mucosa is not visualized especially on conventional radiographic images. Mucosal changes are often discovered as incidental findings on images made for other purposes such as implant planning or TMJ evaluation. When it is possible to visualize, mucosal thickening is seen as well-defined, noncorticated radiopaque band which runs along parallel to the bony wall of the sinus (Fig. 11.27).

The image of thickened sinus mucosa may be uniform or polypoid. In allergic reactions, the mucosa tends to be more lobulated [20] (Fig. 11.28).

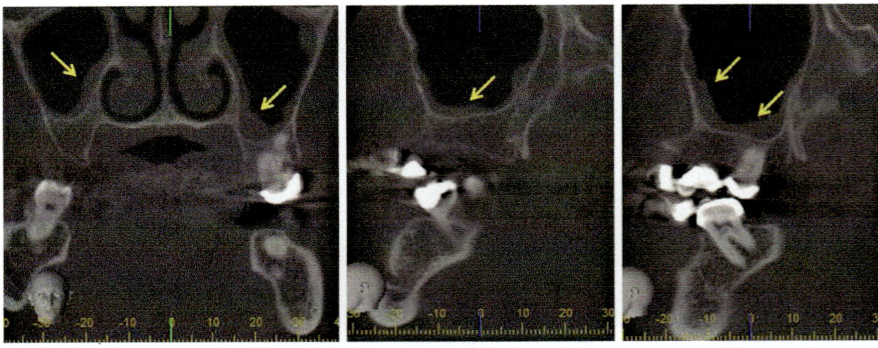

Fig. 11.28 Coronal and sagittal views (right and left) of maxillary sinus with bilateral mucosal thickening (arrows)

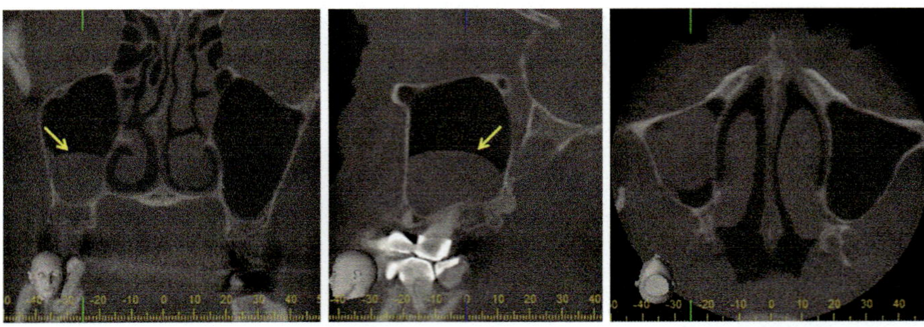

Fig. 11.29 A dome-shaped, well-defined mucous retention cyst in the right maxillary sinus

Mucocele is the lesion which shows certain characteristics such as complete filling of the maxillary sinus and bony expansion. It occurs as a result of blockade of sinus ostium for various reasons such as intra-antral or intranasal inflammation, polyp, or neoplasm. Because of its expansive and destructive character, it is easily diagnosed. Sinus cavity is uniformly radiopaque. Maxillary sinus is rarely affected. Ninety percent of the cases occur in the ethmoid air cells and frontal sinuses. Plain conventional imaging modalities are mostly visualized lesion. But comprehensive evaluation or exact diagnosis is easily made with CT or CBCT [20].

Mucous retention cyst is related to several causes such as humidity, allergens, temperature, or seasonal changes. They are mostly asymptomatic as long as they do not blockade the ostium. They usually visualize as dome-shaped, well-defined, smooth radiopaque masses. They occur mostly on the sinus floor more than the other walls of the sinus (Fig. 11.29). Periapical radiographs of maxillary molar teeth could show a part of mucous retention cyst, but extraoral imaging modalities are most effective. CT or CBCT may be more appropriate for comprehensive evaluation [20]. It will appear as isointense on T1 and hyperintense on T2 images.

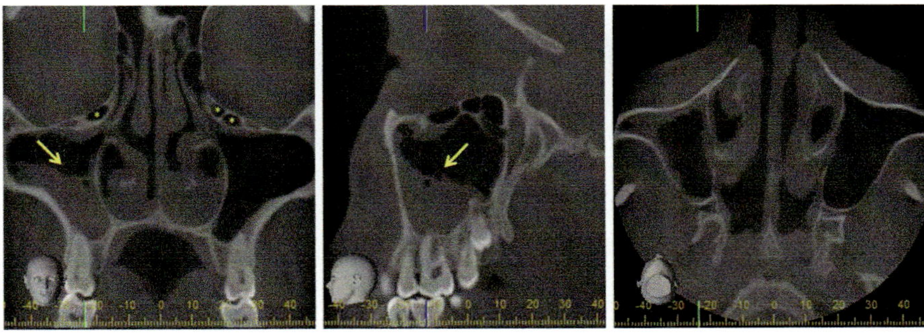

Fig. 11.30 Maxillary sinus with unilateral air-fluid level. Note the clear bubbly foamy-appearing fluid (arrows). Coronal view of CBCT scan also shows bilateral Haller cell (*asterisk*)

Total or partial opacifications occur in inflammatory conditions. Total opacification blockades the ostium and has some symptoms, but partial opacifications are sometimes asymptomatic. They both do not cause expansion or destruction. Sinus cavity is uniformly radiopaque.

Air-fluid level appears in sinus with its characteristic "bubbly or foamy" appearance (Fig. 11.30). An air-fluid level is the most typical imaging finding of acute sinusitis. It will appear as hypointense on T1 and hyperintense on T2 images.

11.3.3 Hypoplasia and Aplasia

The maxillary sinuses are the first developed among paranasal sinuses and lasts its growth at the end of puberty [126, 127]. Hypoplasia is underdevelopment or incomplete development of a tissue or organ. Aplasia is defined as absence of organ or tissue. Etiology of hypoplasia or aplasia includes both embryological and acquired causes like trauma or infection [128].

Hypoplasia of the paranasal sinuses is a rare condition [129]. The frontal and sphenoid sinuses are most frequently involved [130]. The incidence of maxillary sinus hypoplasia ranges between 1.5 and 10% [129]. Hypoplasia of the maxillary sinuses occurs unilaterally in about 1.7% of patients and bilaterally in 7.2%. Hypoplasia of the frontal sinus is a common normal variant, and aplasia of the frontal sinuses is noted in approximately 4% of the population [20].

Conventional radiographs such as panoramic radiography, Water's projection, and intraoral radiography are routinely used in evaluation of maxillary sinus. Because of the complex anatomy of the dentomaxillofacial region, it is difficult to visualize important anatomical structures due to the superimposition [124]. Maxillary sinus hypoplasia can be misdiagnosed with mucosal thickening in infectious disease or neoplasms involving the sinus in conventional radiographs. Maxillary sinus hypoplasia can be seen as a partial opacification, and aplasia appears

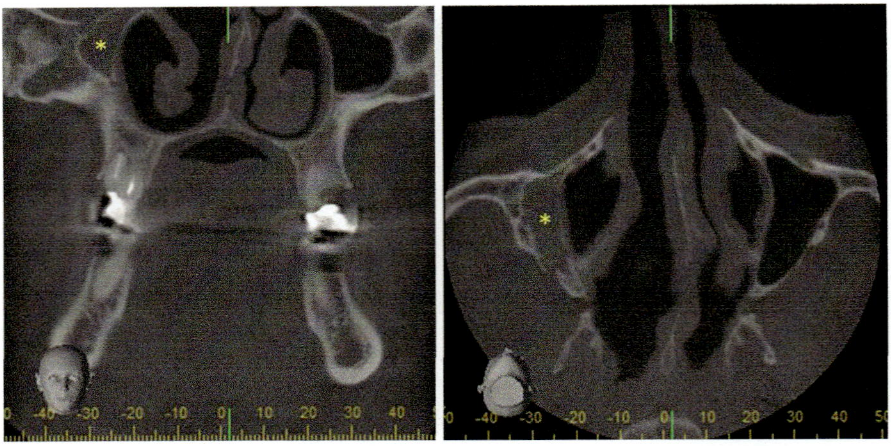

Fig. 11.31 Coronal and axial views of maxillary sinus hypoplasia. It is also seen a total opacification (asterisk)

as a total opacification. CT/CBCT examination is the ideal method for detecting this anatomical variation. Radiological diagnosis of maxillary sinus hypoplasia and aplasia is important to prevent possible complications during endoscopic sinus surgery, such as causing potential harm to the orbit [131] (Fig. 11.31).

11.3.4 Haller Cell

Haller cell is an anatomical variation which is located lateral to the maxillo-ethmoidal suture along the inferomedial orbital floor. They are also known as infraorbital ethmoidal air cells [132]. The prevalence of Haller cells is reported to be between 2% and 68% in the literature [133, 134]. Some reports have shown the Haller cells with larger than 3 mm in diameter, have a precious relationship with maxillary sinusitis [132, 135, 136].

With the increasing popularity of endoscopic sinus surgery, visualization of Haller cell or any anatomical variations became important. Infraorbital ethmoid cells may be visualized by a variety of imaging methods that show a view of the maxillary sinus. Plain radiography or three-dimensional imaging modalities which were performed to evaluate TMJ commonly visualize infraorbital ethmoid cells. CT and CBCT are commonly used for imaging infraorbital ethmoid cells, and they are frequently seen as incidental findings in CT/CBCT examination of paranasal sinuses. It is also possible to detect them by panoramic radiographs [137].

11.3.5 Onodi Air Cell

Sphenoethmoidal air cell, also known as the Onodi air cell, is an anatomic variant of the most posterior ethmoid cell that pneumatized superiorly and laterally to the

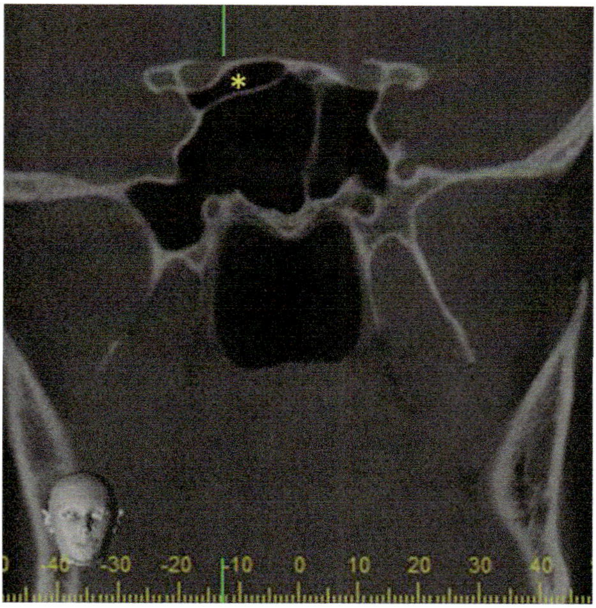

Fig. 11.32 Unilateral Onodi cell (asterisk)

sphenoid sinus and is in close relation to the optic nerve and internal carotid artery. Their importance is the close relationship with optic nerve and internal carotid artery. The damage of these structures causes some important complications during sinus surgery. They are usually asymptomatic, unless complicated by sinus disease. The incidence of Onodi cells on imaging studies is between 4.6% and 65.6% [121, 138]. The possible causes of the variety of prevalence are racial factors and differences of chosen imaging modalities. Using endoscopic dissection, Kainz and Stammberger [139] reported its prevalence was 42%.

Onodi cells are often discovered as incidental findings on radiographic images. CT/CBCT scanning of paranasal sinuses provides valuable information in assessing extent of the air cell and detailed anatomy prior to endoscopic sinus surgery (Fig. 11.32). It is also suggested that, among examination/imaging methods, nasal endoscopy is more sensitive than CT in identifying an Onodi cell [140].

11.3.6 Concha Bullosa

Concha bullosa is generally defined as the pneumatization of the middle turbinate in the nose. However, pneumatization may also be seen in the superior and inferior turbinate [141]. In majority of cases, these variants are asymptomatic. Sometimes it is associated with deviation of the nasal septum. Although it was first described as a rare anatomical variation, Smith et al. [142] reported that incidence rate was 67.5%. In addition to radiologic reports, clinical data from Goldman [143], who encountered pneumatization in 80% of resected middle turbinates from patients undergoing ethmoidectomy for chronic sinusitis, suggested a higher prevalence.

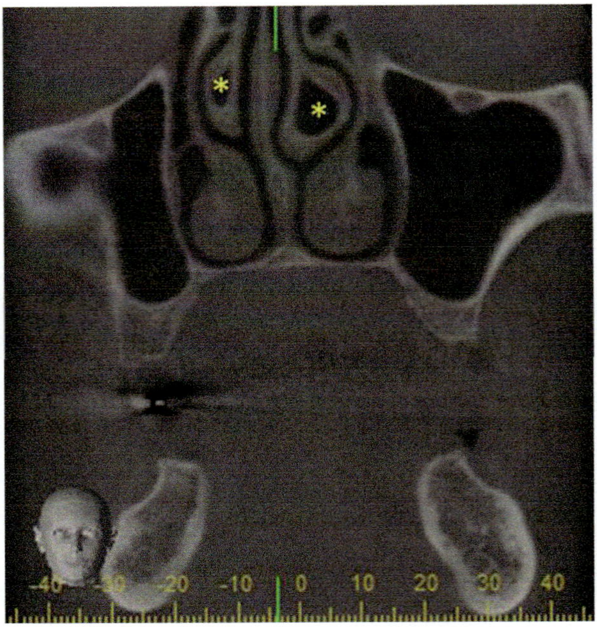

Fig. 11.33 Bilateral concha bullosa (asterisk)

Coronal plane CT/CBCT imaging was used to critically analyze the middle turbinate pneumatization (Fig. 11.33).

11.3.7 Agger Nasi

Agger nasi cells are the most anterior ethmoid air cells and are located anterior, lateral, and inferior to the frontal recess. Presence of some anatomical variations such as Agger nasi may affect the functional drainage pathways and predispose for sinus disease. The recognition of sinonasal anatomic variations is important for the avoidance of surgical complications [144]. The prevalence of Agger nasi cells has previously been reported as wide ranging. In a CBCT examination, Avsever et al. [121] found Agger nasi cells in 2.88% of specimens examined; however, Bolger et al. [145] noted this cell type in 98.5% of their sample. They should not be confused with Haller cells which located along the medial floor of the orbit.

Imaging of Agger nasi with standard sinus radiographic techniques may be failed because of their limitations. Endoscopic visualization is gold standard. High-resolution multisliced multiplanar CT or CBCT scans provide valuable information about anatomical structures or variations [121] (Fig. 11.34).

11.3.8 Accessory Ostium

The maxillary sinuses communicate with the nasal cavity by the ostium, approximately 3–6 mm in diameter and positioned under the posterior aspect of the middle

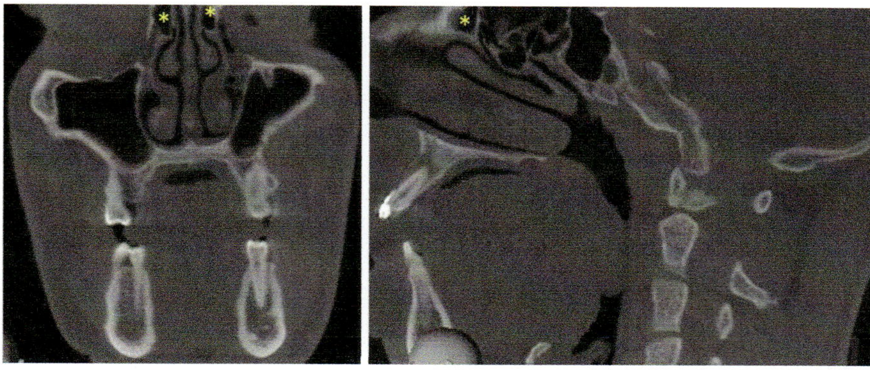

Fig. 11.34 Coronal and sagittal views show bilateral Agger nasi cells (asterisk)

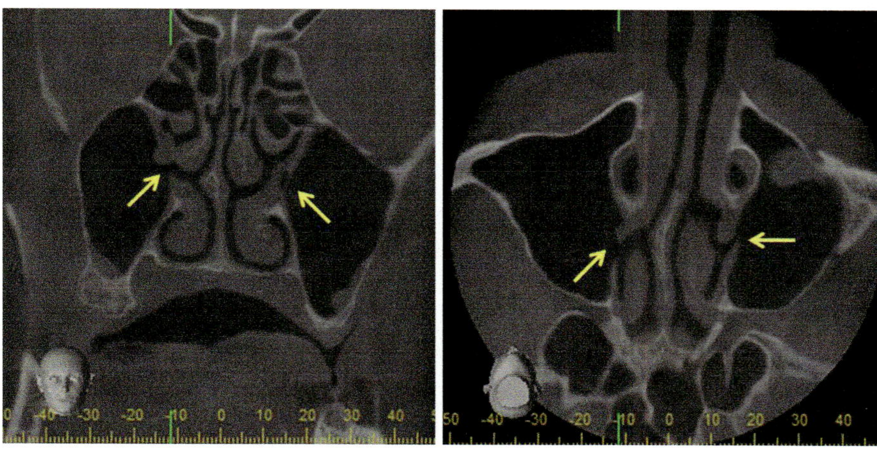

Fig. 11.35 Coronal and axial views of accessory maxillary sinus ostium (arrows)

concha [20]. Accessory maxillary ostium was another variation seen in nearly three-fourths of the cases which opened into membranous meatus inferior to the uncinate process [146]. It is a rare variation of paranasal sinuses. The prevalence of accessory ostium has been reported between 0% and 43% [147–150]. According to CT evaluations in a study, Earwalker [147] reported its prevalence as 14%. Jog and McGarry [148] used a flexible endoscope to investigate accessory ostium, and they reported the prevalence as 4%.

Many radiographic imaging techniques have been employed to study the maxillary sinus. Due to its limitations, plain conventional radiographic techniques are not able to visualize the paranasal variations such as accessory ostium. Obtaining a three-dimensional view using CT is a more accurate method to evaluate the maxillary sinus. In addition, CBCT becomes the first choice to evaluate dentomaxillary area because of its advantages [151] (Fig. 11.35).

Acknowledgments The authors would like to thank to Dr. Murat İçen for providing maxillofacial cysticercosis images.

References

1. Orhan K, Gorurgoz C, Akyol M, Ozarslanturk S, Avsever H. An anatomical variant: evaluation of accessory canals of the canalis sinuosus using CBCT. Folia Morphol (Warsz). 2018. https://doi.org/10.5603/FM.a2018.0003.
2. Kini YK, Kharkar VR, Rudagi BM, Kalburge JV. An unusual occurrence of epidermoid cyst in the buccal mucosa: a case report with review of literature. J Maxillofac Oral Surg. 2013;12(1):90–3.
3. Osborn AG, Preece MT. Intracranial cysts: radiologic-pathologic correlation and imaging approach. Radiology. 2006;239(3):650–64.
4. Park TW, Kim JK, Kim JR. Giant epidermal cyst in the posterior neck developing over 40 years: a case report. Exp Ther Med. 2014;7(1):287–9.
5. Zhou F, Yang Z, Zhu W, Chen L, Song J, Quan K, Li S, Li P, Pan Z, Liu P, Mao Y. Epidermoid cysts of the cavernous sinus: clinical features, surgical outcomes, and literature review. J Neurosurg. 2017;22:1–11.
6. Hu XY, Hu CH, Fang XM, Cui L, Zhang QH. Intraparenchymal epidermoid cysts in the brain: diagnostic value of MR diffusion-weighted imaging. Clin Radiol. 2008;63(7):813–8.
7. Janarthanam J, Mahadevan S. Epidermoid cyst of submandibular region. J Oral Maxillofac Pathol. 2012;16(3):435–7.
8. Garg K, Borkar SA, Kale SS, Sharma BS. Spinal arachnoid cysts - our experience and review of literature. Br J Neurosurg. 2017;31(2):172–8.
9. Logan C, Asadi H, Kok HK, Looby S, O'Hare A, Tornton J, Brennan P. Arachnoid cysts - common and uncommon clinical presentations and radiological features. J Neuroimaging Psychiatry Neurol. 2016;1(2):79–84.
10. Nadgir R, Yousem DM. Neuroradiology: the requisites. 4th ed. Philadelphia: Mosby/Elsevier; 2017.
11. Righi S, Boffano P, Pateras D, Malvè L, Chiodo D, Boson M. Thornwaldt cysts. J Craniofac Surg. 2014;25(5):456–7.
12. Weissman JL. Thornwaldt cysts. Am J Otolaryngol. 1992;13(6):381–5.
13. Ford WJ, Brooks BS, el Gammal T. Thornwaldt cyst: an incidental MR diagnosis. AJNR Am J Neuroradiol. 1987;8(5):922–3.
14. Brennan B. Nasopharyngeal carcinoma. Orphanet J Rare Dis. 2006;26:1–23.
15. Chua MLK, Wee JTS, Hui EP, Chan ATC. Nasopharyngeal carcinoma. Lancet. 2016;387(10022):1012–24.
16. Hsu WM, Wang AG. Nasopharyngeal carcinoma with orbital invasion. Eye (Lond). 2004;18(8):833–8.
17. Shanmugaratnam K, Sobin LH. The World Health Organization histological classification of tumours of the upper respiratory tract and ear. A commentary on the second edition. Cancer. 1993;71(8):2689–97.
18. Hermans R. Head and neck cancer imaging. 1st ed. Berlin: Springer; 2006.
19. Bailey BJ. Head and neck surgery otolaryngology. 3rd ed. Philadelphia: Lippincott Williams and Wilkins; 2001.
20. White CS, Pharoah JM, editors. Oral radiology principles and interpretation. 7th ed. St. Louis: Elsevier; 2014.
21. Rong X, Zhu Q, Ji H, Li J, Huang H. Differentiation of pleomorphic adenoma and Warthin's tumor of the parotid gland: ultrasonographic features. Acta Radiol. 2014;55(10):1203–9.
22. Dumitriu D, Dudea SM, Botar-Jid C, Băciuţ G. Ultrasonographic and sonoelastographic features of pleomorphic adenomas of the salivary glands. Med Ultrason. 2010;12(3):175–83.

23. Klintworth N, Mantsopoulos K, Zenk J, Psychogios G, Iro H, Bozzato A. Sonoelastography of parotid gland tumours: initial experience and identification of characteristic patterns. Eur Radiol. 2012;22(5):947–56.
24. Weidner N, Cote R, Suster S, Weiss L. Modern surgical pathology. 2nd ed. Philadelphia: Saunders; 2009.
25. Sepúlveda I, Platín E, Spencer ML, Mucientes P, Frelinghuysen M, Ortega P, Ulloa D. Oncocytoma of the parotid gland: a case report and review of the literature. Case Rep Oncol. 2014;7(1):109–16.
26. Lee YY, Wong KT, King AD, Ahuja AT. Imaging of salivary gland tumours. Eur J Radiol. 2008;66(3):419–36.
27. Spiro RH. Salivary neoplasms: overview of a 35-year experience with 2,807 patients. Head Neck Surg. 1986;8(3):177–84.
28. Liu XW, Xie CM, Li H, Zhang R, Geng ZJ, Mo YX, Zhao J, Cai MY, Lv YC, Wu PH. Nasopharyngeal adenoid cystic carcinoma: magnetic resonance imaging features in ten cases. Chin J Cancer. 2012;31(1):19–28.
29. Rzepakowska A, Zwierzyńska K, Osuch-Wójcikiewicz E, Niemczyk K. Lymphoid tissue neoplasms in the neck region - epidemiological and clinical analysis over 15 years. Otolaryngol Pol. 2017;71(3):1–9.
30. Weber AL, Rahemtullah A, Ferry JA. Hodgkin and non-Hodgkin lymphoma of the head and neck: clinical, pathologic, and imaging evaluation. Neuroimaging Clin N Am. 2003;13(3):371–92.
31. Ying M, Bhatia KS, Lee YP, Yuen HY, Ahuja AT. Review of ultrasonography of malignant neck nodes: greyscale, Doppler, contrast enhancement and elastography. Cancer Imaging. 2014;13(4):658–69.
32. Louis DN, Perry A, Reifenberger G, von Deimling A, Figarella-Branger D, Cavenee WK, Ohgaki H, Wiestler OD, Kleihues P, Ellison DW. The 2016 World Health Organization classification of tumors of the central nervous system: a summary. Acta Neuropathol. 2016;131(6):803–20.
33. Yue JJ, Guyer RD, Johnson JB, Khoo LT, Hochschuler SH. The comprehensive treatment of the aging spine minimally invasive and advanced techniques. 1st ed. Philadelphia: Elseiver; 2011.
34. Haaga JR, Dogra VS, Forsting M, Gilkeson RC, Kwon Ha H, Sundaram M. CT and MRI of the whole body. 5th ed. Philadelphia: Mosby Elsevier; 2009.
35. Niiro M, Yatsushiro K, Nakamura K, Kawahara Y, Kuratsu J. Natural history of elderly patients with asymptomatic meningiomas. J Neurol Neurosurg Psychiatry. 2000;68(1): 25–8.
36. Surov A, Gottschling S, Mawrin C, Prell J, Spielmann RP, Wienke A, Fiedler E. Diffusion-weighted imaging in meningioma: prediction of tumor grade and association with histopathological parameters. Transl Oncol. 2015;8(6):517–23.
37. Schlosser RJ, Woodworth BA, Gillespie MB, Day TA. Endoscopic resection of sinonasal hemangiomas and hemangiopericytomas. ORL J Otorhinolaryngol Relat Spec. 2006;68(2):69–72.
38. Nikiforova L, Sapundzhiev N, Kolova P, Boyadzhiev G, Bradley P. Fulminant hemangiopericytoma of the larynx - a case report and a review of the literature. Braz J Otorhinolaryngol. 2017; pii: S1808-8694(17)30073.
39. Batsakis JG, Rice DH. The pathology of head and neck tumors: vasoformative tumors, part 9B. Head Neck Surg. 1981;3(4):326–39.
40. Koch M, Nielsen GP, Yoon SS. Malignant tumors of blood vessels: angiosarcomas, hemangioendotheliomas, and hemangioperictyomas. J Surg Oncol. 2008;97:321–9.
41. Persky M, Tran T. Acquired vascular tumors of the head and neck. Otolaryngol Clin North Am. 2018;51(1):255–74.
42. Becker M, Stefanelli S, Rougemont AL, Poletti PA, Merlini L. Non-odontogenic tumors of the facial bones in children and adolescents: role of multiparametric imaging. Neuroradiology. 2017;59(4):327–42.

43. Maniu A, Harabagiu O, Perde Schrepler M, Cătană A, Fănuţă B, Mogoantă CA. Molecular biology of cholesteatoma. Romanian J Morphol Embryol. 2014;55(1):7–13.
44. Preciado DA. Biology of cholesteatoma: special considerations in pediatric patients. Int J Pediatr Otorhinolaryngol. 2012;76(3):319–21.
45. Thompson LD. Update from the 4th edition of the world health organization classification of head and neck tumours: tumours of the ear. Head Neck Pathol. 2017;11(1):78–87.
46. Lingam RK, Connor SEJ, Casselman JW, Beale T. MRI in otology: applications in cholesteatoma and Ménière's disease. Clin Radiol. 2018;73(1):35–44.
47. Widmann G, Henninger B, Kremser C, Jaschke W. MRI sequences in head & neck radiology - state of the art. Rofo. 2017;189(5):413–22.
48. Vaid S, Kamble Y, Vaid N, Bhatti S, Rawat S, Nanivadekar A, Karmarkar S. Role of magnetic resonance imaging in cholesteatoma: the Indian experience. Indian J Otolaryngol Head Neck Surg. 2013;65(Suppl 3):485–92.
49. Lincot J, Veillon F, Riehm S, Babay N, Matern JF, Rock B, Dallaudière B, Meyer N. Middle ear cholesteatoma: compared diagnostic performances of two incremental MRI protocols including non-echo planar diffusion-weighted imaging acquired on 3T and 1.5T scanners. J Neuroradiol. 2015;42(4):193–201.
50. Neville BW, Damm DD, Allen CM, Bouquot JE, editors. Oral and maxillofacial pathology. Pennsylvania: W. B. Saunders; 2002.
51. Orhan K, Kocyigit D, Kisnisci R, Paksoy CS. Rhinolithiasis: an uncommon entity of the nasal cavity. Oral Surg Oral Med Oral Pathol Oral Radiol Endod. 2007;01:e28–32.
52. Orhan K, Orhan AI, Oz U, Pekiner FN, Delilbasi C. Misdiagnosed fibrosarcoma of the mandible mimicking temporomandibular disorder: a rare condition. Oral Surg Oral Med Oral Pathol Oral Radiol Endod. 2007;104(4):e26–9.
53. Sapp JP, Eversole LR, Wysocki GP, editors. Contemporary oral and maxillofacial pathology. St. Louis: Mosby; 2004. p. 302–3.
54. Gobetti JP, Türp JC. Fibrosarcoma misdiagnosed as a temporomandibular disorder: a cautionary tale. Oral Surg Oral Med Oral Pathol Oral Radiol Endod. 1998;85(4):404–9.
55. Wang H, Nie P, Dong C, Li J, Huang Y, Hao D, Xu W. CT and MRI findings of soft tissue adult fibrosarcoma in extremities. Biomed Res Int. 2018;2018:1–7. Article ID 6075705, 7 pages.
56. Nadol JB, Eavey RD. Acute and chronic mastoiditis: clinical presentation, diagnosis, and management. Curr Clin Top Infect Dis. 1995;15:204–9.
57. Orhan K, Nishiyama H, Tadashi S, Shumei M, Furukawa S. MR of 2270 TMJs: prevalence of radiographic presence of otomastoiditis in temporomandibular joint disorders. Eur J Radiol. 2005;55(1):102–7.
58. Som MP, Curtin DH. Head and neck imaging. St. Louis: Mosby; 2011.
59. Chien JH, Chen YS, Hung IF, Hsieh KS, Wu KS, Cheng MF. Mastoiditis diagnosed by clinical symptoms and imaging studies in children: disease spectrum and evolving diagnostic challenges. J Microbiol Immunol Infect. 2012;45(5):377–81.
60. Debnath J, Ravikumar R, Sharma V, Senger KP, Maurya V, Singh G, Sharma P, Khera A, Singh A. 'Empty sella' on routine MRI studies: an incidental finding or otherwise? Med J Armed Forces India. 2016;72(1):33–7.
61. Guitelman M, Garcia Basavilbaso N, Vitale M, Chervin A, Katz D, Miragaya K, Herrera J, Cornalo D, Servidio M, Boero L, Manavela M, Danilowicz K, Alfieri A, Stalldecker G, Glerean M, Fainstein Day P, Ballarino C, Mallea Gil MS, Rogozinski A. Primary empty sella (PES): a review of 175 cases. Pituitary. 2013;16(2):270–4.
62. Agarwal JK, Sahay RK, Bhadada SK, Reddy VS, Agarwal NK. Empty sella syndrome. J Indian Acad Clin Med. 2001;2(3):198–202.
63. Chiloiro S, Giampietro A, Bianchi A, Tartaglione T, Capobianco A, Anile C, De Marinis L. Diagnosis of endocrine disease: primary empty Sella: a comprehensive review. Eur J Endocrinol. 2017;177(6):R275–85.
64. Narula N, Siddiqui F, Katyal N, Avula A, Chalhoub M. Internal carotid artery dissection with lidocaine nerve block injection trauma: a rare case report. Cureus. 2018;10(1):e2027.

65. Provenzale JM. Dissection of the internal carotid and vertebral arteries: imaging features. AJR Am J Roentgenol. 1995;165(5):1099–104.
66. Rodallec MH, Marteau V, Gerber S, Desmottes L, Zins M. Craniocervical arterial dissection: spectrum of imaging findings and differential diagnosis. Radiographics. 2008;28(6):1711–28.
67. English SW, Passe TJ, Lindell EP, Klaas JP. Multiple cranial neuropathies as a presentation of spontaneous internal carotid artery dissection: a case report and literature review. J Clin Neurosci. 2018;50:129–31.
68. Truwit CL. Venous angioma of the brain: history, significance, and imaging findings. AJR Am J Roentgenol. 1992;159(6):1299–307.
69. Wiggins RH, Harnsberger HR, Salzman KL, Shelton C, Kertesz TR, Glastonbury CM. The many faces of facial nerve schwannoma. AJNR Am J Neuroradiol. 2006;27(3):694–9.
70. Garrity JA, Henderson JW. Henderson's orbital tumors. 4th ed. New York: Lippincott Williams and Wilkins; 2007.
71. Younis RT, Gross CW, Lazar RH. Schwannomas of the paranasal sinuses. Case report and clinicopathologic analysis. Arch Otolaryngol Head Neck Surg. 1991;117(6):677–80.
72. Mesolella M, Cimmino M, Di Martino M, Criscuoli G, Albanese L, Galli V. Tonsillolith. Case report and review of the literature. Acta Otorhinolaryngol Ital. 2004;24(5):302–7.
73. Chan J, Rashid M, Karagama Y. An unusual case of a tonsillolith. Case Rep Med. 2012;2012:587503.
74. Dykes M, Izzat S, Pothula V. Giant tonsillolith – a rare cause of dysphagia. J Surg Case Rep. 2012;4:4.
75. de Moura MD, Madureira DF, Noman-Ferreira LC, Abdo EN, de Aguiar EG, Freire AR. Tonsillolith: a report of three clinical cases. Med Oral Patol Oral Cir Bucal. 2007;12(2):E130–3.
76. Alfayez A, Albesher MB, Alqabasani MA. A giant tonsillolith. Saudi Med J. 2018;39(4):412–4.
77. Valdez TA, Vallejo JG. Infectious diseases in pediatric otolaryngology. 1st ed. Basel: Springer; 2016.
78. Centurion BS, Imada TS, Pagin O, Capelozza AL, Lauris JR, Rubira-Bullen IR. How to assess tonsilloliths and styloid chain ossifications on cone beam computed tomography images. Oral Dis. 2013;19:473–8.
79. Oda M, Kito S, Tanaka T, Nishida I, Awano S, Fujita Y, et al. Prevalence and imaging characteristics of detectable tonsilloliths on 482 pairs of consecutive CT and panoramic radiographs. BMC Oral Health. 2013;13:54.
80. Omami G. Soft tissue calcification in oral and maxillofacial imaging: a pictorial review. Int J Dentistry Oral Sci. 2016;03(4):219–24.
81. Altındağ A, Avsever H, Borahan O, Akyol M, Orhan K. Incidental findings in cone-beam computed tomographic images: calcifications in head and neck region. Balk J Dent Med. 2017;21:100–7.
82. Price JB, Thaw KL, Tyndall DA, Ludlow JB, Padilla RJ. Incidental findings from cone beam computed tomography of the maxillofacial region: a descriptive retrospective study. Clin Oral Implants Res. 2012;23:1261–8.
83. Bar T, Zagury A, London D, Shacham R, Nahlieli O. Calcifications simulating sialolithiasis of the major salivary *glan*ds. Dentomaxillofac Radiol. 2007;36(1):59–62.
84. Siddiqui SJ. Sialolithiasis: an unusually large submandibular salivary stone. Br Dent J. 2002;193(2):89–91.
85. Nass Duce M, Talas DU, Ozer C, Yildiz A, Apaydin FD, Ozgür A. Antrolithiasis: a retrospective study. J Laryngol Otol. 2003;117:637–40.
86. Senkal HA, Süslü AE, Ünal ÖF. A rare cause of rhinolithiasis: ectopic. Int J Pediatr Otorhinolaryngol. 2006;70:2129.
87. Karjodkar FR. Textbook of dental and maxillofacial radiology. 2nd ed. Mumbai: Jaypee Brothers Medical; 2009.
88. Ozarslanturk S, Ozturk HP, Senel B, Avsever H, Ozen T. What surprises lie beneath a panoramic radiograph in dental implant planning. Dentistry Adv Res. 2018; DTAR-148.

89. Orhan K, Kocyigit D, Kisnisci R, Paksoy CS. Rhinolithiasis: an uncommon entity of the nasal cavity. Oral Surg Oral Med Oral Pathol Oral Radiol Endod. 2006;101(2):e28–32.
90. Edwards R, Alsufyani N, Heo G, Flores-Mir C. The frequency and nature of incidental findings in large-field cone beam computed tomography scans of an orthodontic sample. Prog Orthod. 2014;15(1):37.
91. Khadija A, Lahlou Y, Chemlali S, Kissa J, Gharibi A, Baite M. Cone beam computed tomography study of intra-sinus calcifications. Glob J Med Res. 2017;17(1):4–13.
92. deShazo RD, Chapin K, Swain RE. Fungal sinusitis. N Engl J Med. 1997;337(4):254–9.
93. Orhan K, Kocyigit D, Turkoglu K, Kartal Y, Arslan A. Illosis of maxillary sinus in immunocompromised patient. Case report. N Y State Dent J. 2012;78(1):46–9.
94. Mossa-Basha M, Ilica AT, Maluf F, Karakoç Ö, Izbudak I, Aygün N. The many faces of fungal disease of the paranasal sinuses: CT and MRI findings. Diagn Interv Radiol. 2013;19(3):195–200.
95. Kishi K, Kawahara K, Moriya I, Komatsu H, Sato M, Aono K. Clinical and radiographic study of multiple miliary osteomas of the skin. Dentomaxillofac Radiol. 1984;13:105–8.
96. Shigehara H, Honda Y, Kishi K, Sugimoto T. Radiographic and morphologic studies of multiple miliary osteomas of cadaver skin. Oral Surg Oral Med Oral Pathol Oral Radiol Endod. 1998;86:121–5.
97. Safi Y, Valizadeh S, Vasegh Z, Aghdasi MM, Shamloo N, Azizi Z. Prevalence of osteoma cutis in the maxillofacial region and classification of its radiographic pattern in cone beam CT. Dermatol Online J. 2016;22(1):2.
98. Eisenkraft BL, Som PM. The spectrum of benign and malignant etiologies of cervical node calcification. Am J Roentgenol. 1999;172:1433–7.
99. Garcia HH, Gonzalez AE, Evans CAW, Gilman RH, Cysticercosis Working Group in Peru. Taenia solium cysticercosis. Lancet. 2003;362(9383):547–56.
100. Chakraborty P, Kumari R, Jain RK, Prasad V, Pradhan S, Joshi P. Solitary head and neck cysticercosis: a series of rare cases. Iran J Otorhinolaryngol. 2017;29(95):347–51.
101. Hosur BM, Byakodi S, Puranik RS, Vanaki SS, Puranik RS, Shivakumar SM. Oral cysticercosis: a case report and review of literature. J Maxillofac Oral Surg. 2015;14(3):853–7.
102. Lustigman S, Prichard KR, Gazzinelli A, Grant NW, Boatin AB, McCarthy SJ, Basáñez GM. A research agenda for helminth diseases of humans: the problem of helminthiases. PLoS Negl Trop Dis. 2012;6(4):e1582.
103. Kanlı A, Özkan G. Yumuşak dokuda radyoopak görüntü veren lezyonlar. Turkiye Klinikleri J Dent Sci Special Topics. 2010;1(2):58–65.
104. Avsever H, Orhan K. Calcifications of jaws and related soft tissues. Turkiye Klinikleri J Oral Maxillofac Radiol Special Topics. 2018;4(1):43–52.
105. Bardouni EA, Boufettal M, Zouaidia F, Kharmaz M, Berrada SM, Mahassini N, Yaacoubi EM. Non-traumatic myositis ossificans circumscripta: a diagnosis trap. J Clin Orthop Trauma. 2014;5(4):261–5.
106. Boffano P, Zavattero E, Bosco G, Berrone S. Myoasperapsitis ossificans of the left medial pterygoid muscle: case report and review of the literature of myositis ossificans of masticatory muscles. Craniomaxillofac Trauma Reconstr. 2014;7(1):43–50.
107. Nemoto H, Sumiya N, Ito Y, Kimura N, Akizuki A, Maruyama N. Myositis ossificans traumatica of the masticatory muscles. J Craniofac Surg. 2012;23(5):e514–6.
108. Goldman AB. Myositis ossificans circumscripta: a benign lesion with a malignant differential diagnosis. Am J Roentgenol. 1976;126:32–40.
109. Amendola MA, Glazer GM, Agha FP, Francis IR, Weatherbee L, Martel W. Myositis ossificans circumscripta: computed tomographic diagnosis. Radiology. 1983;149:775–9.
110. Sedghizadeh PP, Nguyen M, Enciso R. Intracranial physiological calcifications evaluated with cone beam CT. Dentomaxillofac Radiol. 2012;41:675–8.
111. Kıroğlu Y, Çallı C, Karabulut N, Öncel C. Intracranial calcifications on CT. Diagn Interv Radiol. 2010;16:263–9.
112. Kwak R, Takeuchi F, Ito S, Kadoya S. Intracranial physiological calcification on computed tomography (part 1): calcification of the pineal region. No To Shinkei. 1988;40:56–74.

113. Daghighi MH, Rezaei V, Zarrintan S, Pourfathi H. Intracranial physiological calcifications in adults on computed tomography in Tabriz, Iran. Folia Morphol (Warsz). 2007;66:115–9.
114. Mahdian M, Moghaddam EJ, Alzahrani A, Rengasamy K, Tadinada A. Calcification of the stylohyoid ligament in panoramic radiography and cone beam computed tomography among patients referred for dental implant treatment planning. Implant Dent. 2014;23:508–13.
115. Ramadan SU, Gökharman D, Koşar P, Kacar M, Koşar U. The stylohyoid chain: CT imaging. Eur J Radiol. 2010;75:346–51.
116. Lanzer P, Boehm M, Sorribas V, Thiriet M, Janzen J, Zeller T, et al. Medial vascular calcification revisited: review and perspectives. Eur Heart J. 2014;35:1515–25.
117. Tahmasbi-Arashlow M, Barghan S, Kashtwari D, Nair MK. Radiographic manifestations of Mönckeberg arteriosclerosis in the head and neck region. Imaging Sci Dent. 2016;46(1): 53–6.
118. Frazier JJ, Casian R, Benson BW. Mönckeberg medial calcinosis of the infraorbital arteries: a first case report. *Oral Surg Oral Med Oral Pathol Oral Radiol. 2018;125(2):e31–5.*
119. Romano-Sousa CM, Krejci L, Medeiros FMM, Graciosa-Filho RG, Martins MFF, Guedes VN, et al. Diagnostic agreement between panoramic radiographs and color doppler images of carotid atheroma. J Appl Oral Sci. 2009;17:45–8.
120. Damaskos S, Tsiklakis K, Syriopoulos K, van der Stelt P. Extra-and intra-cranial arterial calcifications in adults depicted as incidental findings on cone beam CT images. Acta Odontol Scand. 2015;73:202–9.
121. Avsever H, Gunduz K, Karakoç O, Akyol M, Orhan K. Incidental findings on cone-beam computed tomographic images: paranasal sinus findings and nasal septum variations. Oral Radiol. 2018;34:40–8.
122. Conrad DA, Jenson HB. Management of acute bacterial rhinosinusitis. Curr Opin Pediatr. 2002;14(1):86–90.
123. Zacharisen M, Casper R. Pediatric sinusitis. Immunol Allergy Clin N Am. 2005;25(2): 313–32.
124. Brüllman DD, Schmidtmann I, Hornstein S, Shulze RK. Correlation of cone beam computed tomography (CBCT) findings in the maxillary sinus with dental diagnoses: a retrospective cross-sectional study. Clin Oral Investig. 2012;16:1023–9.
125. Lana JP, Carneiro PM, Machado Vde C, de Souza PE, Manzi FR, Horta MC. Anatomic variations and lesions of the maxillary sinus detected in cone beam computed tomography for dental implants. Clin Oral Implants Res. 2012;23:1398–403.
126. Bassiouny A, Newlands WJ, Ali H, Zaki Y. Maxillary sinus hypoplasia and superior orbital fissure asymmetry. Laryngoscope. 1982;92:441–8.
127. Hupp JR, Ellis E, Tucker MR, editors. Contemporary oral and maxillofacial surgery. 5th ed. St. Louis: Mosby Elsevier; 2008. p. 515–20.
128. Weed DT, Cole RR. Maxillary sinus hypoplasia and vertical dystopia of the orbit. Laryngoscope. 1994;104(6 Pt 1):758–62.
129. Thiagarajan B, Narashiman S. Hypoplasia of all paranasal sinuses: a case series and literature review. Otolaryngol Online J. 2012;2(2):1–5.
130. Erdem T, Aktas D, Erdem G, Miman MC, Ozturan O. Maxillary sinus hypoplasia. Rhinology. 2002;40:150–3.
131. Jafari-Povze N, Sheikhi M, Ataie-Khorasgani M, Jafari-Povze S. Aplasia and hypoplasia of the maxillary sinus: a case series. Dent Res J (Isfahan). 2014;11(5):615–7.
132. Mathew R, Omami G, Hand A, Fellows D, Lurie A. Cone beam CT analysis of Haller cells: prevalence and clinical significance. Dentomaxillofac Radiol. 2013;42:20130055.
133. Alkire BC, Bhattacharyya N. An assessment of sinonasal anatomic variants potentially associated with recurrent acute rhinosinusitis. Laryngoscope. 2010;120:631–4.
134. Lloyd GA. CT of the paranasal sinuses: study of a control series in relation to endoscopic sinus surgery. J Laryngol Otol. 1990;104:477–81.
135. Kainz J, Braun H, Genser P. Haller's cells: morphologic evaluation and clinico-surgical relevance. Laryngorhinootologie. 1993;72:599–604.
136. Milczuk H. Nasal and paranasal sinus anomalies in children with chronic sinusitis. Laryngoscope. 1993;103:247–52.

137. Ahmad M, Khurana N, Jaberi J, Sampair C, Kuba RK. Prevalence of infraorbital ethmoid (Haller's) cells on panoramic radiographs. Oral Surg Oral Med Oral Pathol Oral Radiol Endod. 2006;101(5):658–61.
138. Chmielik LP, Chmielik A. The prevalence of the Onodi cell- most suitable method of CT evaluation in its detection. Int J Pediatr Otorhinolaryngol. 2017;97:202–5.
139. Kainz J, Stammberger H. Danger areas of the posterior rhinobasis. An endoscopic and anatomical-surgical study. Acta Otolaryngol. 1992;112(5):852–61.
140. Badia L, Lund VJ, Wei W, Ho WK. Ethnic variation in sinonasal anatomy on CT-scanning. Rhinology. 2005;443(3):210–4.
141. Koo SK, Kim JD, Moon JS, Jung SH, Lee SH. The incidence of concha bullosa, unusual anatomic variation and its relationship to nasal septal deviation: a retrospective radiologic study. Auris Nasus Larynx. 2017;44(5):561–70.
142. Smith KD, Edwards PC, Saini TS, Norton NS. The prevalence of concha bullosa and nasal septal deviation and their relationship to maxillary sinusitis by volumetric tomography. Int J Dent. 2010;2010:404982.
143. Goldman JL. The principles and practice of rhinology: a text on the diseases and surgery of the nose and paranasal sinuses. New York: Wiley; 1987. p. 405.
144. Türk B, Akpinar M, Mahmutoğlu AS, Uçak I, Coşkun BU. Anatomic variations in paranasal sinuses of patients with sinonasal polyposis: radiological evaluation. J Craniofac Surg. 2016;27:1336–9.
145. Bolger WE, Butzin CA, Parsons DS. Paranasal sinus bony anatomic variations and mucosal abnormalities: CT analysis for endoscopic sinus surgery. Laryngoscope. 1991;101:56–64.
146. Prasanna LC, Mamatha H. The location of maxillary sinus ostium and its clinical application. Indian J Otolaryngol Head Neck Surg. 2010;62(4):335–7.
147. Earwaker J. Anatomic variants in sinonasal CT. Radiographics. 1993;13:381–415.
148. Jog M, McGarry GW. How frequent are accessory sinus ostia? J Laryngol Otol. 2003;117:270–2.
149. May M, Sobol SM, Korzec K. The location of the maxillary os and its importance to the endoscopic sinus surgeon. Laryngoscope. 1990;100:1037–42.
150. Scheaffer JP. Paranasal sinuses, nasolacrimal passageways and olfactory organ in man. Philadelphia: Blakiston; 1920.
151. Tadinata A, Fung K, Thacker S, Mahdian M, Jadhav A, Schincaglia GP. Radiographic evaluation of the maxillary sinus prior to dental implant therapy: a comparison between two-dimensional and three-dimensional radiographic imaging. Imaging Sci Dent. 2015;45:169–74.

Nuclear Medicine in TMJ Imaging

12

Ingrid Różyło-Kalinowska

12.1 Nuclear Medicine

Nuclear medicine deals with diagnostics and therapy using radioactive isotopes emitting beta or gamma radiation. Radiopharmaceuticals are pharmaceuticals containing radioactive isotope as tracer and a ligand, i.e. a molecule, chemical compound or cell (e.g. granulocyte) that has an affinity towards a tissue or organ. When administered to a patient, radioactivity emitted by a radiopharmaceutical is being registered. As various tissues and organs differently accumulate this tracer, changes in radioisotope intake are detectable, especially when tissue metabolism rate is disturbed by a pathological process.

Registration of radiation can be performed by means of a single static gamma camera (also known as a scintillation camera), one or more rotating gamma cameras or multiheaded gamma cameras. Depending on the type of registration device, the imaging methods are divided into scintigraphy, single-photon emission computed tomography (SPECT) and positron emission tomography (PET).

12.2 Scintigraphy

In scintigraphy a single static gamma camera is used to pick up radioisotope emission in a static manner (e.g. bone scintigraphy) or analyse function of an organ in a dynamic way (e.g. sialo-scintigraphy, lymphoscintigraphy or three-phase technique in bone scintigraphy).

Bone scintigraphy is performed using osteotropic tracers, most commonly methylene diphosponate (MDP) linked with radioactive technetium (^{99m}Tc), which is injected into a vein (arm, hand or foot). MDP targets bone tissue, and its uptake

I. Różyło-Kalinowska
Independent Unit of Propaedeutics of Dentomaxillofacial Radiology, Medical University of Lublin, Lublin, Poland

I. Rozylo-Kalinowska, K. Orhan (eds.), *Imaging of the Temporomandibular Joint*, https://doi.org/10.1007/978-3-319-99468-0_12

depends on bone mineralisation, collagen content, vascularisation and bone remodelling. Forming of hydroxyapatite crystals in the areas of production of new osteoid tissue by osteoblasts leads to an increased uptake of tagged MDP; thus these areas accumulate more radioactive tracer and show up as "hot" [1].

In static (single phase) scintigraphy, bone scanning is performed after 2–5 h following the administration of the radiopharmaceutical. Planar scintigraphy of TMJ is performed typically in anterior, posterior, right lateral and left lateral projections with a 500,000 count per each image [2, 3].

Three-phase technique in bone scintigraphy comprises emission of radiation in three stages:

- Perfusion phase—dynamic scanning of blood flow immediately after the administration of the tracer
- Blood pool phase—evaluation of blood supply of soft tissues recorded about 10 min later
- Metabolic phase—similar to static (single phase) scintigraphy, with images acquired after about 2 h from injection of the radiopharmaceutical

The use of bone scintigraphy in TMJ diagnostics is not common in comparison with other diagnostic imaging techniques [4]. Indications for a static bone scan include osteomyelitis, especially in early phase and evaluation of its progress and bone remodelling, synovitis, bone metastasis diagnostics and treatment follow-up, aseptic bone necrosis and metabolic diseases (such as fibrous dysplasia or Paget's disease) [5]. Kim et al. [6] evaluated usefulness of bone scintigraphy in diagnostics of TMJ osteoarthritis. There were significant differences in uptake ratios between the osteoarthritis and non-osteoarthritis groups thus leading to a conclusion that bone scans may help to diagnose osteoarthritis when uptake ratios are increased. Open-mouth bone scintigraphy was proved to be better than closed-mouth bone scan in patients with temporomandibular osteoarthritis as it is difficult to differentiate physiologic bone uptake in a condyle and glenoid fossa of temporal bone in closed-mouth position [7].

Bone scintigraphy is very sensitive, but not specific. Detailed patient's history must be recorded before the scan, including recent fractures, as areas with increased tracer concentration may not be new pathological lesions, but rather areas of bone healing with increased metabolism rate. Specificity of diagnostics of inflammatory lesions may be increased by application of dedicated radiopharmaceutical such as nanocolloid, labelled polyclonal human immunoglobulin G (^{99m}Tc-IgG), labelled granulocytes and gallium citrate (^{67}Ga or ^{68}Ga) [8]. Labelled granulocytes and immunoglobulins accumulate in areas of inflammatory process. Gallium has an affinity to mucopolysaccharides within an inflamed tissue and is used to label granulocytes, while nanocolloid demonstrates increased permeability of blood vessels.

Patients should be well-hydrated before and after bone scan in order to increase diuresis and elimination of radiopharmaceutical from organism, thus decreasing time of exposure to radiation emitted by radioisotopes. In pregnant and breast-feeding females, benefits of the scan must outweigh possible consequences of irradiation. Mean effective dose to a patient derived from bone scintigraphy is about 4 mSv.

12.3 Single-Photon Emission Computed Tomography (SPECT)

SPECT is based on registration of emission of radiation by means of a rotating gamma camera to obtain projections from multiple angles. Typically either a full 360-degree rotation is performed by one gamma camera or 180-degree rotation when two gamma cameras are used, and projections are acquired every 3–6°. After completed acquisition lasting for about 15 min, the data is reconstructed providing a three-dimensional data set and tomographic images (Fig. 12.1).

SPECT uses the same radiopharmaceuticals as scintigraphy, but the acquired images are more precise regarding localisation of areas of tracer uptake. Further precision is gained when SPECT is combined with a CT scanner (SPECT/CT). SPECT/CT scanners can provide quantitative date on voxel values of kilobecquerels

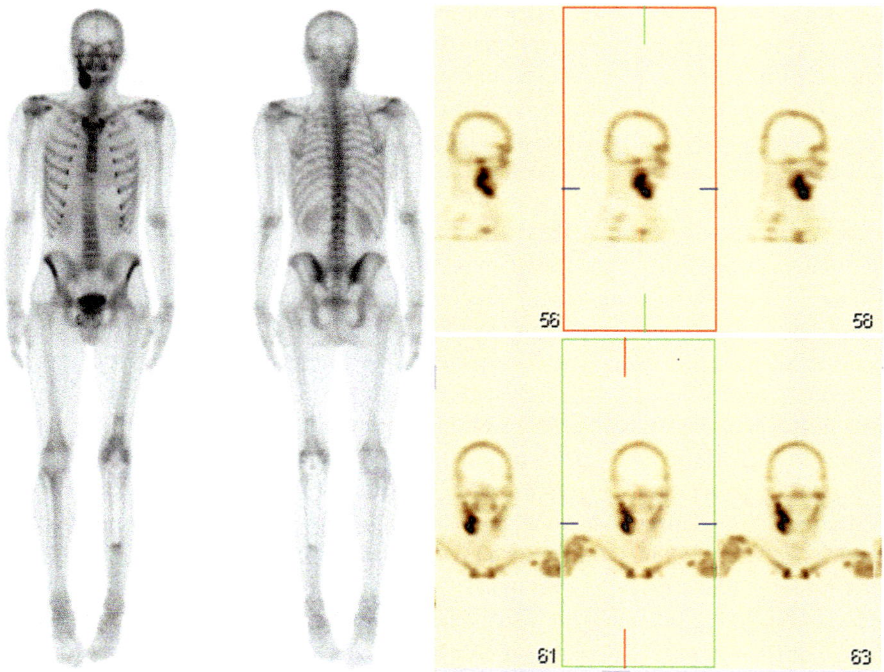

Fig. 12.1 SPECT examination after administration of ^{99m}Tc-MDP obtained in a male patient aged 20 as follow-up to osteosarcoma of left tibia treated by resection and implantation of an endoprothesis. Differential diagnosis of the area of increased accumulation of radiotracer in the right mandible included osteomyelitis, osteosarcoma and fibrous dysplasia (the images are reproduced courtesy of Prof. Leszek Królicki, Head of the Department of Nuclear Medicine of the Medical University of Warsaw, Poland)

per millilitre. Patient preparation and precautions in pregnant and breast-feeding patients are similar to those for a bone scan [7].

The following applications of SPECT in TMJ imaging were reported:

- Unilateral condylar hyperplasia [9–11]
- Bone tracer uptake in patients suffering from TMJ pain [12]
- Osteoarthritis [2, 7]
- Quantitative evaluation of temporomandibular joint disorder (TMD) [13]
- Evaluation of the effects of functional orthopaedic treatment of TMJ [14, 15]

12.4 Positron Emission Tomography (PET)

In PET scans a special gamma camera and different types of radiopharmaceuticals are used. The applied radioisotopes are characterised by a deficit of neutrons in the nuclei; thus there is an additional proton in each nucleus. This imbalance forces each additional proton to emit a positron and a neutrino (positive beta decay). Following this emission the proton changes to a missing neutron. In turn the arising positrons soon are annihilated when collide with electrons in vicinity. The annihilation produces two gamma photons characterised by energy of 511 keV that travel in opposite directions at 180°, which are detected by a scintillator producing photons of light. Only pairs reaching the scintillator within a few nanoseconds are registered. Detection of only this type of radiation increases sensitivity and specificity of the scan by elimination of detection of scattered radiation; however, there is always a slight direction error [16].

Radioisotopes applied in PET examinations have a very short half-life (from 2 min to approximately 2 h). There are numerous PET tracers with affinity to different target molecules and metabolic processes, but due to their short half-lives, they should be produced in a cyclotron located close to PET facilities, which increases costs of examination. However, the most commonly applied radiopharmaceutical is 2-fluoro-2-deoxyglucose labelled with fluorine-18 (^{18}FDG), with half-life of 110 min, which makes it feasible to be manufactured in other locations and transported to PET centres. FDG is an analogue of glucose and is uptaken by areas characterised by an increased metabolism rate such as neoplastic lesions, inflammatory lesions and granulation tissue in wound healing. This way it is possible to differentiate lesions with high metabolic rate and areas with lower glucose uptake [16].

Currently PET scans are combined with CT PET-CT and MRI as PET-MRI, which is called hybrid imaging and is gaining more and more importance due to higher precision of examination as information on metabolism is overlapped on morphological images [16].

Patient preparation for an FGD PET scan is essential. Patients must refrain from eating for at least 6 h before a PET scan, and baseline glucose blood level should be lower than 120 mg/dl. A patient must be well-hydrated in order to increase diuresis, this way eliminating free FDG with urea. During 1–2 days before the scan, intensive physical activity should be avoided as it increases metabolic rate in skeletal muscles and will result in FDG uptake during the scan producing bias in image interpretation. PET scanning should be performed at least 3 months after surgery, radiotherapy, biopsy or endoscopy as FDG is accumulated in inflammatory areas induced by these procedures. Also at least 10 days to 3 months delay in PET scanning should be applied in case of chemotherapy as it may cause temporary inhibition of accumulation of radiopharmaceutical. Sensitivity of FDG PET is much lower in diabetic patients [16].

After intravenous administration of FDG, a patient must remain reclined in a dimmed room with decreased exposure to stimuli in order to decrease uptake of FDG by the brain and muscles. Activity of the head and neck should be limited as well in order to avoid FDG accumulation in muscles working during jaw movements and thus false-positive results. Within the head and neck FDG is physiologically accumulated to a various extent in the brain, salivary glands, bone marrow, skeletal muscles, brown fat tissue in the neck and lymphatic tissue. The PET scanning itself lasts for about 20–30 min [16].

Indications for PET scanning of TMJ area are mostly related to diagnostics and treatment follow-up of malignant tumours. They include early diagnostics of neoplasms; staging of some tumours, e.g. lymphoma; planning of radiotherapy; and location of an unknown primary tumour with known metastases, response to treatment, follow-up and differentiation between recurrent tumour and post-treatment lesions induced by, e.g. radiotherapy [16–20] (Fig. 12.2).

Other applications are far less common [21]. The first study to evaluate the clinical utility of FDG-PET/CT in patients with TMD was published in 2013 by Lee et al. [2]. They concluded that PET/CT showed high TMJ uptake rations in

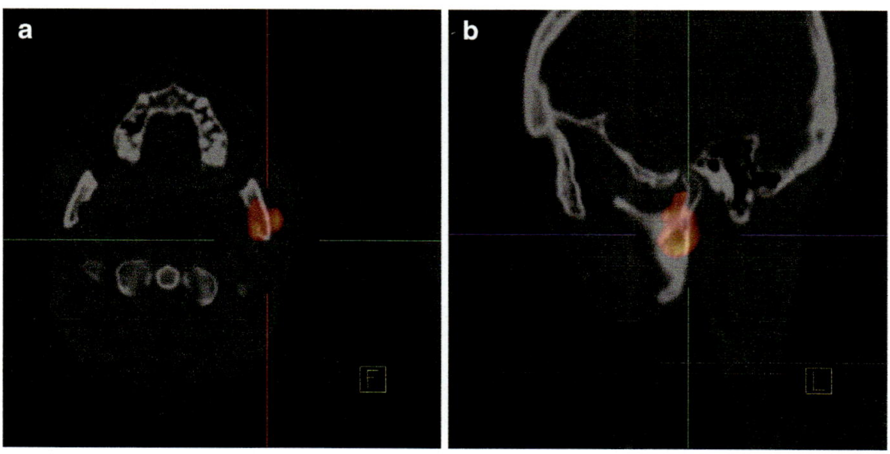

Fig. 12.2 18F-FDG PET-CT scan demonstrating increased uptake in primary lymphoma of the left mandibular ramus and left masseter muscle. (**a**) Axial image, (**b**) coronal slice (the images are reproduced courtesy of Prof. Leszek Królicki, Head of the Department of Nuclear Medicine of the Medical University of Warsaw, Poland)

patients with osteoarthritis, while accuracy and sensitivity were higher than in conventional bone scintigraphy.

Suh et al. [13] investigated patients with temporomandibular joint disorder (TMD) by means of PET-CT with ^{8}F-sodium fluoride (NaF) as tracer and found out that this imaging modality was useful in arthralgic TMJ and TMD osteoarthritis and a correlation with the patients' response to splint therapy was ascertained.

Lindell and Thor [22] described the use of FDG PET-CT in a young patient who experienced progressive ankyloses following a glenoid fossa fracture with condyle displacement into the middle cranial fossa and underwent total joint replacement at the age of 18 with a custom-made alloplastic TMJ prosthesis. PET-CT revealed that there were no signs of increased remodelling or pathology after the reconstruction. The resolution of FDG PET for bone fractures is comparable with this of skeletal scintigraphy.

Saridin et al. [23] assessed bone growth and blood flow in the condylar region in patients with unilateral condylar hyperactivity (UCH) by means of PET scan, which demonstrated that there were no evidences of hypervascularization or an abnormally high rate of bone growth in the affected condylar region in UCH patients. Instead, the rate of bone growth was reduced in the contralateral condylar region.

PET scan evaluation requires thorough correlation with patient's medical history and other examinations—physical, laboratory and diagnostic imaging. In PET report there are assessed standardised uptake values (SUV), which are semi-quantitative measurements of the uptake in a tumour normalised on the basis of a distribution volume [3, 13].

Mean effective dose for a PET scan is from 3 to 4 mSv, while simultaneous use of CT scanning will increase the total dose by the radiation from the CT examination. For a whole body PET/CT, the dose may reach 14–17 mSv. Like in case of bone scintigraphy, the use of PET and PET/CT in pregnant and breast-feeding females should be limited to patients in whom the examinations cannot be rescheduled after birth and benefits from the study would outweigh potential foetal risks [16, 24–26].

References

1. Choi BH, Yoon SH, Song SI, Yoon JK, Lee SJ, An YS. Comparison of diagnostic performance between visual and quantitative assessment of bone scintigraphy results in patients with painful temporomandibular disorder. Medicine (Baltimore). 2016;95(2):e2485. https://doi.org/10.1097/MD.0000000000002485.
2. Lee JW, Lee SM, Kim SJ, Choi JW, Baek KW. Clinical utility of fluoride-18 positron emission tomography/CT in temporomandibular disorder with osteoarthritis: comparisons with 99mTc-MDP bone scan. Dentomaxillofac Radiol. 2013;42(2):29292350. https://doi.org/10.1259/dmfr/29292350.
3. Suh MS, Lee WW, Kim Y-K, Yun P-Y, Kim SE. Maximum standardized uptake value of ^{99m}Tc hydroxymethylene diphosphonate SPECT/CT for the evaluation of temporomandibular joint disorder. Radiology. 2016;280(3):890–6.
4. Epstein JB, Rea A, Chahal O. The use of bone scintigraphy in temporomandibular joint disorders. Oral Dis. 2002;8(1):47–53.
5. Hayashi D, Roemer FW, Katur A, Felson DT, Yang SO, Alomran F, Guermazi A. Imaging of synovitis in osteoarthritis: current status and outlook. Semin Arthritis Rheum. 2011;41(2):116–30.

6. Kim JH, Kim YK, Kim SG, Yun PY, Kim JD, Min JH. Effectiveness of bone scans in the diagnosis of osteoarthritis of the temporomandibular joint. Dentomaxillofac Radiol. 2012;41(3):224–9.
7. Park KS, Song HC, Cho SG, Kang SR, Kim J, Jun HM, Song M, Jeong GC, Park HJ, Kwon SY, Min JJ, Bom HH. Open-mouth bone scintigraphy is better than closed-mouth bone scintigraphy in the diagnosis of temporomandibular osteoarthritis. Nucl Med Mol Imaging. 2016;50(3):213–8.
8. de Bois MH, Tak PP, Arndt JW, Kluin PM, Pauwels EK, Breedveld FC. Joint scintigraphy for quantification of synovitis with 99mTc-labelled human immunoglobulin G compared to histological examination. Clin Exp Rheumatol. 1995;13(2):155–9.
9. Martin-Granizo R, Garcia-Rielo JM, De la Sen O, Maniegas L, Berguer A, De Pedro M. Correlation between single photon emission computed tomography and histopathologic findings in condylar hyperplasia of the temporomandibular joint. J Craniomaxillofac Surg. 2017;45(6):839–44.
10. Portelli M, Gatto E, Matarese G, Militi A, Catalfamo L, Gherlone E, Lucchese A. Unilateral condylar hyperplasia: diagnosis, clinical aspects and operative treatment. A case report. Eur J Paediatr Dent. 2015;16(2):99–102.
11. Rushinek H, Tabib R, Fleissig Y, Klein M, Tshori S. Evaluation of three analysis methods for ^{99m}Tc MDP SPECT scintigraphy in the diagnosis of unilateral condylar hyperplasia. Int J Oral Maxillofac Surg. 2016;45(12):1607–13.
12. Ahn BC, Kim HJ, Lee SW, Yoo J, Choi JK, Lee J. New quantitative method for bone tracer uptake of temporomandibular joint using Tc-99m MDP skull SPECT. Ann Nucl Med. 2009;23(7):651–6.
13. Suh MS, Park SH, Kim YK, Yun PY, Lee WW. ^{18}F-NaF PET/CT for the evaluation of temporomandibular joint disorder. Clin Radiol. 2018;73(4):414.e7–414.e13. pii: S0009-9260(17)30527-5. https://doi.org/10.1016/j.crad.2017.11.008.
14. Güner DD, Oztürk Y, Sayman HB. Evaluation of the effects of functional orthopaedic treatment on temporomandibular joints with single-photon emission computerized tomography. Eur J Orthod. 2003;25(1):9–12.
15. Hersek N, Canay S, Caner B, Ulutuncel N. Bone SPECT imaging of patients with internal derangement of temporomandibular joint before and after splint therapy. Oral Surg Oral Med Oral Pathol Oral Radiol Endod. 2002;94(5):576–80.
16. Boellaard R, Delgado-Bolton R, Oyen WJG, Giammarile F, Tatsch K, Eschner W, Verzijlbergen FJ, Barrington SF, Pike LC, Stroobants S, Delbeke D, Donohoe KJ, Holbrook S, Graham MM, Testanera G, Hoekstra OS, Zijlstra J, Visser E, Hoekstra CJ, Pruim J, Willemsen A, Arends B, Kotzerke J, Bockisch A, Beyer T, Chiti A, Krause BJ. FDG PET and PET/CT: EANM procedure guidelines for tumour PET imaging: version 2.0. Eur J Nucl Med Mol Imaging. 2015;42:328–54.
17. Hu Y, Kuang B, Chen Y, Shu J. Imaging features for diffuse-type tenosynovial giant cell tumor of the temporomandibular joint: a case report. Medicine (Baltimore). 2017;96(26):e7383. https://doi.org/10.1097/MD.0000000000007383.
18. Shintaku WH, Venturin JS, Yepes JF. Application of advanced imaging modalities for the diagnosis of metastatic adenocarcinoma of the lungs in the temporomandibular joint. Oral Surg Oral Med Oral Pathol Oral Radiol Endod. 2009;107(6):e37–41. https://doi.org/10.1016/j.tripleo.2009.02.027.
19. Shintaku WH, Venturin JS, Langlais RP, Clark GT. Imaging modalities to access bony tumors and hyperplasic reactions of the temporomandibular joint. J Oral Surg. 2010;68(8):1911–21.
20. Terzic A, Becker M, Wissmeyer M, Scolozzi P. 18F-DOPA PET/CT unravels malignant paraganglioma mimicking temporomandibular joint disorder. Dentomaxillofac Radiol. 2011;40(5):315–9.
21. Rice DD, Abramovitch K, Roche S, Cora CA, Torralba KD, Christensen HL, Christiansen EL. Undiagnosed, chronic temporomandibular joint pain: making a case for FDG-PET/CT. Int J Rheum Dis. 2017;20(12):2122–6.
22. Lindell B, Thor A. A case of glenoid fossa fracture, progressive ankylosis, total joint reconstruction with alloplastic prosthesis to normalized function including evaluation with F18-PET/CT-a four year follow-up. Craniomaxillofac Trauma Reconstr. 2017;10(1):60–5.

23. Saridin CP, Raijmakers PG, Kloet RW, Tuinzing DB, Becking AG, Lammertsma AA. No signs of metabolic hyperactivity in patients with unilateral condylar hyperactivity: an in vivo positron emission tomography study. J Oral Maxillofac Surg. 2009;67(3):576–81.
24. Bural GG, Laymon CM, Mountz JM. Nuclear imaging of a pregnant patient: should we perform nuclear medicine procedures during pregnancy? Mol Imaging Radionucl Ther. 2012;21(1):1–5.
25. Kaushik A, Jaimini A, Tripathi M, D'Souza M, Sharma R, Mondal A, Mishra AK, Dwarakanath BS. Estimation of radiation dose to patients from ^{18}FDG whole body PET/CT investigations using dynamic PET scan protocol. Indian J Med Res. 2015;142(6):721–31.
26. Takalkar AM, Khandelwal A, Lokitz S, Lilien DL, Stabin MG. 18F-FDG PET in pregnancy and fetal radiation dose estimates. J Nucl Med. 2011;52(7):1035–40.

TMJ Disc Disorders and Osteoarthritis

13

Tore A. Larheim, Bjørn B. Mork-Knutsen, Caroline Hol, Anna-Karin Abrahamsson, Margareth Kristensen Ottersen, and Linda Z. Arvidsson

13.1 Disc Disorders

13.1.1 Disc Displacement in Adults

The disc is seen on MR images as a low signal structure between the articular eminence/fossa and the condylar head. It is defined as anteriorly displaced or dislocated when located in an anterior or ventral position relative to the condylar head, compared to the disc position in a normal (healthy) joint. However, there is no consensus as to how much displacement is considered abnormal [1], although attempts were made to define the normal range of disc position [2]. According to Schiffman et al. [3], the disc is considered anteriorly displaced when the posterior band of the disc is located anterior to the 11:30 position and the intermediate zone of the disc is anterior to the condylar head on oblique sagittal images in the maximum intercuspal position (Fig. 13.1).

Disc displacement is reported to occur in up to about 80% in TMD patients referred for diagnostic TMJ imaging [4–8] and seems to be the most common TMJ pathology. Displacements in directions other than anteriorly are unusual.

Functional Types of Disc Displacement and Value of Clinical Examination for the Diagnosis According to Schiffman et al. [3], there are four functional disc disorders: (1) disc displacement with reduction, (2) disc displacement with reduction with intermittent locking, (3) disc displacement without reduction with limited mouth opening, and (4) disc displacement without reduction without limited mouth opening.

T. A. Larheim (✉) · B. B. Mork-Knutsen · C. Hol · A.-K. Abrahamsson · M. K. Ottersen
L. Z. Arvidsson
Department of Maxillofacial Radiology, Faculty of Dentistry, University of Oslo, Oslo, Norway
e-mail: t.a.larheim@odont.uio.no; b.b.mork-knutsen@odont.uio.no; caroline.hol@odont.uio.no; a.k.johansen@odont.uio.no; m.k.ottersen@odont.uio.no; l.z.arvidsson@odont.uio.no

I. Rozylo-Kalinowska, K. Orhan (eds.), *Imaging of the Temporomandibular Joint*, https://doi.org/10.1007/978-3-319-99468-0_13

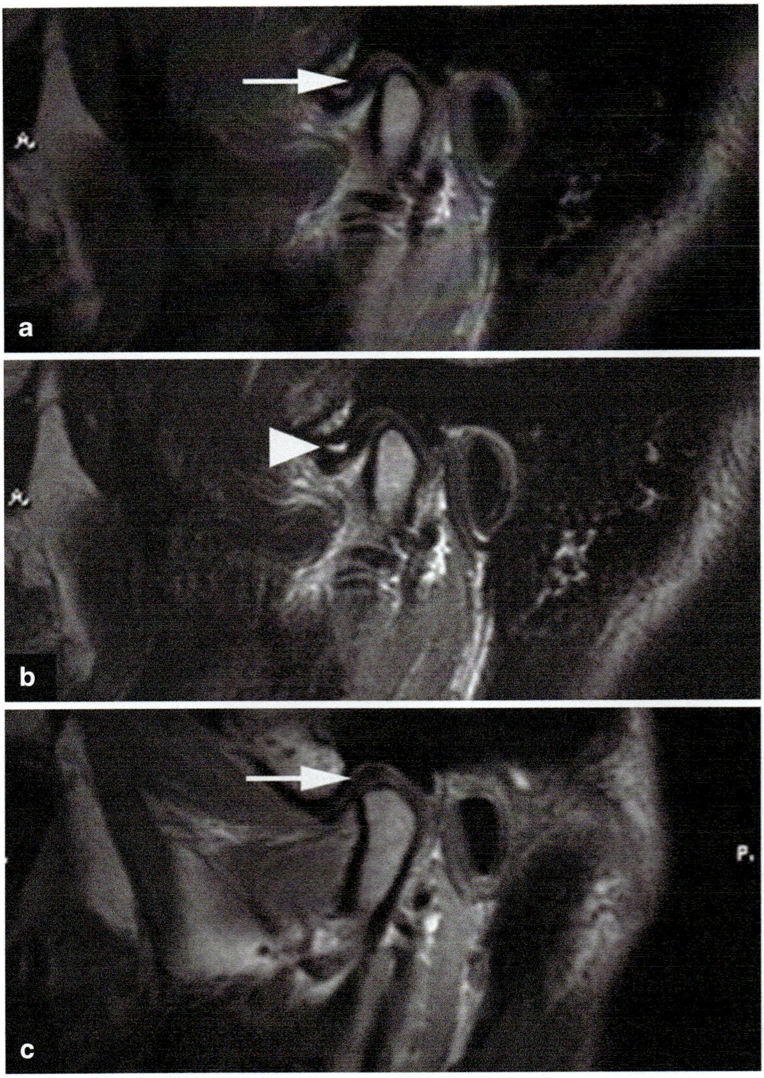

Fig. 13.1 Disc displacement and normal bone in the right joint (**a**, **b**). Normal disc position and normal bone in the left joint (**c**). (**a**) Oblique sagittal PD-weighted MRI shows posterior band (*arrow*) anterior to the condyle. (**b**) Oblique sagittal T2-weighted MRI shows minimal (normal) joint fluid (*arrowhead*). (**c**) Oblique sagittal PD-weighted MRI shows posterior band (*arrow*) superior to the condyle. Reproduced with permission from Larheim T.A., Westesson P-L. A. Maxillofacial Imaging (Springer 2018)

Clinical examination provides relatively limited information with respect to the articular disc status, with MRI used as a reference method. However, the value of the clinical examination varies substantially with the functional disc status. The sensitivity/specificity obtained with the clinical examination to diagnose disc displacement with reduction or intermittent locking is 0.34/0.92 and 0.38/0.98, respectively. The clinical diagnosis of disc displacement without reduction without limited mouth opening is only slightly better (0.54/0.79). On the other hand, clinical examination of disc displacement without reduction with limited mouth opening has high sensitivity/specificity (0.80/0.97) [3]. Thus, of the four functional disc disorder conditions, only the latter can be reliably diagnosed by clinical examination.

Imaging Necessary for Disc Displacement Diagnosis Diagnostic imaging is necessary to make a reliable assessment of the disc status, if needed. MRI is the only method that can depict the disc satisfactorily.

Before the era of diagnostic imaging, the dislocation of the articular disc relative to the mandibular condyle was considered a well-known pathologic condition based on symptoms such as clicking sounds and impaired mouth opening [9]. When soft-tissue imaging of the TMJ became possible, dislocation of the disc was frequently confirmed in adult TMD patients [4]. Many authors considered the displaced disc being the main cause of pain [10].

However, when MRI was performed on asymptomatic volunteers, disc displacement was found in as many as one third [5, 7, 8, 11]. Since then there has been a controversy whether disc displacement is a pathologic condition or a normal variant [11, 12].

Differences Between Symptomatic Patients and Asymptomatic Volunteers Regarding Disc Displacement There are documented differences between these groups of individuals regarding both the disc function and the type of displacement. In all studies of asymptomatic volunteers, the anteriorly displaced disc is reported to normalize (reduce) on open-mouth images in almost all joints examined [5, 6, 8, 11, 13, 14].

In addition to a satisfactory disc function, another feature also contributes to the disc displacement being less severe in volunteers than in patients. Larheim et al. reported that 90% of the displaced discs in volunteers were partially displaced [8], supporting a study of Rammelsberg et al. [14]. Partial disc displacement is here defined as displacement only in one portion of the joint [15]. The same observation was made in a study of schoolchildren without symptoms [16]. Partial disc displacement has also been documented in autopsy specimens [6].

Partial and Complete Disc Displacement Since then, little attention has been paid to the differentiation between partial and complete disc displacement although it is mentioned in some recent studies [1, 17]. In the comprehensive imaging study on diagnostic criteria by Ahmad et al. [18], all sections through each joint were analyzed. When there were different findings in the different sections, however, the "worst case" scenario was scored. If the disc was anteriorly displaced only in one section and not in other sections, the diagnosis was recorded as anterior disc displacement [18]. No differentiation was made between partial and complete disc displacement. Thus, the authors "lost" the proportion of partially displaced discs. In the study by Larheim et al. [8], partial disc displacement occurred with the same frequency (about 22%) in volunteers and patients

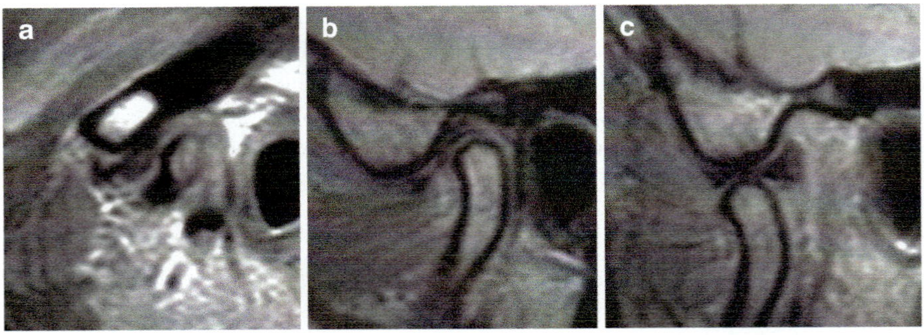

Fig. 13.2 Partial disc displacement (disc displaced only in one part of the joint) with reduction (normalization) and normal bone in an asymptomatic volunteer. (**a**) Oblique sagittal PD-weighted MRI shows displaced disc in the lateral section of the joint, (**b**) normal disc position in the medial section, and (**c**) normal disc position in the open-mouth image. Reproduced with permission from Larheim et al. [8]

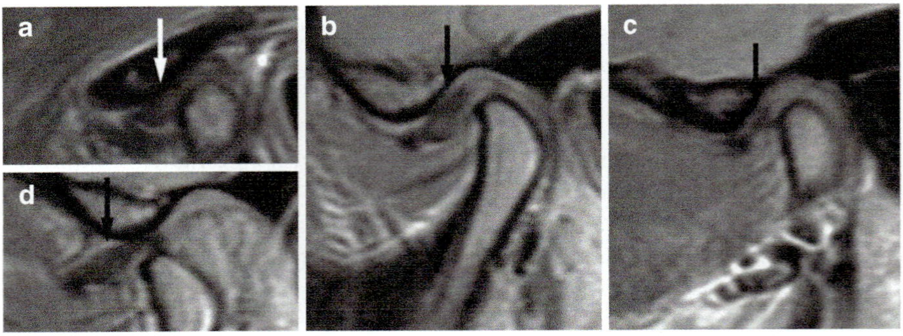

Fig. 13.3 Complete anterior disc displacement (disc displaced throughout the joint) without reduction (normalization) and normal bone. (**a**–**c**) Oblique sagittal PD-weighted MRI shows displaced and deformed disc (*arrow*) in lateral (**a**), central (**b**), and medial section (**c**). (**d**) Oblique sagittal open-mouth MRI shows anteriorly displaced disc (*arrow*). Reproduced with permission from Larheim et al. [8]

(Fig. 13.2). On the other hand, complete disc displacement, i.e., a disc being anteriorly displaced in all sections throughout the joint (Fig. 13.3), almost exclusively occurred in patients [8]. Other types of disc displacements such as sideways displacements may occur (Fig. 13.4), but are rare unless combined with an anterior displacement [6, 8].

Inflammatory Abnormalities Accompanying Disc Displacement We know that disc displacement even complete displacement without reduction may be asymptomatic. Other abnormalities such as increased fluid in the joint compartment (joint effusion) and signal alterations in the condyle marrow (marrow edema and osteonecrosis (marrow necrosis)) have been investigated to try to explain why disc displacement sometimes is symptomatic and sometimes is not.

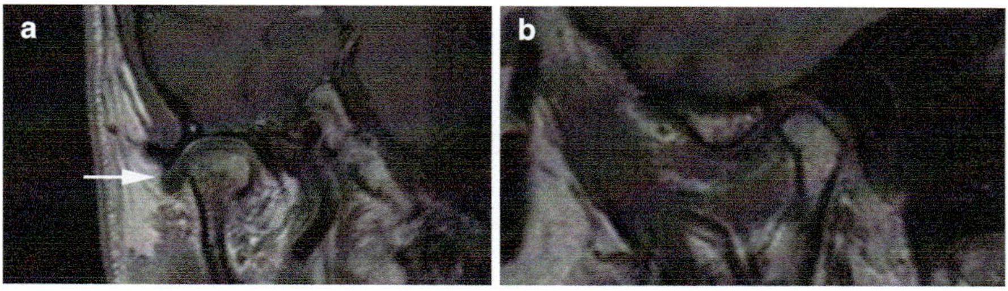

Fig. 13.4 Partial disc displacement and normal bone. (**a**) Oblique coronal T1-weighted post-Gd MRI shows laterally displaced disc (*arrow*). (**b**) Oblique sagittal T1-weighted MRI shows apparently normal disc position. Reproduced with permission from Larheim T.A., Westesson P-L. A. Maxillofacial Imaging (Springer 2018)

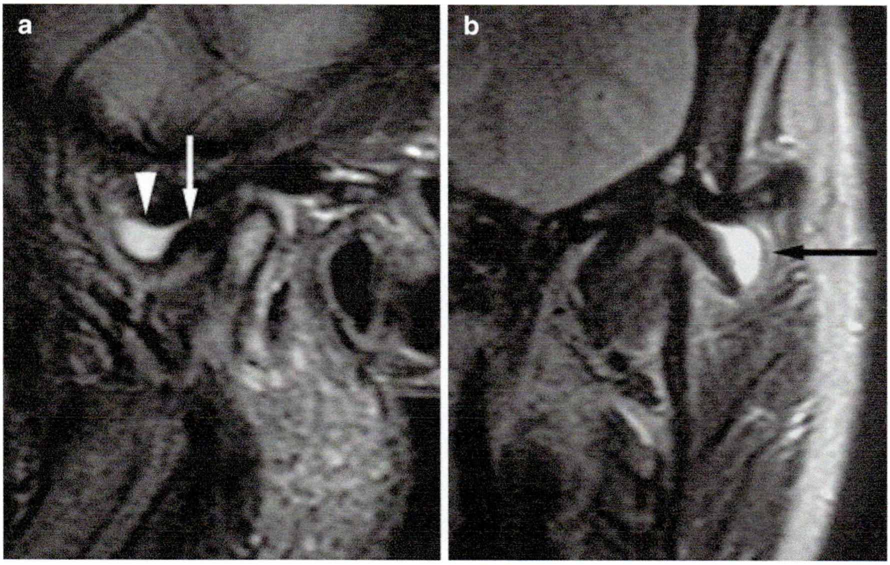

Fig. 13.5 Anterolateral disc displacement and joint effusion. (**a**) Oblique sagittal T2-weighted MRI shows anteriorly displaced disc (*arrow*) and joint effusion (*arrowhead*) in anterior recess of the upper compartment. (**b**) Oblique coronal T2-weighted MRI shows joint effusion in lateral part of the upper joint compartment (*arrow*). Reproduced with permission from Larheim T.A., Westesson P-L. A. Maxillofacial Imaging (Springer 2018)

Joint effusion, diagnosed as high T2 signal from the joint compartments, has been demonstrated in a number of studies. Typically, the effusion is located in the anterior recess of the upper joint compartment and laterally in the joint (Fig. 13.5). However, fluid is found in about half of asymptomatic volunteers [19] and may be rather evident (Fig. 13.6). If effusion is defined as more fluid than seen in any asymptomatic volunteer, only about 13% in a consecutive series of more than 500 patients with TMD had effusion [20]. Almost all these patients also had disc

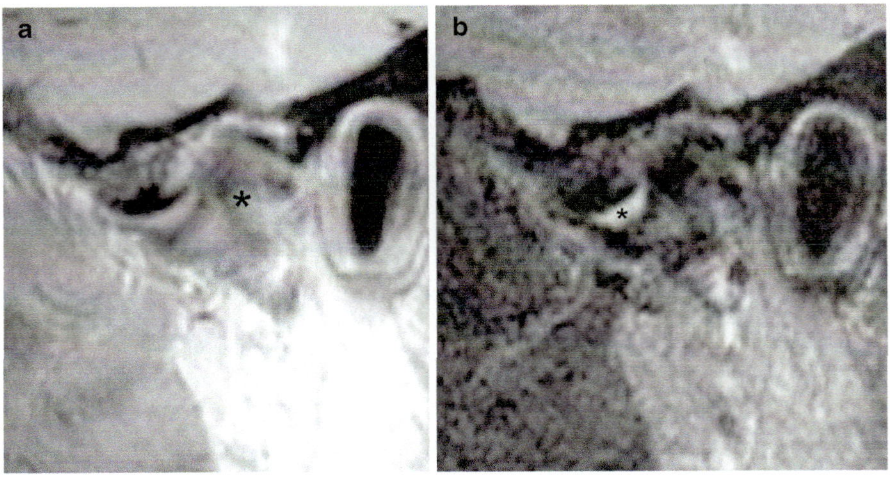

Fig. 13.6 Joint fluid in an asymptomatic volunteer. (**a**) PD-weighted (condyle is shown with *asterisk*) and (**b**) Corresponding T2-weighted MRI. Increased T2-signal consistent with fluid (*asterisk*) in the anterolateral recess of upper compartment. This was the maximum amount of fluid seen among asymptomatic volunteers. Reproduced with permission from Larheim et al. [19]

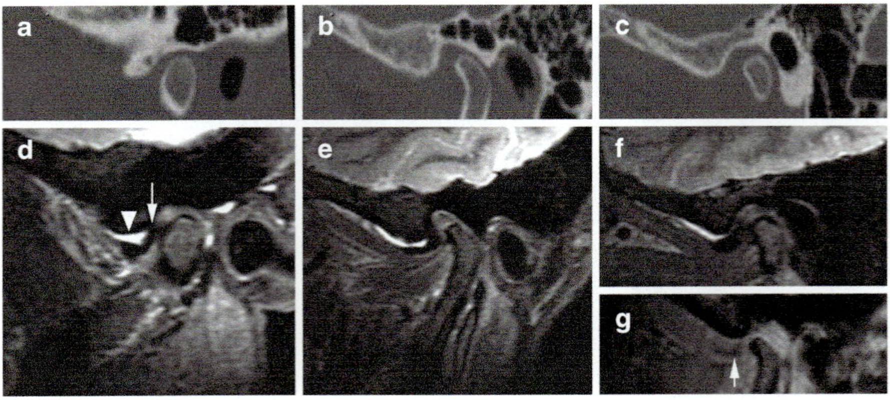

Fig. 13.7 Complete anterior disc displacement without reduction and normal bone. (**a**–**c**) Oblique sagittal CT images show normal bone in lateral, central, and medial sections. (**d**–**f**) Oblique sagittal STIR MRI shows anteriorly displaced disc (*arrow*) in lateral, central, and medial sections and joint effusion (arrowhead) throughout the joint. (**g**) Oblique sagittal open-mouth MRI shows displaced disc (*arrow*) and reduced condylar translation. Reproduced with permission from Larheim T.A., Westesson P-L. A. Maxillofacial Imaging (Springer 2018)

displacement. Joint effusion was found in patients with normal cortical bone (Fig. 13.7) and in patients with osteoarthritis.

MRI studies have suggested that osteonecrosis (avascular or aseptic necrosis) can affect the mandibular condyle marrow, based on signal alterations similar to those seen in the femoral head [21, 22]. However, this has been a controversial subject until histologically documented [23]. In a series of 50 TMJs in 44 patients in whom MRI and surgery were performed for painful disc displacements, a core

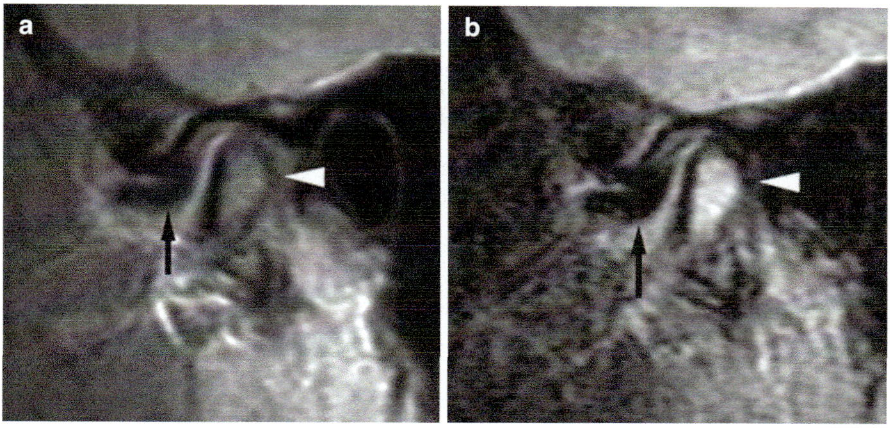

Fig. 13.8 Anterior disc displacement, bone marrow edema, and normal cortical bone. (**a**) Oblique sagittal MRI shows anteriorly displaced disc (*arrow*) and intermediate signal in condyle marrow (*arrowhead*). (**b**) Oblique sagittal T2-weighted MRI shows displaced disc (*arrow*) and increased signal in the condyle marrow consistent with edema (*arrowhead*). Reproduced with permission from Larheim et al. [20]

biopsy specimen was obtained from the marrow of the mandibular condyles at the time of surgery. This highly selected material from surgically treated patients showed that histologically abnormal bone marrow occurred in more than one third (36%) of the joints. Half of these joints showed marrow edema only and half of the joints showed osteonecrosis, with or without marrow edema. Abnormal bone marrow was found both in joints with normal cortical bone (Fig. 13.8) and in joints with osteoarthritis.

Internal Derangement Disc function seems to be essential for patient symptomatology, more so than the displaced disc per se. Thus, disc displacement without reduction is definitely a pathologic condition that is hardly seen in asymptomatic volunteers. The condition should preferably be named internal derangement. This orthopedic term, defined as a localized mechanical fault that interferes with the smooth action of the joint [24], should not be used synonymously with disc displacement in general as many do. Internal derangement may be used on a displaced disc that is reducing on mouth opening, but only if the joint function is altered. A fixed disc, normally located but not moving with the condyle due to fibrous adhesions [25], is also an internal derangement (Fig. 13.9).

13.1.2 Disc Displacement in Children and Adolescents

TMD may also occur in young people. A systematic review and meta-analysis concluded that one in six children and adolescents has clinical signs of TMJ disorders, with clicking as the most prevalent sign [26]. Disc displacement has been documented by imaging for a long time in this age group [27]. In pre-orthodontic patients with TMD aged 6–15 years, the prevalence was as high as 74%. The prevalence and

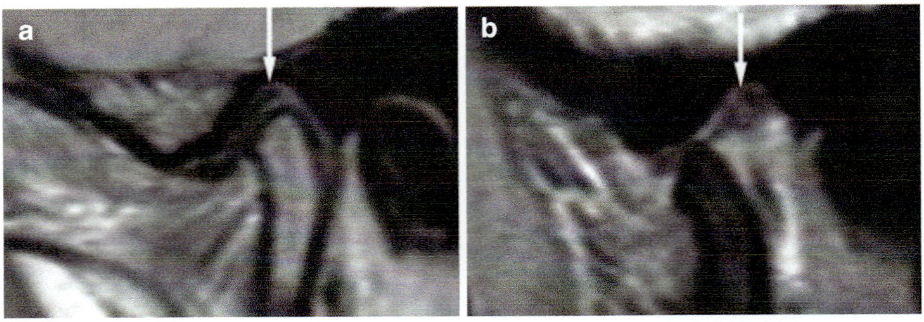

Fig. 13.9 Stuck (fixed) disc and normal bone. (**a**) Oblique sagittal MRI shows disc (arrow) in normal position. (**b**) Oblique sagittal open-mouth MRI shows disc (arrow) in same position and no motion of disc with the condyle, probably due to fibrous adhesions. Reproduced with permission from Larheim T.A., Westesson P-L. A. Maxillofacial Imaging (Springer 2018)

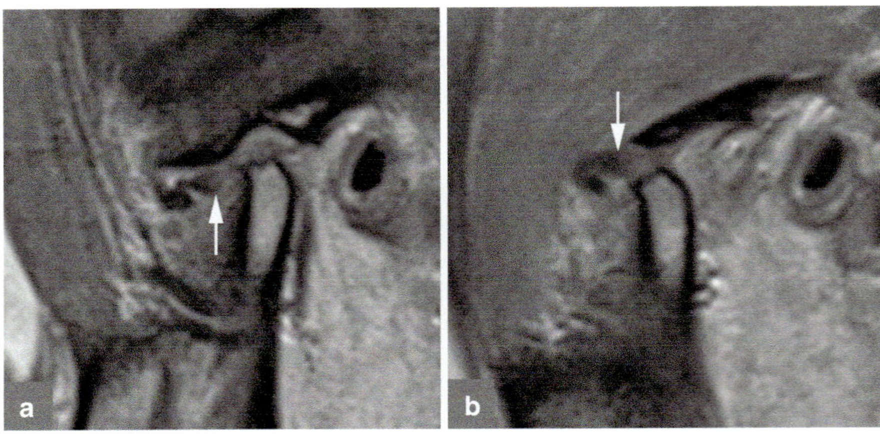

Fig. 13.10 Juvenile osteoarthritis and disc displacement, 18-year-old female (**a**) Closed-mouth and (**b**) Open-mouth oblique sagittal PD-weighted MRI shows anteriorly displaced disc (*arrow*) and condylar flattening with defect. Similar disc abnormalities in contralateral joint (not shown). Reproduced with permission from Larheim T.A., Westesson P-L. A. Maxillofacial Imaging (Springer 2018)

severity increased with age [28]. Also in asymptomatic young individuals (schoolchildren), the disc may be anteriorly displaced. As in asymptomatic adults, the disc displacement is usually partial [16]. An anteriorly displaced disc without reduction is demonstrated in an 18-year-old girl (Fig. 13.10).

To investigate whether disc displacement is solely an acquired condition, or may be congenital, a study of the disc position in infants aged 2 months to 5 years was performed [29]. Having observed normally located discs in all joints, the authors concluded that disc displacement seems to develop later in life, being an acquired condition. However, since sedation was required during the examinations and the joints seem to have been imaged in an open-mouth position only, this study could have included possible cases of disc displacement with reduction not recognized in the open-mouth images. Thus, in our opinion the question whether disc displacement is an acquired or a congenital condition is still not resolved.

13.2 Osteoarthritis

13.2.1 Osteoarthritis in Adults

Osteoarthritis can be defined as a degenerative disorder of synovial joints, primarily affecting articular cartilage and subchondral bone, initiated by deterioration of articular soft-tissue cover and exposure of bone. The disease was previously thought of as noninflammatory and was called osteoarthrosis, but is now accepted as an inflammatory condition that involves all components of the joint [30, 31]. In medical literature, the term osteoarthrosis is therefore regarded as a misnomer [31]. Osteoarthritis is usually considered a low-grade inflammatory disease, in contrast to the high-grade inflammatory diseases discussed in Chap. 14.

Osteoarthritis is the most common degenerative joint disease and a major cause of pain and disability in adult individuals. Worldwide, about 10% of all men and 18% of all women over 60 years are estimated to have symptomatic osteoarthritis [32]. The joints most commonly affected are the knee, hip, and hand joints, but the TMJ can also be involved. In a recent study of a cohort of patients with hand osteoarthritis, i.e., a population with increased osteoarthritis susceptibility, 67% of the individuals had TMJ osteoarthritis based on CBCT findings [33]. As in other joints, the TMJs of women are more frequently affected than in men, and the frequency increases with age [34].

Value of Clinical Examination for Diagnosing Osteoarthritis The validity of clinical examination and patient history is relatively limited in the diagnosis of osteoarthritis, using CT as reference method. According to Schiffman et al. [3], the sensitivity/specificity obtained with clinical information is 0.55/0.61, and crepitation is the only criterion. Thus, clinical diagnostics will underestimate the occurrence of osteoarthritis compared to CT diagnostics. TMJs with osteoarthritis can be painful, with impaired function, but may also be asymptomatic and well-functioning.

In the Diagnostic Criteria for TMD (DC/TMD), degenerative TMJ disease is divided into osteoarthritis (in a patient with arthralgia) and osteoarthrosis (in a patient without arthralgia). With regard to the imaging diagnosis, this nomenclature can be confusing, and it is not being used for other joints. Being an inflammatory condition [35–37] we are consistently applying osteoarthritis in this chapter. However, degenerative joint disease, osteoarthrosis, and osteoarthritis are used in the expanded DC/TMD [38] and more recently by Ahmad and Schiffman [39].

Value of Imaging for Diagnosing Osteoarthritis In cases where the clinical diagnosis needs to be confirmed, diagnostic imaging is necessary. MRI may show the presence of disc displacement and of osteoarthritis. Since both soft tissue and bone abnormalities can be assessed, MRI has been the primary imaging modality for TMJ diagnostics [40]. However, for bone details CT is generally accepted as superior to MRI. In the comprehensive study of diagnostic imaging criteria, Ahmad et al. [18] compared panoramic and MR examinations with CT to assess their validity for detecting osteoarthritis. The results indicated that about 40% of CT-diagnosed osteoarthritis were undetected using MRI [18]. They wrote "In our validation assessment study, we considered the CT findings to be the reference standard for diagnosing osteoarthritis using images," by referring to Westesson et al. [41] and Larheim [4]. Interestingly, the inter-observer reliability (with three observers) for diagnosing osteoarthritis was poor (kappa 0.16) when based on the panoramic images, better when based on MRI (kappa 0.47) and clearly better when based on CT (kappa 0.71) [18].

CBCT is increasingly used to assess the TMJ. It is convincingly documented that the diagnostic accuracy of CBCT, with lower radiation dose, is comparable with CT for TMJ diagnostics [42]. CBCT has an acceptable accuracy for diagnosing osseous abnormalities with fairly high sensitivity (in the range 0.7–0.9), although smaller cortical defects might be missed. In most studies, high specificity was also reported. However, it was emphasized that there are differences in image quality depending on imaging protocol and CBCT device [42].

Imaging Characteristics of Osteoarthritis CT/CBCT is an excellent imaging modality to visualize the cortical bone abnormalities that characterize TMJ osteoarthritis [43, 44], and CT definitions for osteophyte, sclerosis, surface erosion, and subcortical cyst have been published [18]. The diagnostic criteria can surely be applied on CBCT images as well [42].

For osteoarthritis in general, bone-productive changes usually dominate [45]. Although erosions are not typical, they may be a dominant feature of the disease; patients with bone-erosive disease report more pain than those with bone-productive disease [46].

Also in the TMJ, the bone may show productive features (osteophyte formation, sclerosis) or destructive features (erosion, subcortical cyst), in addition to remodeling (flattening). TMJ osteoarthritis may be predominantly bone-productive (Fig. 13.11) or predominantly bone-destructive (Fig. 13.12), or it may show a combination of both (Fig. 13.13). Additional findings may be loose bodies (Fig. 13.14). Osteoarthritis imaging features at CT and MRI are illustrated in Fig. 13.15.

Inflammatory Abnormalities Accompanying Osteoarthritis Joints with osteoarthritis may show inflammatory features on images such as effusion (Fig. 13.16) and bone marrow abnormalities. In addition, enhancement of the synovial membrane after intravenous injection of contrast agent may also been seen, similar to contrast enhancement in joints with rheumatoid arthritis and related diseases [47, 48]. A case with disc displacement, osteoarthritis, marrow edema, joint effusion, and contrast enhancement in the synovial membrane is shown in Fig. 13.17. Osteonecrosis has also been documented in joints with osteoarthritis [23], illustrated in Fig. 13.18.

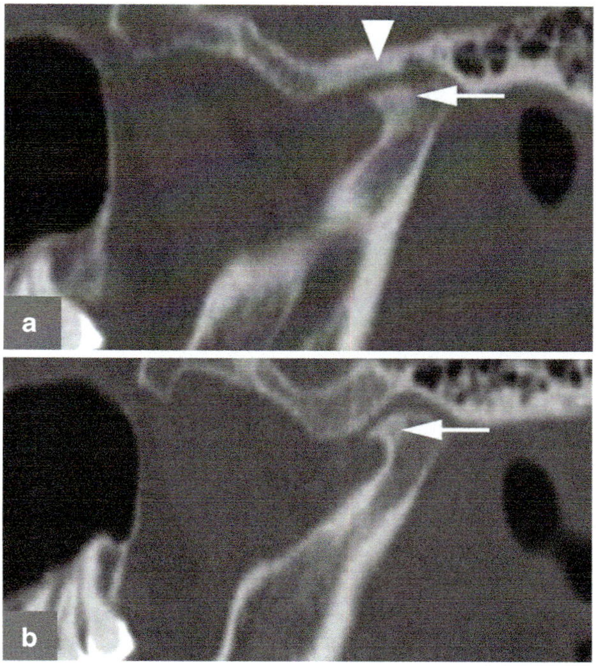

Fig. 13.11 Osteoarthritis, bilateral, with predominantly bone-productive changes. (**a**) Right joint. (**b**) Left joint. Oblique sagittal CT images show flattened articular surfaces and large condylar osteophyte/sclerosis (*arrow*) and sclerosis in fossa/eminence (*arrowhead*). Reproduced with permission from Larheim T.A., Westesson P-L. A. Maxillofacial Imaging (Springer 2018)

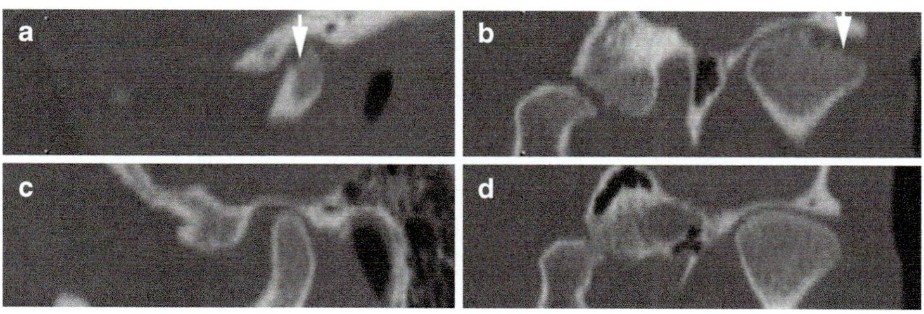

Fig. 13.12 Osteoarthritis with predominantly bone-destructive changes in right joint (**a, b**) and normal bone in left joint (**c, d**). (**a**) Oblique sagittal and (**b**) Oblique coronal CT images show bone erosion in lateral part of the condyle (*arrow*). (**c**) Oblique sagittal and (**d**) Oblique coronal CT images show normal bone. Reproduced with permission from Larheim T.A., Westesson P-L. A. Maxillofacial Imaging (Springer 2018)

13.2.2 Osteoarthritis in Children and Adolescents

Although osteoarthritis traditionally affects adults and elderly people, a similar condition is known to occur in the TMJ of symptomatic children and adolescents, mostly females in their late teens. In studies of large series of TMD patients in this age group, frequencies in the range 27–41% have been reported [49–51]. The

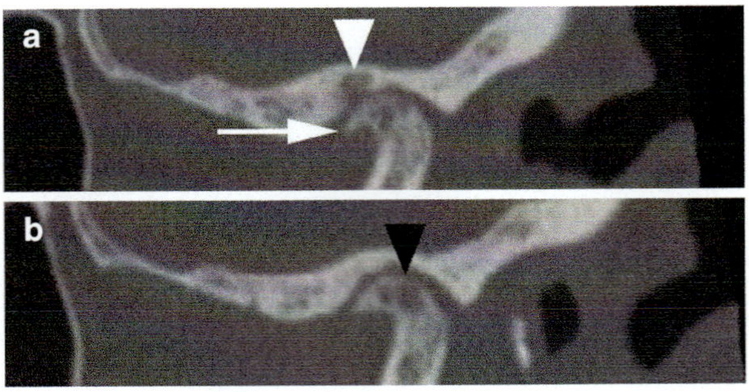

Fig. 13.13 Osteoarthritis with bone-destructive and bone-productive changes. (**a**) Oblique sagittal CT image shows large condylar osteophyte (*arrow*) and severe erosion in temporal bone (*arrowhead*). (**b**) Another section shows subcortical cysts in the condyle (*black arrowhead*). Reproduced with permission from Larheim T.A., Westesson P-L. A. Maxillofacial Imaging (Springer 2018)

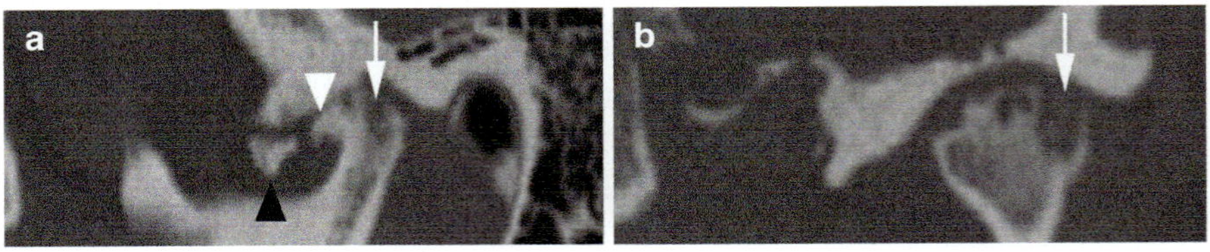

Fig. 13.14 Osteoarthritis with both bone-destructive and bone-productive changes and a loose body. (**a**) Oblique sagittal and (**b**) oblique coronal CT images show severe erosion (*arrow*), large osteophyte (*arrowhead*), and loose body (*black arrowhead*). Reproduced with permission from Larheim T.A., Westesson P-L. A. Maxillofacial Imaging (Springer 2018)

condition can also be found in asymptomatic individuals (controls) but significantly less frequently than in symptomatic patients [50, 51].

Different names have been used for this condition, such as degenerative arthritis, degenerative joint disease, osteoarthrosis, osteoarthritic changes, condylar degeneration, condylar bony changes, osteoarthritis, and juvenile osteoarthritis [42] (see also next section: idiopathic condylar resorption).

There are no generally accepted clinical criteria for this condition, and the diagnosis is based on imaging. Bone erosion (Fig. 13.19) and remodeling are characteristic radiologic features. Osteophyte formation is less common than in adult osteoarthritis [52]. Surface destruction seems associated with clinical symptoms such as pain [50].

Identifying bone abnormalities in young individuals may be challenging since the cortical outline of the articular surfaces in the TMJ starts to develop around the age of 12. It is not completed until after the age of 20 [53].

It may also be a challenge to differentiate the condition from juvenile idiopathic arthritis, which also features bone erosion and remodeling. Rheumatologic evaluation should always be considered in young patients, especially when destructive bone changes are present.

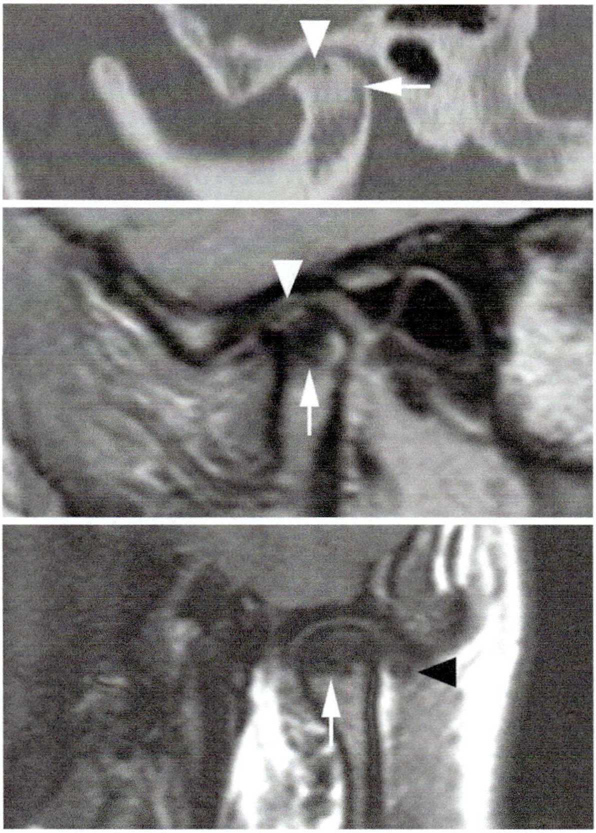

Fig. 13.15 Osteoarthritis with condylar erosion and condylar sclerosis shown with both CT (**a**) and MRI (**b, c**). (**a**) Oblique sagittal CT, (**b**) Oblique sagittal PD-weighted MRI, and (**c**) Oblique coronal T1-weighted MRI show sclerosis as reduced signal intensity in the condyle (*arrow*), condylar erosion (*white arrowhead*), and laterally displaced disc (*black arrowhead*). Reproduced with permission from Larheim T.A., Westesson P-L. A. Maxillofacial Imaging (Springer 2018)

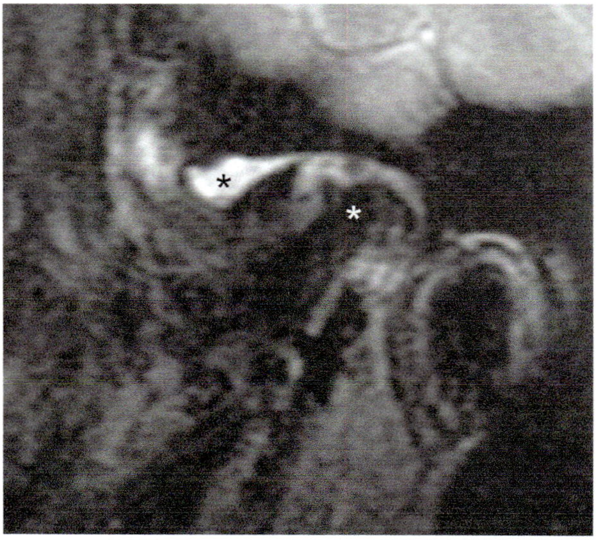

Fig. 13.16 Advanced osteoarthritis, anterior disc displacement, and joint effusion. Oblique sagittal T2-weighted MRI shows anteriorly displaced, deformed disc, large joint effusion (*black asterisk*) in anterior recess of upper compartment, and possible bone fragment superior to condyle. The condyle has cortical irregularities and is completely sclerotic (*white asterisk*). Reproduced with permission from Larheim et al. [20]

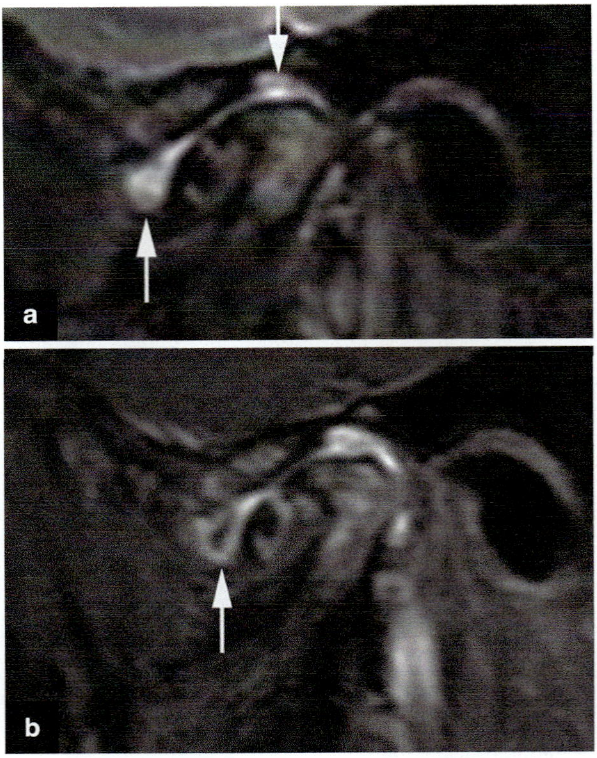

Fig. 13.17 Advanced osteoarthritis, anterior disc displacement, marrow edema, joint effusion, and synovial contrast enhancement. (**a**) Oblique sagittal T2-weighted MRI shows large joint effusion in anterior and posterior recesses (*arrows*) of upper joint compartment. (**b**) Oblique sagittal T1-weighted fat sat post-Gd MRI shows evident contrast enhancement in synovial membrane (synovitis) surrounding effusion in the anterior recess (*arrow*). Note contrast enhancement in the condyle marrow consistent with edema. Reproduced with permission from Larheim T.A., Westesson P-L. A. Maxillofacial Imaging (Springer 2018)

13.2.3 Idiopathic Condylar Resorption

This is an uncommon condition considered a severe form of osteoarthritis mainly affecting female adolescents and young female adults bilaterally. It leads to loss of condylar height resulting in progressive mandibular retrusion and anterior open bite [38, 54]. Condylar resorption should be suspected in any patient with an acquired and progressive open bite, increasing overjet or class II malocclusion and mandibular retrognathia [55]. A number of different names have been proposed for this condition, including arthrosis deformans juvenilis introduced by Boering in 1966 [56], progressive condylar resorption, condylysis, adolescent internal condylar resorption [57], and osteonecrosis (for review see Kristensen et al. [58]).

The affected TMJ is radiographically characterized by condylar destruction and remodeling [59, 60] and small condyles [58]. The condition was first reported in 1961 as condylar hypoplasia [61], and in 1977 its destructive nature was recognized [62]. It is now considered inflammatory in nature [60].

A patient with bilateral osteoarthritis/idiopathic condylar resorption and anterior bite opening is shown in Fig. 13.20.

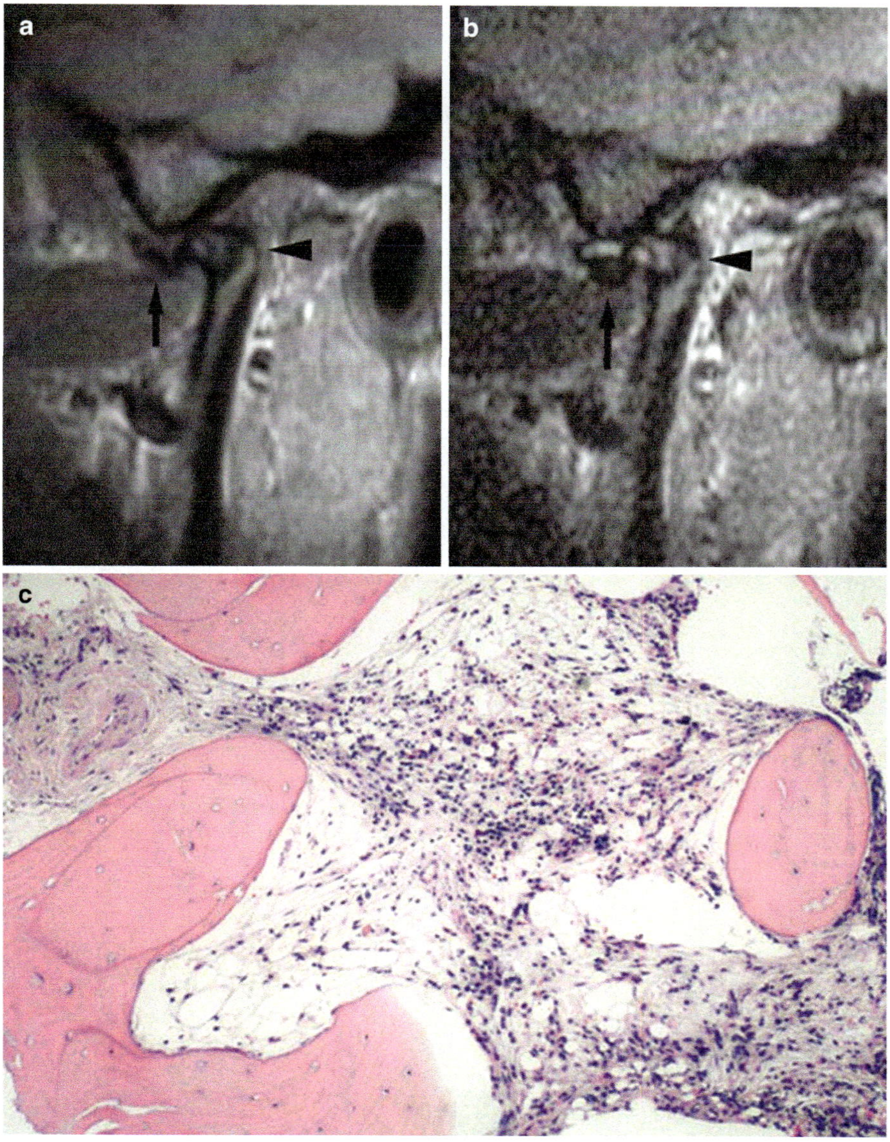

Fig. 13.18 Osteonecrosis (characteristic MRI findings), anterior disc displacement, osteoarthritis. (**a**) Oblique sagittal open-mouth MRI shows anteriorly displaced, deformed disc (*arrow*), condyle osteophyte, and reduced signal in condyle marrow (*arrowhead*), consistent with sclerosis or fibrosis. (**b**) Oblique sagittal open-mouth T2-weighted MRI shows fluid in anterior recess of upper compartment above disc (*arrow*) and characteristic MRI findings of osteonecrosis: both increased signal in condyle marrow, marrow edema and reduced signal in condyle marrow, marrow sclerosis, or fibrosis (*arrowhead*). (**c**) Histologic section of condyle marrow shows osteonecrosis, complete loss of hematopoietic marrow, with evidence of inflammatory cell infiltrate (hematoxylin eosin; original magnification ×50). Reproduced with permission from Larheim et al. [23]

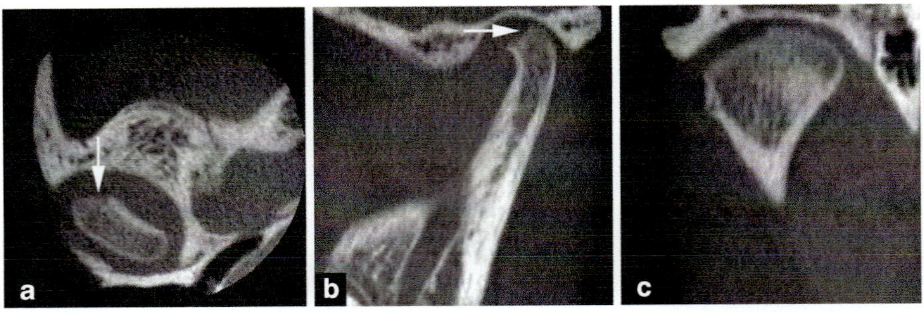

Fig. 13.19 Juvenile osteoarthritis, 12-year-old female. (**a**) Axial, (**b**) Oblique sagittal, and (**c**) Oblique coronal CBCT images show erosive changes of the condyle (*arrow*). Reproduced with permission from Larheim T.A., Westesson P-L. A. Maxillofacial Imaging (Springer 2018)

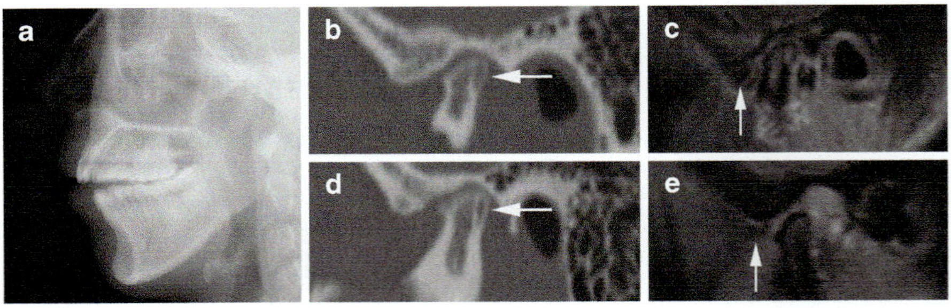

Fig. 13.20 Juvenile osteoarthritis, 21-year-old female. (**a**) Lateral cephalogram shows open bite. (**b**) Oblique sagittal CT of left joint (**d**) Oblique sagittal CT of right joint show remodeled condyles (flattened with posterior bone apposition) (*arrow*). (**c**) Oblique sagittal closed-mouth T1-weigted post-Gd MRI and (**e**) Oblique sagittal gradient echo open-mouth MRI of left joint show anteriorly displaced disc (*arrow*). Similar MRI findings in right joint (not shown). Reproduced with permission from Larheim T.A., Westesson P-L. A. Maxillofacial Imaging (Springer 2018)

Condylar destruction may be seen in different diseases, in particular rheumatic diseases such as juvenile idiopathic arthritis. Other conditions must have been excluded when the diagnosis of idiopathic condylar resorption is made. Condylar resorption has also been associated with orthodontic treatment and orthognathic surgery [55].

References

1. Morales H, Cornelius R. Imaging approach to temporomandibular joint disorders. Clin Neuroradiol. 2016;26(1):5–22.
2. Drace JE, Enzmann DR. Defining the normal temporomandibular joint: closed-, partially open, and open-mouth MR imaging of asymptomatic subjects. Radiology. 1990;177(1):67–71.
3. Schiffman E, Ohrbach R, Truelove E, Look J, Anderson G, Goulet JP, et al. Diagnostic Criteria for Temporomandibular Disorders (DC/TMD) for Clinical and Research Applications: recommendations of the International RDC/TMD Consortium Network* and Orofacial Pain Special Interest Groupdagger. J Oral Facial Pain Headache. 2014;28(1):6–27.

4. Larheim TA. Current trends in temporomandibular joint imaging. Oral Surg Oral Med Oral Pathol Oral Radiol Endod. 1995;80(5):555–76.
5. Katzberg RW, Westesson PL, Tallents RH, Drake CM. Anatomic disorders of the temporomandibular joint disc in asymptomatic subjects. J Oral Maxillofac Surg. 1996;54(2):147–53. discussion 53–5
6. Tasaki MM, Westesson PL, Isberg AM, Ren YF, Tallents RH. Classification and prevalence of temporomandibular joint disk displacement in patients and symptom-free volunteers. Am J Orthod Dentofac Orthop. 1996;109(3):249–62.
7. Ribeiro RF, Tallents RH, Katzberg RW, Murphy WC, Moss ME, Magalhaes AC, et al. The prevalence of disc displacement in symptomatic and asymptomatic volunteers aged 6 to 25 years. J Orofac Pain. 1997;11(1):37–47.
8. Larheim TA, Westesson P, Sano T. Temporomandibular joint disk displacement: comparison in asymptomatic volunteers and patients. Radiology. 2001;218(2):428–32.
9. Annandale T. On displacement of the inter-articular cartilage of the lower jaw, and its treatment by operation. Lancet. 1887;129(3313):411.
10. Farrar WB, McCarty WL Jr. Inferior joint space arthrography and characteristics of condylar paths in internal derangements of the TMJ. J Prosthet Dent. 1979;41(5):548–55.
11. Kircos LT, Ortendahl DA, Mark AS, Arakawa M. Magnetic resonance imaging of the TMJ disc in asymptomatic volunteers. J Oral Maxillofac Surg. 1987;45(10):852–4.
12. Turp JC, Schlenker A, Schroder J, Essig M, Schmitter M. Disk displacement, eccentric condylar position, osteoarthrosis - misnomers for variations of normality? Results and interpretations from an MRI study in two age cohorts. BMC Oral Health. 2016;16(1):124.
13. Westesson PL, Eriksson L, Kurita K. Reliability of a negative clinical temporomandibular joint examination: prevalence of disk displacement in asymptomatic temporomandibular joints. Oral Surg Oral Med Oral Pathol. 1989;68(5):551–4.
14. Rammelsberg P, Pospiech PR, Jager L, Pho Duc JM, Bohm AO, Gernet W. Variability of disk position in asymptomatic volunteers and patients with internal derangements of the TMJ. Oral Surg Oral Med Oral Pathol Oral Radiol Endod. 1997;83(3):393–9.
15. Kerstens HC, Golding RP, Valk J, van der Kwast WA. Magnetic resonance imaging of partial temporomandibular joint disc displacement. J Oral Maxillofac Surg. 1989;47(1):25–9.
16. Tominaga K, Konoo T, Morimoto Y, Tanaka T, Habu M, Fukuda J. Changes in temporomandibular disc position during growth in young Japanese. Dentomaxillofac Radiol. 2007;36(7):397–401.
17. Hasegawa Y, Kakimoto N, Tomita S, Fujiwara M, Ishikura R, Kishimoto H, et al. Evaluation of the role of splint therapy in the treatment of temporomandibular joint pain on the basis of MRI evidence of altered disc position. J Cranio-Maxillofac Surg. 2017;45(4):455–60.
18. Ahmad M, Hollender L, Anderson Q, Kartha K, Ohrbach R, Truelove EL, et al. Research diagnostic criteria for temporomandibular disorders (RDC/TMD): development of image analysis criteria and examiner reliability for image analysis. Oral Surg Oral Med Oral Pathol Oral Radiol Endod. 2009;107(6):844–60.
19. Larheim TA, Katzberg RW, Westesson PL, Tallents RH, Moss ME. MR evidence of temporomandibular joint fluid and condyle marrow alterations: occurrence in asymptomatic volunteers and symptomatic patients. Int J Oral Maxillofac Surg. 2001;30(2):113–7.
20. Larheim TA, Westesson PL, Sano T. MR grading of temporomandibular joint fluid: association with disk displacement categories, condyle marrow abnormalities and pain. Int J Oral Maxillofac Surg. 2001;30(2):104–12.
21. Schellhas KP, Wilkes CH. Temporomandibular joint inflammation: comparison of MR fast scanning with T1- and T2-weighted imaging techniques. AJR Am J Roentgenol. 1989;153(1):93–8.
22. Schellhas KP, Wilkes CH, Fritts HM, Omlie MR, Lagrotteria LB. MR of osteochondritis dissecans and avascular necrosis of the mandibular condyle. AJR Am J Roentgenol. 1989;152(3):551–60.
23. Larheim TA, Westesson PL, Hicks DG, Eriksson L, Brown DA. Osteonecrosis of the temporomandibular joint: correlation of magnetic resonance imaging and histology. J Oral Maxillofac Surg. 1999;57(8):888–98. discussion 99

24. Hamblen DL, Simpson AHRW, Adams JC, Raby N. Adams's outline of orthopaedics. 14th ed. Edinburgh: Churchill Livingstone Elsevier; 2010.
25. Rao VM, Liem MD, Farole A, Razek AA. Elusive "stuck" disk in the temporomandibular joint: diagnosis with MR imaging. Radiology. 1993;189(3):823–7.
26. da Silva CG, Pacheco-Pereira C, Porporatti AL, Savi MG, Peres MA, Flores-Mir C, et al. Prevalence of clinical signs of intra-articular temporomandibular disorders in children and adolescents: a systematic review and meta-analysis. J Am Dent Assoc. 2016;147(1):10–8.e8.
27. Katzberg RW, Tallents RH, Hayakawa K, Miller TL, Goske MJ, Wood BP. Internal derangements of the temporomandibular joint: findings in the pediatric age group. Radiology. 1985;154(1):125–7.
28. Ikeda K, Kawamura A, Ikeda R. Prevalence of disc displacement of various severities among young preorthodontic population: a magnetic resonance imaging study. J Prosthodont. 2014;23(5):397–401.
29. Paesani D, Salas E, Martinez A, Isberg A. Prevalence of temporomandibular joint disk displacement in infants and young children. Oral Surg Oral Med Oral Pathol Oral Radiol Endod. 1999;87(1):15–9.
30. Loeser RF, Goldring SR, Scanzello CR, Goldring MB. Osteoarthritis: a disease of the joint as an organ. Arthritis Rheum. 2012;64(6):1697–707.
31. Berenbaum F. Osteoarthritis as an inflammatory disease (osteoarthritis is not osteoarthrosis!). Osteoarthr Cartil. 2013;21(1):16–21.
32. World Health Organization (WHO). Chronic diseases and health promotion 2017. Available from: http://www.who.int/chp/topics/rheumatic/en/
33. Abrahamsson AK, Kristensen M, Arvidsson LZ, Kvien TK, Larheim TA, Haugen IK. Frequency of temporomandibular joint osteoarthritis and related symptoms in a hand osteoarthritis cohort. Osteoarthr Cartil. 2017;25(5):654–7.
34. Alexiou K, Stamatakis H, Tsiklakis K. Evaluation of the severity of temporomandibular joint osteoarthritic changes related to age using cone beam computed tomography. Dentomaxillofac Radiol. 2009;38(3):141–7.
35. Stegenga B. Osteoarthritis of the temporomandibular joint organ and its relationship to disc displacement. J Orofac Pain. 2001;15(3):193–205.
36. Larheim TA, Westesson P-LA. Maxillofacial imaging. Berlin: Springer; 2018.
37. Wang XD, Zhang JN, Gan YH, Zhou YH. Current understanding of pathogenesis and treatment of TMJ osteoarthritis. J Dent Res. 2015;94(5):666–73.
38. Peck CC, Goulet JP, Lobbezoo F, Schiffman EL, Alstergren P, Anderson GC, et al. Expanding the taxonomy of the diagnostic criteria for temporomandibular disorders. J Oral Rehabil. 2014;41(1):2–23.
39. Ahmad M, Schiffman EL. Temporomandibular joint disorders and orofacial pain. Dent Clin North Am. 2016;60(1):105–24.
40. Larheim TA. Role of magnetic resonance imaging in the clinical diagnosis of the temporomandibular joint. Cells Tissues Organs. 2005;180(1):6–21.
41. Westesson PL, Katzberg RW, Tallents RH, Sanchez-Woodworth RE, Svensson SA. CT and MR of the temporomandibular joint: comparison with autopsy specimens. AJR Am J Roentgenol. 1987;148(6):1165–71.
42. Larheim TA, Abrahamsson AK, Kristensen M, Arvidsson LZ. Temporomandibular joint diagnostics using CBCT. Dentomaxillofac Radiol. 2015;44(1):20140235.
43. Larheim TA, Kolbenstvedt A. High-resolution computed tomography of the osseous temporomandibular joint. Some normal and abnormal appearances. Acta Radiol Diagn (Stockh). 1984;25(6):465–9.
44. Koyama J, Nishiyama H, Hayashi T. Follow-up study of condylar bony changes using helical computed tomography in patients with temporomandibular disorder. Dentomaxillofac Radiol. 2007;36(8):472–7.
45. Jacobson JA, Girish G, Jiang Y, Sabb BJ. Radiographic evaluation of arthritis: degenerative joint disease and variations. Radiology. 2008;248(3):737–47.

46. Haugen IK, Slatkowsky-Christensen B, Boyesen P, van der Heijde D, Kvien TK. Cross-sectional and longitudinal associations between radiographic features and measures of pain and physical function in hand osteoarthritis. Osteoarthr Cartil. 2013;21(9):1191–8.
47. Smith HJ, Larheim TA, Aspestrand F. Rheumatic and nonrheumatic disease in the temporomandibular joint: gadolinium-enhanced MR imaging. Radiology. 1992;185(1):229–34.
48. Farina D, Bodin C, Gandolfi S, De Gasperi W, Borghesi A, Maroldi R. TMJ disorders and pain: assessment by contrast-enhanced MRI. Eur J Radiol. 2009;70(1):25–30.
49. Sanchez-Woodworth RE, Katzberg RW, Tallents RH, Guay JA. Radiographic assessment of temporomandibular joint pain and dysfunction in the pediatric age-group. ASDC J Dent Child. 1988;55(4):278–81.
50. Cho BH, Jung YH. Osteoarthritic changes and condylar positioning of the temporomandibular joint in Korean children and adolescents. Imaging Sci Dent. 2012;42(3):169–74.
51. Wang ZH, Jiang L, Zhao YP, Ma XC. Investigation on radiographic signs of osteoarthrosis in temporomandibular joint with cone beam computed tomography in adolescents. Beijing Da Xue Xue Bao. 2013;45(2):280–5.
52. Lei J, Han J, Liu M, Zhang Y, Yap AU, Fu KY. Degenerative temporomandibular joint changes associated with recent-onset disc displacement without reduction in adolescents and young adults. J Craniomaxillofac Surg. 2017;45(3):408–13.
53. Lei J, Liu MQ, Yap AU, Fu KY. Condylar subchondral formation of cortical bone in adolescents and young adults. Br J Oral Maxillofac Surg. 2013;51(1):63–8.
54. Arnett GW, Milam SB, Gottesman L. Progressive mandibular retrusion--idiopathic condylar resorption. Part I. Am J Orthod Dentofac Orthop. 1996;110(1):8–15.
55. Papadaki ME, Tayebaty F, Kaban LB, Troulis MJ. Condylar resorption. Oral Maxillofac Surg Clin North Am. 2007;19(2):223–34, vii.
56. Nickerson JW, Boring G. Natural course of osteoarthrosis as it relates to internal derangement of the temporomandibular joint. Oral Maxillofac Surg Clin North Am. 1989;1:27–45.
57. Wolford LM, Galiano A. Adolescent internal condylar resorption (AICR) of the temporomandibular joint, part 1: a review for diagnosis and treatment considerations. Cranio. 2017. https://doi.org/10.1080/08869634.2017.1386752.
58. Kristensen KD, Schmidt B, Stoustrup P, Pedersen TK. Idiopathic condylar resorptions: 3-dimensional condylar bony deformation, signs and symptoms. Am J Orthod Dentofac Orthop. 2017;152(2):214–23.
59. Arnett GW, Gunson MJ. Risk factors in the initiation of condylar resorption. Semin Orthod. 2013;19(2):81–8.
60. Hatcher DC. Progressive condylar resorption: pathologic processes and imaging considerations. Semin Orthod. 2013:19(2):97–105.
61. Burke PH. A case of acquired unilateral mandibular condylar hypoplasia. Proc R Soc Med. 1961;54:507–10.
62. Rabey GP. Bilateral mandibular condylysis-a morphanalytic diagnosis. Br J Oral Surg. 1977;15(2):121–34.

High-Grade Inflammatory TMJ Diseases and Traumatic TMJ Conditions

14

Linda Z. Arvidsson, Bjørn B. Mork-Knutsen, Caroline Hol, Anna-Karin Abrahamsson, Margareth Kristensen Ottersen, and Tore A. Larheim

14.1 High-Grade Inflammatory Joint Diseases

A number of inflammatory conditions may affect the TMJ. Perhaps the most well known are the rheumatic diseases, which are autoimmune and chronic and may be progressive and disabling. Rheumatoid arthritis is the most common to involve the TMJ, but also the seronegative spondyloarthropathies such as psoriatic arthritis, ankylosing spondylitis, and reactive arthritis can involve this synovial joint. The imaging signs are similar; hence, the final diagnosis cannot be made by radiology alone. Often the patient's history and general condition will be decisive for the final diagnosis. Occasionally the TMJ is the first or the only joint to be affected.

14.1.1 Rheumatoid Arthritis (RA)

The prevalence of RA is around 0.5–1.0%, but can be much higher in certain populations [1]. Women are twice to three times as likely to develop RA as men [2]. The most common disease onset age is between 40 and 60 years. The proximal joints of the hands and feet are most often involved, but also the wrists, ankles, knees, hips, shoulders, elbows, neck, and TMJ are commonly affected, often symmetrically. Most studies show that at least 50% of RA patients develop a clinical involvement of the TMJ [3], but in patients with long disease duration, four out of five showed

L. Z. Arvidsson (✉) · B. B. Mork-Knutsen · C. Hol · A.-K. Abrahamsson · M. K. Ottersen
T. A. Larheim
Department of Maxillofacial Radiology, Faculty of Dentistry, University of Oslo, Oslo, Norway
e-mail: l.z.arvidsson@odont.uio.no; b.b.mork-knutsen@odont.uio.no; caroline.hol@odont.uio.no; a.k.johansen@odont.uio.no; m.k.ottersen@odont.uio.no; t.a.larheim@odont.uio.no

I. Rozylo-Kalinowska, K. Orhan (eds.), *Imaging of the Temporomandibular Joint*, https://doi.org/10.1007/978-3-319-99468-0_14

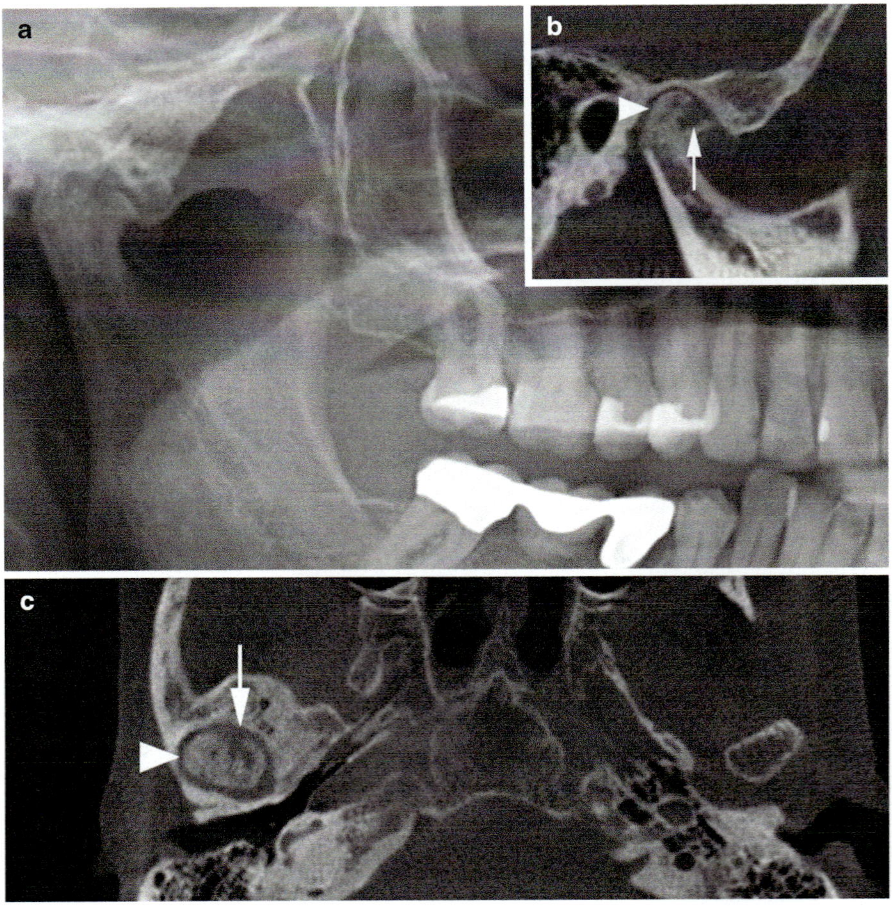

Fig. 14.1 Rheumatoid arthritis; 59-year-old female with variable right-sided TMJ pain and mouth opening problems. (**a**) Panoramic view, (**b**) oblique sagittal, and (**c**) axial CBCT images show punched-out destruction (*arrow*) in the right condyle with sclerosis (*arrowhead*). Reproduced with permission from Larheim T.A., Westesson P-L. A. Maxillofacial Imaging (Springer 2018)

TMJ involvement [4]. Synovial inflammation, the cardinal sign of RA, may lead to damage of the cartilage and bone, deformities, and loss of function. TMJ with RA involvement is shown in Fig. 14.1.

14.1.2 Psoriatic Arthritis (PA)

This disease typically occurs in people with skin psoriasis. It may also occur without psoriasis in those who have relatives with the disease. Between 5% and 24% of those with psoriasis will develop PA [5], and onset is usually between 30 and 50 years of age. In most people, the skin disease will precede the arthritis, but the opposite may

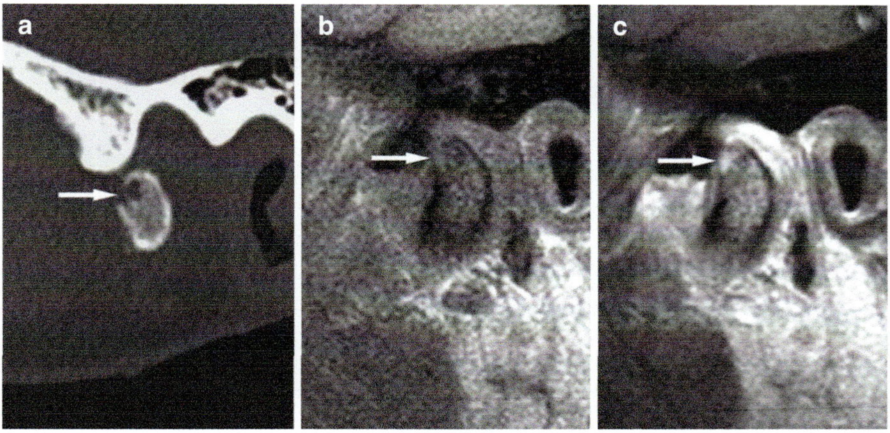

Fig. 14.2 Psoriatic arthropathy. (**a**) Sagittal CT image shows punched-out erosion (*arrow*). (**b**) Oblique sagittal T1-weighted pre-Gd and (**c**) oblique sagittal T1-weighted post-Gd MRI show contrast enhancement within the bone erosion (*arrow*) and in joint space, consistent with thickened synovium/pannus formation. Reproduced with permission from Larheim T.A., Westesson P-L. A. Maxillofacial Imaging (Springer 2018)

also occur. Men and women are affected equally. Like other spondyloarthropathies, PA is associated with the HLA-B27 factor. The disease typically affects the knees, ankles, distal joints of fingers and toes, the back and sacroiliac joints of the pelvis, and sometimes the TMJ. PA involvement in the TMJ is shown in Fig. 14.2.

14.1.3 Ankylosing Spondylitis (AS)

The prevalence of AS is less than 1% in Europeans, but varies in different populations. Men are more frequently affected than women [2]. The disease affects people often at an age younger than 30 years [6]. There is a strong association with genetic factors, especially HLA-B27. Extra-articular manifestations may occur. The insertion of ligaments and capsules into bone is the primary site of inflammation, unlike RA, which has its primary site in the synovium. The vertebral column and the sacroiliac joints are the most common sites primarily affected, and progress of the inflammation includes fibrosis and ossification with impaired joint function. Peripheral joints may be involved, also the TMJ, but with variable frequency [7]. AS involvement in the TMJ is shown in Fig. 14.3.

14.1.4 Reactive Arthritis

Reactive arthritis is a sterile inflammatory arthritis following an infectious process at a remote site. The arthritis is commonly triggered by enteric or urogenital infection [8]. Reiter's syndrome is a subtype of reactive arthritis characterized by large

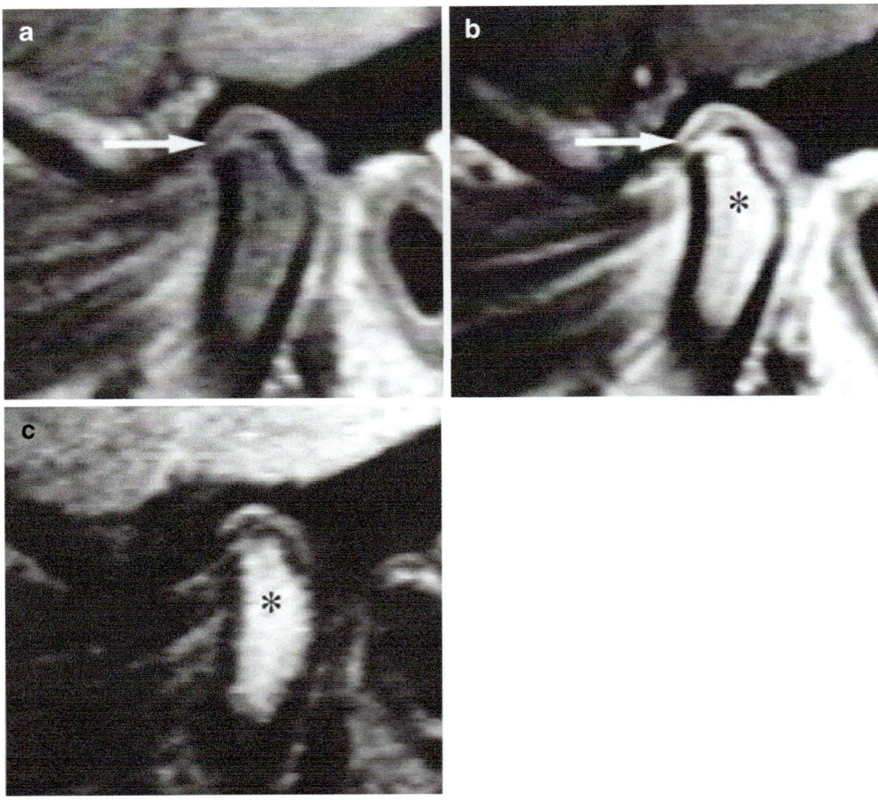

Fig. 14.3 Ankylosing spondylitis. (**a**) Oblique sagittal T1-weighted pre-Gd and (**b**) oblique sagittal T1-weighted post-Gd MRI show cortical erosion, deformed, thin disc in normal position (*arrow*), and contrast enhancement in the upper and lower compartment, consistent with thickened synovium/synovitis, and in the condyle marrow consistent with edema (*asterisk*). (**c**) Oblique sagittal T2-weighted MRI shows high signal in condyle marrow consistent with bone marrow edema in the entire condyle (*asterisk*). Reproduced with permission from Larheim T.A., Westesson P-L. A. Maxillofacial Imaging (Springer 2018)

joint oligoarthritis, urogenital tract infection, and conjunctivitis or uveitis. There is a strong association between the HLA-B27 antigen and reactive arthritis, which is most common in young adults between 20 and 40 years of age and often affects large joints in the lower extremities. Smaller joints may also be affected, including the TMJ, and a number of additional symptoms can be found [9].

14.2 High-Grade Inflammatory TMJ Disease: Imaging and Clinical Characteristics

In CT and CBCT, the sign of active arthritis is the destructive bone changes or erosions. Those are typically seen as punched out destructions on the joint surface and, if massive, as loss of the entire cortex of the articulating surface. As a consequence the condyles may show loss of height and be severely flattened and pencillike or even be completely destroyed. The seronegative spondyloarthropathies are generally more prone to feature bone proliferation like sclerosis and periostitis, whereas in RA there is usually a lack of bone proliferation. Later, and secondarily to the inflammatory arthritis, bone production may be more prominent. Sclerosis and osteophytes may develop, making it difficult to separate the condition from the more common osteoarthritis [10]. Fibrous or osseous ankylosis may occur in joints with inflammatory conditions but are rare. In contrast to other joints where the joint space is used as a reliable indicator of disease, the joint space in the TMJ is frequently asymmetric in asymptomatic (healthy) individuals, both in children [11] and adults [12]. Thus, narrowing or widening of the joint space should not be used as a diagnostic criterion for TMJ disease when found as the only sign.

The synovial thickening, characteristic for arthritis, can be shown with contrast-enhanced MRI. The intravenous contrast will make it possible to differentiate between synovitis and effusion [13]. Effusion and bone marrow edema may also be visible on MRI without contrast and can be good indicators of inflammatory activity [14].

The disc may often be affected by the disease and become thin, perforated, or destroyed [14]. Occasionally the disc is displaced. As primary disc displacement also can be accompanied by synovitis, it is difficult to distinguish between this condition and early arthritis, in particular if bone changes are absent [15, 16].

As emphasized in the beginning of this chapter, the different rheumatic diseases in the TMJ cannot be differentiated from each other by diagnostic imaging alone.

Reduced mouth opening, palpation tenderness in the TMJ, crepitation, and masticatory muscle tenderness are frequent in patients with TMJ arthritis. Anterior open bite is a possible consequence of severe TMJ involvement of rheumatic disease [4]. Only the posterior teeth will be in contact at occlusion.

14.3 Rheumatic Disease in Children

14.3.1 Juvenile Idiopathic Arthritis (JIA)

Several rheumatic diseases may affect children and adolescents. The most common is JIA with onset between 1 and 3 years of age or before puberty. The disease includes several subtypes and is more frequent in girls than in boys, the ratio varying between 3:2 and 2:1. In contrast to adult rheumatoid arthritis affecting small joints in the hands and feet, childhood arthritis predominantly involves large joints like knees, wrists, and ankles [17]. The TMJ is commonly involved in JIA with reported frequencies between 40% and 90% [18, 19].

The typical clinical signs of arthritis are pain, swelling, and reduced mobility. However, in children, the symptoms from the TMJs may be few or vague. Therefore, imaging is necessary for diagnostic assessment of the TMJs. MRI can show active inflammation and synovitis [16, 20] like in adult arthritis. Disc abnormalities can occur already in an early phase of TMJ arthritis with normal bone, but also in late stages of the disease [16]. The efficacy of ultrasound is being debated [21].

Temporomandibular bone surface changes can be better assessed with CT and CBCT than with MRI. The characteristic changes are deformed joint surfaces like flattening and widening of the condylar head and the fossa, but often without obvious erosions (Fig. 14.4). The TMJ changes could be viewed as remodeling or growth disturbances rather than destructions [18]. Imaging with open and closed mouth can show reduced condylar translation.

A consequence of JIA in the TMJ is growth disturbances like facial asymmetry (Fig. 14.5) or underdevelopment of the mandible (Fig. 14.6) [22]. Low-grade inflammatory activity in the TMJs may persist into adulthood [15] like in other joints [23].

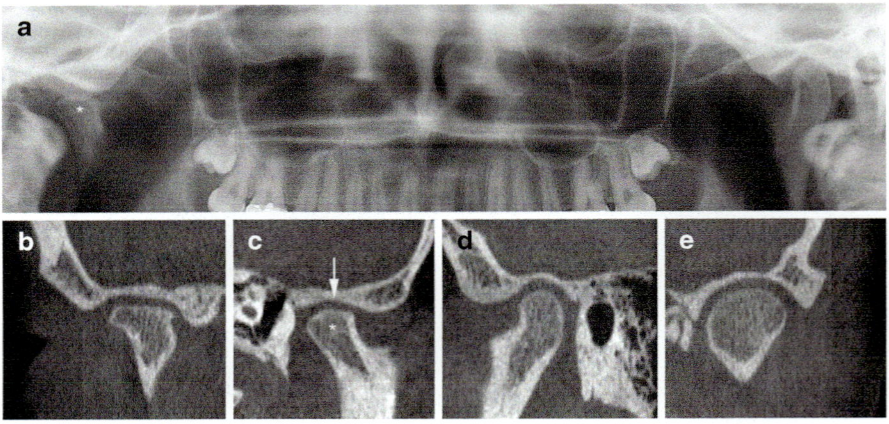

Fig. 14.4 Juvenile idiopathic arthritis; 17-year-old female. (**a**) Panoramic view, (**b**) oblique coronal, and (**c**) oblique sagittal CBCT images show abnormal right TMJ with rather flat condyle (*asterisk*) and rather flat fossa/eminence (*arrow*) without erosion. (**d**) Oblique sagittal and (**e**) oblique coronal CBCT images show normal contralateral joint

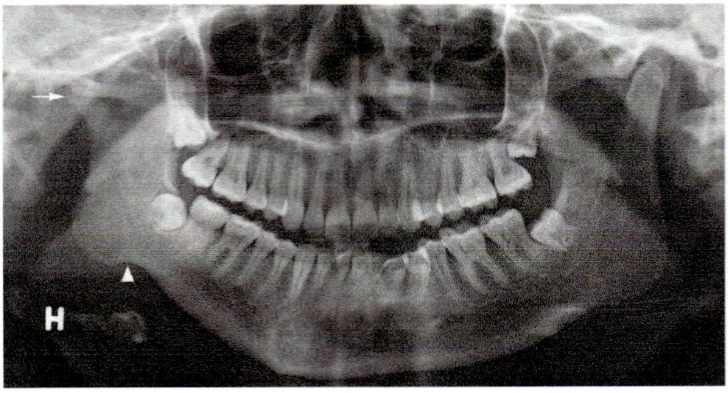

Fig. 14.5 Juvenile idiopathic arthritis, facial asymmetry; 17-year-old female. Panoramic view shows jaw asymmetry; underdevelopment of right side with antegonial notching (*arrowhead*) and small, flat condyle (*arrow*). Reproduced with permission from Larheim T.A., Westesson P-L. A. Maxillofacial Imaging (Springer 2018)

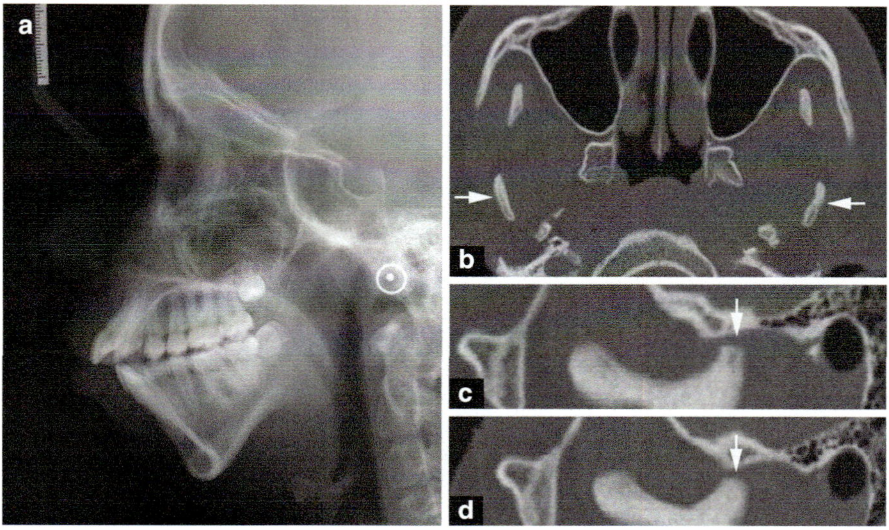

Fig. 14.6 Juvenile idiopathic arthritis, micrognathia; 13-year-old female. (**a**) Lateral view show micrognathia (retruded chin). (**b**) Axial CT image shows abnormal long axis angulation of both, thin condyles (*arrows*). (**c, d**) Oblique sagittal CT images of right (**c**) and left (**d**) joints show almost flat eminence and rudimentary condyle (*arrow*) anteriorly located in fossa, almost at apex of eminence, in closed-mouth images (these could be mistaken for open-mouth images). Reproduced with permission from Larheim T.A., Westesson P-L. A. Maxillofacial Imaging (Springer 2018)

14.4 Other Types of Arthritis

The different types of arthritis have similar imaging features. In this part, we will emphasize the imaging findings that are unique for the different conditions.

14.4.1 Infectious Arthritis (IA)

Bacteria or, more seldom, virus or fungus may cause infectious or septic arthritis. In the TMJ, IA is a possible complication of the systemic diseases tuberculosis, syphilis, and gonorrhea. Being a very rare condition in the developed countries, IA might be subject to misdiagnosis and underreporting. Septic arthritis in children may account for a significant percentage of cases of mandibular ankyloses. In a retrospective study of 41 children with TMJ ankylosis, the etiology was septic in 54% of the cases [24]. Ankylosis may cause underdevelopment of the mandible and facial asymmetry. Infectious arthritis can involve the TMJ by direct extension of local odontogenic infections. It may also be caused by osteomyelitis in the mandible or originate from parotid, ear, or throat infections. Direct infections may also occur during traumatic injury or surgery, also including implant placement in the TMJ.

The patient presents with fever and clinical cardinal signs of inflammation, usually involving a single joint. Deviation of the mandible to the contralateral side will occur secondary to increased amount of joint fluid. The imaging signs are similar to other types of arthritis, but destruction may be more rapid. Left untreated the infectious arthritis may cause complete destruction of the condylar cartilage and bone.

14.4.2 Gout

Gout is a metabolic disorder that leads to elevated serum uric acid levels (hyperuricemia) and hard painless deposits of uric acid crystals known as tophi which are pathognomonic for the disease. The prevalence increases with age. More than 90% of the patients with primary gout are men. The onset is earlier in men than in women, who rarely develop the disorder before menopause. In women, the disease often presents as secondary gout. The fact that gout mainly affects men is in contrast to other diseases involving the TMJ. Gouty arthritis and RA rarely coexist. The reason for this is not known. Gout in the TMJ should be included as a differential diagnosis for joint disorders, though it rarely affects the TMJ alone [25]. Only a few cases have been described in the literature [26].

Characteristic imaging changes usually occur years after the onset of the gout. On MRI a majority of lesions seems to be characteristically heterogeneously hypointense on T2-weighted images with tophi enhancement on post-contrast T1-weighted images. On ultrasound examinations, tophi tend to be circumscribed, hyper- and/or hypoechoic, and heterogeneous, although the appearance may vary [27]. The tophi can be multiple, grouped, and surrounded by anechoic halos. CBCT is recommended for diagnosis only in advanced cases as it takes years before the urate crystals reach a density high enough to be radiographically detectable in the TMJs. CT and CBCT may show bone destruction in the condyle and fossa as well as coalescent foci of crystal growth [25].

14.4.3 Pseudogout

Pseudogout (chondrocalcinosis, pyrophosphate arthropathy) is a metabolic disease that often occurs in association with other metabolic diseases such as hyperparathyroidism [28]. It is characterized by the deposition of calcium pyrophosphate in soft tissues and cartilage. The prevalence of pseudogout in the TMJ is uncertain; it affects people above 40 years of age and has an equal sex predilection. The clinical presentation of pseudogout is the same as for gout. Unlike gout, pseudogout is associated with an elevation of uric acid only in a third of the patients.

Osseous tophi within the joint and calcification of the disc may be demonstrable in radiographs [29]. The crystal deposits may have a punctate or linear appearance. Pseudogout involvement in the TMJ is shown in Figs. 14.7 and 14.8.

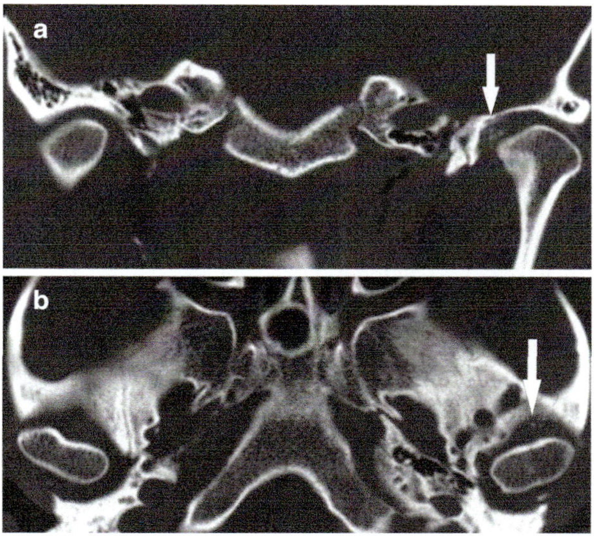

Fig. 14.7 Pseudogout, early stage. (**a**) Coronal and (**b**) axial CT images show subtle calcifications within the joint space (*arrows*). Reproduced with permission from Larheim T.A., Westesson P-L. A. Maxillofacial Imaging (Springer 2018)

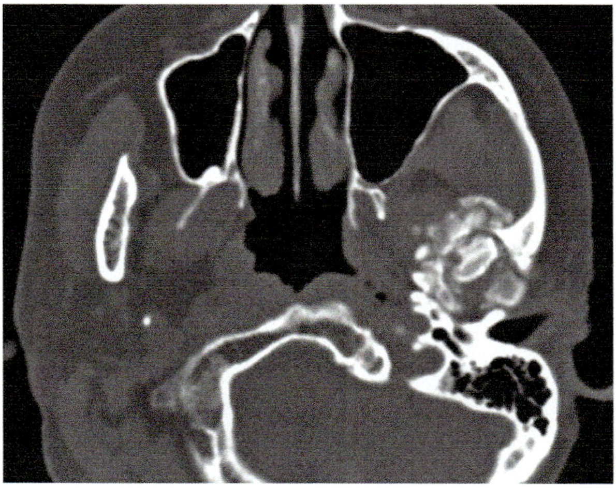

Fig. 14.8 Pseudogout, late stage. Axial CT image shows extensive calcifications in the left TMJ. Courtesy of Lado Lako Loro and Tore Bjørnland (Norway)

14.4.4 Pigmented Villonodular Synovitis (PVNS)

PVNS or tenosynovial giant cell tumor of diffuse type (TGCT-d) is a rare benign condition affecting the synovial membranes of joints, bursae, or tendons [30]. It is resulting from possibly neoplastic synovial proliferation with villous and nodular projections and hemosiderin deposition. It is most commonly found in the joints of the long bones, but rarely in the TMJ. When present, it may extend intracranially [31]. Histopathology and imaging evaluation are important for the diagnosis of PVNS, which should be included in the differential diagnosis of preauricular aggressive swellings. Another clinical sign may be restricted mandibular movement [31].

On imaging the synovial proliferation may be seen as an enlarging mass extending away from the joint on MRI. The hemosiderin deposition may be depicted as "blooming" on gradient-echo images or as prominent hypointensity on T2-weighted images, which is typical for PVNS [32]. Figure 10.35 in Chap. 10, page 198 shows a 62-year-old female with pain and swelling in the right TMJ. The right condyle is expanded, and CT shows well-defined multilocular radiolucencies with homogenous inner structure, and an almost cystic outline. The MRI shows very low signal in the entire condyle on the T1 sequence, and lateral effusion, which is confirmed by the ultrasound examinations.

14.4.5 Traumatic Arthritis and Traumatic TMJ Conditions

Facial trauma, in particular to the mandible or TMJ region, may lead to fractures that can be extracapsular, frequently of the mandibular neck (Fig. 14.9a), or intracapsular (Fig. 14.9b). However, TMJ pathology may also be the result of a non-fracture trauma. Traumatic arthritis can be defined as an intracapsular tissue response to a single (major) trauma or repetitive episodes of (minor) trauma. In traumatic arthritis, conventional radiologic examination or CT and CBCT can show the condylar head out of fossa at closed mouth position (Fig. 14.10a). The patient reports that the teeth do not fit together. With MRI the occurrence of joint effusion will confirm the traumatic arthritis diagnosis (Fig. 14.10b, c). Traumatic arthritis can also be found in patients with mandibular fracture (Fig. 14.11).

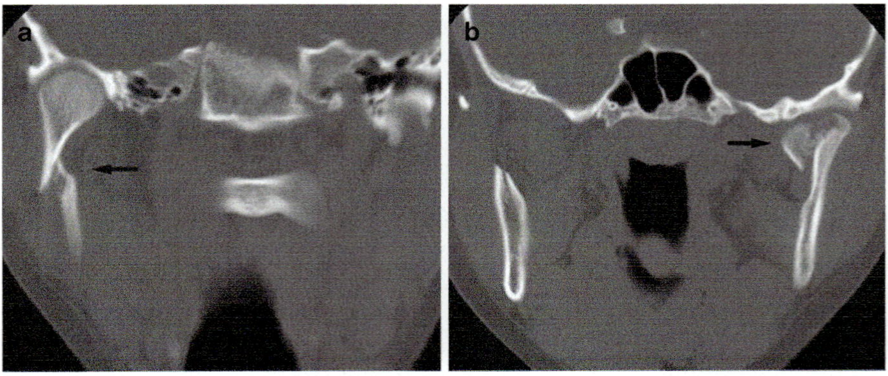

Fig. 14.9 Mandibular fractures, bilateral. (**a**) Mandibular neck fracture (*arrow*) and (**b**) condylar head fracture (*arrow*). Reproduced with permission from Larheim T.A., Westesson P-L. A. Maxillofacial Imaging (Springer 2018)

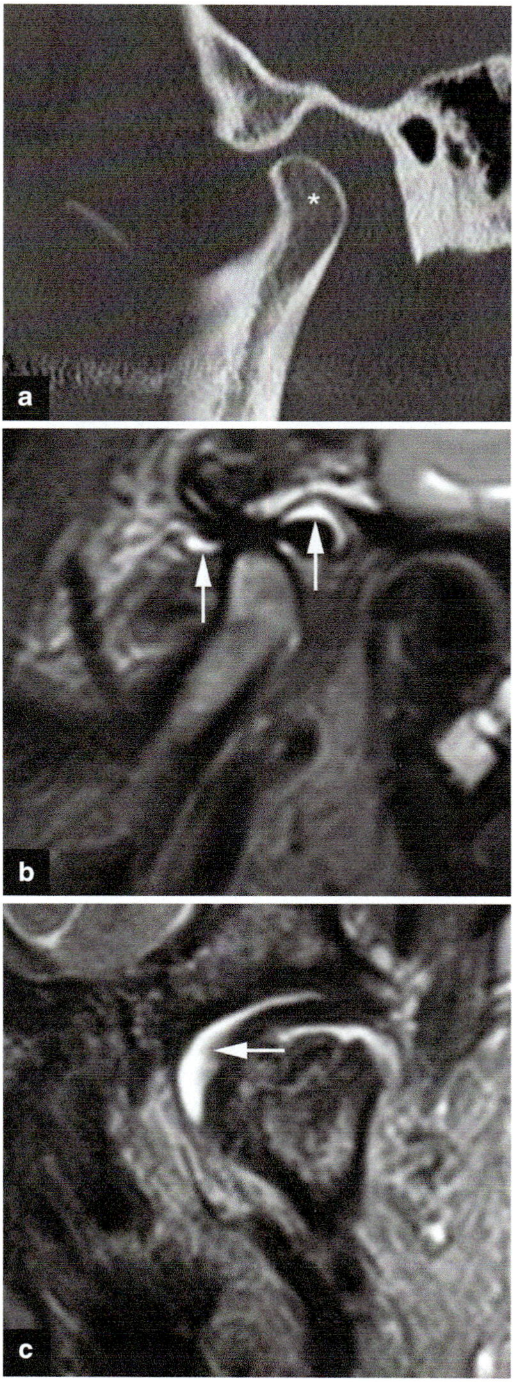

Fig. 14.10 Traumatic arthritis due to non-fracture trauma to the mandible. (**a**) Oblique sagittal CT image shows the condyle (*asterisk*) located "out of fossa." (**b**) Oblique sagittal T2-weighted image confirms abnormal condyle position and additionally shows joint effusion in both anterior and posterior joint recesses of upper compartment (*arrows*). (**c**) Oblique coronal T2 image confirms joint effusion (*arrow*). Reproduced with permission from Larheim T.A., Westesson P-L. A. Maxillofacial Imaging (Springer 2018)

Trauma in the TMJ area can lead to jaw luxation (Fig. 14.12) and probably also to disc displacement (Fig. 14.13). One late sequela of trauma is osteoarthritis. Another is fibrous ankylosis due to hemarthrosis causing contractions and adhesions between the joint components. An even more serious complication is fibro-osseous ankylosis (Fig. 14.14), leading to a significantly impaired joint function. If occurring in young age, mandibular growth disturbances may be a consequence.

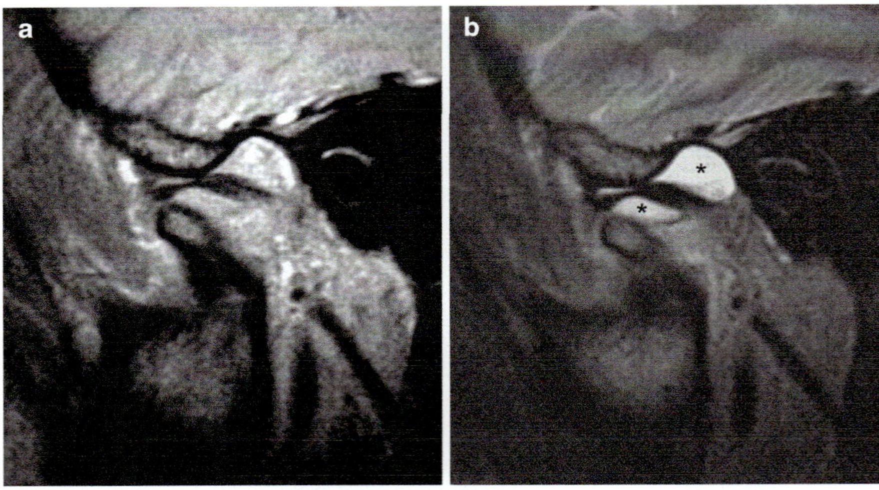

Fig. 14.11 Traumatic arthritis due to mandibular neck fracture, unilateral. Severe pain and severely impaired mouth-opening capacity immediately after trauma. (**a**) Oblique sagittal PD-weighted and (**b**) oblique sagittal T2-weighted MRI show condyle and disc in abnormal position and large effusion in both upper and lower joint compartments (*asterisk*). Reproduced with permission from Larheim T.A., Westesson P-L. A. Maxillofacial Imaging (Springer 2018)

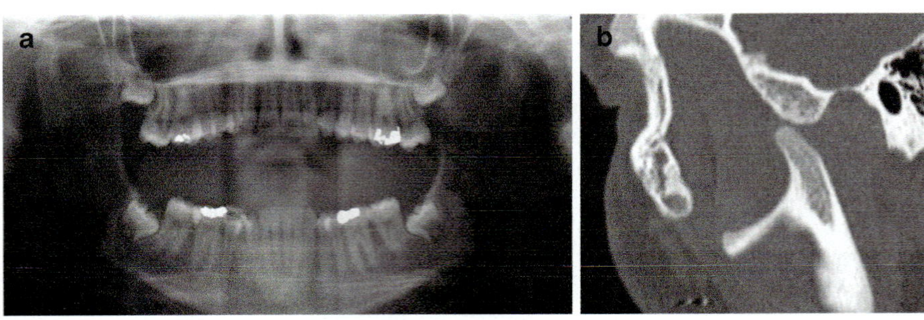

Fig. 14.12 Non-fracture trauma to the mandible with jaw luxation. (**a**) Panoramic view and (**b**) oblique sagittal CT image show the condyle in front of the eminence. Reproduced with permission from Larheim T.A., Westesson P-L. A. Maxillofacial Imaging (Springer 2018)

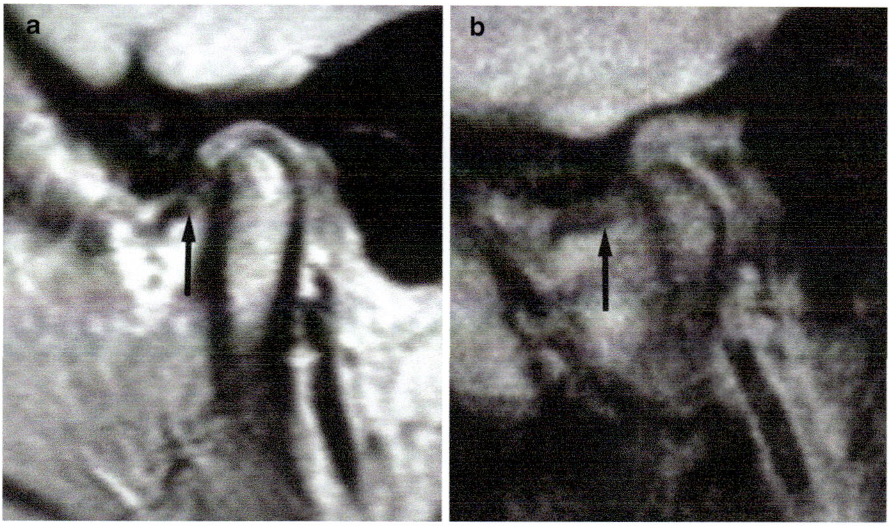

Fig. 14.13 Disc displacement without reduction probably due to non-fracture trauma to the mandible; 2 months after trauma with pain and limited mouth-opening capacity, and without joint sound (before trauma there had been a clicking joint). (**a**) Oblique sagittal MRI at closed and (**b**) at opened-mouth shows anteriorly displaced disc (*arrow*). Reproduced with permission from Larheim T.A., Westesson P-L. A. Maxillofacial Imaging (Springer 2018)

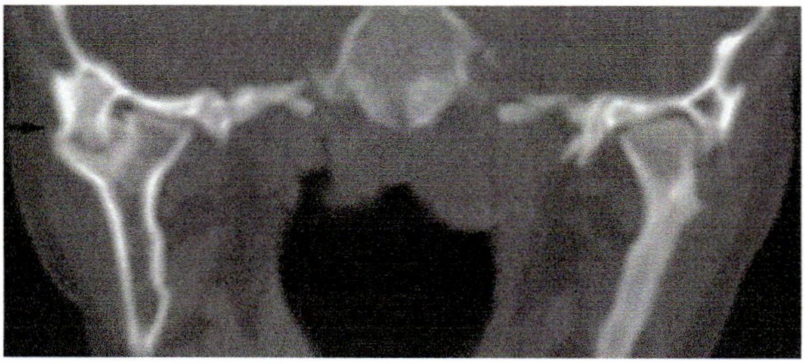

Fig. 14.14 Ankylosis after fracture. Coronal CT shows ankylosis of right joint (*arrow*) 4 years after head trauma, but mandibular fracture not diagnosed at that time. Previous fracture of the left mandibular neck as well. Reproduced with permission from Larheim T.A., Westesson P-L. A. Maxillofacial Imaging (Springer 2018)

References

1. Silman AJ, Pearson JE. Epidemiology and genetics of rheumatoid arthritis. Arthritis Res. 2002;4(Suppl 3):S265–72.
2. Ngo ST, Steyn FJ, McCombe PA. Gender differences in autoimmune disease. Front Neuroendocrinol. 2014;35(3):347–69.
3. Witulski S, Vogl TJ, Rehart S, Ottl P. Evaluation of the TMJ by means of clinical TMD examination and MRI diagnostics in patients with rheumatoid arthritis. Biomed Res Int. 2014;2014:328560.

4. Larheim TA, Storhaug K, Tveito L. Temporomandibular joint involvement and dental occlusion in a group of adults with rheumatoid arthritis. Acta Odontol Scand. 1983;41(5):301–9.
5. Badel T, Savic Pavicin I, Krapac L, Zadravec D, Rosic D. Psoriatic arthritis and temporomandibular joint involvement - literature review with a reported case. Acta Dermatovenerol Croat. 2014;22(2):114–21.
6. Braun J, Sieper J. Ankylosing spondylitis. Lancet. 2007;369(9570):1379–90.
7. Arora P, Amarnath J, Ravindra SV, Rallan M. Temporomandibular joint involvement in ankylosing spondylitis. BMJ Case Rep. Published online: 2 May 2013.
8. Klecker RJ, Weissman BN. Imaging features of psoriatic arthritis and Reiter's syndrome. Semin Musculoskelet Radiol. 2003;7(2):115–26.
9. Selmi C, Gershwin ME. Diagnosis and classification of reactive arthritis. Autoimmun Rev. 2014;13(4-5):546–9.
10. Larheim TA, Westesson P-LA. Maxillofacial imaging. Berlin: Springer; 2018.
11. Larheim TA. Temporomandibular joint space in children without joint disease. Acta Radiol Diagn (Stockh). 1981;22(1):85–8.
12. Pullinger AG, Hollender L, Solberg WK, Petersson A. A tomographic study of mandibular condyle position in an asymptomatic population. J Prosthet Dent. 1985;53(5):706–13.
13. Smith HJ, Larheim TA, Aspestrand F. Rheumatic and nonrheumatic disease in the temporomandibular joint: gadolinium-enhanced MR imaging. Radiology. 1992;185(1):229–34.
14. Larheim TA, Smith HJ, Aspestrand F. Rheumatic disease of the temporomandibular joint: MR imaging and tomographic manifestations. Radiology. 1990;175(2):527–31.
15. Arvidsson LZ, Smith HJ, Flato B, Larheim TA. Temporomandibular joint findings in adults with long-standing juvenile idiopathic arthritis: CT and MR imaging assessment. Radiology. 2010;256(1):191–200.
16. Kirkhus E, Arvidsson LZ, Smith HJ, Flato B, Hetlevik SO, Larheim TA. Disk abnormality coexists with any degree of synovial and osseous abnormality in the temporomandibular joints of children with juvenile idiopathic arthritis. Pediatr Radiol. 2016;46(3):331–41.
17. Petty RE, Laxer RM, Wedderburn LR. Chapter 15 - Juvenile idiopathic arthritis. Philadelphia: Elsevier; 2016. p. 188–204.e6.
18. Larheim TA, Doria AS, Kirkhus E, Parra DA, Kellenberger CJ, Arvidsson LZ. TMJ imaging in JIA patients-an overview. Semin Orthod. 2015;21(2):102–10.
19. Arvidsson LZ, Flato B, Larheim TA. Radiographic TMJ abnormalities in patients with juvenile idiopathic arthritis followed for 27 years. Oral Surg Oral Med Oral Pathol Oral Radiol Endod. 2009;108(1):114–23.
20. Kellenberger CJ, Junhasavasdikul T, Tolend M, Doria AS. Temporomandibular joint atlas for detection and grading of juvenile idiopathic arthritis involvement by magnetic resonance imaging. Pediatr Radiol. 2018;48(3):411–26.
21. Hechler BL, Phero JA, Van Mater H, Matthews NS. Ultrasound versus magnetic resonance imaging of the temporomandibular joint in juvenile idiopathic arthritis: a systematic review. Int J Oral Maxillofac Surg. 2017;47(1):83–9.
22. Stabrun AE, Larheim TA, Hoyeraal HM, Rosler M. Reduced mandibular dimensions and asymmetry in juvenile rheumatoid arthritis. Pathogenetic factors. Arthritis Rheum. 1988;31(5):602–11.
23. Flato B, Lien G, Smerdel A, Vinje O, Dale K, Johnston V, et al. Prognostic factors in juvenile rheumatoid arthritis: a case-control study revealing early predictors and outcome after 14.9 years. J Rheumatol. 2003;30(2):386–93.
24. Lopez EN, Dogliotti PL. Treatment of temporomandibular joint ankylosis in children: is it necessary to perform mandibular distraction simultaneously? J Craniofac Surg. 2004;15(5):879–84; discussion 84–5.
25. Bhattacharyya I, Chehal H, Gremillion H, Nair M. Gout of the temporomandibular joint: a review of the literature. J Am Dent Assoc. 2010;141(8):979–85.
26. Oliveira IN, Gomes RC, Dos Santos RR, Oliveira Tde P, Pereira LL, Mainenti P. Gout of the temporomandibular joint: report of a case. Int Arch Otorhinolaryngol. 2014;18(3):316–8.

27. Yuan Y, Liu C, Xiang X, Yuan TL, Qiu L, Liu Y, et al. Ultrasound scans and dual energy CT identify tendons as preferred anatomical location of MSU crystal depositions in gouty joints. Rheumatol Int. 2018;38(5):801–11.
28. Abhishek A, Doherty M. Epidemiology of calcium pyrophosphate crystal arthritis and basic calcium phosphate crystal arthropathy. Rheum Dis Clin N Am. 2014;40(2):177–91.
29. Ishida T, Dorfman HD, Bullough PG. Tophaceous pseudogout (tumoral calcium pyrophosphate dihydrate crystal deposition disease). Hum Pathol. 1995;26(6):587–93.
30. O'Sullivan TJ, Alport EC, Whiston HG. Pigmented villonodular synovitis of the temporomandibular joint. J Otolaryngol. 1984;13(2):123–6.
31. Romanach MJ, Brasileiro BF, Leon JE, Alves DB, de Almeida OP, Vargas PA. Pigmented villonodular synovitis of the temporomandibular joint: case report and review of the literature. Oral Surg Oral Med Oral Pathol Oral Radiol Endod. 2011;111(3):e17–28.
32. Morales H, Cornelius R. Imaging approach to temporomandibular joint disorders. Clin Neuroradiol. 2016;26(1):5–22.

Other Pathologic Conditions of the TMJ

15

Linda Z. Arvidsson, Bjørn B. Mork-Knutsen, Caroline Hol, Anna-Karin Abrahamsson, Margareth Kristensen Ottersen, and Tore A. Larheim

A number of benign tumors and tumorlike conditions, all of them rare, may occur in the TMJ [1–3]. Some of the conditions are unlikely to originate within the TMJ, but extension of the lesions from the mandibular ramus may result in condylar involvement. In the present chapter, we mainly discuss conditions that we have been able to illustrate. Thus, many conditions are not included here, such as hemangioma or vascular malformation, aneurysmal bone cyst, giant cell granuloma, non-ossifying fibroma, and chondroblastoma.

15.1 Synovial Chondromatosis

Synovial chondromatosis is characterized by synovitis and/or joint effusion and cartilaginous metaplasia of the synovial membrane, producing small nodules of cartilage. The nodules separate from the membrane to become loose bodies that may ossify. Usually synovial chondromatosis is monoarticular, developing in large joints, in particular the knee [4]. It seems to be the most frequently reported benign lesion in the TMJ presenting with characteristics of a tumor. A swelling without pain is the common clinical sign. In the TMJ it is mostly confined to the upper joint compartment [5]. However, it can be locally aggressive; the first case with extension through the base of the skull into the middle cranial fossa was reported in 1987 [6]. The disc and the condyle may be intact. The relative merits of CT and MRI for depicting the bone and soft tissue abnormalities have been nicely demonstrated [7].

L. Z. Arvidsson (✉) · B. B. Mork-Knutsen · C. Hol · A.-K. Abrahamsson · M. K. Ottersen
T. A. Larheim
Department of Maxillofacial Radiology, Faculty of Dentistry, University of Oslo, Oslo, Norway
e-mail: l.z.arvidsson@odont.uio.no; b.b.mork-knutsen@odont.uio.no; caroline.hol@odont.uio.no; a.k.johansen@odont.uio.no; m.k.ottersen@odont.uio.no; t.a.larheim@odont.uio.no

I. Rozylo-Kalinowska, K. Orhan (eds.), *Imaging of the Temporomandibular Joint*, https://doi.org/10.1007/978-3-319-99468-0_15

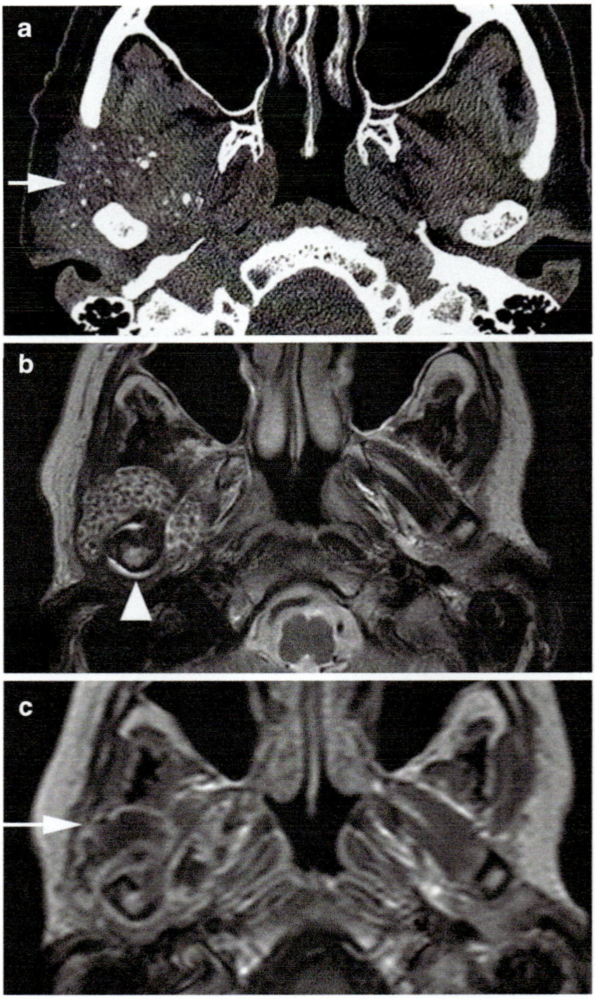

Fig. 15.1 Synovial chondromatosis. (**a**) Axial CT image shows several small calcifications (*arrow*). (**b**) Axial T2-weighted MRI shows multiple small low signal nodules and joint effusion (*arrowhead*). (**c**) Axial T1-weighted post-Gd MRI shows contrast enhancement in thin rim (synovial membrane) (*arrow*) throughout the right joint consistent with synovitis. Reproduced with permission from Larheim T.A., Westesson P-L. A. Maxillofacial Imaging (Springer 2018)

CT shows the calcifications which usually are multiple, and MRI shows the cartilage nodules, as well as the synovitis (Fig. 15.1).

15.2 Unilateral Condylar Hyperplasia

Unilateral condylar hyperplasia is characterized by a nonneoplastic overgrowth of the condyle and the mandible, frequently detected due to facial asymmetric development. It has a female predominance [8]. The condition is self-limiting and is

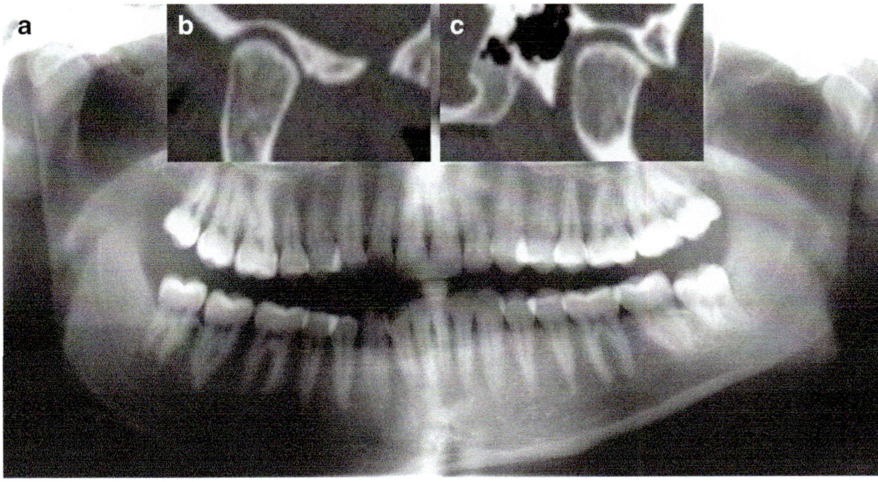

Fig. 15.2 Condylar hyperplasia and facial asymmetry. (**a**) Panoramic radiography shows jaw asymmetry due to unilateral mandibular overgrowth (right side). (**b**) Oblique coronal and (**c**) oblique sagittal CT images show the right condyle with abnormal shape and size but normal bone structure. Reproduced with permission from Larheim T.A., Westesson P-L. A. Maxillofacial Imaging (Springer 2018)

observed as an acceleration of growth during a certain period, usually in the late teens to mid-20s [9]. Condylar hyperplasia is radiologically characterized by a large condyle with normal bone structure as shown in Fig. 15.2. To assess the metabolic activity in the joint for the surgical planning, nuclear medicine such as scintigraphy is valuable. In the majority of cases, when the patient seeks treatment, the condition has already become metabolically quiescent [10].

15.3 Osteochondroma

Osteochondroma, also known as osteocartilaginous exostosis, is defined as a cartilage-capped bony projection arising on the external surface of bone, continuous with underlying bone [11]. It is rare in the TMJ; of 2186 cases of benign and malignant cysts/tumors of the maxillofacial region, 8 osteochondromas of the mandibular condyle were identified [12]. It is often found incidentally but may be detected because of facial asymmetry. Osteochondroma is characterized as a type of overgrowth that can occur where cartilage forms bone. Radiologically the cortical outline and internal structure may be irregular as shown in Fig. 15.3, but the cortical outline may also be smooth. It may be difficult to distinguish between condylar hyperplasia and osteochondroma radiologically and even histologically [13].

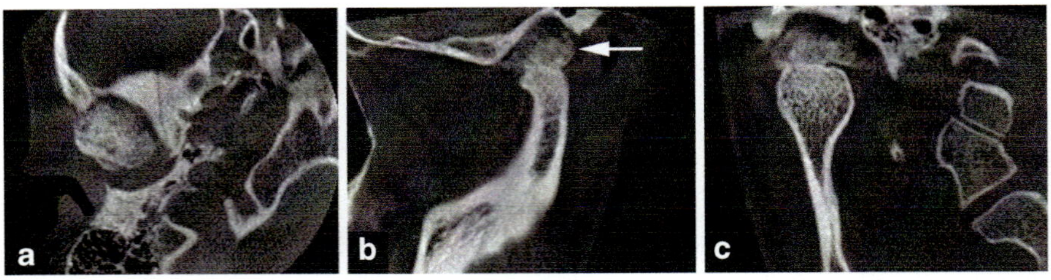

Fig. 15.3 Osteochondroma; 26-year-old female with some jaw asymmetry. (**a**) Axial, (**b**) oblique sagittal, and (**c**) oblique coronal CBCT images show cranial outgrowth with irregular outline on the condyle (*arrow*). Reproduced with permission from Larheim T.A., Westesson P-L. A. Maxillofacial Imaging (Springer 2018)

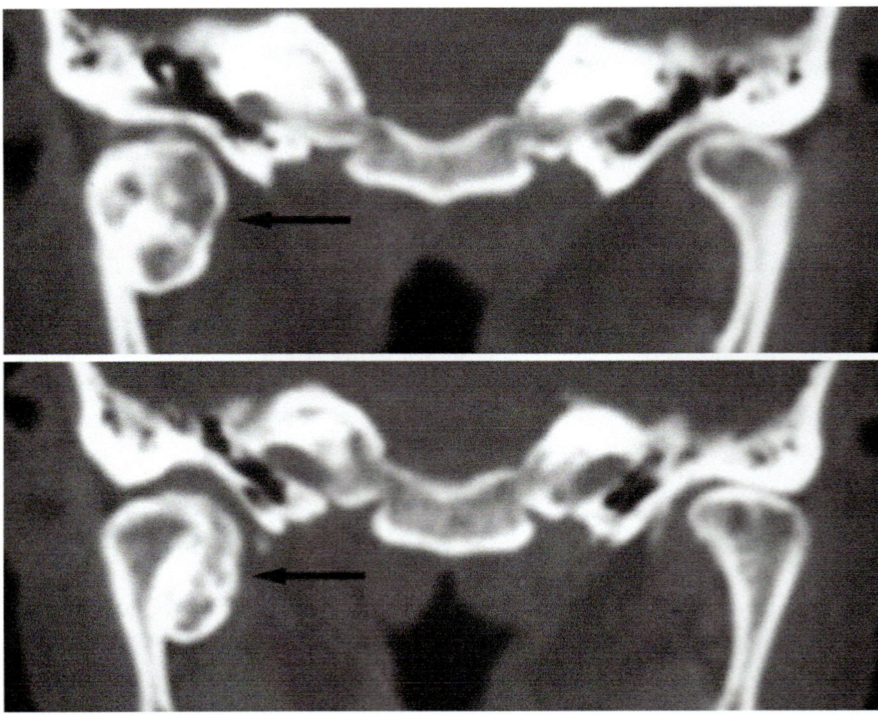

Fig. 15.4 Osteoma, incidental finding. Two coronal CT images show bony outgrowth (*arrow*) of medial aspect of the condyle. Reproduced with permission from Larheim T.A., Westesson P-L. A. Maxillofacial Imaging (Springer 2018)

15.4 Osteoma

Osteoma is defined as a benign neoplasm composed of mature bone, limited almost exclusively to the craniofacial bones [14]. It is the most common benign neoplasm in the nose and paranasal sinuses and often asymptomatic. Radiologically the osteoma is characterized by normal cortical bone and marrow, as shown in Fig. 15.4.

15.5 Osteoid Osteoma

Osteoid osteoma is defined as a benign bone-forming tumor characterized by limited growth potential [14]. The majority of patients complain of nocturnal pain. It is histologically identical to osteoblastoma, but is smaller, usually not exceeding 2 cm. Radiologically, it is characterized by a nidus surrounded by a zone of sclerotic bone [15]. To distinguish the condition from osteomyelitis with sequestrum formation, sodium 18-fluoride positron-emission tomography combined with low-dose computed tomography (Na-18F PET-CT) is highly valuable. Osteoid osteoma is demonstrated as a localized hot spot due to intense metabolic activity [16].

15.6 Synovial Cyst and Ganglion Cyst

Synovial cyst and ganglion cyst are para-articular cysts most commonly found in the wrist, ankle, and knee joints, but may also occur in the TMJ [17] where it is difficult to clinically distinguish between them [18]. The terms have been used synonymously when diagnosing a para-articular cyst. However, synovial cysts are true cysts containing synovial fluid and are lined by synoviocytes. They may or may not communicate with the joint compartment [19]. Ganglion cysts are pseudocysts with an acellular fibrous tissue lining, which do not communicate with the joint compartment [18]. On MRI both cyst types are well-defined with a homogeneous and very high T2 signal (Fig. 15.5).

15.7 Simple Bone Cyst

Simple bone cyst is defined as an intraosseous cavity that is devoid of an epithelial lining. It is either empty or filled with serous or sanguineous fluid [11]. Radiologically, the simple bone cyst is a well-defined radiolucency with or without a cortex-like

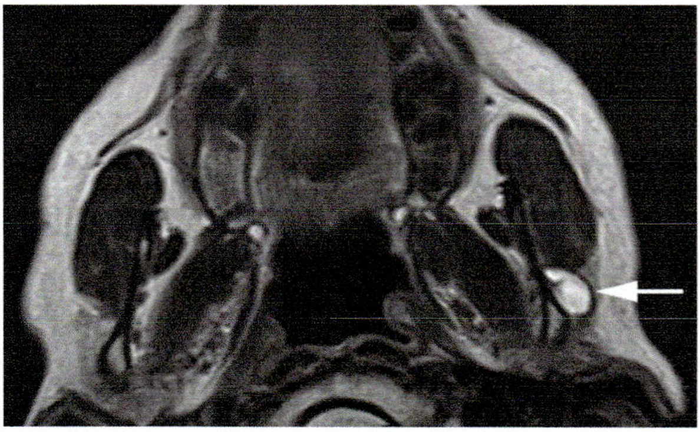

Fig. 15.5 Synovial cyst. Axial T2-weighted MRI shows well-defined lesion with high, homogeneous signal intensity (*arrow*). Reproduced with permission from Larheim T.A., Westesson P-L. A. Maxillofacial Imaging (Springer 2018)

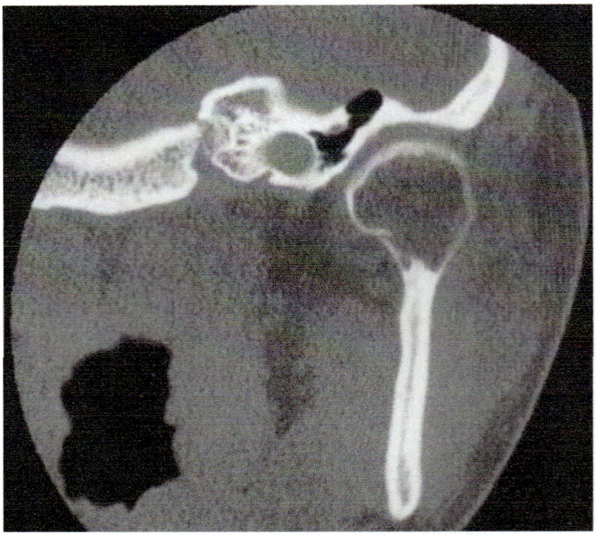

Fig. 15.6 Simple bone cyst. Coronal CT image shows enlarged condyle with radiolucency and intact cortical bone. Reproduced with permission from Larheim T.A., Westesson P-L. A. Maxillofacial Imaging (Springer 2018)

outline. The condition has occasionally been demonstrated in the mandibular condyle [20, 21] also with recurrence after surgery [21]. A simple bone cyst was found incidentally, when a 14-year-old female was examined for fracture after a facial trauma (Fig. 15.6).

15.8 Coronoid Hyperplasia

Coronoid hyperplasia can be defined as a coronoid enlarged to 1 cm above the zygomatic arch (Fig. 15.7). Restricted mouth opening can have several causes, most frequently related to the masticatory muscles (trismus) and/or nonreducing disc displacement. However, one cause of restricted mouth opening that may be overlooked because the examination is generally focused on joint abnormalities is elongation of the coronoid process. In a series of 163 consecutive patients referred for radiographic examination of the TMJ, 5% had restricted mouth opening caused by coronoid process hyperplasia [22]. For detailed evaluation of the impingement between the malar bone and the coronoid process, three-dimensional CT is highly valuable [23]. This is illustrated in Fig. 15.8.

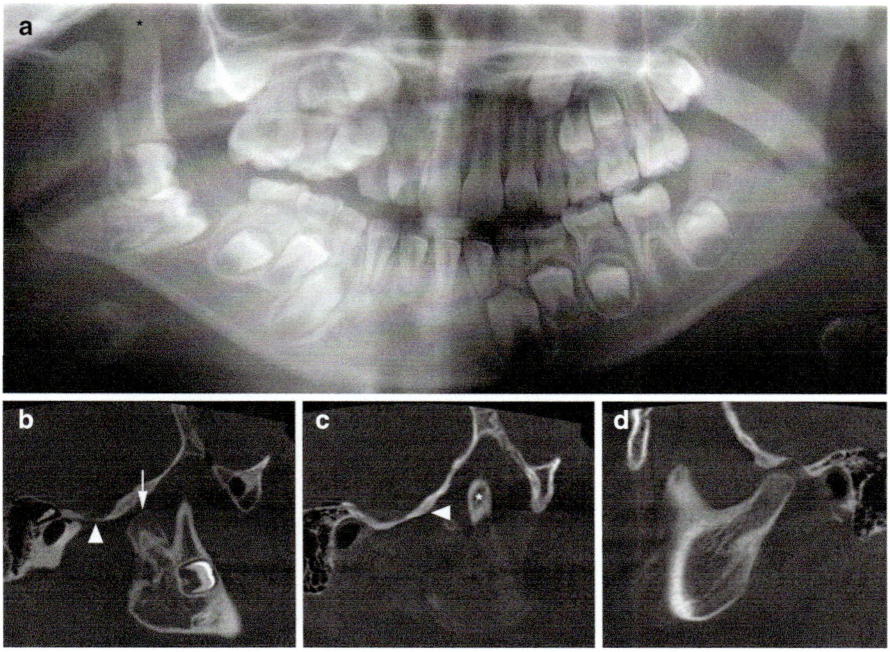

Fig. 15.7 Facial asymmetry; 7-year-old male with underdeveloped right mandible (probably due to neonatal fracture(s); use of forceps during delivery). (**a**) Panoramic view shows underdeveloped right mandible with short condylar process and enlarged coronoid process (*asterisk*) and the characteristic appearance of a partly opened pair of scissors. (**b**) Oblique sagittal CBCT image (at closed mouth) shows abnormal condylar process (*arrow*) located anterior to flat (underdeveloped) articular fossa/eminence (*arrowhead*). (**c**) Oblique sagittal CBCT image (lateral to B) shows enlarged coronoid process (asterisk) and flat eminence/fossa (*arrowhead*). (**d**) Oblique sagittal CBCT image (at closed mouth) shows normal contralateral joint. Note in particular the well-developed fossa/eminence. Reproduced with permission from Larheim T.A., Westesson P-L. A. Maxillofacial Imaging (Springer 2018)

Fig. 15.8 Coronoid hyperplasia in a patient with micrognathia. 3D CT image shows both coronoid processes are locking against zygomatic arch (*arrows*) at mouth opening (impaired). Reproduced with permission from Larheim T.A., Westesson P-L. A. Maxillofacial Imaging (Springer 2018)

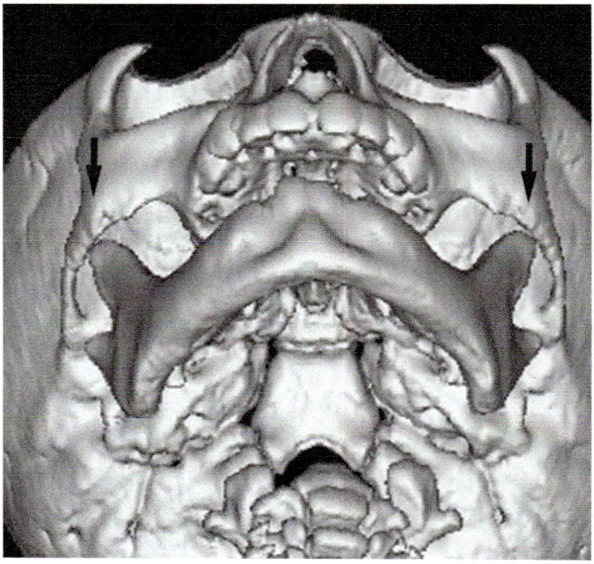

15.9 Malignant Tumors

Malignant tumors may occasionally occur in the TMJ, such as different types of sarcomas, multiple myeloma, and metastases [3] such as from the lung [24]. Usually there is a swelling but symptoms may simulate a more common condition. Metastatic osteosarcoma is shown in Fig. 15.9 and metastasis from lung cancer in Fig. 15.10.

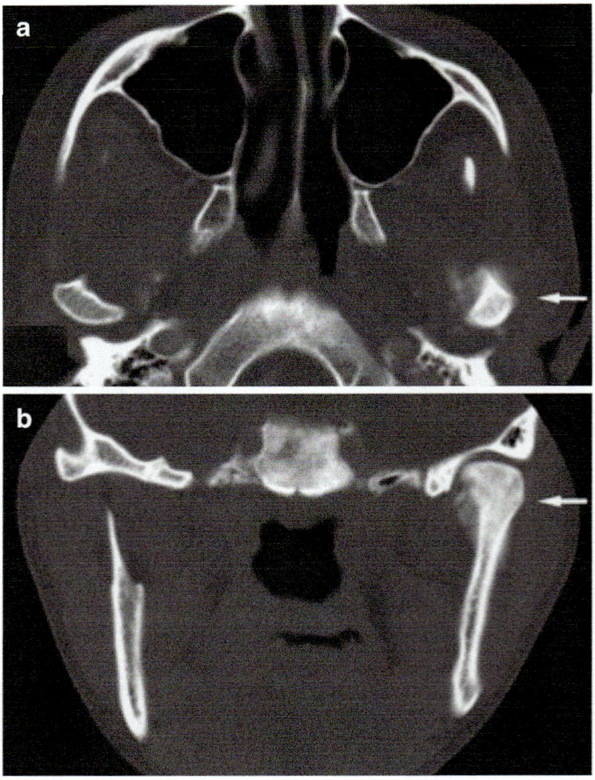

Fig. 15.9 Metastatic osteosarcoma, 18-year-old female with terminal widespread osteosarcoma (2.5-year history). (**a**) Axial and (**b**) coronal CT images show sclerotic condyle and intense periosteal bone production in condyle (*arrow*), but no evident bone destruction. Reproduced with permission from Larheim T.A., Westesson P-L. A. Maxillofacial Imaging (Springer 2018)

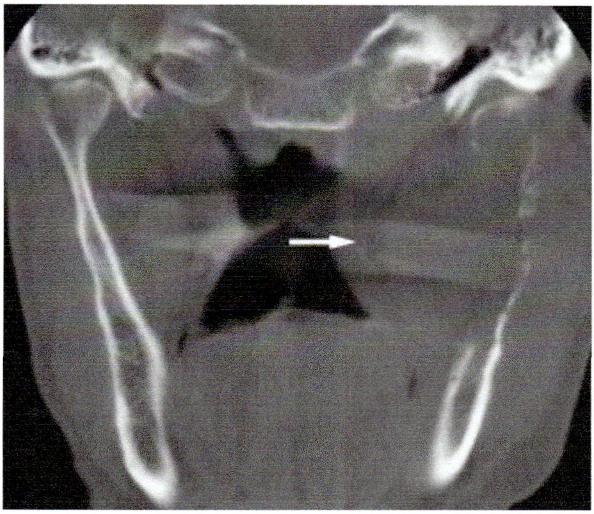

Fig. 15.10 Metastatic tumor, mandible, lung cancer spread. Coronal CT image shows destruction of ramus and condyle, and soft tissue mass (*arrow*). Reproduced with permission from Larheim T.A., Westesson P-L. A. Maxillofacial Imaging (Springer 2018)

References

1. Warner BF, Luna MA, Robert NT. Temporomandibular joint neoplasms and pseudotumors. Adv Anat Pathol. 2000;7(6):365–81.
2. Bouloux GF, Roser SM, Abramowicz S. Pediatric tumors of the temporomandibular joint. Oral Maxillofac Surg Clin North Am. 2018;30(1):61–70.
3. Stern D. Benign and malignant tumors. In: Laskin DM, Greene CS, Hylander WL, editors. Temporomandibular disorders : an evidence-based approach to diagnosis and treatment. Chicago: Quintessence; 2006. p. 319–33.
4. von Lindern JJ, Theuerkauf I, Niederhagen B, Berge S, Appel T, Reich RH. Synovial chondromatosis of the temporomandibular joint: clinical, diagnostic, and histomorphologic findings. Oral Surg Oral Med Oral Pathol Oral Radiol Endod. 2002;94(1):31–8.
5. Kim DH, Lee EH, Cho ES, Kim JY, Jeon KJ, Kim J, et al. Temporomandibular joint synovial chondromatosis extending to the temporal bone: a report of two cases. J Korean Assoc Oral Maxillofac Surg. 2017;43(5):336–42.
6. Nokes SR, King PS, Garcia R Jr, Silbiger ML, Jones JD 3rd, Castellano ND. Temporomandibular joint chondromatosis with intracranial extension: MR and CT contributions. AJR Am J Roentgenol. 1987;148(6):1173–4.
7. Herzog S, Mafee M. Synovial chondromatosis of the TMJ: MR and CT findings. AJNR Am J Neuroradiol. 1990;11(4):742–5.
8. Raijmakers PG, Karssemakers LH, Tuinzing DB. Female predominance and effect of gender on unilateral condylar hyperplasia: a review and meta-analysis. J Oral Maxillofac Surg. 2012;70(1):e72–6.
9. Rodrigues DB, Castro V. Condylar hyperplasia of the temporomandibular joint: types, treatment, and surgical implications. Oral Maxillofac Surg Clin North Am. 2015;27(1):155–67.
10. Cisneros GJ, Kaban LB. Computerized skeletal scintigraphy for assessment of mandibular asymmetry. J Oral Maxillofac Surg. 1984;42(8):513–20.

11. El-Naggar AK, Chan JKC, Grandis JR, Takata T, Slootweg PJ. WHO classification of head and neck tumours. 4th ed. International Agency for Research on Cancer: Lyon; 2017.
12. Ord RA, Warburton G, Caccamese JF. Osteochondroma of the condyle: review of 8 cases. Int J Oral Maxillofac Surg. 2010;39(6):523–8.
13. Ji H, Li J, Shao J, He D, Liu Y, Fei W, et al. Histopathologic comparison of condylar hyperplasia and condylar osteochondroma by using different staining methods. Oral Surg Oral Med Oral Pathol Oral Radiol. 2017;123(3):320–9.
14. Larheim TA, Westesson P-LA. Maxillofacial imaging. Berlin: Springer; 2018.
15. Nielsen GP, Rosenberg AE. Update on bone forming tumors of the head and neck. Head Neck Pathol. 2007;1(1):87–93.
16. Deferm JT, Steens SCA, Vriens D, Bekers EM, Kalaykova SI, Borstlap WA. Chronic temporomandibular joint pain: two cases of osteoid osteoma and a review of the literature. Int J Oral Maxillofac Surg. 2017;46(9):1130–7.
17. Spinzia A, Panetta D, Russo D, Califano L. Synovial cyst of the temporomandibular joint: a case report and literature review. Int J Oral Maxillofac Surg. 2011;40(8):874–7.
18. Partridge JC, Cipriani N, Faquin WC, Chuang SK, Keith DA, Lahey ET. Periarticular cysts of the temporomandibular joint are more frequently synovial than ganglion. J Oral Maxillofac Surg. 2016;74(7):1396–402.
19. Goudot P, Jaquinet AR, Richter M. Cysts of the temporomandibular joint. Report of two cases. Int J Oral Maxillofac Surg. 1999;28(5):338–40.
20. Tanaka H, Westesson PL, Emmings FG, Marashi AH. Simple bone cyst of the mandibular condyle: report a case. J Oral Maxillofac Surg. 1996;54(12):1454–8.
21. Kim K-A, Koh K-J. Recurrent simple bone cyst of the mandibular condyle: a case report. Imaging Sci Dent. 2013;43(1):49.
22. Isberg A, Isacsson G, Nah KS. Mandibular coronoid process locking: a prospective study of frequency and association with internal derangement of the temporomandibular joint. Oral Surg Oral Med Oral Pathol. 1987;63(3):275–9.
23. Takahashi A, Hao-Zong W, Murakami S, Kondoh H, Fujishita M, Fuchihata H. Diagnosis of coronoid process hyperplasia by three-dimensional computed tomographic imaging. Dentomaxillofac Radiol. 1993;22(3):149–54.
24. Guarda-Nardini L, Stellini E, Di Fiore A, Manfredini D. A rare case of misdiagnosed silent lung cancer with solitary metastasis to the temporomandibular joint condyle. J Oral Facial Pain Headache. 2017;31(2):180–5.

Arthrography of the Temporomandibular Joint and Arthrography-Guided Steroid Treatment

16

Eva Levring Jäghagen and Jan Ahlqvist

16.1 Introduction

This chapter describes arthrography as a method for diagnosing soft tissue derangements of the temporomandibular joint (TMJ). We will also present arthrography as an aid for intervention when mixing iodine contrast media with corticosteroids.

Clinicians with access to magnetic resonance imaging (MRI) who have not practiced or experienced arthrography might wonder when this invasive method can be useful. An explanation to that as well as a description of the method will be presented in this chapter.

MRI as a method for diagnosing soft tissue derangements of the TMJ has been described in Chap. 10, and is the most common method used for that purpose. However, for some patients MRI is not feasible, e.g. when:

- the patient has loose ferromagnetic objects in the body,
- the patient has metal object in the head and neck area causing disturbances in the images, e.g. orthodontic devices,
- the patient suffers from claustrophobia.

These patients need another method for diagnosing possible disc displacement.

Electronic Supplementary Material The online version of this chapter (doi:10.1007/978-3-319-99468-0_16) contains supplementary material, which is available to authorized users.

E. Levring Jäghagen (✉) · J. Ahlqvist
Oral and Maxillofacial Radiology, Department Odontology, Umeå University, Umeå, Sweden
e-mail: eva.levring.jaghagen@umu.se

I. Rozylo-Kalinowska, K. Orhan (eds.), *Imaging of the Temporomandibular Joint*, https://doi.org/10.1007/978-3-319-99468-0_16

16.1.1 Instances where Arthrography is Superior to MRI

1. Presence of soft tissue perforations in the disc or the posterior attachment.

In cases with perforations, the contrast media leaks from one joint compartment to the other during injection, which is simultaneously seen during fluoroscopy.

2. Adherences between the disc or the posterior attachment and the condyle or the temporal bone can be revealed during the real-time dynamic assessment.

After injection of contrast media, the TMJ movements are examined during fluoroscopy that will show the actual movement and continuously reveal the relations between the TMJ components. This is an advantage compared to assessments of single images at different levels of movement acquired in MRI, in the so-called cine sequences.

3. Like for all types of injections into the joint, filling of the joint compartment can contribute to loosening adherences.

4. The anaesthesia preceding the injection of contrast media can confirm origin of pain.

The examination is initiated with injection of anaesthesia. This can also be used as part of diagnosing. If the patient experiences pain relief after injection of anaesthesia, it is confirmed that the pain is originating from the TMJ.

5. Splint therapy follow-up.

During the examination, it is possible to verify that the design of an occlusal splint is correct. After inserting the splint into the mouth of the patient, the intended function to keep the condyle in a position where the disc is reduced can be assessed.

6. As guidance for intervention with corticosteroids.

When performing arthrography, there is a possibility to administer different therapeutic agents. One example is corticosteroids that can be mixed with contrast media, which will serve as guidance and simultaneously allow for diagnosing soft tissue derangements of the joint. This is an area where more research could be valuable to further elucidate whether injection of steroids with guidance that makes the location of the injection precise is more effective compared to the “free hand” injection performed by clinicians without fluoroscopic guidance.

At our department, approximately 20% of all examinations of TMJ soft tissue are performed with arthrography. Of these, more than 80% are arthrography-guided corticosteroid injections.

16.1.2 Drawbacks

There are some drawbacks with arthrography. The method is invasive and requires use of ionising radiation. It is not possible to make a reliable diagnosis regarding sideway disk displacement unless a CBCT examination is performed immediately after the contrast is injected. Finally, injection of a fluid into the joint can limit the joint function during examination.

16.2 Background

Arthrography for diagnosing the TMJ soft tissues was first introduced in the early 1940s by Zimmer [1]. Some years later, in 1944, professor Flemming Nørgaard described the technique and possibilities of the method for diagnosing soft tissue derangements of the TMJ [2]. However, it was not until the 1970 that the method was widely recognised when image-intensifying techniques were introduced that lowered the dose and facilitated simultaneous viewing of the injection and the joint dynamics [3, 4]. At that time, anterior disc displacement was recognised as a common cause of TMJ pain and dysfunction, and both surgical and conservative treatment methods were developed that required thorough assessment of TMJ function [5, 6]. Double contrast examinations were introduced in the 1960s [7] and interventional examination with steroids in combination with contrast media in the beginning of the 1990s [8]. At that time, MRI was getting more available and special coils for the TMJ and inner ear were developed. MRI slowly replaced arthrography when it came to diagnosing disc displacement. The method is superior in many aspects since it does not require radiation, sideways disc displacement can be assessed and MRI is not invasive. However, there are still several types of soft tissue derangements of the TMJ that cannot be assessed by MRI. As discussed in the introduction, the possibility to diagnose perforations and adherences, to study real-time dynamics, to verify successful splint treatment and to accurately perform corticosteroid intervention implies that arthrography still has a position in the arsenal of modalities for TMJ diagnostics.

16.3 Arthrography

16.3.1 Indications for Arthrography

The indications for arthrography of the TMJ are partly the same as for MR examinations, with some exceptions. Arthrography is justified when there is a need for:

- assessment of the soft tissues of the TMJ, i.e. to determine the configuration, position and function of the disc when MRI is contraindicated
- diagnosing perforations in the disk or posterior attachment
- verifying suspected adherences
- real-time dynamic assessment of the function

- dynamic assessment or verification of the position of the disc and condyle during use of an occlusal splint
- identification of loose bodies in the TMJ
- guided intra-articular therapeutic injections of, e.g. corticosteroids

16.3.2 Contraindication to Arthrography [9]

- Previous severe reaction to iodine contrast media (can be performed with corticosteroid premedication)
- Anticoagulant medication or bleeding disorders
- Patient anxiety
- Infection in the preauricular area

In case of uncertainty, consultation with the treating physician is recommended.

16.3.3 Fluoroscopy

Fluoroscopy is used in many examinations or procedures for diagnostic purposes or treatment including arthrography and administration of, e.g. corticosteroids. The radiation source and the detector are connected with a C-shaped arm that can be manoeuvred in all three dimensions (Fig. 16.1). Fluoroscopy enables continuous X-ray imaging, mostly presented on a monitor. An image intensifier or flat panel detector captures a conventional central projection. The radiation dose can thereby be kept relatively low, allowing for extended exposure that facilitates functional studies. It also enables detailed control of the administration of, e.g. contrast media and during manoeuvring of different tools for interventions.

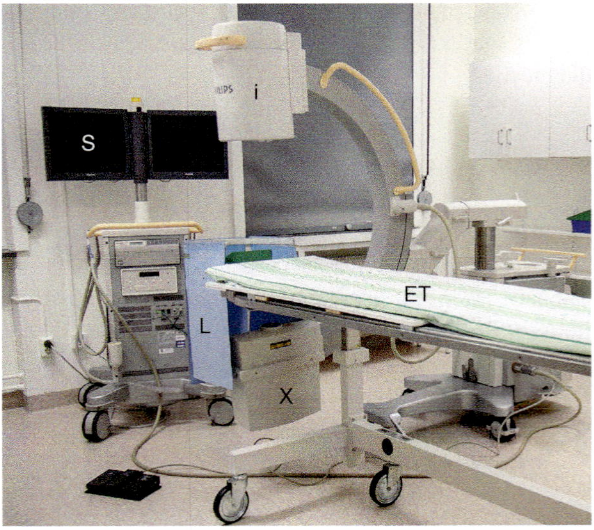

Fig. 16.1 Equipment for fluoroscopy. C-arm with the X-ray source (X) positioned under the trimmed head support of the exam table (ET). The X-ray source is surrounded with lead shields (L) for radiation protection of the radiologist and assisting personnel. The image intensifier (i) is positioned above the patient's head. Screen (S) for monitoring the examination

The examinations are performed with pulsed fluoroscopy (in the complementary videos the frame rate is 12 frames/sec) and automatised exposure. A normal fluoroscopic exposure time per joint is 1.5–2.5 min. The dose is dependent on exposure time and field of view. It is important to limit these parameters.

16.3.4 Contrast Media for Arthrography

In order to visualise the soft tissues of the TMJ, injection of contrast media into the TMJ compartments is necessary. For this purpose, iodine-containing contrast media is used, the same or similar to the contrast media used for enhancement in CT imaging (see Chap. 7). The iodine has higher attenuation compared to the surrounding tissues, which is beneficial for diagnostics. The amount of contrast media needed for arthrography is very small, maximum 1.5–2.0 mL in total, and since the purpose is to inject the contrast into the joint compartments and not the vascular system, the risk of idiosyncratic reactions is low. Since the amount of contrast media that can be injected is limited, it is important to have a high concentration of iodine, e.g. 300 mg iodine/mL.

16.3.5 Preparation of the Patient

To avoid risks of infection of the joint due to the invasive procedure, a highly antiseptic approach is necessary. Disinfection of the equipment, sterile preparation of the field and use of sterile instruments are mandatory. A wad of unrefined cotton wool is placed in the external auditory meatus to prevent incidental leakage of chlorhexidine-ethyl alcohol (5 mg/mL) when the preauricular skin covering the TMJ is cleaned (Fig. 16.2). The upper half of the patient is covered in sterile drape sheets except the skin surface of the TMJ of interest (Figs. 16.3 and 16.4). The radiologist wears sterile

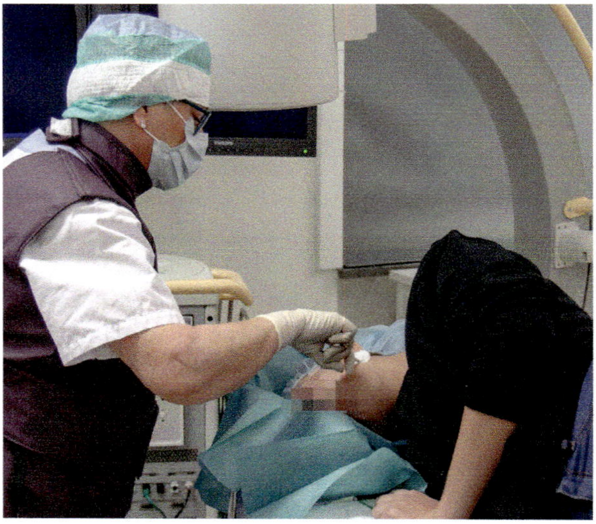

Fig. 16.2 The patient is positioned on the exam table according to Figs. 16.6 and 16.7 with the head resting on a sterile drape sheet. The preauricular skin area is thoroughly disinfected. A wad of unrefined cotton wool is placed in the external auditory meatus to prevent leakage of the disinfection solution into the external auditory canal. After disinfection, the upper half of the patient is covered with sterile drape sheets

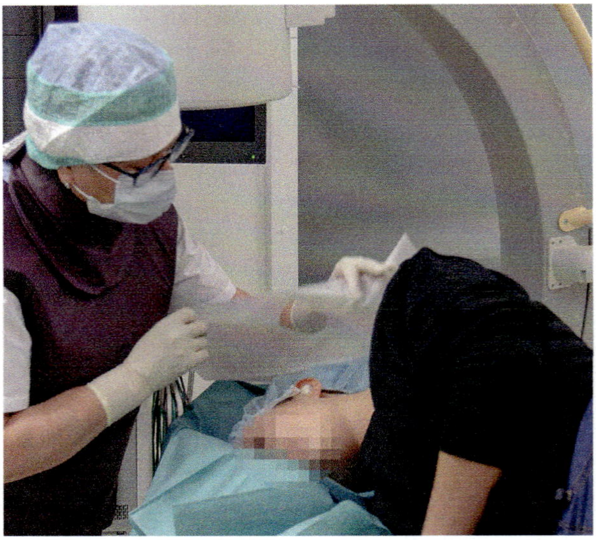

Fig. 16.3 After disinfection, a sterile adhesive drape sheet with an aperture for the intervention area is placed over the patient's cheek

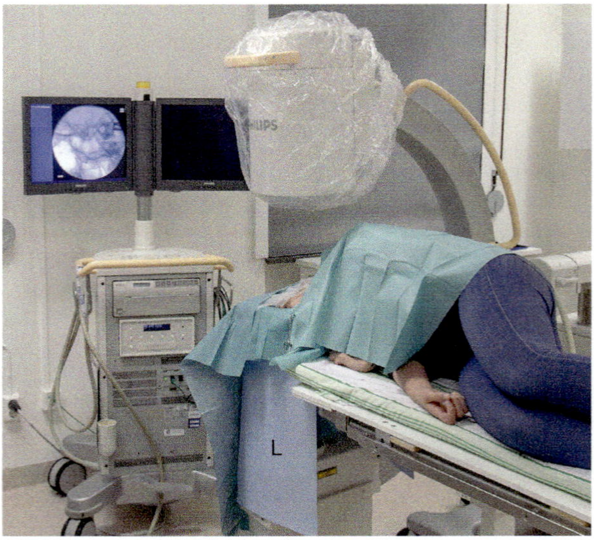

Fig. 16.4 Patient prepared for examination. The upper half of the patient is covered with sterile drape sheets. The image intensifier is covered with a sterile cap allowing the radiologist to adjust the projections during the examination. Under the head support, a lead shield (L) prevents secondary radiation from the exam table and the inferior parts of the patient to reach the radiologist and assisting personnel

gloves, a sterile arm sleeve on the operating arm and a surgical cap and face mask to prevent contamination. The image intensifier of the C-arm is covered with a sterile cap to facilitate projection changes during the examination without contamination.

After the examination, a sterile translucent film dressing is placed over the perforated preauricular skin for protection for a minimum of 8 h before removal. If the patient is unable to close the eyelid due to unintended anaesthesia of the facial nerve, a surgical tape can be placed over the eyelid to protect the eye from drying out during the anaesthetic palsy that can last up to 2 h. The patient should be informed that pain can appear when the anaesthesia ceases and advised to avoid food that demands hard chewing during 2–7 days. Conventional analgesics (e.g. paracetamol) can give pain relief. If the patient has an occlusal splint for treatment of TMJ symptoms, the patient can continue to use it.

16.3.6 Brief Repetition of the Anatomy (Fig. 16.5)

The upper compartment of the TMJ is superiorly limited by the articular fossa and the articular tubercle. Inferiorly, it is limited by the disc and its attachment to the articular capsule that surrounds the joint and superiorly attaches to the temporal bone. Anteriorly, the articular capsule attaches ventral to the articular tubercle and posteriorly it attaches cranioventral to the middle ear and the external auditory canal. Medially and laterally, it attaches to the edges of articular fossa. The lower joint compartment is superiorly limited by the disc and its attachment to the articular capsule that inferiorly tapers into a funnel shape and attaches to the neck of the mandible, a little further down on its posterior part. From the lateral part of the articular tubercle, extending posteriorly/inferiorly, the capsule is thickened in a band called the temporomandibular ligament or external lateral ligament. This ligament prevents the mandible to extend its movement backwards beyond the articular fossa.

16.3.7 Positioning of the Patient and Radiographic Projection

The patient is examined in a supine position, lying prone or on the side on the examination table with the lateral side of the face and the joint of interest positioned upwards. The head should be slightly tilted (hanging) towards the table and slightly rotated upwards (Fig. 16.6). This facilitates vertical positioning of the C-arm for a

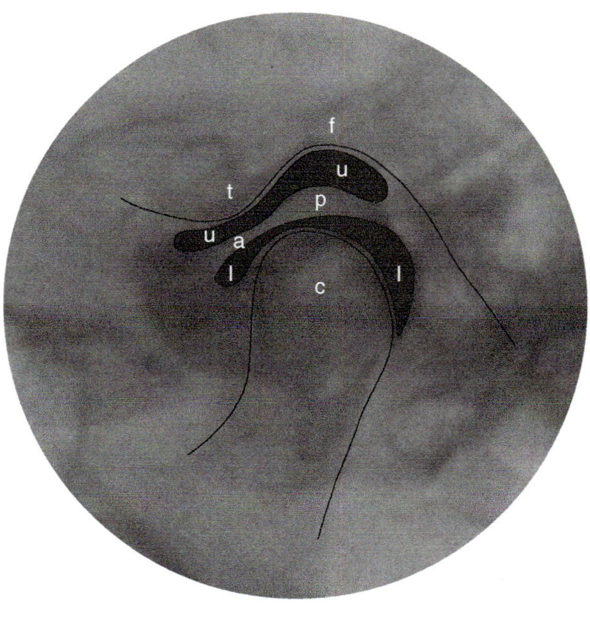

Fig. 16.5 Arthrography of the left TMJ showing normal disc position with joint components outlined and contrast media highlighted. The letters mark the following anatomical structures: (f) articular fossa, (t) articular tubercle, (c) condyle, (u) upper joint compartment, (l) lower joint compartment, (a) anterior band of the disc, and (p) posterior band of the disc

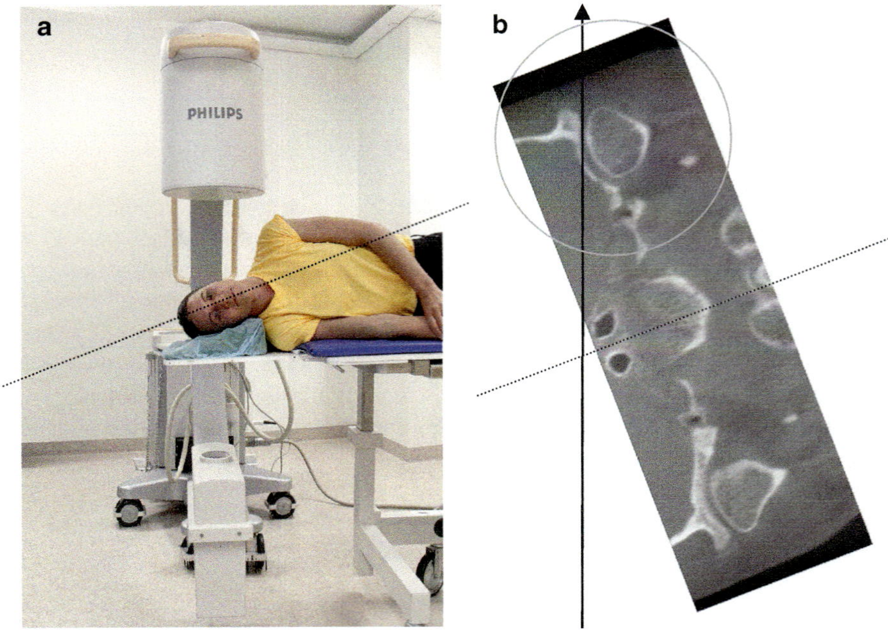

Fig. 16.6 Beam direction in oblique transcranial projection illustrated as in the clinical set-up (**a**), also illustrated in a coronal slice from a CBCT examination of the TMJ's (**b**). The patient's head is tilted towards the examination table allowing for a vertical beam direction. In the coronal plane, the beam is angled in a caudal direction relative to the patient's head. Thereby, the dense petrous part of the temporal bone on the contralateral side is not superimposed on the region of interest. As a result, the image of the joint will show the lateral part of the joint (circle in CBCT)

lateral oblique transcranial projection of the TMJ of interest, with the X-ray source positioned under the exam table. The image intensifier/flat panel detector is placed above the examination table and head of the patient and TMJ (Fig. 16.6). This projection is used to avoid the dense petrous part of the temporal bone on the contralateral side from being superimposed on the joint of interest. This projection also implies that the X-ray beam is inclined anteriorly to align with the long axis of the condyle being depicted (Fig. 16.7).

Images exposed with lateral oblique transcranial projection represent lateral parts of the joint components (Fig. 16.8). The central and medial parts of the joint are projected inferiorly relative to the visualised lateral part and are not possible to assess in this projection. Therefore, the first projection should be complemented with a projection visualising the medial part of the joint (Fig. 16.5 and 16.9). There the dynamic assessment is repeated, and differences in disc position between the lateral and medial part of the joint can indicate a rotational component of a disc displacement (Fig. 16.10 and Complementary Videos 16.1 and 16.2).

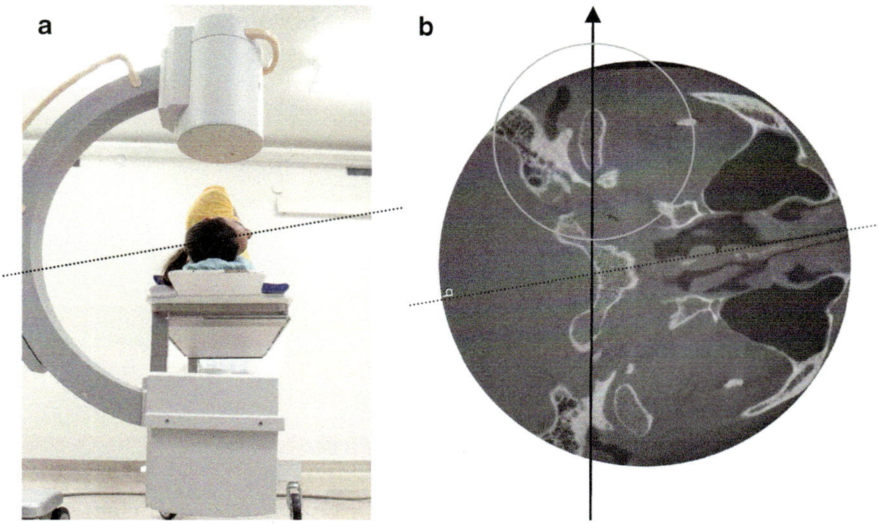

Fig. 16.7 Beam direction in oblique transcranial projection illustrated as in the clinical set-up (**a**) and in an axial slice of a CBCT examination of the TMJ's (**b**). In the axial plane, the beam should be angled in a ventral direction relative to the patient's head for the beam to coincide with the long axis of the condyle for depiction in a modified sagittal view (circle in CBCT). By asking the patient to slightly turn the face upward, the condyles long axis will be aligned in the vertical beam direction and depicted in a modified sagittal projection

16.3.8 Materials Needed for Arthrography

A number of items are needed when preparing for an arthrography with an aseptic approach. In addition to contrast media, anaesthesia and if applicable corticosteroids, please find an example of necessary items in Fig. 16.11.

16.3.9 Single Contrast Arthrography

16.3.9.1 Anaesthesia

Before insertion of the needle for anaesthesia, the tip of the needle is placed on the skin under fluoroscopy in a correct position to ensure accurate insertion. The needle is inserted in alignment with the central beam of the oblique lateral transcranial projection towards the posterior surface of the lateral pole of the condyle (Fig. 16.12a). During a slow retraction of the needle, anaesthesia is administrated from the lateral pole of the condyle to the surface of the skin. The needle is then redirected for injection of anaesthesia for access to the upper joint compartment, anteriorly to the condyle, aiming at the upper part of the posterior surface of articular tubercle (Fig. 16.12b). Again, the anaesthesia is injected whilst slowly retracting

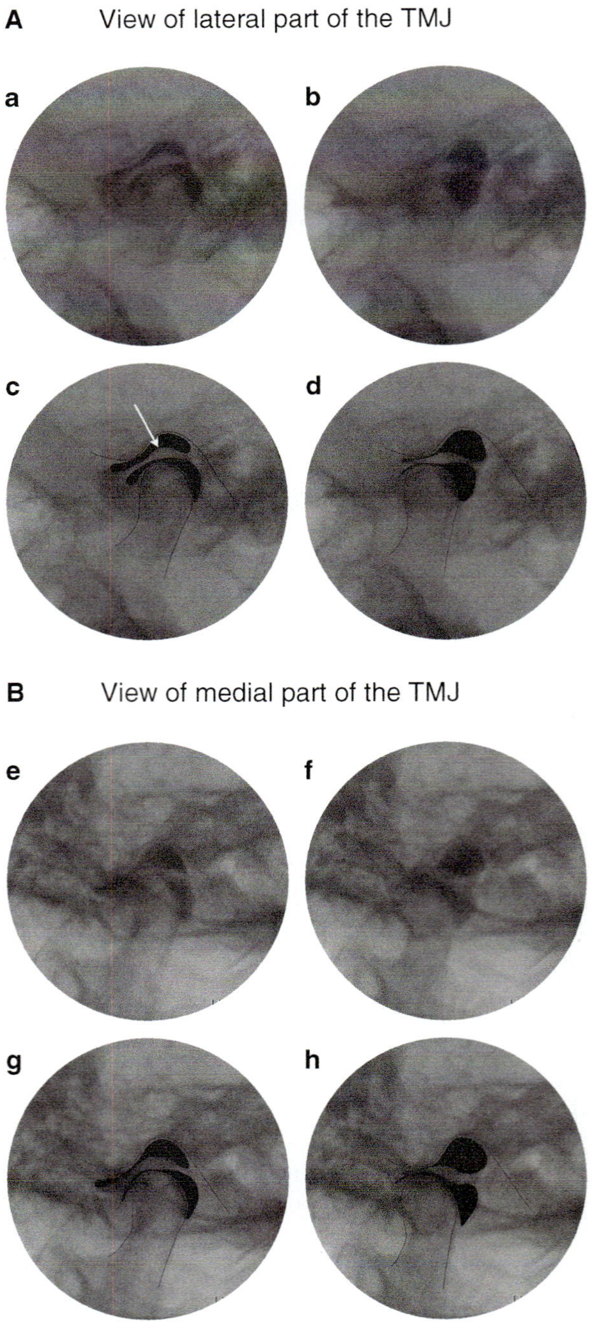

Fig. 16.8 (A and B) Arthrography of the left TMJ showing normal disc position (A): (**a**–**d**) Oblique transcranial projection revealing the lateral part of the joint. Contrast media injected into the upper and lower joint compartment indirectly revealing the disc and its attachments. (**c**, **d**) Corresponding images with joint components outlined and contrast media highlighted. (**a** and **c**) Mouth closed and disc in normal position with its posterior band between caput and the fossa (arrow). (**b** and **d**) Mouth open and disc in normal position (B): (**e**, **f**) Oblique transcranial projection with the beam angled cranially revealing the medial part of the joint, the mouth is closed (**e**) and open (**f**) and the disc position is normal. (**g**, **h**) Corresponding images with joint components outlined and contrast media highlighted. In the complementary material, there is a video showing the real-time movement in an arthrography of the left TMJ showing normal disc position in the lateral part of the joint (Complementary Video 16.1) and medial part of the joint (Complementary Video 16.2)

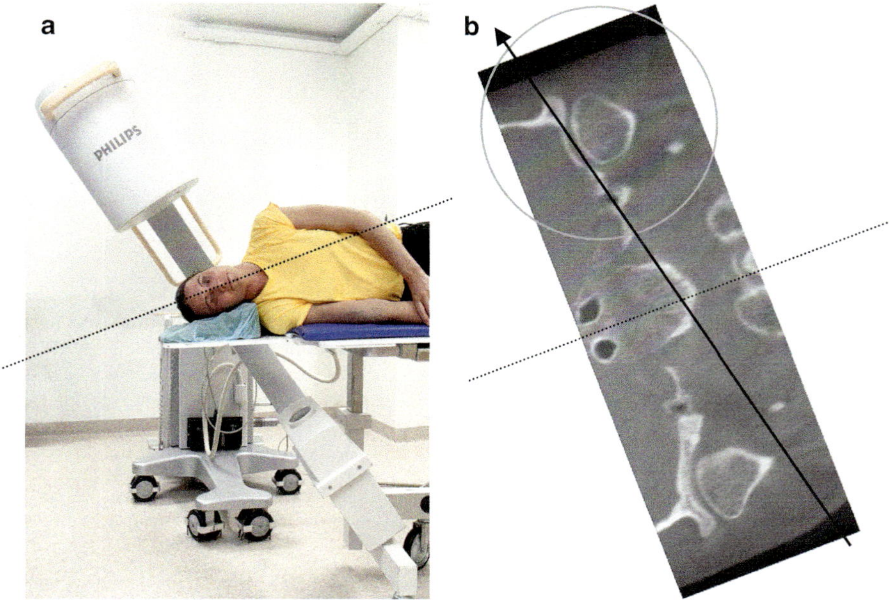

Fig. 16.9 Beam direction in oblique transcranial projection for depiction of the medial part of the left TMJ shown as in the clinical set-up (**a**) and in a coronal slice from a CBCT examination (**b**). In the coronal plane, the beam is angled in a cranial direction relative to the patient's head. Thereby, the dense petrous part of the temporal bone on the contralateral side is not superimposed on the region of interest. As a result, the image of the joint will show the medial part of the joint (circle in CBCT)

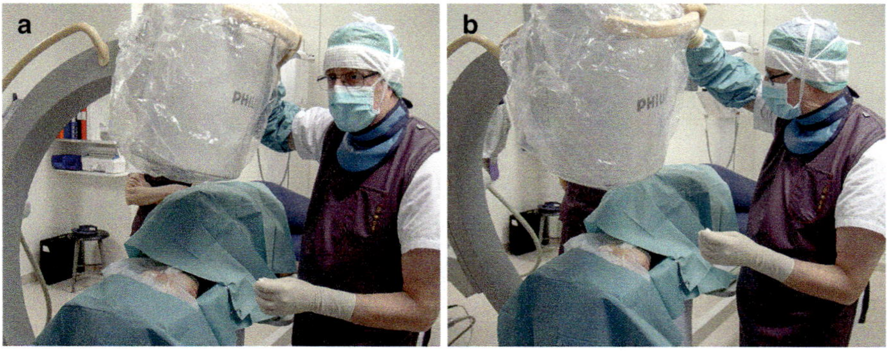

Fig. 16.10 Examination of the left TMJ. (**a**) Oblique transcranial projection revealing the lateral part of the left condyle. The patient's head is tilted (hanging) towards the exam table allowing for a vertical beam direction. In the coronal plane, the beam is angled in a caudal direction relative to the patient's head. (**b**) Adjusted projection for depiction of the medial part of the left TMJ. In the coronal plane, the projection is angled in a cranial direction relative to the patient's head. As a result, the image of the joint will be defined by the medial part of the joint

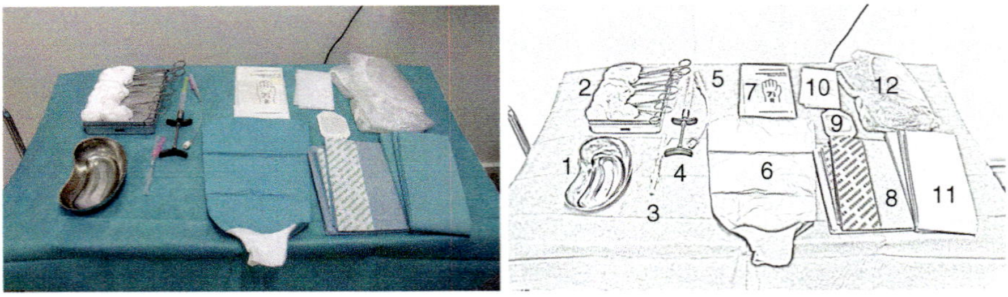

Fig. 16.11 Materials used for arthrography. (1) Basin for disinfection solution (chlorhexidine-ethyl alcohol, 5 mg/mL). (2) Gauze sponge for cleaning. (3) Syringe for contrast media. (4) Syringe for anaesthetics. (5) Tube with needle for administration of contrast media. (6) Sterile arm sleeve. (7) Sterile gloves. (8) Sterile adhesive operation towel for covering the patient's head. (9) Sterile transparent film dressing for postoperative covering of the penetrated skin over the TMJ. (10) Sterile adhesive drape with aperture to cover the surroundings of the entrance area. (11) Sterile drape sheet for covering the patient. (12) Sterile plastic cap for covering the image intensifier

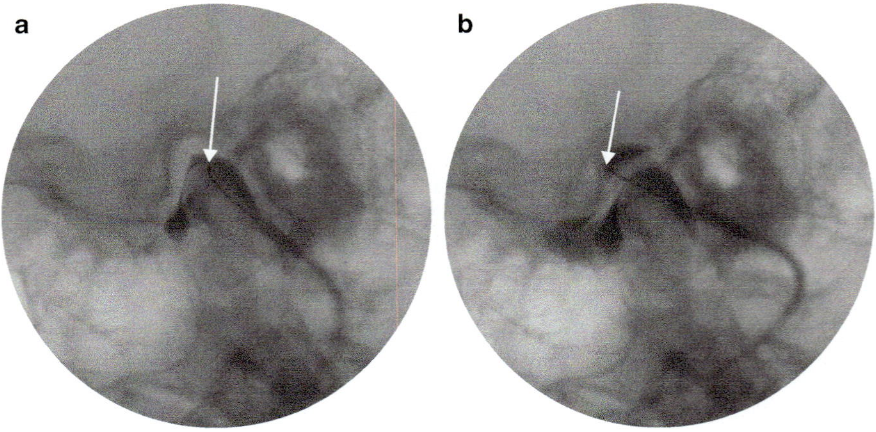

Fig. 16.12 (**a**, **b**) Needle positioning during injection for arthrography of a left TMJ. (**a**) For contrast filling of the lower joint compartment, the needle is positioned in close relation to the upper posterior part of the lateral pole of the condyle (arrow). (**b**) For contrast filling of the upper joint compartment, the needle is positioned in close relation to the upper part of the posterior surface of the articular tubercle (arrow)

the needle from the target position to the surface of the skin. The guided management of the needle during short fluoroscopy allows for deposition of small amounts of anaesthetics with high accuracy. It accomplishes infiltration anaesthesia in a corridor from each joint compartment to the surface of the skin, corresponding to the planned insertion path of the needle for injection of contrast media [8]. Optimal anaesthesia is normally obtained with common dental local anaesthesia after injection of 1.0–1.8 mL of, e.g. Citanest Dental/Octapressin 30 mg/mL + 0.54 μg/mL. There is always a risk that the anaesthesia affects other nerves than intended, most commonly transient facial nerve palsy with an inability to close the eyelid on the affected side. The risk increases with injected amount of anaesthesia.

Contraindications of anaesthesia are the same as for use in other parts of the body. Local anaesthetic failure can be due to inflammation in the joint.

16.3.9.2 Guiding the Needle and Injection of Contrast Media

For contrast media injection, a 2-mL syringe with a 15-mm extension tube and an attached needle with dimension 0.40 × 38 mm is used. It is important that any air bubbles are eliminated in the syringe and extension tube, to avoid simulation of loose bodies in the joint. In accordance with the insertion of anaesthesia, the needle for injection of contrast in the lower compartment is directed towards the posterior surface of the lateral pole of the condyle under fluoroscopy in lateral oblique transcranial projection of the TMJ (Figs. 16.12a and 16.13). During cannulation, the bevel of the needle should face the surface of the condyle to diminish unnecessary damage to the condyle and facilitate injection. It is important to observe changes in resistances appearing when the needle passes through different tissue types. High resistance indicates penetration of the joint capsule and when passed could indicate that the needle is positioned in the joint compartment. With a sensation of the needle rubbing the surface of the condyle, the position is likely to be correct. In addition, the patient can be asked to slowly and restrictedly open the mouth under fluoroscopy, and if the needle follows the condyle the location in the joint compartment is further confirmed. The final confirmation of a correct intra-articular position is when contrast medium can be injected with low resistance and the immediate distribution of the contrast media into the joint compartment can be observed under fluoroscopy. However, it is important to make the first attempt of injection with a small amount of contrast media. This ensures that all the contrast media is not injected into a vessel and if a diffuse appearance is noticed, the position of the needle is in

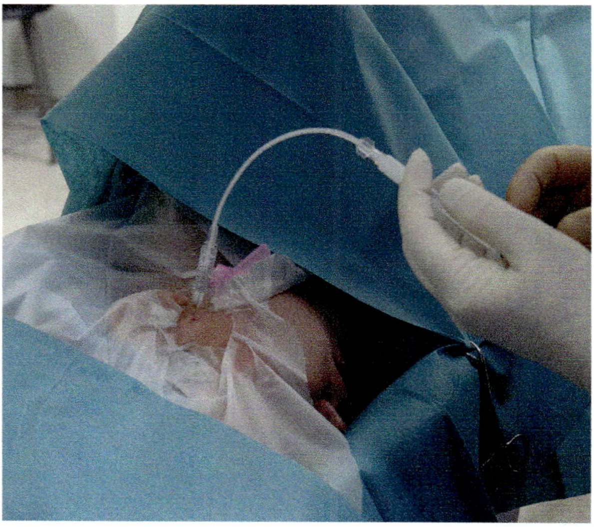

Fig. 16.13 The needle for injection of contrast media and corticosteroids has been inserted in position, first filling the lower compartment followed by redirection of the needle and filling of the upper compartment. The needle is inserted under fluoroscopic guidance using an oblique lateral transcranial projection

the soft tissue outside the joint and an adjustment should be made, aiming at the compartment.

If filling the lower compartment is performed without signs of perforation in the disc or posterior attachment (implying leakage of contrast media into the upper compartment), a second syringe and needle can be used for separate injection into the upper joint compartment. The insertion is performed in accordance with cannulation for anaesthesia and with the bevel of the needle positioner towards the temporal bone (Fig. 16.12b). The choice of two syringes allows for supplementary injection of contrast media after successful cannulation of both compartments. This is particularly useful if an arthrotomography is planned after the arthrography.

16.3.9.3 Diagnosing in Arthrography

Disc Displacement with and Without Reduction

When both joint compartments are filled with contrast media, the disc appears. The first step in diagnosing is then to define the shape and position of the disc in closed mouth position. The shape of the disc can be biconcave or deformed. The biconcave-shaped disc can be normal or, e.g. the posterior band can be thickened, which can prevent a displaced disc from reducing if the resistance of the extension is too pronounced. A deformed disc can vary from slightly to extensively deformed (Fig. 16.14). Next step is to locate the position of the disc. In the starting position of the C-arm during arthrography, the lateral part of the TMJ can be assessed. To determine the medial part of the TMJ, the projection is changed to a slightly cranial beam direction in relation to the patient's head (Fig. 16.9). Sideway disc displacement can only be assessed with an additional CBCT examination (Fig. 16.15). Anterior disc displaced in relation to the condyle can be detected in the sagittal projection. During opening of the mouth, the disc either reduces (Fig. 16.16 and Video 16.4), or is pushed forward during opening in a permanent displaced position, i.e. non-reducing (Fig. 16.14 and Video 16.3).

In patients with anterior disc displacement with reduction, the function of an occlusal splint designed to prevent disc displacement at rest can be checked. The splint is placed in the mouth during full mouth opening to ensure disc reduction before inserting the splint. The position of the disc with mouth closed and the splint in place is assessed under fluoroscopy. For optimal function, the disc should now maintain in a normal position (Fig. 16.17).

Adhesions, Cartilage Missing

Adhesions can be detected during the dynamic examination when the disc does not move in relation to the condyle or the temporomandibular fossa or tuberculum, i.e. to the structure that it is attached to. The arthrography can be complemented with an arthrotomography. In these images, the cartilage covering the joint surfaces can be assessed since the projection can be adjusted for specific areas of the joint surfaces, the resolution is higher and the superimposition of contrast has less impact on the image (Fig. 16.18).

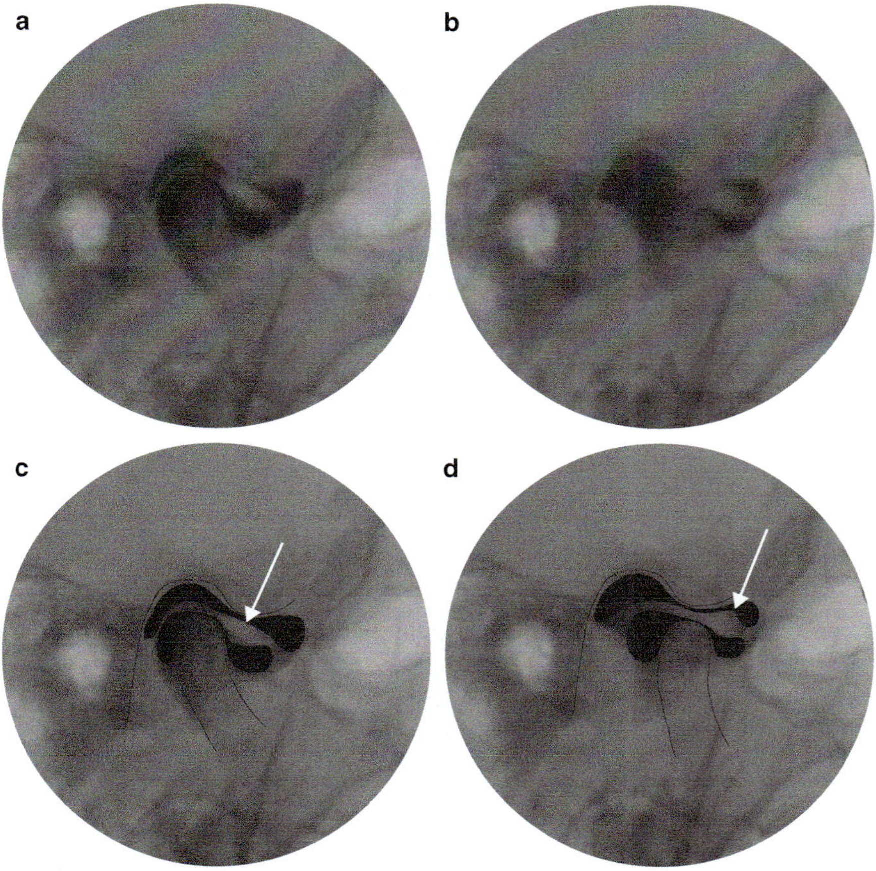

Fig. 16.14 Arthrography of the right TMJ showing anterior disc displacement without reduction. (**a**, **b**) Oblique transcranial projection revealing the lateral part of the joint. (**c**, **d**) Corresponding images with joint components outlined and contrast media highlighted. (**a** and **c**) Mouth closed, anteriorly displaced and deformed disc with a thickened posterior band anterior to the caput (arrow). (**b** and **d**) Mouth open, disc including the posterior band still displaced anterior to the caput (arrow). In the complementary material, there is a video showing the real-time movement of the described frames (Complementary Video 16.3)

Perforation/Rupture of the Disc or Posterior Attachment

Perforation in the disc or the posterior attachment of the disc is concluded when contrast media leaks from the lower compartment to the upper compartment during the initial filling of the lower compartment (Fig. 16.19 and Video 16.5). Sometimes, the perforation can be iatrogenic if several attempts to locate the compartments have been made.

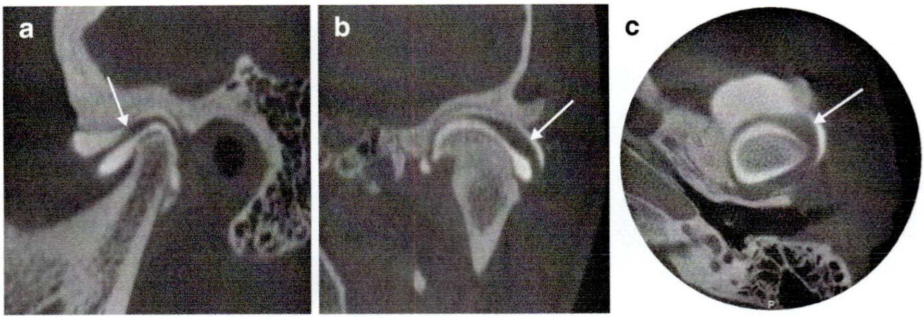

Fig. 16.15 Arthrotomography of the left TMJ in three planes showing both sagittal and sideway displacement of the disc. (**a**) The disc is anteriorly displaced in the sagittal plane with the posterior band (arrow) placed anterior to the condyle, (**b**) the disc is laterally displaced (arrow) in the coronal plane and in (**c**) the axial plane the anterolateral disc displacement (arrow) is depicted

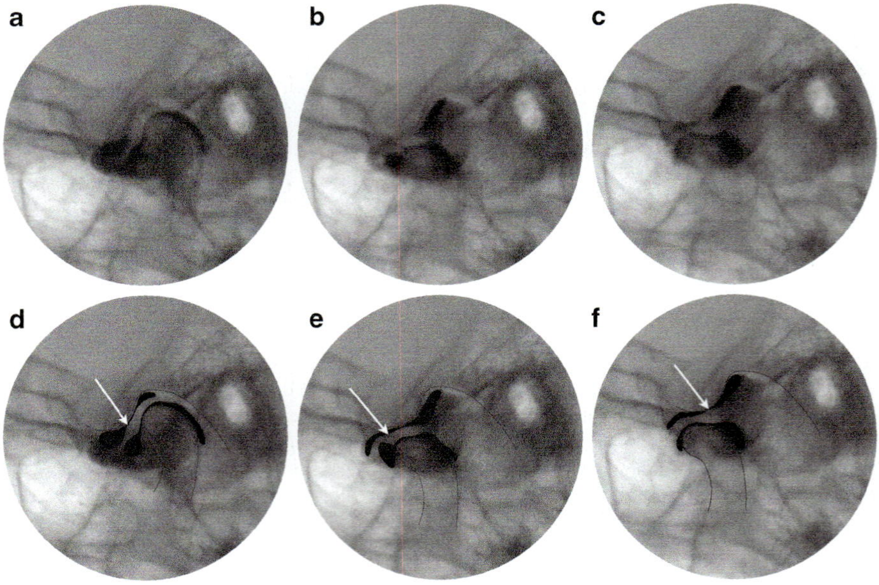

Fig. 16.16 Arthrography of the left TMJ showing anterior disc displacement (ADD) with late reduction. (**a**–**c**) Oblique transcranial projection revealing the lateral part of the joint. (**d**–**f**) Corresponding images with joint components outlined and contrast media highlighted. (**a** and **d**) The mouth is closed and the disk is anteriorly displaced with the posterior band anterior to the caput (arrow). (**b** and **e**) During the first part of mouth opening, the disc is still displaced with the posterior band anterior to the caput (arrow). (**c** and **f**) At full mouth opening, the disk and its posterior band has reduced to a normal position in relation to the joint components (arrow). In the complementary material, there is a video showing the real-time movement of the described frames (Complementary Video 16.4)

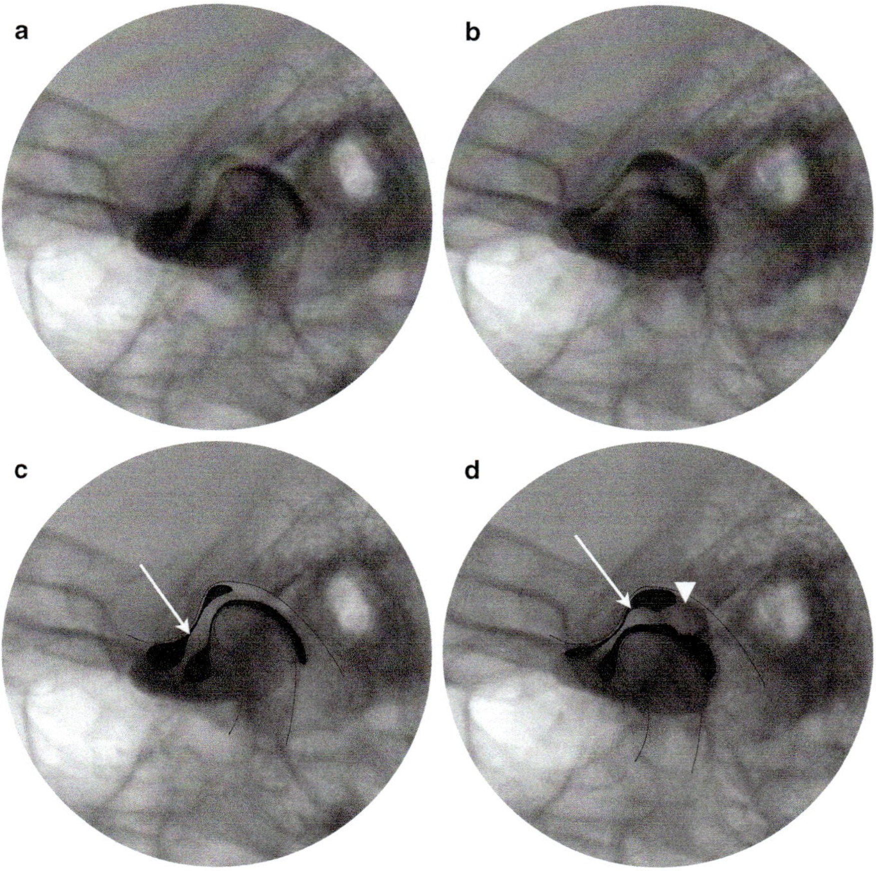

Fig. 16.17 Arthrography of the left TMJ with closed mouth without (**a**) and with (**b**) occlusal splint designed to prevent disk displacement at rest. (**a**, **b**) Oblique transcranial projection revealing the lateral part of the joint. (**c**, **d**) Corresponding images with joint components outlined and contrast media highlighted. (**a** and **c**) Mouth closed without splint. Anteriorly displaced disc with the posterior band anterior to the caput (arrow). (**b**, **c**) Mouth closed with occlusal splint in place. Disc and its posterior band in normal position (arrow). The previously stretched posterior ligament is now crumpled behind the posterior band (arrow head). In the complementary material, there is a video showing the real-time movement of the described frames (Complementary Video 16.4)

16.4 Double Contrast Technique

Double contrast examination of the TMJ implies the use of a combination of high (iodine) and low (air) attenuating contrast media [10, 11]. Venous catheters are used to prepare access to the joint compartments. The compartments are filled with iodine contrast media as in conventional arthrography. The catheter allows drainage of the contrast media. Thereafter, air is injected into the joint compartments. The amount of dense

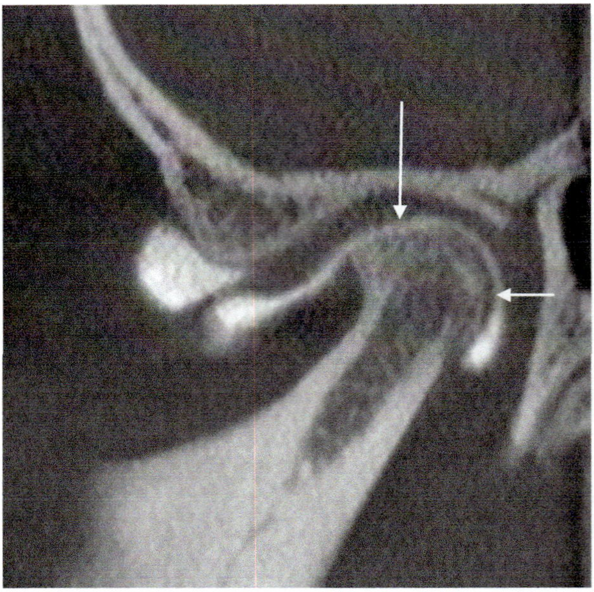

Fig. 16.18 Arthrotomography of the left TMJ depicted in sagittal plane. The disc is anteriorly displaced. Loss of cartilage superior on the condyle (long arrow) is found since the contrast media is in direct contact with the bone. Posterior on the condyle, the cartilage is still present since there is a gap between the contrast media and the outlining of the bone (short arrow)

iodine contrast media is then smaller compared to conventional arthrography. With this technique, the surfaces of the joint components are covered with thin layers of radiopaque contrast media separated by air. The technique enables visualisation of adhesions, small loose bodies in the joint and loss of cartilage on the condyle and temporal bone without superimposition of contrast media as in arthrography [9]. This possibility of visualisation increases further if combined with a CBCT examination of the TMJ, performed in closed and sometimes also in open mouth position. In a study including cryosections of the TMJ, it was shown that the diagnostic outcome of double compared to conventional contrast arthrography is rather similar [12]. The technique also increases the demands on the radiologist's skill [13] and it extends the exposure time and thereby radiation dose, especially if combined with CBCT examinations. The risks with the technique are, however, low and the same as for arthrography. The risk of emboli due to injection of air is insignificant, aspiration before injection should be performed to prevent that any content is injected into a blood vessel.

16.5 Arthrotomography

When conventional or double contrast arthrography is combined with CBCT imaging of the TMJ, visualisation of the disc position in both the sagittal and the coronal planes is provided (Fig. 16.20). Further, e.g. adhesions, small loose bodies in the

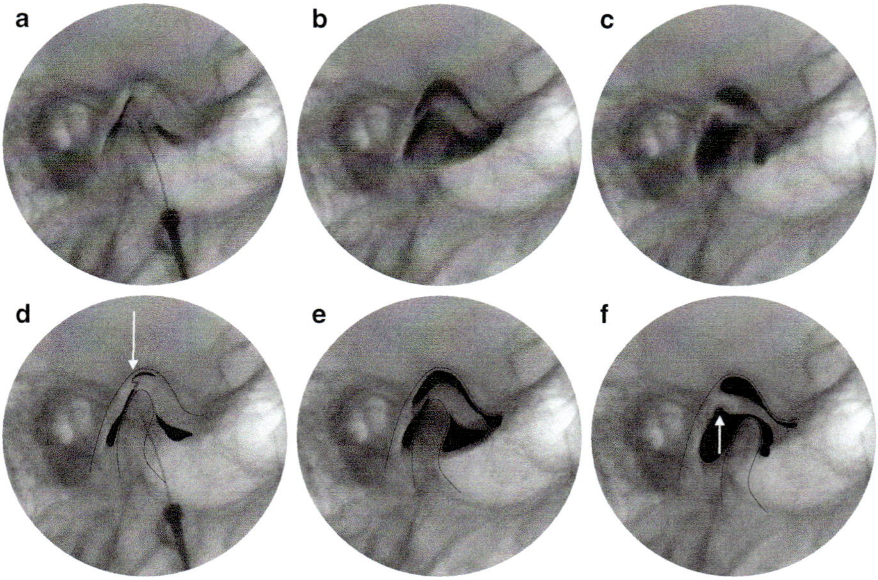

Fig. 16.19 Perforation and ADD with reduction. Arthrography of the right TMJ showing anterior disc displacement with reduction and perforation of the posterior attachment. (**a**–**c**) Oblique transcranial projection revealing the lateral part of the joint. (**d**–**f**) Corresponding images with joint components outlined and contrast media highlighted. (**a** and **d**) Mouth closed. During filling of the lower joint compartment, contrast media is leaking into the upper compartment through a perforation in the posterior attachment of the disc (arrow). (**b** and **e**) Mouth closed, both compartments are filled with contrast, the disc is anteriorly displaced. (**c** and **f**) Mouth open. The disc is reduced and a defect in the posterior attachment where caput was positioned in (**a**, **b**) is visualised (arrow). In the complementary material, there is a video showing the real-time movement of the described frames (Complementary Video 16.5)

joint and loss of cartilage (Fig. 16.18) on the condyle and temporal bone are easily visualised and detected.

CBCT examination in both closed and open mouth position increases the dose and should not replace the fluoroscopic examination of function since the advantage of a true dynamic examination would then be lost. Therefore, CBCT examinations after arthrography are only performed when refined and extra detailed diagnostics is needed prior to, e.g. surgery.

16.6 Arthrography-Guided Steroid Treatment

In addition to diagnostic purposes, image-guided joint access, performed with the same technique as arthrography, can be used for therapeutic injections. Therapeutic injections most commonly imply anti-inflammatory treatment with corticosteroids, but also anaesthetics or viscosupplements such as hyaluronic acid. Corticosteroids

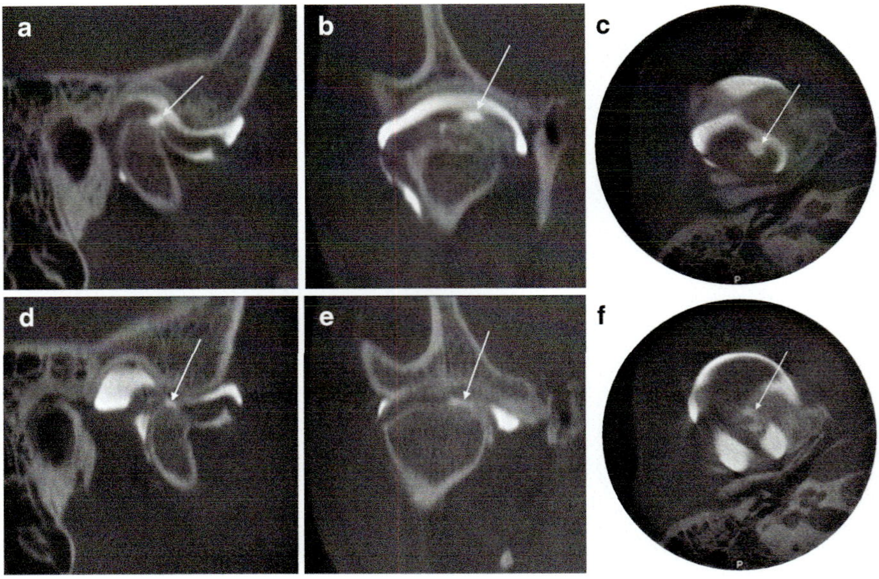

Fig. 16.20 Arthrotomography of the right TMJ in three projections: (**a**) sagittal plane, (**b**) coronal plane and (**c**) axial plane with closed mouth and (**d–f**) in the same projections with open mouth. (**a–c**) There is a perforation in the posterior attachment of the disc, contrast has leaked from the lower to the upper compartment during contrast injection (arrows in all planes), the disc is deformed and anteriorly displaced. (**d–f**) Arthrotomography of the joint with open mouth, no reduction of the disc and the perforation can still be detected (arrows in all planes)

are generally safe for both short- and long-term treatment of TMJ pain [14–17]. Steroid injections can be beneficial for patients with TMJ arthritis-related symptoms and/or MRI-verified signs of TMJ inflammation [18]. Injection of anaesthesia is used both for the therapeutic effect and as a diagnostic tool [19]. If the patients get a relief of pain after injection, the pain most likely originates from the TMJ and is less likely related to the ear or myalgia. Even if the main purpose of the injection of anaesthesia is to facilitate continued examination with arthrography or injection of corticosteroids or other intervention, the patient should, for diagnostic purpose, be asked if there is a pain relief.

In order to achieve the desired therapeutic effect of corticosteroids, administration into the joint compartments is necessary. This can be facilitated with image guidance of the injection as described for arthrography.

Mixing contrast media with therapeutic agents and injecting it under fluoroscopy is a procedure that largely increases the accuracy of correct administration to the target region in anatomically complicated areas, e.g. at cervical epidural injections [20, 21]. The technique has also been applied for the accurate administration of corticosteroids in the TMJ [8]. Relatively insoluble steroids are preferable for intra-articular injections in order to increase the duration of the treatment. A corticosteroid, e.g. 1.0 mL metylprednisolonacetat (Depo-Medrol 40 mg/mL) is mixed with an equal amount of iohexol contrast media (Omnipaque 300 mg I/mL). In total,

1.2–1.6 mL of the mixture is deposited in the joint compartments, i.e. 24–32 mg metylprednisolonacetat. The contrast enhancement obtained with the mixture is more than sufficient and the proportion of contrast media relative the corticosteroid can be altered if needed. However, the recommendation is to inject maximum 40 mg metylprednisolonacetat into the TMJ. The recommendations differ for different joints in the body.

Sodium hyaluronate is also indicated for treatment of osteoarthritis and has been shown to have similar effect on function as corticosteroids [22]. A complication reported for sodium hyaluronate was pain that could be due to extra-articular injection into the soft tissues surrounding the TMJ. Injection guidance with fluoroscopy was not used.

Complications in connection with intra-articular injections are rare. Local complications such as bleeding and pain can occur and are easily remediated. To avoid complications, injections should not be performed on patients with psoriasis or infections in the skin. Previous severe reaction to any component in the injection solutions is a contraindication. Systemic effects in connection with intra-articular steroid injections have been reported [23]. Transient increase in pain (steroid flare), mild headache and facial flushing can occur. Patients with diabetes can expect a short spike in blood glucose level. The majority of systemic effects are, however, transient and significant adverse effects are infrequent.

Acknowledgments We would like to express our sincere gratitude to Dr. Per Erik Legrell and research engineer Magnus Johansson for their contributions to the illustrations.

References

1. Zimmer EA. Die Röntgenologie des kiefergelenkes. Schweiz Monatsschr Zahnheilkd. 1941;51:12–24.
2. Nørgaard F. Athrography of the Mandibular Joint. Acta Radiol. 1944;25(5–6):679–85.
3. Katzberg RW, Dolwick MF, Bales DJ, Helms CA. Arthro tomography of the temporomandibular joint: new technique and preliminary observations. AJR Am J Roentgenol. 1979;132:949–55.
4. Wilkes CH. Arthrography of the temporomandibular joint in patients with the TMJ pain-dysfunction syndrome. Minn Med. 1978;61:645–52.
5. Dolwick MF, Riggs RR. Diagnosis and treatment of internal derangements of the temporomandibular joint. Dent Clin N Am. 1983;27:561–72.
6. Lundh H, Westesson P-L, Kopp S, Tillström B. Anterior repositioning splint in the treatment of temporomandibular joints with reciprocal clicking. Comparison with a flat occlusal splint and an untreated control group. Oral Surg. 1985;60:131–6.
7. Arnaudow M, Haage H, Pflaum I. Die doppelkontrast arthrographie des kiefergelenkes. Dtsch Zahnartztl Z. 1968;23:390–3.
8. Ahlqvist J, Legrell PE. A technique for the accurate administration of corticosteroids in the temporomandibular joint. Technical report. DMFR. 1993;22:211–3.
9. Katzberg RW, Westesson PL. Diagnosis of the temporomandibular joint. Philadelphia: WB Saunders; 1993.
10. Westesson P-L, Omnell KÅ, Rohlin M. Double-contrast tomography of the temporomandibular joint: a new technique based on autopsy specimen examinations. Acta Radiol. 1980;21:777–84.

11. Westesson P-L. Double-contrast arthrotomography of the temporomandibular joint: introduction of an arthrographic technique for visualization of the disk and articular surfaces. J Oral Maxillofac Surg. 1983;41:163–72.
12. Westesson P-L, Bronstein SL. Temporomandibular joint: comparison of single- and double-contrast arthrography. Radiology. 1987;164:65–70.
13. Ahlqvist J, Isberg A. Radiographic imaging. In: Isberg A, editor. Temporomandibular joint dysfunction: A practitioners guide p 187. Oxford: ISIS Medical Media Ltd; 2001. ISBN 1901865444.
14. Hollander JL, Brown EM Jr, Jessar RA, Brown CY. Hydrocortisone and Cortisone injected into arthritic joints. Comparative effects of and use of hydrocortisoe as a local antiarthritic agent. J Am Med Assoc. 1951;147(17):1629–35.
15. Kopp S, Wennerberg B. Effects of occlusal treatment and intraarticular injections on temporomandibular joint pain and dysfunction. Acta Odontol Scand. 1981;39(2):87–96.
16. Kopp S, Akerman S, Nilner M. Short-term effects of intra-articular sodium hyaluronate, glucocorticoid, and saline injections on rheumatoid arthritis of the temporomandibular joint. J Craniomandib Disord. 1991;5(4):231–8.
17. Vallon D, Akerman S, Nilner M, Petersson A. Long-term follow-up of intra-articular injections into the temporomandibular joint in patients with rheumatoid arthritis. Swed Dent J. 2002;26(4):149–58.
18. Stoustrup P, Kristensen KD, Verna C, Kuseler A, Pedersen TK, Herlin T. Intra-articular steroid injections for temporomandibular joint arthritis in juvenile idiopathic arthritis: A systematic review on efficacy and safety. Semin Arthritis Rheum. 2013;43(1):63–70.
19. Tjakkes G-HE, TenVergert EM, de Bont LGM, Stegenga B. The effect of intra-articular injection of ultracain in the temporomandibular joint in patients with preauricular pain. A randomized prospective double-blind placebo-controlled crossover study. Clin J Pain. 2007;23:233–6.
20. Renfrew DL, Moore TE, Kathol MH, El-Khoury GY, Lemke JH, Walker CW. Correct placement of epidural steroid injections: Fluoroscopic guidance and contrast administration. AJNR. 1991;12:1003–7.
21. Stojanovic MP, Vu T-N, Caneris O, Slezak J, Cohen SP, Sang CN. The role of fluoroscopy in cervical epidural steroid injections. Spine. 2002;27(5):509–14.
22. Björnland T, Gjaerum AA, Möystad A. Osteoarthritis of the temporomandibular joint: An evaluation of the effects and complications of corticosteroid injection compared with injection with sodium hyaluronate. J Oral Rehabil. 2007;34:583–9.
23. Habib GS. Systemic effects of intra-articular corticosteroids. Clin Rheumatol. 2009;28(7):749–56.

Connection Between the Temporomandibular Joint and Temporal Bone

17

Kaan Orhan and Franciszek Burdan

17.1 Anatomical Connections Between the TMJ and Middle Ear

The temporal bone is a crucial structure, not only for the temporomandibular joint (TMJ) and brain, but also for the ear, since it surrounds the internal, middle, and – partially – external ear. Owing to their common origin and development, as well as nearby location, the temporal bone and TMJ may modify each other and share similar pathologies.

17.1.1 Development of Temporal Bone and Mandible

The temporal bone consists of elements of both the chondrocranium and the visceral/pharyngeal arch cartilages (endoskeleton). The paraxial mesenchyme differentiates into the parachondral cartilages, such as the trabeculae cranii, and the nasal, optic, and otic capsules, which surround the hypophysis and the olfactory, visual, and hearing organs, respectively. All these elements are supported by the ala temporalis and synotic tecta, and by structures that develop from the visceral arches, mostly the first and second ones [1–4]. The mesenchymal part of the temporal bone is well formed in the fifth gestational week (GW), while its cartilaginous transformation starts in the second month of gestation. At first, there are a number of separate foci that later fuse into a single but complex chondrocranium, which is divided into occipital, otic, sphenoidal, and ethmoidal parts (areas). The otic parts

K. Orhan (✉)
Department of Dentomaxillofacial Radiology, Ankara University, Faculty of Dentistry, Ankara, Turkey

F. Burdan
Department of Radiology, St. John's Cancer Centre, Lublin, Poland

Department of Human Anatomy, Medical University of Lublin, Lublin, Poland

I. Rozylo-Kalinowska, K. Orhan (eds.), *Imaging of the Temporomandibular Joint*, https://doi.org/10.1007/978-3-319-99468-0_17

(capsules) are multiple and are joined by basicochlear commissures, but each otic capsule is divided into cochlear and canalicular parts, constituted of the mastoid/parietal/nuchal plate. On the rostral surfaces, otic vesicles, the internal carotid artery, the facial (cranial nerve; CN VII) and vestibule-cochlear nerves (CN VIII) are attached, later surrounding the temporal bone and finally forming the bony/osseous labyrinth and walls of the internal acoustic meatus and facial and carotid canals. It is important that, before the anterior cartilaginous chondrocranium is fully formed, ossification in the posterior (occipital) parts starts, taking place at the end of the second month [4]. Much later, the formation of the facial skeleton and mandible is initiated [5, 6].

At the end of the fourth GW, visceral arches appear at the level of the stomodeum. The first arch elongates from the otic capsule, and extends to the floor of the mouth. It forms upper, lower, and medial enlargements called the maxillary, mandibular, and frontonasal processes. In the fifth GW, the last process and its surrounding mesenchyme split into a medial part, which forms the so-called intermaxillary segment of the head (anterior part of the nose, upper lip, primary palate) and a lateral part, which joins the maxillary process and differentiates into the lateral part of the nose, cheek, and palatine shelves, which, at the end of the eighth GW, join to form the secondary palate. In the classical description, the proximal cartilaginous part of the first pharyngeal arch in the endochondral ossifications forms the malleus and incus. On the lateral aspect of Meckel's cartilage, the mesenchyme finally forms a membranaceus structure that later differentiates into half of the mandible, including the condyloid process, that forms the head of the TMJ. The cartilage itself disappears and its only remnant is a mylohyoid groove on the internal surface of the bone. The second visceral arch (Reichert's, hyoid arch) differentiates into the stapes and the styloid process of the temporal bone. The remaining arches are related only to hyoid, laryngeal, and tracheal formation, and are not directly involved in the TMJ [4–7]. However, according to Hanson and co-workers [8, 9], the first arch differentiates only into the head of the malleolus, as well as the body and short crus of the incus, while the remaining part of both bones and the head and crura of the stapes develop from the second arch. The anterior process of the malleolus and the footplate of the stapes arise from separate mesenchyme of the otic capsule.

It is worth mentioning that, in the fourth to fifth GWs, the tympanic cavity and auditory tube develop from the tubotympanic recess that arises from the primitive pharynx, which involves the first and second pharyngeal pouches [4, 5, 10]. The first pharyngeal pouch also differentiates into the external auditory meatus. The two pouches are initially separated by developing auditory ossicles. Five weeks later (tenth GW), ossification, in a poorly defined tympanic ring, starts between the manubrium of the malleolus and the remaining part of Meckel's cartilage. At the same time ossification may be visible in the auditory ossicles and bony labyrinth. Similar advance remodeling of the capsular part of the petrous temporal bone starts and is accelerated at the 24th to 30th GWs. The tympanic cavity may be visible in a shape typical for adults at GW 30, but the full enclosing of the facial canal takes place at the end of the first year of postnatal life. On the other hand, in GW 35 a pneumatization process starts. It accelerates postnatally, but initially air replaces the amniotic fluid and forms the main groups of cells: antral, tubarian, and main tympanic [1, 4, 5, 10, 11].

Ossification of the temporal squama starts at GWs 7–8 but accelerates from the 9th to 20th GW, when it is visible radiologically [12]. The center (zygomatico-squamal suture) is located at the base of the zygomatic process. The second ossification (squamomastoid) may be seen posteriorly in some cases, but usually they form a unit together. At about GW 20 the mandibular fossa may be visible in the posterior part of the zygomatic process. Its postero-inferior process—the scutum—becomes pneumatized and later unites with the tegmentum tympani. At GW 35 most of the ossification is highly advanced and the temporal ring fuses with the squama superiorly and with the zygomatic arch anteriorly and posteriorly (by the scutum). The anterior aspect of the ring is free and is separated from the base of the petrosal part by the petrotympanic fissure. In the late fetal period, the changes are less intensive. Postnatally, fusion between each ossification centers, styloid and mastoid process downward growth; as well, rapid pneumatization changes the morphology of the temporal bone. It is worth mentioning that the mastoid process is the only part of the temporal bone that shows high sexual dimorphism [4]. It is bigger and has its peak growth at age 7 and later at ages 11–19 years in males, while these features are shown at ages 7 and 9–15 years in females [13].

As noted above, the mandible develops from the right and left parts of the mesenchyme on the lateral aspect of both Meckel's cartilages. Initially, at GWs 6–7, there are two parts; these fuse together at the eighth GW—small anterosuperior part forms the coronoid process and elongated posterior one constitutes the main part of the body and ramus mandibula. The formation of the proper condylar process, as well as the mental ossicles, takes place at GWs 12–14 from secondary cartilage; the end of this process initiates deciduous tooth germs. It is notable that proper mandibular ossification, which starts at the sixth GW, requires direct contact with the epithelium of the mandibular arch and the inferior alveolar nerve that lies between the medial and lateral pterygoid muscle. The right and left part of the mandible fuse in the early postnatal period [4].

In summary, the chondrocranium differentiates into the pterygoid (pyramid) and mastoid parts of the temporal bone. The same mesenchyme is responsible for the development of the tympanic and squamal parts, which are formed by way of intramembranous ossification. The arches are responsible for the endochondral development of the auricular ossicles and the styloid process. The last, upper part of the bone—the squama—is the only part that originates from a membranous vault.

17.1.2 Anatomy of the Temporal Bone

The morphology of the TMJ is explained in detail in Chap. 1, and for this reason the main goal of this section is to describe the structures located nearby and/or related to the stomatognathic system.

The mandibular fossa is divided by the petrotympanic fissure into the anterior part (articular fossa), which is covered by the fibrous cartilage that, together with its continuation of its posterior aspect on the articular tubercle, forms the socket for the TMJ, while the posterior part is covered by the periosteum. The fissure itself is separated by the inferior process of the tegmen tympani into the anteriorly located and cartilage-covered petrosquamal fissure and posteriorly, the proper petrotympanic fissure. The internal opening is located on the lateral (membranaceus) wall of the tympanic cavity just in front of the tympanic ring (tympanic membrane). The lower part transmits the anterior tympanic artery, tympanic veins, chorda tympani, and anterior malleolar ligament. The upper part is covered by the anterior malleolar process. The external acoustic meatus is located more posteriorly. Its external opening (porus) is limited superiorly by the suprameatal spine, and inferiorly by the sheath of the styloid process and the process itself. Posteriorly, it is separated from the mastoid process by the tympanomastoid fissure, which transmits the auricular branch of the vagus nerve (CN X) from the retroauricular space to the jugular fossa by the mastoid canaliculus. The carotid and musculotubarius canals, as well as the tympanic cavity, are located medially to the fossa. The first two canals arise on an interior aspect of the temporal pyramid and run in front of the anterior (carotid) wall of the cavity. The carotid canal terminates in the middle cranial fossa and transmits the internal carotid artery, which is surrounded by the autonomic carotid plexus. On the upper wall, a few small openings for small caroticotympanic nerves and arteries are seen. They open at the junction between the inferior (jugular) and anterior wall of the tympanic cavity, slightly below the upper opening of the musculotubarius canal.

The musculotubarius canal is a bony structure divided by a horizontal plate into the tubarius and muscular semi-canals—the lower and upper parts, respectively. The septum of the musculotubarius canal penetrates deeply into the tympanic cavity and continues on the medial (labyrinthine) wall, where it ends with the cochlear process—the structure located between the promontory of the tympanic cavity and the proximal openings of the lesser palatine canal and the eminence of the facial canal. The cochlear process forms a trochlea for a tendon of the tensor tympanic muscle. The belly of this muscle occupies the muscular semi-canal, whose walls, plus the externally located cartilage of the auditory tubes, form its proximal attachment [14–16].

The tympanic cavity is a narrow space surrounded by the tympanic part of the temporal bone. It has a lateral and inferior wall, as explained above. On the inferior (jugular) wall, besides the mentioned caroticotympanic openings, there is also a superior opening of the tympanic canal, the tympanic groove that transmits the tympanic nerve from the canal on the promontory, located on the medial (labyrinthine) wall, where it splits and forms the tympanic plexus. At the junction between the inferior and posterior (mastoid) walls a styloid eminence is visible. It is formed by the elevation of the base of the styloid processes. The biggest foramen on the posterior wall is a triangular-shape opening to the mastoid cavity. It is located in the epitympanic part of the cavity, laterally to the eminence of the facial canal and laterally to the semi-circular canal, which continues on the medial wall as well. Below, on the posterior wall, there is also a pyramidal eminence for the stapedius muscle, the opening for the chorda tympani, and the seldom visible incus fossa.

The most difficult to visualize medial (labyrinthinel) wall in the inferior part of the tympanic cavity has a promontory—an elevation formed by the basilar curve of the cochlea with oval and round windows, which are covered by the footplate of the stapes and the secondary tympanic membrane, respectively. All other structures located above the promontory have been mentioned before. The posterior wall (tegmental) has a small depression that is partially or almost completely covered by mucosa, consisting of tegmental/tympanic semi-cells or cells, respectively. A similar structure may be visible in the mastoid process or in the septum of the musculotubarius canal [14, 15, 17]. The above-mentioned tympanic membrane divides the tympanic cavity into the epi-, meso- and hypotympanum, which are located above the tympanic membrane, on the same level, and below it, respectively. Because of its clinical importance, the so-called protympanum (bony portion of the auditory tube) is also distinguished. This section lies anterior to the mesotympanum, confluent with the epitympanum superiorly and with the hypotympanum inferiorly. The space is limited superiorly by the tegmen tympani and the entire tensor tympani canal. Inferiorly, it extends from the protiniculum (an oblique bony ridge demarcating the transition from the hypotympanum) posteriorly, extending anteriorly with the possible presence of protympanic air cells, with an anterior extension of the hypotympanic cell complex. The main anterior border of the protympanum is formed by confluence with the junctional and then the cartilaginous portion of the auditory tube and posteriorly, by confluence with the mesotympanum. The medial border is limited medially by the lateral wall of the carotid canal, extending from the caroticocochlear recess anteriorly, with caroticotympanic vessels and nerves, including anterior branches from the tympanic branch of the glossopharyngeal nerve, and more anteriorly by false passages whose morphology depends on pneumatization patterns. The lateral border consists of a bony wall separating the space from the mandibular fossa and extending to the anterior annulus, from the level of the protiniculum inferiorly to the anterior limit of the notch of Rivinus at the anterior tympanic spine [18].

It should be noted that that the medial, anterior, and lateral parts of the auricular capsule of the TMJ are directly attached to the lateral pterygoid, temporalis, and masseter muscles, respectively. The posterior part of the auricular capsule of the TMJ is covered by the upper process of the deep part of the parotid gland [14, 15, 17].

17.1.3 Anatomical Connection Between the TMJ and Temporal Bone

17.1.3.1 Pneumatization: The Mastoid and Zygomatic Bones

Inside the skull are many air-filled cavities (termed pneumatization). In addition to the major paranasal sinuses, accessory air cells, especially in the mastoid air cells, may arise at numerous locations in the skull, including the temporal bone [19–21]. The development of complete adult pneumatization can be divided into three stages: the infantile, from birth to 2 years of age; the transitional, from 2 to 5 years; and thereafter the adult. In the infantile stage, the mastoid (squamomastoid) undergoes gradual enlargement, with the migration of air cells toward the periphery. The air cells, which vary in size and shape, become more distinct with time because of progressive calcification of their walls. Pneumatization ceases during the adult stage [22].

Tremble, in 1934, first reported ten locations within the temporal bone where accessory air cells could be found, including one in the zygomatic process of the temporal bone [23]. Allam, in 1969, proposed a simpler classification of pneumatization of the temporal bone [24]. According to Allam, pneumatization of the temporal bone can be divided into five regions, which, in turn, are subdivided into areas. The primary regions consist of the middle ear, mastoid (squamomastoid), perilabyrinthine, petrous apex, and accessory. The mastoid consists of two key areas of pneumatization: the mastoid antrum and the peripheral area. The mastoid antrum lies superior. Inferiorly and laterally the antrum extends downward in the direction of the mastoid tip, forming an oblong space called the central tract. Immediately surrounding the antrum are the periantral cells. These cells can be classified as tegmental, sino-dural, facial, sinal, and tip cells. The tegmental cells lie in the tegmen mastoideum above the mastoid antrum. The more posterior sinodural air cells are located in the posterosuperior angle of the pyramid. The sinal cells lie at the level of the external auditory canal and mastoid process. Lying ventrally, but separated from them by the central tract, are the facial cells. More inferiorly, below the central tract, are the tip cells, in the mastoid process and tip. The accessory regions include the squamous, occipital, and the styloid. The sinal cells may extend into the occipital squamous process and the tip cells into the styloid process, and are then called occipital and styloid cells. Tegmental cells may pass upward into the squamous temporal process or extend into the zygomatic arch toward the articular eminence, which is called the pneumatic articular eminence (PAT). The phrase of PAT is described as an accessory air cells that occur in the root of the zygomatic arch and in the articular eminence of the temporal bone which is similar to air cells in the mastoid process and ethmoid bone [25]. In the literature, several cases of an abnormality of the TMJ, termed an "unusual bony lesion of the zygomatic arch" or pneumatization, were described for PAT during surgical removal of the articular eminence [20]. Tyndall and Matteson [25] first identified the common characteristics of the PAT of the temporal bone as: (1) an asymptomatic radiolucent defect in the zygomatic process of the temporal bone with an appearance similar to that of mastoid air cells, (2) the defect extended anteriorly as far as the articular eminence but not beyond the zygomaticotemporal suture, and (3) there was no enlargement or cortical destruction of the zygoma (Fig. 17.1).

Previously, it was pointed out that the accessory air cells began to pneumatize after puberty and achieved full size after several years, as with mastoid air cells proper [26]. In contrast to this statement, Hofmann et al. [27] and Orhan et al. [20] detected cases of PAT in children at 7 and 11 years of age, before the second half of the second decade of life; this can be interpreted as the pneumatization of accessory air cells beginning before puberty Moreover, a relatively high rate of PAT was observed among people with orthodontic malocclusions, i.e., class II and class III,

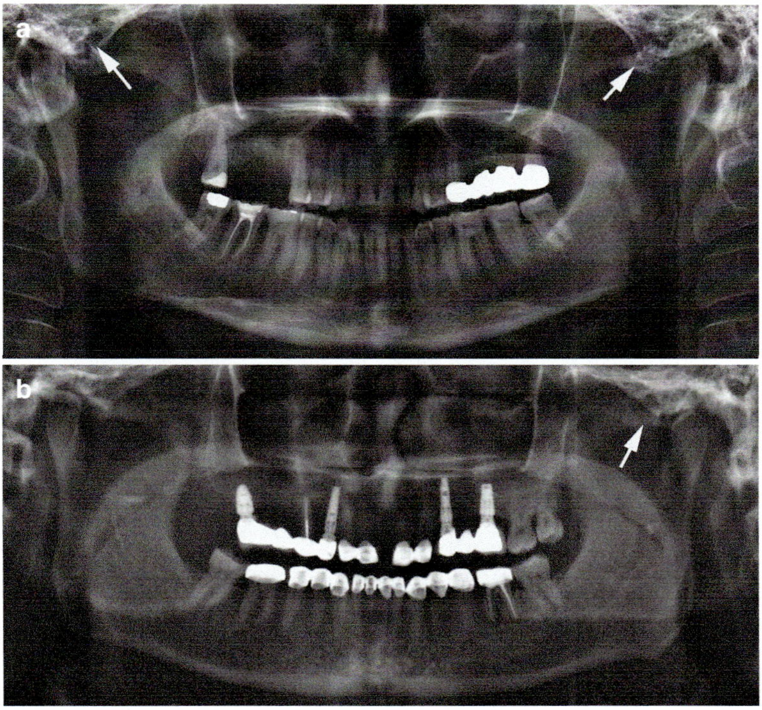

Fig. 17.1 Panoramic images of pneumatic articular eminence (PAT) showing (**a**) bilateral and (**b**) unilateral multilocular appearance

when compared with general population studies [21] (Fig. 17.2). The mastoid air cell system has been recognized as an important contributor to and pathway of suppuration in mastoid infections. Tumors of the mastoid process and ear may extend into the TMJ, and otitis or otomastoiditis may involve the TMJ and can even result in ankylosis [28, 29].

A panoramic radiograph is a useful technique to display PAT of the temporal bone [21], since the posterior aspect of the zygomatic arch is usually displayed. Transorbital or transmaxillary radiographs could be adjunctive projections in the visualization of PAT. Other radiographic projections, such as transcranial views for the TMJ, the submentovertex view, the Towne projection, and Waters' view do not provide adequate visualization of the posterior aspect of the zygomatic arch for this purpose [19].

Computed tomography (CT) is also considered as a method of choice for the assessment of bony structures and air spaces in the base of the skull. Since CT is not subject to superimposition, it exceeds the diagnostic accuracy of plain radiographs in the evaluation of temporal air spaces. Furthermore, less superficially located structures (such as the medial portion of the articular eminence) and the air cells adjacent to the TMJ may only be visible on CT. Cone beam CT (CBCT) can also be used to evaluate the TMJ and it has a substantially lower radiation dose than CT

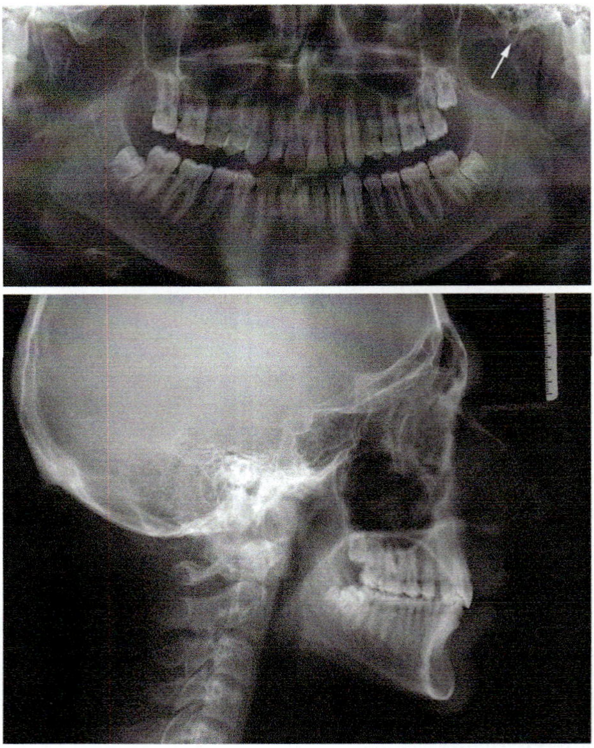

Fig. 17.2 Panoramic and cephalometric image of a unilateral PAT in the same patient as the one whose features are shown in Fig. 17.1

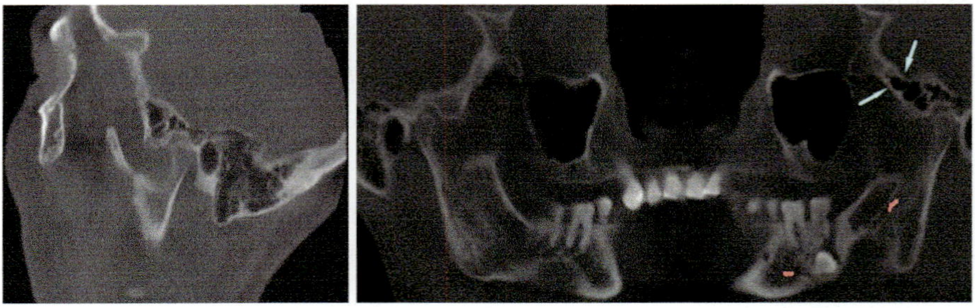

Fig. 17.3 Sagittal and panoramic reconstructed cone beam computed tomography (CBCT) image showing multilocular pneumatic articular eminence

(Fig. 17.3). CBCT is useful for TMJ evaluation, without superimposition and distortion, for bone morphology analysis. The diagnostic efficacy of CBCT is as good as that of conventional CT and is better than that of panoramic radiography. More accurate images and a lower radiation dose enable CBCT to be the commonly preferred modality for the evaluation of the anatomical structures noted above [30] (Fig. 17.4). Besides CT, magnetic resonance imaging (MRI) can also be used to visualize the pneumatization of mastoid air cells.

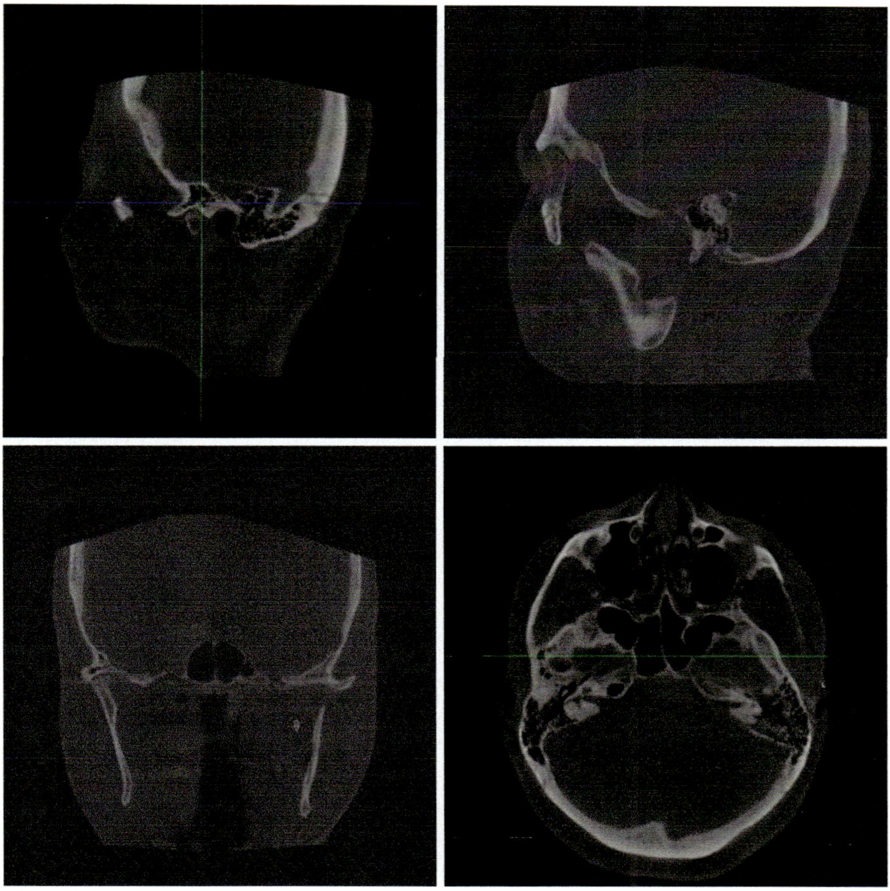

Fig. 17.4 CBCT image showing extensive pneumatization

On MRI, the identification of an area of low signal within the temporal bone overlying the glenoid fossa will likely represent extensive pneumatization of the mastoid air cells; in particular, it can be stated that an area of low signal overlying the glenoid fossa on a T2-weighted image shows extensive temporal bone pneumatization of the mastoid air cells [31] (Fig. 17.5). Although MRI is an excellent tool for evaluation of the soft tissues of the TMJ, high-resolution CBCT (Fig. 17.6) or CT remains the method of choice for the assessment of defects in bony structures and pneumatic spaces, as CT is more sensitive than panoramic radiography in the diagnosis of these defects. However, due to their low cost and widespread availability, panoramic radiographs and plain radiographs are considered the initial method for the diagnosis of these defects.

The differential diagnosis of radiolucencies within the zygomatic arch includes aneurismal bone cyst, osseous hemangioma, chondroblastoma, fibrous dysplasia, giant cell tumor, eosinophilic granuloma, metastatic tumor, and

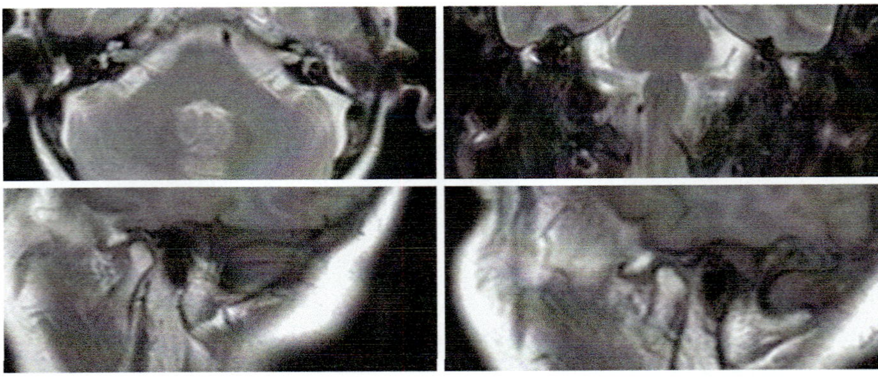

Fig. 17.5 Magnetic resonance (MR) images of otomastoiditis in the patient with articular eminence and mastoid process, showing, on T2-weighted images, bright signal areas, and increased signal intensity, and on T1-weighted images, low to iso signal intensity

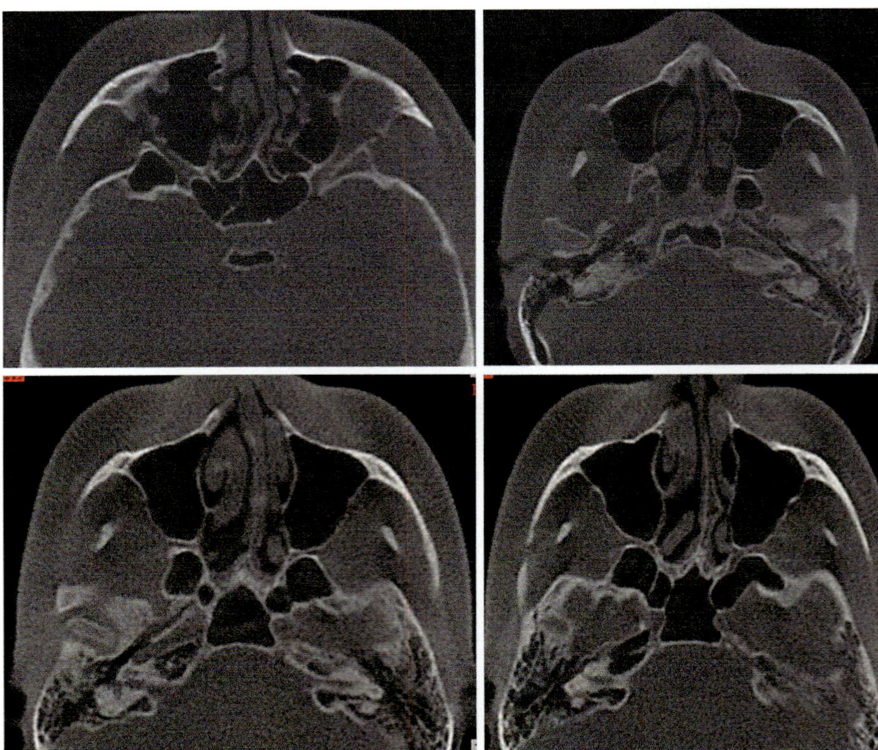

Fig. 17.6 Axial CBCT image showing extensive pneumatization in the temporal and sphenoid bones, distributed along the skull base

PAT. Only PAT can be visualized incidentally on radiographs; without nonexpansile, nondestructive characteristics. The other conditions would be characterized by enlarged and usually painful, bony expansions with cortical destruction [32].

17.1.3.2 Foramen Tympanicum (Foramen of Huschke) and the TMJ

The foramen tympanicum or foramen of Huschke is a persistent anatomical malformation of the temporal bone due to a defect in ossification in normal bone physiology in the neonatal or postnatal period [33]. The foramen tympanicum represents a developmental defect or malformation in the anteroinferior aspect of the external auditory canal (EAC), posteromedial to the TMJ, and is an unusual condition in human skulls [34]. Foramen tympanicum occurs during the embryological development of the viscero-cranial bone, and was described first by Emil Huschke [35]. In general, the foramen tympanicum gradually becomes smaller and completely closes before the age of 5 years, but it occasionally persists. An anomaly of the tympanic ring during embryogenesis could lead to an abnormal ossification of the tympanic bone and to a persistent foramen tympanicum. Also, genetic factors may lead to delays in ossification. Tympanic bone dehiscence present at the precise point of fusion of the two prominences (i.e. one anterior and one posterior) should be considered an anatomical variant only after the age of 5 years [36].

Foramen tympanicum may be associated with salivary discharge into the EAC during joint movements, or it can be associated with a symptomatic TMJ herniation into the EAC [37, 38]. In the literature, it was reported that foramen tympanicum may lead to the extension of infections from the infratemporal fossa to the EAC, and from the EAC to the infratemporal fossa or TMJ cavity [28]. Tumors of the mastoid process and ear may extend into the TMJ, and otitis or otomastoiditis may involve the TMJ and can even result in ankylosis [39, 40]. Moreover, EAC injury into the EAC during athroscopy or athrography can result in otologic complications [41, 42]. These anatomical variations can be detected in clinical practice using radiography.

The current literature describes the foramen tympanicum as an oval opening [43] and suggests that that its size is larger in patients with class II malocclusion because of the condyle position that causes pressure to the retrodiscal tissue and to the foramen tympanicum [33]. Many factors can influence the ossification process of the tympanic bone; mostly environmental or acquired aspects of the process cause the occurrence of foramen tympanicum and its persistence or enlargement.

Conventional radiographs have several drawbacks, including errors of projection and errors of identification. Conventional radiographic techniques collapse a three-dimensional (3D) structure onto a two-dimensional plane. The resulting superimposition of anatomical structures complicates image interpretation and landmark identification, and this distortion and magnification may lead to errors of identification [44]. Thus, the detection of anatomical variations can be done efficiently using CT or CBCT (Fig. 17.7).

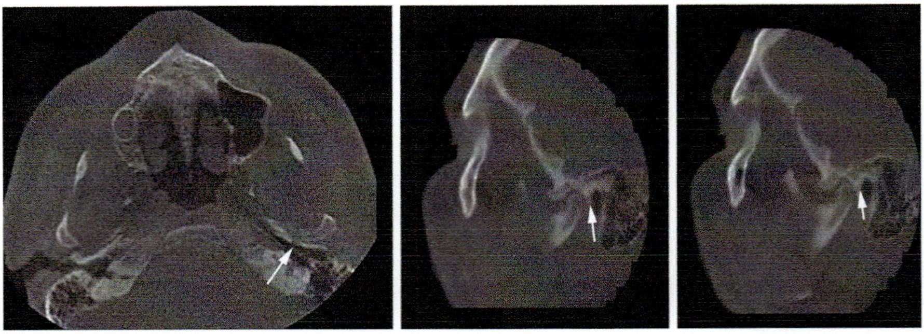

Fig. 17.7 Axial and sagittal CBCT image showing the foramen tympanicum. Note the direct communication between the temporomandibular joint (TMJ) and temporal bone

17.1.3.3 Petrotympanic Fissure, Malleolar Ligaments, and the TMJ

The TMJ is the smallest but the most complex joint of the human body; it participates in all jaw movements, chewing, swallowing, breathing, and speech functions. The literature has clearly revealed that there are close relationships between the TMJ and the structure of the middle ear [45–50]. These relationships have been explained by the presence of the discomalleolar ligament (DML), sphenomandibular ligament (SML), and the anterior malleolar ligament (AML) [51, 52].

The petrotympanic fissure (squamotympanic fissure, Glaserian fissure) is a fissure in the temporal bone that runs from the TMJ to the tympanic cavity. The mandibular fossa is bounded, in front, by the articular tubercle; behind, by the tympanic part of the bone, which separates it from the external acoustic meatus; it is divided into two parts by a narrow slit, the petrotympanic fissure. It opens just above and in front of the ring of bone into which the tympanic membrane is inserted; in this situation it is a mere slit about 2 mm in length. It lodges the anterior process and anterior ligament of the malleus, and gives passage to the anterior tympanic branch of the internal maxillary artery. The contents of the fissure include the communications of CN VII and IX to the infratemporal fossa. A branch of CN VII, the chorda tympani, runs through the fissure to join with the lingual nerve, providing special sensory (taste) innervation to the tongue. The tympanic nerve branches off CN IX to pass through the fissure as the lesser petrosal nerve, which passes through the foramen ovale and joins V3 of the trigeminal nerve and synapses in the otic ganglion, to provide parasympathetic innervation to the parotid gland ([53], accessed 11.01.2018).

The petrotympanic fissure, located at the mandibular fossa of the temporal bone, is crossed by two ligaments connecting the TMJ to the middle ear, each adherent individually to the collum mallei. The DML extends from the retrodiscal region of the articular capsule to the malleus ossicle and the anterior ligament of the malleus, which becomes continuous to the SML [54]. These ligaments are assumed to be related to otological symptoms, as well TMJ symptoms, because of the involvement of the middle ear, which is determined by the anterior displacement of the TMJ disc or by excessive mandibular movements, which would cause excessive traction of the DML [54]. The petrotympanic fissure can be classified as consisting of four main types: type 1, a wide tunnel-shaped structure; type 2, a tunnel-shaped structure with a wide opening in the entrance of the petrotypanic fissure to the mandibular fossa and gradually thinning out in the tympanic cavity; type 3, a tunnel-shaped structure with a wide opening in the entrance of the middle region of the mandibular fossa, with a flat tunnel-shaped structure and narrow exit in the tympanic cavity; and type 4, a tunnel-shaped structure with a wide opening in the entrance of the mandibular fossa, gradually thinning to a narrow exit in the tympanic cavity [55, 56] (Fig. 17.8).

The DML, which is part of the anterior ligament of the malleus, shares a common origin with the AML, and runs through a narrow bony space of the petrotympanic fissure that joins the articular disc of the TMJ and the malleus in the tympanic cavity. The AML, the malleus, and the incus develop from the dorsal end of Meckel's cartilage. Some investigators consider the DML to be a continuation of the lateral pterygoid muscle, and not a separate structure. However, further studies have indicated that the DML is not a residue or a degenerated structure, noting that it is a separate anatomical structure that links the malleus to the joint disc and capsule [52]. Adult cadaver studies have shown that the DML and AML are two distinct ligamentous structures [57]. The AML continues as the SML after passing through the petrotympanic fissure. The malleus connections of the SML, AML, and DML are different. However, the detailed structure of the temporomandibular ligaments is connected with the tympanic cavity from the petrotympanic fissure (Fig. 17.9). Studies have shown that there is a close relationship between the TMJ and the ear in relation to the anatomical and functional aspects of the DML, malleomandibular ligament, and the SML through the petrotympanic fissure [51, 52] (Fig. 17.10).

There are many radiological imaging techniques available for examining the petrotympanic fissure. Because of superimposition, the use of conventional radiography to visualize these structures is limited. CT and CBCT can be used for the visualization of these small structures. CBCT especially allows the evaluation of the bone components, joint space, and pathology of the TMJ joint in three dimensions without superimposition. CBCT provides increased spatial resolution as compared with multislice CT (MSCT). Moreover, due to volume averaging and resolution limits, MSCT may overestimate morphological evaluations such as semicircular canal dehiscences and temporal bone evaluations. Hence, the possibilities of the use of and increasing access to CBCT imaging, especially for surgeons, mean that this modality is of increasing value [58]. Diagnostic imaging of the lateral skull base requires high resolution because the anatomical structures of interest are small; however, pathological changes to these structures can have a large impact on health, including diminished hearing and balance. It is also difficult to interpret the petrotympanic fissure because of its narrow anatomical structure and the ligaments passing through it. An understanding of the anatomy of their location is gaining importance with the rising popularity of endoscopic procedures with high visibility, for which CBCT and high-resolution CT can be the first choice for evaluation [51].

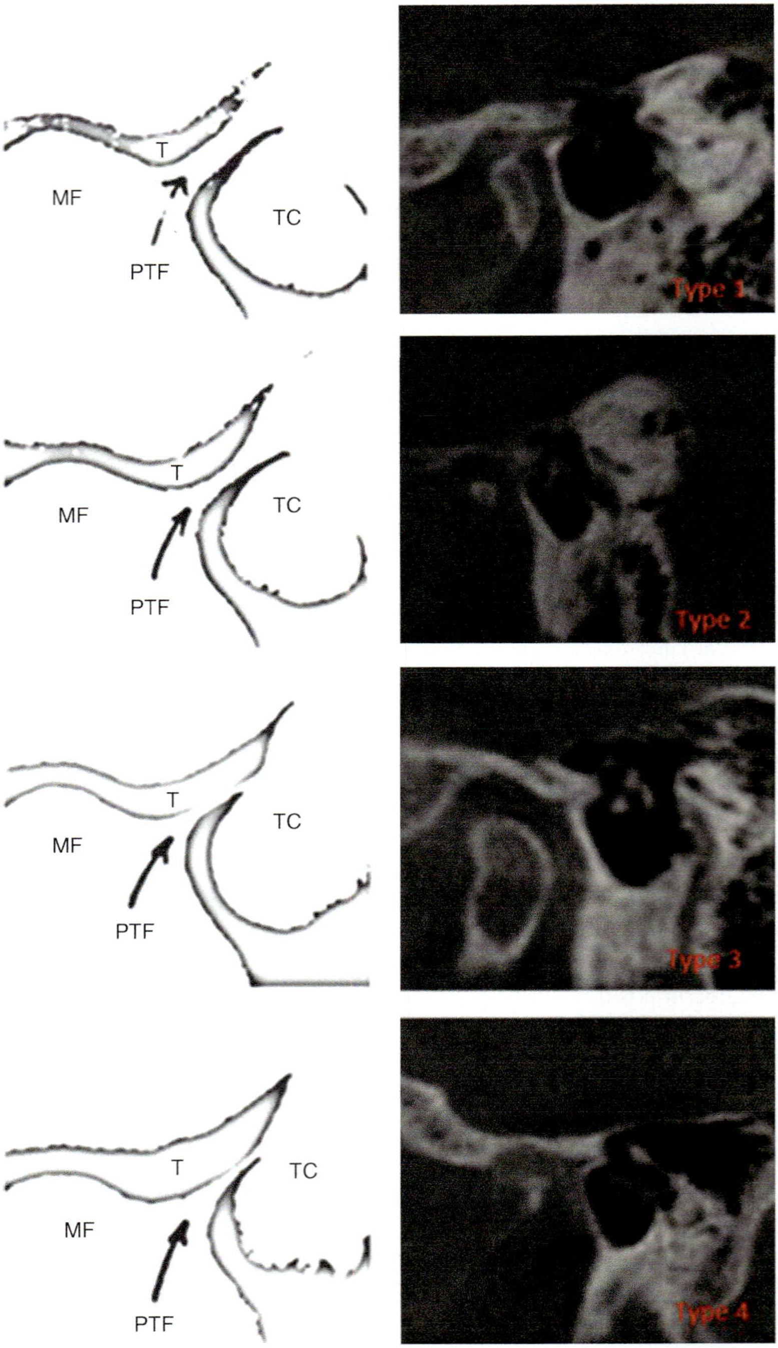

Fig. 17.8 Sagittal CT images showing petrotympanic fissure types. *TC* Tympanic cavity, *PTF* petrotympanic fissure, *T* tuberculum articulare, *MF* mandibular fossa

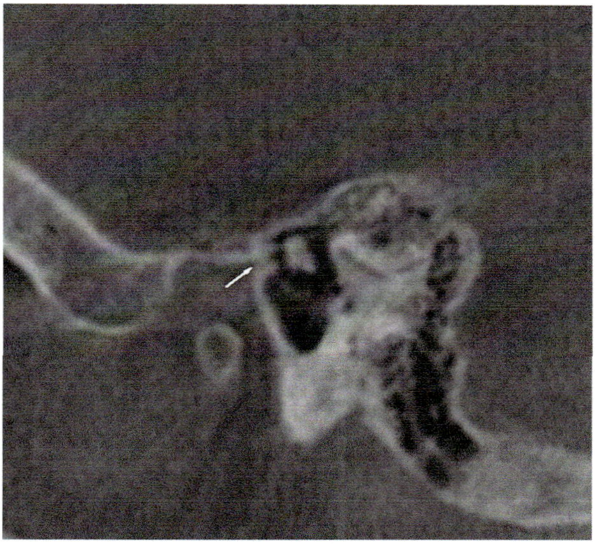

Fig. 17.9 Sagittal CT image showing malleolus and attached ligaments with petrotympanic fissure

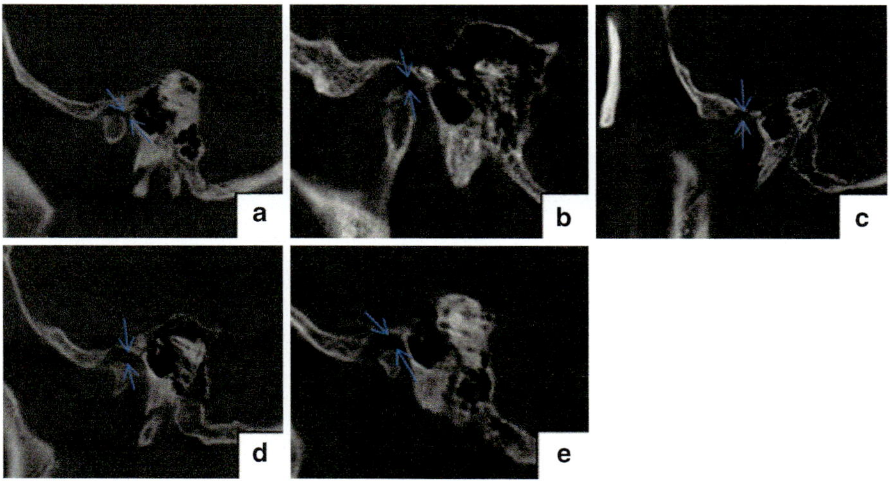

Fig. 17.10 Images showing connection of (**a**) and (**b**) discomalleolar ligament (DML), (**c**) and (**d**) anterior malleolar ligament (AML), and (**e**) DML

17.1.3.4 Semicircular Canals and the TMJ

Clinical imaging of the temporal bone, especially the middle and inner ear portion, is an integral element for anatomical evaluation in terms of medical considerations. Many incidental anatomical variations can be found in the temporal anatomy and identifying these variations can be crucial, especially before surgical procedures. The semicircular canals are one of the elements that show variation; they are defined as three canals; namely, the superior, posterior, and lateral semicircular canals [59, 60] (Fig. 17.11).

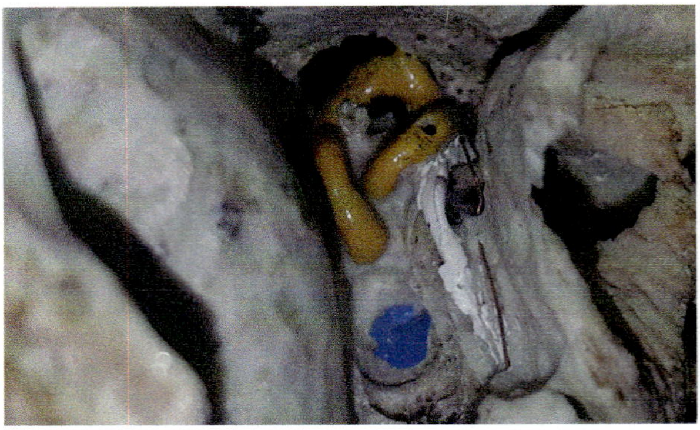

Fig. 17.11 Colored dry skull images showing dissected semicircular canals

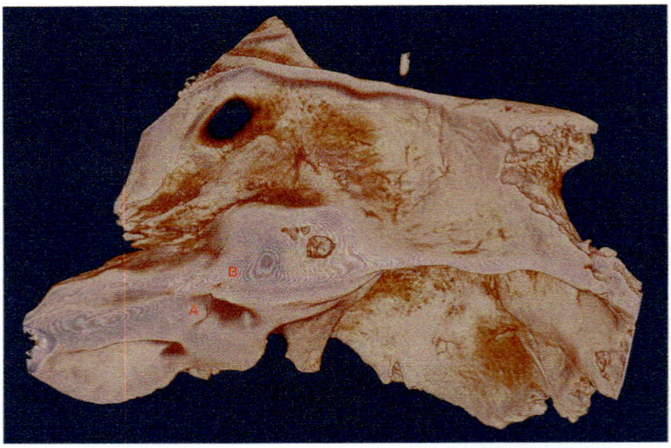

Fig. 17.12 Three-dimensional (3D) micro-CT image of the temporal bone. (*A*) Meatus acusticus internus, (*B*) eminentia arcuata

It is generally accepted that the three semicircular canals are set at right angles to each other and the lateral semicircular canal is smaller than the anterior and posterior semicircular canals. Precise knowledge of the size and spatial relationships of the semicircular canals is vital. Variation in the morphology of these canals correlates with locomotor agility and affects surgical interventions [61–63] (Fig. 17.12).

The semicircular canals are a component of the bony labyrinth. The three semicircular canals are continuous with the vestibule. Each of the canals makes about two-thirds of a circle and measures about 1 mm in cross-sectional diameter. The superior and posterior semicircular canals are oriented vertically at right angles to each other. The lateral semicircular canal is at about a 30° angle from the horizontal plane [59] (Fig. 17.13).

Each canal is enlarged anteriorly by an ampulla. The non-ampulated ends of the superior and posterior semicircular canals join to form the bony common crus. A portion of the superior semicircular canal is closely related to a ridge (arcuate eminence) on the anterior surface of the petrous bone (the posterior delimitation of the middle cranial fossa).

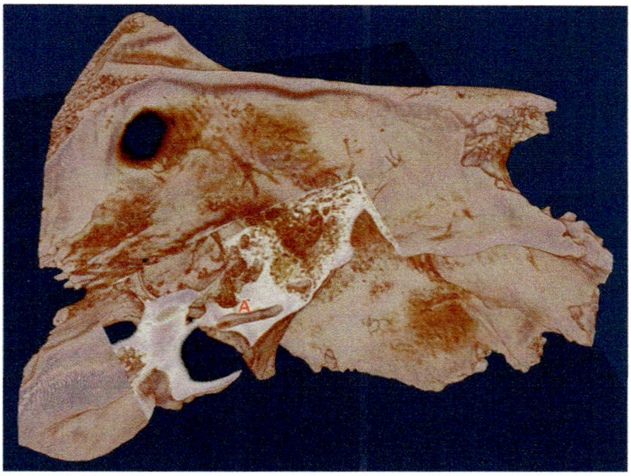

Fig. 17.13 3D Micro-CT image of the temporal bone. (*A*) Lateral semicircular canal

17.1.3.5 Horizontal Semicircular Canal

The lateral or horizontal canal (external semicircular canal) is the shortest of the three canals. This canal is responsible for conveying rotational motion of the head around the vertical axis (i.e., the neck), or, in other words, rotation in the transverse plane. It measures approximately 15 mm, and its arch is directed horizontally backward and laterally; thus, each semicircular canal stands at right angles to the other two. Its ampullated end corresponds to the upper and lateral angle of the vestibule, just above the oval window, where it opens close to the ampullated end of the superior canal; its opposite end opens at the upper and back part of the vestibule. The radius of curvature of the lateral semicircular canal is approximately 20% smaller than those of the anterior (superior) and posterior semicircular canals [64].

17.1.3.6 Posterior Semicircular Canal

The superior and posterior semicircular canals are both arranged in a vertical orientation at approximately right angles to one another. The superior canal is directed anterolaterally at an angle of about 45° to the mid-sagittal plane, and the posterior canal is directed posterolaterally at a corresponding angle [59]. The posterior semicircular canal is directed superiorly, as per its nomenclature, and posteriorly, nearly parallel to the posterior surface of the petrous bone. The vestibular aqueduct is immediately medial to this canal. The posterior canal is part of the bony labyrinth and is used by the vestibular system to detect rotations of the head in the coronal plane (Figs. 17.11 and 17.14).

17.1.3.7 Superior Semicircular Canal

The superior (anterior) semicircular canal detects rotations of the head around the lateral axis in the sagittal plane. It is approximately 10–15 mm in length, and is placed transversely to the long axis of the petrous part of the temporal bone, on the anterior surface of which its arch forms a round projection [65]. The angles of the vertical canals are oriented within both temporal bones so that the superior semicircular canal of one side has the same orientation as the posterior canal of the opposite side. The roof of the vestibule receives the ampullated limb of the superior semicircular canal. The petrous portion also forms the superior surface of the temporal bone. The superior semicircular canal has a close relation with the arcuate eminence which is an anatomical and surgical landmark that identifies the location of this canal. The canal opens into the upper part of the vestibule; the opposite end joins with the upper part of the posterior canal to form the crus commune, which opens into the upper and medial part of the vestibule [66] (Fig. 17.15).

The imaging study of the semicircular canals began in 1943 with Chaussé. Throughout the following decades, new projections were described, such as those of Schüller II (petrous bones in the orbits), Towne (semi-axial), Stenvers (occipitozygomatic), and others [67]. The most commonly accepted imaging study for the diagnosis of semicircular canal dehiscence (SCD) syndrome is high-resolution CT of the temporal bone. The accuracy of CT is paramount because the finding of superior semicircular canal dehiscence (SSCD) on CT in a patient with debilitating

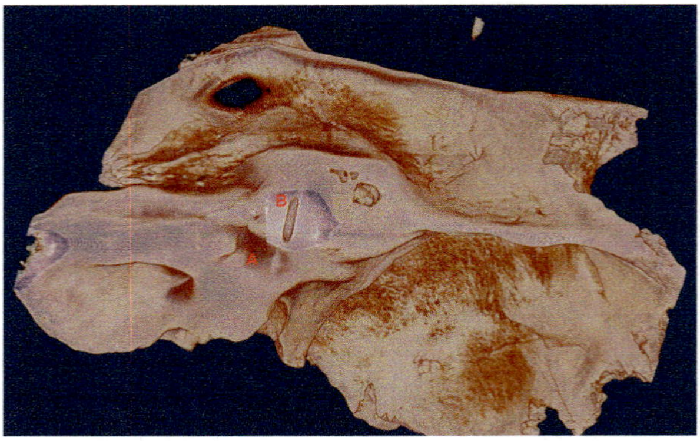

Fig. 17.14 3D Micro-CT image of the temporal bone. (*A*) Meatus acusticus internus (*B*) superior semicircular canal

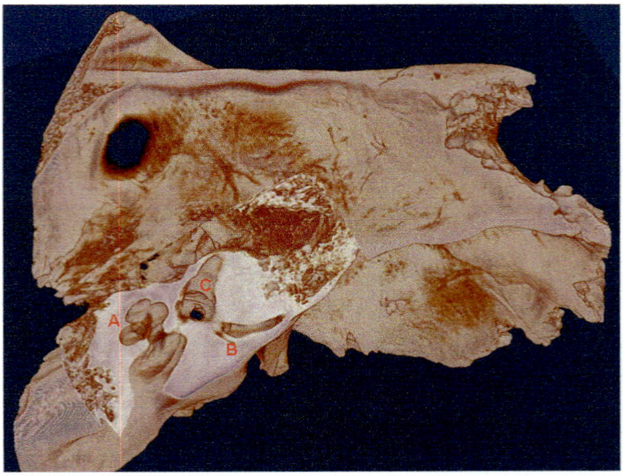

Fig. 17.15 3D Micro-CT image of the temporal bone. (*A*) Cochlea (*B*) posterior semicircular canal (*C*) vestibulum

symptoms may lead to a craniotomy or other surgical approach for repair. However, several studies have indicated that current CT imaging overestimates the prevalence of SSCD, and that CT imaging shows a higher prevalance of dehiscence than other imaging techniques. Moreover, it was stated that it is still difficult to analyze complex middle ear anatomy when using CT imaging only [19]. CT has been of great value in evaluating the condition of the middle ear cavity and labyrinth, but despite the use of very thin adjacent slices, CT is not yet a perfect technique [51, 68]. However, it should be noted that, due to volume averaging and resolution limits, MSCT may overestimate the morphological evaluations of various defects, especially SCD [51, 69, 70]. Recently, it was also noted that CBCT could replace MSCT, especially for preoperative temporal bone surgery, because of its low radiation dose levels and its smaller voxel size and because it enables the use of images with smaller slice thickness for examination.

17.2 Pathways of Connection from the TMJ to the Temporal Bone

17.2.1 Congenital Anomalies of the Ear and Temporal Bone

Due to the complex development of the temporomandibular region, its malformations and developmental variations are complicated, and are often limited to a uni- or bilateral element of the mandible and/or the external and middle ear exclusively. Of note, a higher incidence of otic anomalies is noted in males and there is a higher incidence on the right side [71, 72]. Such lesions are often part of various developmental syndromes such as the Treacher-Collins, Franceschetti-Klein, Pierre Robin, Klippel-Feil, Hanhart, Apert-Crouzon, and DiGeorge syndromes [73, 74].

The pinna is the area mostly affected by anomalies. It may be duplicated, or may show hypoplasia (microtia) or agenesis [73]. Different cysts, which histologically meet the criteria of dermoid cysts, are often visible in this region as a partial reduplication of the external acoustic meatus. Type I cysts occupy the postauricular region and are connected to the sinus, located parallel to the meatus, and end in a blind pouch, while type II cysts are below the angle of the mandible, connected with the parotid gland, and empty into the cartilaginous bony junction of the meatus, close to the tympanic cavity [73]. However, external ear malformations are usually not related to TMJ abnormalities [4, 73–75].

The most common developmental abnormality, well visible during CT examination, is a lack of the short process, or both processes, of the incus [76]. Moreover, such changes, limited to the long and/or lenticular process, may develop postnatally as a remodeling, secondary to various middle ear diseases or related to advanced age [77]. In the stapes, lack of ossification of the footplate, as well as partial or complete absence of the bones, has been described [76]. Base fusion with an oval window may be either congenital, or more commonly, acquired, as a complication of middle ear inflammation—(when it is frequently observed in children) and as a complication of

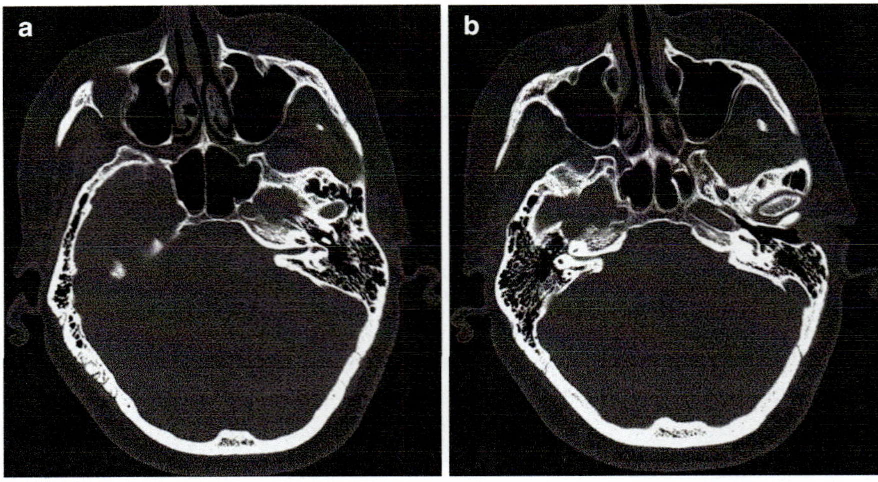

Fig. 17.16 Extensive pneumatization of the (**a**) tympanic part and (**b**) zygomatic process of the temporal bone

otosclerosis (when it is frequently observed in adults). The middle ear may also present vascular and neuronal abnormalities, e.g., persistent stapedial artery and abnormal bulging of the carotid artery and CN VII into the tympanic cavity. Lack of the tympanic membrane and ossification of the whole lateral wall of the tympanic cavity, as well as ankylosis of the auricular ossicles, have also been noted [73].

As mentioned above, there may be extensive pneumatization of the tympanic part and the squama of the temporal bone, but as long this does not impair the morphology and function of the TMJ, the change in the bone itself cannot be classified as a congenital malformation; rather, it is classified as a developmental variation (Fig. 17.16).

17.2.1.1 Superior Semicircular Canal Dehiscence and the TMJ

Superior semicircular canal dehiscence (SSCD) was first described in 1998 by Minor et al. [62] as a phenomenon that results from the thinning or absence of bone overlying the superior semicircular canal. The etiology of SSCD is unclear and it is also a controversial issue in the head and neck region. Some studies have stated that that congenital, developmental, and genetic factors are the primary factors leading to SSCD, but other possibilities for the occurrence of this entity may be a sudden change in middle ear pressure, or pulsatile high mid-cranial pressure, pulsations of the superior petrosal sinuses or sigmoid, or arachnoid granulations (such as those produced by head trauma or direct injury of the superior semicircular canal) during adulthood, especially in obese patients [78, 79].

In the radiological case series reported by Minor et al. [62], SSCD was classified in terms of patterns of the thinning of bone overlying the superior semicircular canal; they classified patterns as normal (amount of overlying bone thickness ranging from 0.6 to –1.7 mm); fine (bone thickness < 0.5 mm); thick (thickness > 1.8 mm);

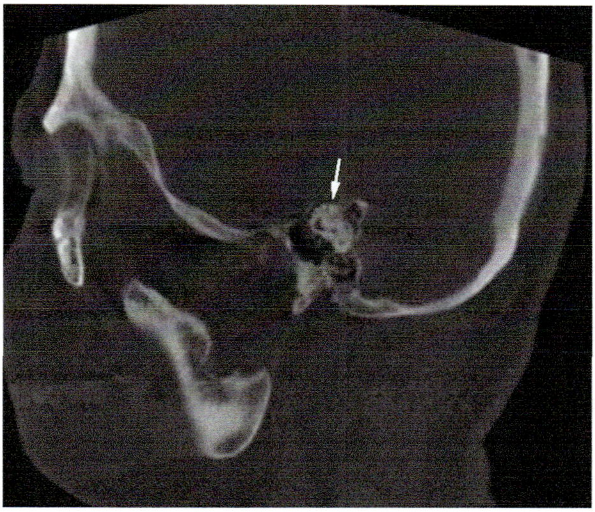

Fig. 17.17 Sagittal CBCT image showing superior semicircular canal pneumatized pattern

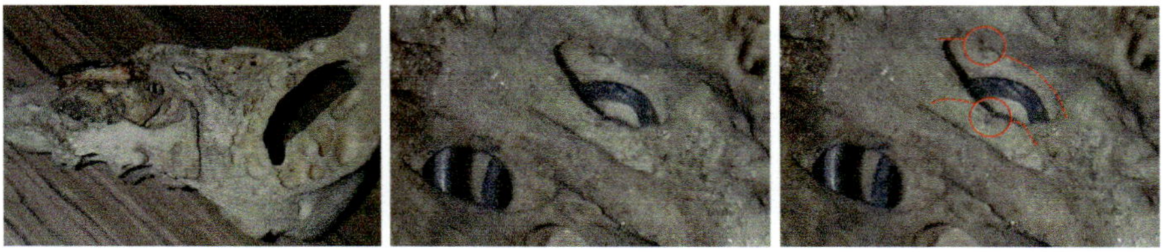

Fig. 17.18 Dissected skull images showing semicircular canals with dehiscence

pneumatized (Fig. 17.17), in which the roof of the canal is occupied by multiple supralabyrinthine cells, making it look like a woven structure (bone thickness > 2.5 mm); and dehiscent, characterized by showing a continuum in the bone cover of the canal an absence of continuum in the bone cover [67]. It was also found that the thinning of bone overlying the semicircular canals was much greater in young individuals than in adults [78] (Fig. 17.18).

Patients with superior SSCD syndrome may have symptoms such as vertigo and/or nystagmus, oscillopsia (Tullio phenomenon), autophony, disequilibrium due to loud noise, fistula symptoms, conductive hearing loss, tinnitus, or vestibular symptoms [51, 80–83]). It was recently found that SSCD may contribute to TMJ symptoms. The most common symptoms in SSCD patients were scattered pain in the TMJ and ear area following tinnitus. The disequilibrium due to loud noise may also contribute to the clinical picture, with clicking, crepitus, restriction of motion, and shape irregularities of the TMJ condyle in the joint region.

Alternatively, SSCD may result from disturbance in bone deposition during the development of the individual [78, 79, 81, 84].

In the developmental or genetic stages, the structure of the TMJ and all of the ear compartments interact with the formation of the malleolar ligaments. Thus, these attached or connected ligaments may be an etiologic factor which cause the ear and

TMJ related pain or other symptoms [52]. Recently, SSCD was found to be associated with alteration of the TMJ. A relationship between the presence of dehiscence and the thickness of the bone covering the semicircular canal and the roof of the glenoid fossa was defined, with an explanation of the embryological development of these structures. The embryological origin and endochondral ossification of the SSC and of part of the tegmen tympani are shared in common. There are solid embryological arguments linking the development and closure of the tegmen tympani to the development of the TMJ, this relationship being based on the role played by the DML. The development of these anatomical landmarks appears to be the bridging element linking the development of the TMJ and development of the superior semicircular canal [85–87]. It should be noted that when clinicians detect any symptom of SSCD, TMJ symptoms should be taken into account/investigated, or vice-versa (Figs. 17.19 and 17.20).

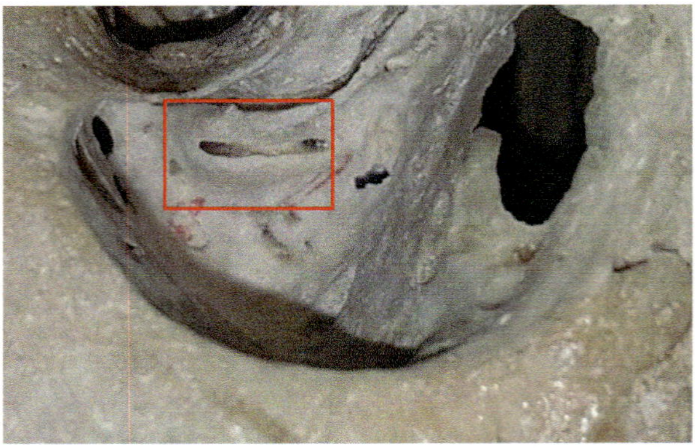

Fig. 17.19 Dry skull images showing semicircular canal dehiscence

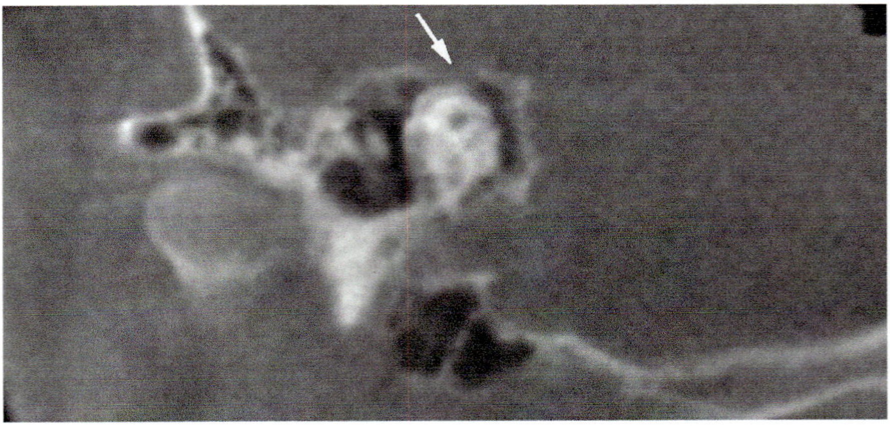

Fig. 17.20 Coronal CBCT image showing superior semicircular canal dehiscence

17.2.2 Fractures of the Temporal Bone

Fractures of the temporal bone are usually part of a serious head injury and involve the petrous part (with or without the squama), auricular ossicle, and internal ear damage. The incidence of these fractures is estimated to account for 14–22% of all skull fractures and 3% of all trauma patients [88]. In most cases, a periauricular swelling, Battle's sign (post-auricular ecchymosis), and bleeding from the external auditory meatus (otorrhagia) may be seen. These signs may be observed concomitantly with an intracranial hemorrhage, hearing loss, vertigo, balance disturbance, diffuse axonal injury, or damage of the facial nerve [89–91].

In clinical practice, fractures of the temporal bone are classified according to the involvement of the otic capsule and/or more commonly according to the involvement of the long axis of the petrous part, which runs obliquely from the apex posterolaterally through the mastoid air cells [88, 91]. Radiologically, longitudinal, transverse, and mixed fractures are recognized. Longitudinal fractures (70–90%) occur parallel to the axis of the temporal bone (Fig. 17.21a). The fracture line runs from the temporal squama through the mastoid, into the lateral wall of the middle ear; passing behind, through, or in front of the external auditory meatus and terminating in a middle cranial fossa, near the foramen spinosum or the foramen lacerum. In transverse temporal bone fractures (20–30%), the fracture line runs perpendicular to the axis; such fractures are associated with an injury of the frontal or occipital bone (Fig. 17.21b) [88]. Unlike longitudinal fractures, transverse fractures normally cross the facial canal and otic capsule and are complicated by facial nerve palsies, sensorineural hearing

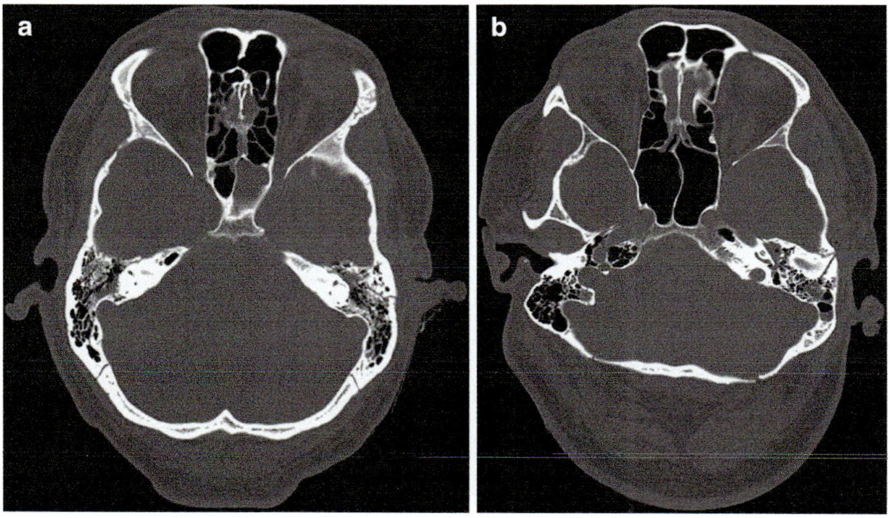

Fig. 17.21 Axial bone CT showing extralabyrinthine longitudinal (**a**) and transverse (**b**) fractures of the petrous part of the left temporal bone with concomitant hemotympanum and hemorrhage in the mastoid cells. Fracture of the occipital squama is also visible (**b**)

loss, vertigo, and injury to the internal carotid artery and/or jugular vein. In tegmen tympani involvement, cerebrospinal fluid otorrhea can be observed. The longitudinal fractures are complicated by tympanic membrane rupture, ossicular injury (incudostapedial dislocation), conductive hearing loss, and pneumocephalus. Displacement of the temporal lobe by fracture may also be visible. Mixed temporal bone fractures are a combination of longitudinal and transverse types, and most frequently involve the otic capsule [89].

17.2.3 Inflammatory Diseases of the Temporal Bone

Acute and chronic infections of the mastoid are still relatively common despite the introduction of antimicrobials in the 1930s [92]. Acute otitis media remains as one of the most common clinical problems for the mastoid area. It is estimated that 30 million cases occurred every year [93]. Although each case of acute otitis media demonstrates an inflammatory process in the communicating mastoid compartment, acute otomastoiditis is defined as an acute infection that results in pyogenic granulation in the mastoid and middle ear and osteolysis of its bony trabeculae [92].

Despite their obvious relationship, acute otomastoiditis and chronic otomastoiditis should be considered as two different diseases. Acute otomastoiditis is the result of bacterial infection. It can, infrequently, be a complication of leukemia, mononucleosis, sarcoma of the temporal bone, and Kawasaki disease. Chronic otomastoiditis is the result of Eustachian tube dysfunction. It is classified as chronic active otitis media with/without cholesteatoma and as chronic inactive otitis media that generally begins as acute suppurative otitis media [59] (Fig. 17.22).

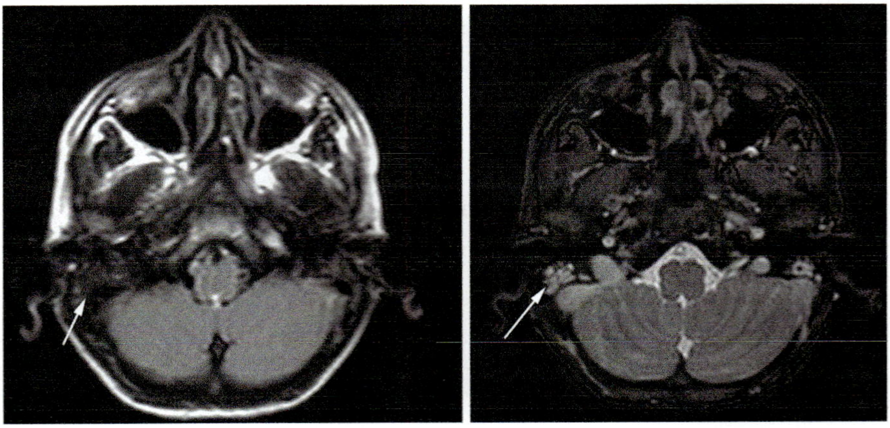

Fig. 17.22 T2- Fluid attenuation inversion recovery (FLAIR) and balanced turbo field echo (B-TFE) MR images show acute otomastoiditis in the mastoid process (*white arrows*)

17.2.3.1 Acute Otitis Media/Otitis Media with Effusion

Acute otitis media is a primary disease in newborns and children. The symptoms are fever, earache, and tympanic membrane flushing. The primary causes of the pathology are *Streptococcus* species and *Haemophilus influenzae*. For uncomplicated cases imaging is not necessary. However, if the infection extends to the mastoid antrum and aditus, the distal tubule of the middle ear can be closed after infection [94]. The pulse that accumulates under pressure causes tympanic membrane inflammation and lateral bulging. Perforation of the membrane leads to a mucopurulent discharge in the external acoustic meatus. Drainage reduces pressure and pain in the middle ear. The release of the mucopurulent flow leads to perforation in the nose as well [94]. High-resolution CT and, recently, CBCT, can be recommended for evaluating the extension of the inflammation. Cortical erosion is a typical finding in mastoid air cells [94].

Otitis media with effusion is the accumulation of non-purulent fluid of various viscosities within the middle ear cavity, usually accompanied by malfunction (occlusion) of the Eustachian tube. Allergic conditions or mucosal edema in response to infection predispose to congestive blockage. An additional pressure increase occurs in the middle ear with transmucosal gas exchange. This increase in pressure increases mucosal secretion and produces middle ear effusion. The Eustachian tube closes, because of vacuum effect due to stretched of the muscles. The persistence of middle ear effusion also affects the tympanic membrane, and hearing loss develops as a consequence of the prevention of vibration, and the persistent effusion provides a favorable environment for bacterial proliferation [16].

The symptoms of the disease are severe and pulsating earache, nasal congestion, sore throat, cough, runny nose, and hearing loss; a tinnitus sensation may also occur [95]. There is a wide variety of complications of otitis media; namely, extracranial (intratemporal or extratemporal) and intracranial complications. With the extratemporal complication of acute otitis media, zygomatic abscess ([59] or scattered pain in the TMJ area can be seen. Differential diagnosis for the pathology is broad, including vagus neuralgia and neuralgia of the glossopharyngeal nerve, which can be related to Eagle syndrome (calcification in the styloideus processus); TMJ pain; and cervicofacial syndrome (C4–C5) [95].

17.2.3.2 Acute and Chronic Otomastoiditis

Clinically, postauricular erythema, tenderness, and edema are seen with both acute and chronic otomastoiditis. With these signs, imaging is important to exclude complications [96]. Mastoiditis is a dangerous and life-threatening condition resulting from the spread of bacterial infection to the tympanic cavities, mastoid antrum, and air cells [16, 20]. In particular, infection may result in the spread of bacterial infection to the tympanic middle cranial fossa dura mater. This may result in dura mater necrosis and infection forming a subdural empyema in the subarachnoid space, or abscess formation in the adjacent temporal lobe and in the posterior cranial fossa [97]. The infection may spread to the cortical lateral wall of the mastoid process and may occupy the sternocleidomastoid muscle and it may also spread from the cortical bone—in the case of a subperiosteal postauricular abscess (Bezold's abscess)—or the end of the mastoid process [16].

There are various types of otomastoiditis: masked mastoiditis, acute mastoiditis, and coalescent mastoiditis. Masked mastoiditisis a chronic inflammation of the mucous membrane lining of pneumatized cells without abscess formation; clinically there are nonspecific complaints, and rarely pain or fever. Acute mastoiditis becomes clinically apparent a few days to 1 or 2 weeks after the onset of acute otitis media. There is postauricular subperiosteal swelling, and tenderness develops in the planum mastoideum. Pain is common, and may be scattered to the TMJ area; the complications can include facial nerve palsy, which is a rare complication of acute mastoiditis. High-resolution CT or CBCT will be the first choice for imaging. On CT the appearance of the mastoid air cells is opaque and they are filled with fluid and soft-tissue density owing to the presence of purulent fluid, a swollen mucous membrane, and granulation tissue. In coalescent mastoiditis, cell partitions become indistinct [95].

The very young are most at risk of suppurative otologic infections due to their immature Eustachian tube function, and because bony development of the temporal bone, glenoid fossa, and TMJ is still incomplete. Because of these factors, this age group is at high risk for the spread of infections between these two anatomically distinct regions (i.e., the temporal bone and the TMJ) [98, 99]. It is critical that the close anatomical relationship between the middle ear, mastoid cavity, glenoid fossa, and the TMJ is appreciated in order to correctly diagnose otomastoiditis when the presenting symptoms, physical examination, or radiographic evaluation implicate TMJ disorders (TMDs) [20]. Temporomandibular disorders were generally presumed to be a condition affecting adults; however, epidemiological studies have reported that signs and symptoms are as frequent in children as in adults [100, 101]. Among the more common signs and symptoms of TMD are TMJ sounds, impaired movement of the mandible, limitation in mouth opening, preauricular pain, facial pain, headache, and earache (otalgia), which have been reported either alone or in combination. Therefore, medical professionals have to be aware of this disease and should keep in mind that children who are admitted for TMJ symptoms can be affected by otitis media or otomastoiditis. Hence, certain patients with ear symptoms have to be examined meticulously by an otolaryngologist and TMJ consultant in order to avoid misdiagnosis and mistreatment [20, 102, 103] (Fig. 17.23).

Chronic inflammation of the middle ear, or mastoid bone, is also known as chronic otomastoiditis. A wide variety of symptoms and physical signs can be seen in the middle ear, with long-term destruction of bone by infection and inflammation. The most important causes of chronic otitis media development are trauma, Eustachian tube dysfunction and tympanic membrane perforation [97]. Chronic otitis media may lead to granulation tissue, cholesterol granuloma, and cholesteoma as sequelae and must be monitored. However, it should be noted that all these lesions have a similar appearance on CT images [96].

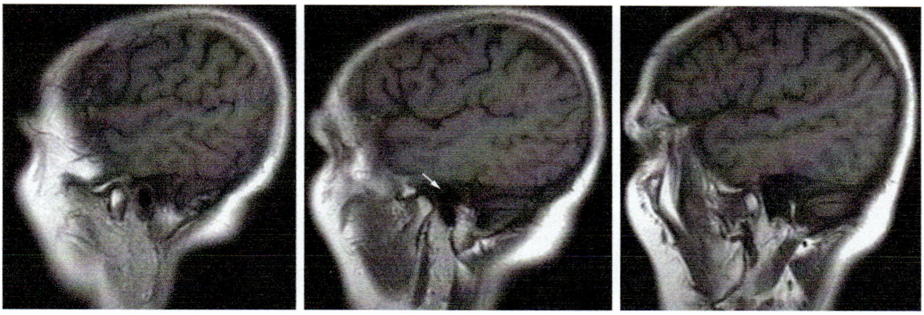

Fig. 17.23 MR images showing a well-pneumatized articular eminence and otomastoiditis close to the TMJ area (*arrow*)

Complications of long-standing chronic inflammation of the middle ear are ossicular resorption (most frequently seen in the long process of the incus) and/or ossicular fixation (most frequently seen in the malleus head). Tympanosclerosis, with tympanic membrane perforation, can also be seen as a complication. High-resolution CT or CBCT will be the first choice for imaging. MRI can be used; however, the diagnosis of infection related to the mastoid region solely with MRI is difficult. The MRI characteristics of acute otomastoiditis are nonspecific debris within the middle ear and mastoid, possibly with several fluid levels, which can be seen as bright signal areas on T2-weighted images. For chronic otomastoiditis with cholesteatoma, MR signal characteristics are nonspecific; ordinarily, both T1 and T2 relaxation times are relatively long [32, 59] (Fig. 17.24).

17.2.3.3 Granulations/Cholesterol Granuloma/Cholesteatoma

Granulation tissue can commonly be seen in the middle ear. A soft-tissue density is seen, with no ossicular displacement or bone erosion. Cholesterol granuloma can occur as a result of anterior tubal dysfunction and negative pressure and the vacuum phenomenon in the middle ear. These lesions may be asymptomatic, or the patient may experience vertigo, dizziness, or nonspecific findings of neuropathies in CN V, CN VI, CN VII, and CN VIII. Enlarged lesions can be seen on CT with indeterminate bone borders [65] (Fig. 17.25).

The distinction between granulation tissue and cholesteatoma can be made with contrast-enhanced MRI. Granulation tissue is usually quite vascular and is enhanced intensely on contrast-enhanced, T1-weighted images, while cholesteatoma is not enhanced [59].

Cholesteatoma is another important complication of chronic otitis media. It is characterized by the accumulation of desquamated keratin epithelium in the pneumatized areas of the ear or temporal bone. Cholesteatoma of the middle ear is relatively frequent and may arise at any time throughout life. A cholesteatoma may be classified as either acquired or congenital. Acquired middle ear cholesteatoma is the one most commonly seen and can result from chronic otitis media. Acquired cholesteatomas usually develop owing to chronic Eustachian tube

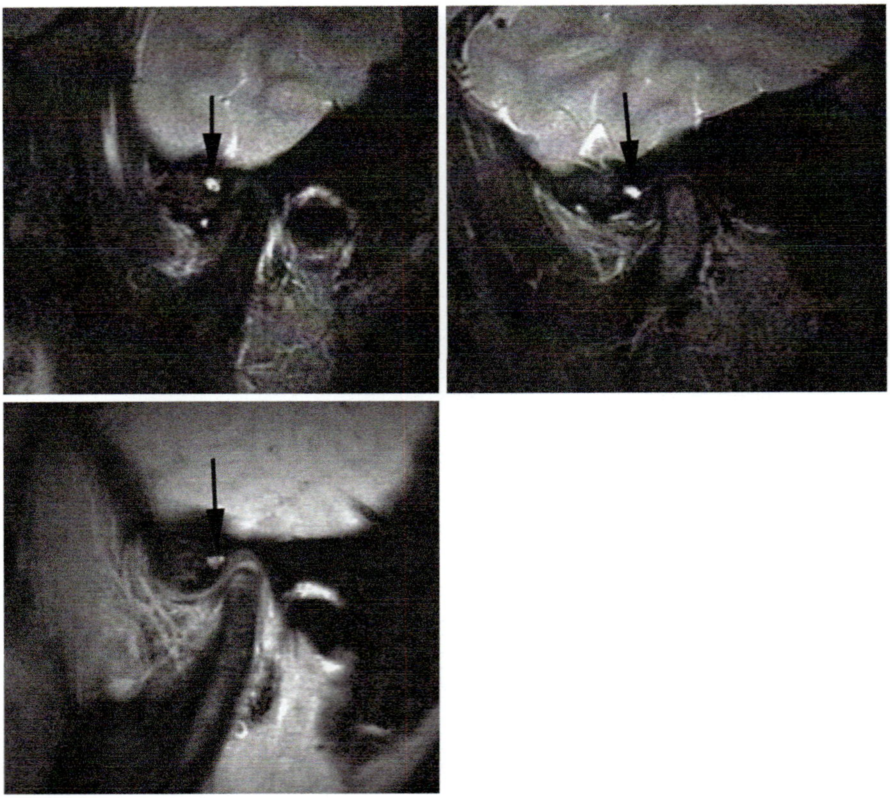

Fig. 17.24 MR images of three patients with acute otomastoiditis, localized at the articular eminence (*black arrows*) (derived from [32])

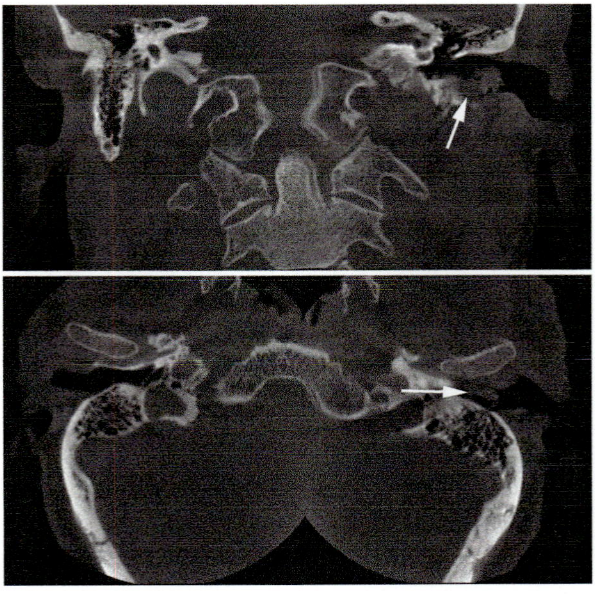

Fig. 17.25 CBCT images showing a case of cholesteatoma with surrounding bone resorption

dysfunction, which is responsible for prolonged negative pressure inside the tympanic cleft, with retraction of the tympanic membrane. The symptoms include otorrhea, bleeding, earache, hearing loss, tinnitus, dizziness, and headache [95]. The underlying formation of acquired cholesteatoma is not fully understood, i.e. the mechanism of osteoclasts and erosion of bone produced by soft tissue epithelial proliferation and soft tissue infection. Depending on the hearing loss, vestibular and semicircular canal damage caused by bone involvement, and damage to the inner ear, acquired cholesteatoma may cause balance problems; Bell's palsy due to ischemia of the facial sinus or necrosis; and intracranial sepsis. Microsurgical removal of the epithelial extension is involved in treatment [17, 104].

Chronic otomastoiditis is the result of Eustachian tube dysfunction, which can be classifed as chronic active otitis media with/without cholesteatoma and chronic inactive otitis media that generally begins as acute suppurative otitis media. The mastoid air cell system has been recognized as an important contributor to and pathway of mastoid infection suppuration. Tumors of the mastoid process and ear may extend into the TMJ, whereas otitis or otomastoiditis may involve the TMJ and can even result in ankylosis [32] (Fig. 17.26).

CBCT or MSCT can localize the cholesteatoma and provide important information on the integrity of the ossicular chain, lateral semicircular canal, and cortical bone of the middle and posterior fossa. On a coronal CT scan, blunting of the scutum, as well as intrapetrous invasion can be seen. Pars flaccida cholesteatoma on CT is associated with erosion and medial displacement of small bones and scutum erosion in Prussak's space, while a round expanding lesion is observed. Congenital cholesteatoma usually resides in the anterior-superior quadrant of the middle ear cavity at the opening of the ostium tube [94, 104, 105]. Most cases tend to be idiopathic or spontaneous, and lesions may develop as a result of a trauma and secondary to surgery or radiation. Due to most of the cases are caused by unilateral ear infection, ear pain is experienced. CT images are seen as focal soft tissue, which is located in the inferior part of the external auditory canal, causing erosion and periostitis in the lesion [96, 106] (Fig. 17.27).

CT of the temporal bone is a useful imaging modality for the diagnosis, description of extension, and possible complications of middle ear cholesteatoma. This modality, however, cannot differentiate between inflammatory/granulomatous tissue and cholesteatoma. It is also difficult, on CT, to diagnose recurrent or residual cholesteatoma after surgery. For cholesteatomatous tissue, MRI shows an intermediate to hypointense signal on T1-weighted images and appears hyperintense on the corresponding T2-weighted images. This hyperintensity is, however, significantly less than that seen in inflammatory lesions [107]. Diffusion-weighted MRI (DWI) is particularly sensitive to cholesteatoma tissue, especially for the diagnosis of intracranial and extracranial epidermoid cysts; as middle ear cholesteatomas have similar histopathological characteristics to epidermoid cysts, this MR sequence should be used for the evaluation of such pathologies [108, 109]. Non-echo planar DWI for cholesteatoma diagnosis can be performed on either 1.5-T or 3-T scanners. High sensitivity and negative predictive value and relatively lower specificity and positive predictive value are achieved with a single non-echo planar DWI protocol [110] (Fig. 17.28).

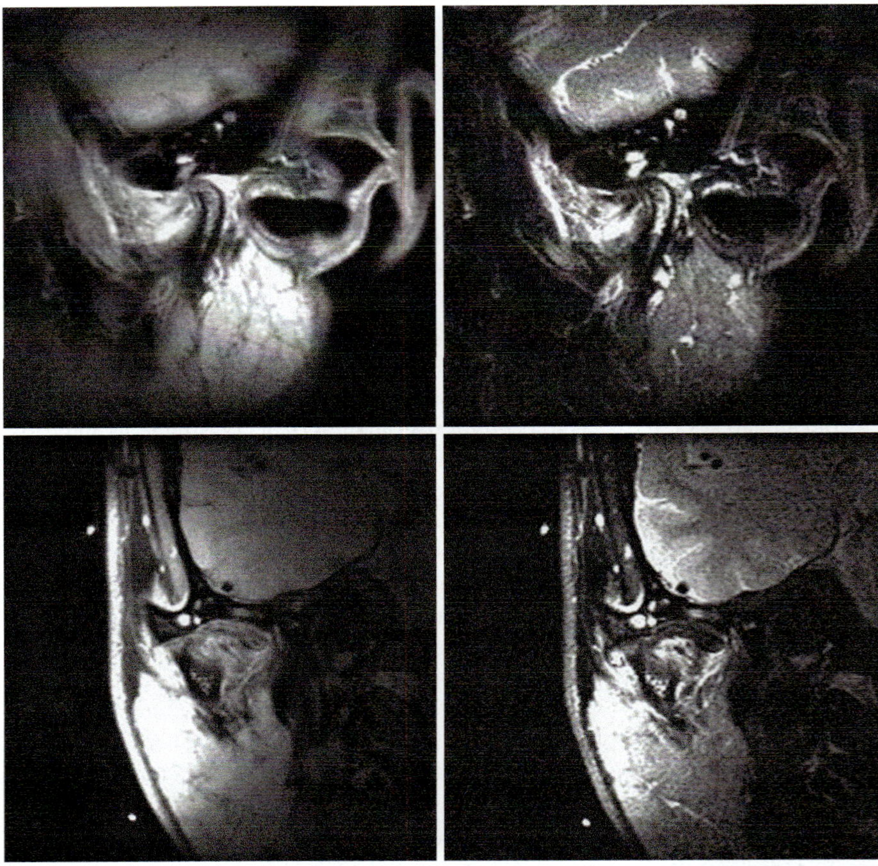

Fig. 17.26 Sagittal, coronal T2-, and proton-weighted MR images of chronic active otitis media with cholesteatoma in the middle ear, which spread through a pneumatized articular eminence and the TMJ area (derived from [19])

As noted above, for chronic otomastoiditis with cholesteatoma, the MR signal characteristics are nonspecific; ordinarily, both T1 and T2 relaxation times are relatively long. On MRI for the TMJ these findings can also be seen, although with a limited field of view, with an increased signal intensity on T2-weighted images and isointense signal intensity on T1-weighted images [32] (Table 17.1) (Fig. 17.29).

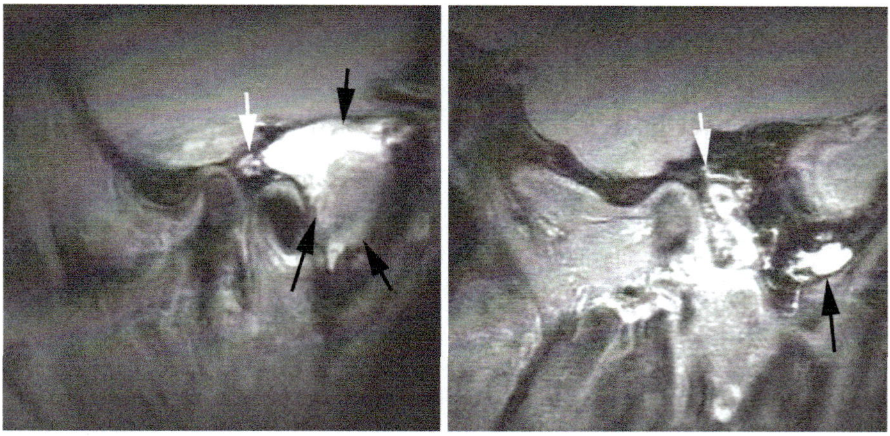

Fig. 17.27 Sagittal T2- and proton-weighted MR images showing acute otomastoiditis in the mastoid process in two patients (*arrows*) (derived from [32])

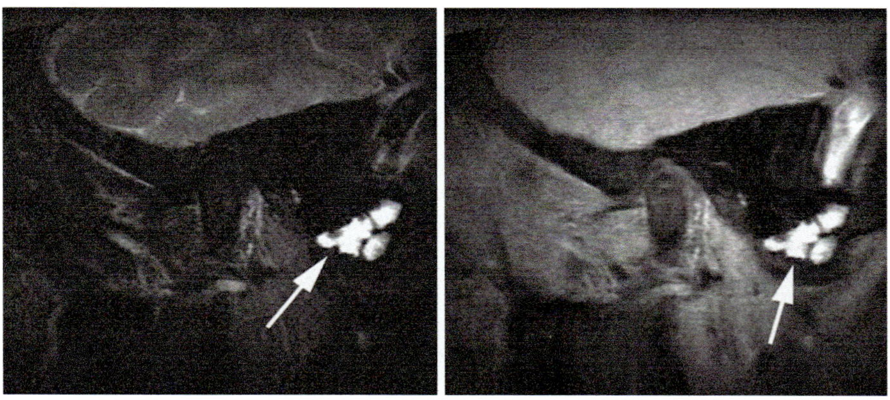

Fig. 17.28 Connection of temporal bone and TMJ; otomastoiditis in both the mastoid process and at the articular eminence on MR images (*arrows*) (derived from [32])

Table 17.1 Imaging of Temporal/TMJ-related pathologies

Temporal/TMJ-related pathologies	Conventional radiography (panoramic, Schüeller's view etc.)	CBCT	CT	MRI
Pneumatization	++	+++	+++	+
Cholesteatoma	+	+++	+++	+
SSCD	+	+++	++	–
Otomastoiditis	+	++	++	+
Chronic otitis media	–	++	++	+
Fractures	++	+++	+++	–

TMJ temporomandibular joint, *CBCT* cone bem computerized tomography, *CT* computerized tomography, *MRI* magnetic resonance imaging, *SSCD* superior semicircular canal dehiscence

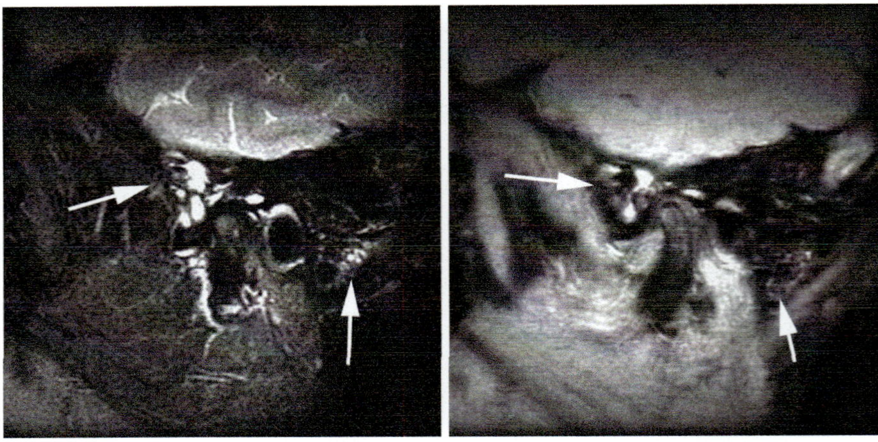

Fig. 17.29 T2- and proton-weighted MR images show bilateral acute otomastoiditis in both the mastoid process (*black arrows*) and at the articular eminence (*white arrows*) (derived from [32])

References

1. Ikari Y, Katori Y, Ohtsuka A, Rodríguez-Vázquez JF, Abe H, Kawase T, Murakami G, Abe S. Fetal development and variations in the cartilages surrounding the human external acoustic meatus. Ann Anat. 2013;195:128–36.
2. McBratney-Owen B, Iseki S, Bamforth SD, Olsen BR, Morriss-Kay GM. Development and tissue origins of the mammalian cranial base. Dev Biol. 2008;322:121–32.
3. Ricciardelli EJ. Embryology and anatomy of the cranial base. Clin Plast Surg. 1995;22:361–72.
4. Scheuer L, Black S. The head, neck and dentition. In: Cunningham C, Scheuer L, Black S, editors. Developmental juvenile osteology. San Diego: Elsevier Academic Press; 2000. p. 36–169.
5. Skarzyński H, Kukwa A, Jegliński W, Skarzyńska B. Degree of middle ear malformation in developmental defects of the I and II branchial arches. Otolaryngol Pol. 1990;44:297–301.
6. Whyte J, Cisneros A, Yus C, Fraile J, Obón J, Vera A. Tympanic ossicles and pharyngeal arches. Anat Histol Embryol. 2009;38:31–3.
7. Cisneros Gimeno AI, Whyte Orozco JR, Obón Nogues JA, Yus Gotor C, Crovetto De La Torre MA, Whyte Orozco A. Contribution to morphological knowledge of the development of the human incudomalleal joint. Acta Otolaryngol. 2009;129:1380–7.
8. Hanson JR, Anson BJ, Strickland EM. Branchial sources of the auditory ossicles in man. II. Observations of embryonic stages from 7 mm. to 28 mm. (CR length). Arch Otolaryngol. 1962;76:200–15.
9. Hanson JR, Anson BJ. Development of the malleus of the human ear. Illustrated in atlas series. Q Bull Northwest Univ Med Sch. 1962;36:119–37.
10. Krmpotić-Nemanić J, Padovan I, Vinter I, Jalsovec D. Prenatal and postnatal development of the tympanic portion of the temporal bone. Ann Anat. 1999;181:593–5.
11. Tóth M, Medvegy T, Moser G, Patonay L. Development of the protympanum. Ann Anat. 2006;188:267–73.
12. Bach-Petersen S, Kjaer I. Ossification of lateral components in the human prenatal cranial base. J Craniofac Genet Dev Biol. 1993;13:76–82.
13. Eby TL, Nadol JB Jr. Postnatal growth of the human temporal bone. Implications for cochlear implants in children. Ann Otol Rhinol Laryngol. 1986;95(4 Pt1):356–64.
14. Bochenek A, Raicher M. Human Anatomy. Warsw: PZWL; 2007.

15. Kurlej WL, Gworys B, Burdan F. Anatomy for dentists. Elsevier Urban & Partner: Wroclaw; 2011.
16. Standring S. Gray's Anatomy, the anatomical basis of clinical practice. 40th ed. Madison: Elsevier; 2008a. p. 615–34.
17. Standring S. Head and neck. In: Standring S, editor. Gray's Anatomy: the anatomical basis of clinical practice, expert consult. 40th ed. London: Elsevier Churchill Livingstone; 2008b. p. 395–705.
18. Jufas N, Marchioni D, Tarabichi M, Patel N. Endoscopic anatomy of the protympanum. Otolaryngol Clin N Am. 2016;49:1107–19.
19. Orhan K, Delilbasi C, Cebeci I, Paksoy C. Prevalence and variations of pneumatized articular eminence: a study from Turkey. Oral Surg Oral Med Oral Pathol Oral Radiol Endod. 2005a;99(3):349–54.
20. Orhan K, Delilbasi C, Orhan AI. Radiographic evaluation of pneumatized articular eminence in a group of Turkish children. Dentomaxillofac Radiol. 2006;35(5):365–70.
21. Orhan K, Oz U, Orhan AI, Ulker AE, Delilbasi C, Akcam O. Investigation of pneumatized articular eminence in orthodontic malocclusions. Orthod Craniofac Res. 2010;13(1):56–60.
22. Virapongse C, Sarwar M, Bhimani S, Sasaki C, Shapiro R. Computed tomography of temporal bone pneumatization: 1. normal pattern morphology. AJNR. 1995;6:551–9.
23. Tremble GJ. Pneumatization of the temporal bone. Arch Odontolaryngol. 1934;9:172.
24. Allam AF. Pneumatization of the temporal bone. Ann Otol Rhinol Laryngol. 1969;78:48–64.
25. Tyndall DA, Matteson RS. Radiographic appearance and population distribution of the pneumatized articular eminence of the temporal bone. J Oral Maxillo Fac Surg. 1985;43:493–7.
26. Hollinshead WH. Anatomy for surgeons: the head and neck. 2nd ed. New York: Harper and Row; 1968.
27. Hofmann T, Friedrich RE, Wedl JS, Schmelzle R. Pneumatization of the zygomatic arch on pantomography. Mund Kiefer Gesichtschir. 2001;5:173–9.
28. Thomson HG. Septic arthritis of the temporomandibular joint complicating otitis externa. J Laryngol Otol. 1989;103:319–21.
29. Youniss S. The relationship between craniomandibular disorders and otitis media in children. Cranio. 1991;9:169–73.
30. Delilbasi C, Orhan K, Icen M, Aksoy S, Horasan S, Kenan KS. Evaluation of articular eminence pneumatization using cone beam computed tomography. Minerva Stomatol. 2013 Oct;62(10):349–54.
31. Wong K, Mung LP. Magnetic resonance imaging of the temporomandibular joint: diagnostic difficulty caused by extensive pneumatization of the mastoid air cells. Skelet Radiol. 1999;28:577–80.
32. Orhan K, Nishiyama H, Tadashi S, Shumei M, Furukawa S. MR of 2270 TMJs: prevalence of radiographic presence of otomastoiditis in temporomandibular joint disorders. Eur J Radiol. 2005b;55(1):102–7.
33. Akbulut N, Kursun S, Aksoy S, Kurt H, Orhan K. Evaluation of foramen tympanicum using cone-beam computed tomography in orthodontic malocclusions. J Craniofac Surg. 2014;25(2):e105–9.
34. Lacout A, Marsot-Dupuch K, Smoker WR, Lasjaunias P. Foramen tympanicum, or foramen of Huschke: pathologic cases and anatomic CT study. Am J Neuroradiol. 2005;26(6): 1317–23.
35. Fusconi M, Benfari G, Franco M, Deriu D, Dambrosio F, Antonio G, et al. Foramen of Huschke: case report and experimental procedure for diagnosis of spontaneous salivary fistula. J Oral Maxillofac Surg. 2009;67:1747–51.
36. Wang RG, Bingham B, Hawke M, Kwok P, Li JR. Persistence of the foramen of Huschke in the adult: an osteological study. J Otolaryngol. 1991;20:251–3.
37. Nakasato T, Nakayama T, Kikuchi K, Ehara S, Ohtsuka H, Fukuda K, Sato H. Spontaneous temporomandibular joint herniation into the external auditory canal through a persistent foramen tympanicum (Huschke): radiographic features. J Comput Assist Tomogr. 2013;37(1):111–3.

38. Prowse SJ, Kelly G, Agada F. Temporomandibular joint herniation and the foramen of Huschke: an unusual external auditory canal mass. J Laryngol Otol. 2011;125(12):1279–81.
39. Dingle AF. Fistula between the external auditory canal and the temporomandibular joint: a rare complication of otitis externa. J Laryngol Otol. 1992;106:994–5.
40. Faerber TH, Ennis RL, Allen GA. Temporomandibular joint ankylosis following mastoiditis: report of a case. J Oral Maxillofac Surg. 1990;48:866–70.
41. Applebaum EL, Berg LF, Kumar A. Otologic complications following temporomandibular joint arthroscopy. Ann Otol Rhinol Laryngol. 1988;97:675–9.
42. Herzog S, Fiese R. Persistent foramen of Huschke: possible risk factor for otologic complications after arthroscopy of the temporomandibular joint. Oral Surg Oral Med Oral Pathol. 1989;68:267–70.
43. Tozoglu U, Caglayan F, Harorli A. Foramen tympanicum or foramen of Huschke: anatomical cone beam CT study. Dentomaxillofac Radiol. 2012;41(4):294–7.
44. Kalender A, Orhan K, Aksoy U. Evaluation of the mental foramen and accessory mental foramen in Turkish patients using cone-beam computed tomography images reconstructed from a volumetric rendering program. Clin Anat. 2012;25(5):584–92.
45. Furstman L. The early development of the human temporomandibular joint. Am J Orthod. 1963;49:672–82.
46. Perry HT, Xu Y, Forbes DP. The embryology of the temporomandibular joint: a study. Cranio. 1985;3:125–32.
47. Pinto OF. A new structure related to the temporomandibular joint and middle ear. J Prosthet Dent. 1962;12:95–103.
48. Toledo FJL, Zorzetto NL, Caldas NJA. Structures and relationships of the temporomandibular joint. J Oral Maxillofac Surg. 1985;43:565–9.
49. Wong GB, Weinberg S, Symington JM. Morphology of the developing articular disc of the human temporomandibular joint. J Oral Maxillofac Surg. 1985;43(8):565–9.
50. Yuodelis RA. The morphogenesis of the human temporomandibular joint and its associated structures. J Dent Res. 1966;45:182–91.
51. Kurt H, Orhan K, Aksoy S, Kursun S, Akbulut N, Bilecenoglu B. Evaluation of the superior semicircular canal morphology using cone beam computed tomography: a possible correlation for temporomandibular joint symptoms. Oral Surg Oral Med Oral Pathol Oral Radiol. 2014;117:280–8.
52. Sencimen M, Yalçin B, Doğan N, Varol A, Okçu KM, Ozan H, Aydintuğ YS. Anatomical and functional aspects of ligaments between the malleus and the temporomandibular joint. Int J Oral Maxillofac Surg. 2008;37:943–7.
53. https://www.imaios.com/en/e-Anatomy/Anatomical-Parts/Petrotympanic-fissure.
54. Monteiro JC, Ennes JP, Zorzatto JR. Ossification of the petrotympanic fissure: morphological analysis and clinical implications. Cranio. 2011;29(4):284–90.
55. Arai H, Sato I. Anatomical study of the human discomallear ligament using cone beam computed tomography imaging and morphological observations. Okajimas Folia Anat Jpn. 2011;88:89–101.
56. Sato I, Arai H, Asaumi R, Imura K, Kawai T, Yosue T. Classifications of tunnel-like structure of human petrotympanic fissure by cone beam CT. Surg Radiol Anat. 2008;30:323–6.
57. Kim HJ, Jung HS, Kwak HH, et al. The discomallear ligament and the anterior ligament of malleus: an anatomic study in human adults and fetuses. Surg Radiol Anat. 2004;26:39–45.
58. Barghan S, Tetradis S, Mallya SM. Application of cone beam computed tomography for assessment of the temporomandibular joints. Aust Dent J. 2012;57:109–18.
59. Curtin HD, Gupta R, Bergeron TR. Embryology, anatomy, and imaging of temporal bone. In: Som PM, Curtin HD, editors. Head and neck imaging. 5th ed. St. Louis: Mosby; 2011. p. 1072.
60. Dieterich M, Brandt T. Vestibular system: anatomy and functional magnetic resonance imaging. Neuroimaging Clin N Am. 2001;11(2):263–73.
61. Minor LB. Clinical manifestations of superior semicircular canal dehiscence. Laryngoscope. 2005;115:1717–27.

62. Minor LB, Solomon D, Zinreich JS, Zee DS. Sound- and/or pressure-induced vertigo due to bone dehiscence of the superior semicircular canal. Arch Otolaryngol Head Neck Surg. 1998;124:249–58.
63. Romo LV, Casselman JW, Robson CD. Congenital anomalies of the temporal bone. In: Som PM, Curtin HD, editors. Head and neck imaging. 5th ed. St. Louis: Mosby; 2011. p. 1113.
64. Lee JY, Shin KJ, Kim JN, Yoo JY, Song WC, Koh KS. A morphometric study of the semicircular canals using micro-CT images in three-dimensional reconstruction. Anat Rec. 2013;296(5):834–9.
65. Ozdil NY, Temporal kemiğin ve komşuluklarinin konik işinli bilgisayarli tomografide farkli fov ve voksel büyüklüklerinde anatomik ve morfolojik retrospektif değerlendirilmesi, Ankara University, MSc (Specialization Thesis), 2016. In Turkish.
66. Lane JI, Witte RJ. Temporal Bone: An Imaging Atlas. Berlin: Springer; 2010.
67. Cisneros AI, Whyte J, Martínez C, Gracia-Tello B, Whyte A, Obón J, Crovetto R, Crovetto MA. Radiological patterns of the posterior semicircular canal. Surg Radiol Anat. 2013;35:61.
68. Stimmer H, Hamann KF, Zeiter S, Naumann A, Rummeny EJ. Semicircular canal dehiscence in HR multislice computed tomography: distribution, frequency, and clinical relevance. Eur Arch Otorhinolaryngol. 2012;269:475–80.
69. Cloutier JF, Belair M, Saliba I. Superior semicircular canal dehiscence: positive predictive value of high-resolution CT scanning. Eur Arch Otorhinolaryngol. 2008;265:1455–60.
70. Siqueira SM, Whiting BR, Shimony JS, et al. Accuracy of computed tomography detection of superior canal dehiscence. Otol Neurotol. 2011;32:1500–5.
71. De la Cruz A, Linthicum FH Jr, Luxford WM. Congenital atresia of the external auditory canal. Laryngoscope. 1985;95:421–7.
72. De la Cruz A, Teufert KB. Congenital aural atresia surgery: long-term results. Otolaryngol Head Neck Surg. 2003;129:121–7.
73. Kos M. Head and neck congenital malformations. Act Clin Croat. 2004;43:195–201.
74. Nargozian C. The airway in patients with craniofacial abnormalities. Paediatr Anaesth. 2004;14:53–9.
75. Swartz JD, Faerber EN. Congenital malformations of the external and middle ear: high-resolution CT findings of surgical import. AJR Am J Roentgenol. 1985;144:501–6.
76. Donaldson I, Snow DG. A five year follow up of incus transposition in relation to the first stage tympanoplasty technique. J Laryngol Otol. 1992;106:607–9.
77. Lannigan FJ, O'Higgins P, Oxnard CE, McPhie P. Age-related bone resorption in the normal incus: a case of maladaptive remodelling? J Anat. 1995;186(Pt3):651–5.
78. Hagiwara M, Shaikh JA, Fang Y, Fatterpekar G, Roehm PC. Prevalence of radiographic semicircular canal dehiscence in very young children: an evaluation using high-resolution computed tomography of the temporal bones. Pediatr Radiol. 2012;42:1456–64.
79. Nadgir RN, Ozonoff A, Devaiah AK, Halderman AA, Sakai O. Superior semicircular canal dehiscence: congenital or acquired condition? AJNR Am J Neuroradiol. 2011;32(5):947–9.
80. Boeddinghaus R. Re: Measurement of defect angle in superior semicircular canal dehiscence. Clin Radiol. 2010;65(10):853–4.
81. Crovetto de la Torre MA, Whyte Orozco J, Cisneros Gimeno AI, et al. Superior semicircular canal dehiscence syndrome. Embryological and surgical consideration. Acta Otorrinolaringol Esp. 2005;56:6–11.
82. Lip G, Nichols DM. Measurement of defect angle in superior semicircular canal dehiscence. Clin Radiol. 2009;64(12):1210–3.
83. Mondina M, Bonnard D, Barreau X, Darrouzet V, Franco-Vidal V. Anatomo-radiological study of the superior semicircular canal dehiscence of 37 cadaver temporal bones. Surg Radiol Anat. 2013;35(1):55–9.
84. Carney AS, Ward V, Malluci CL, O'Donoghue GM, Robertson I, Baldwin DL, Maw AR, Coakham HB. Meningiomas involving the internal auditory canal: a diagnostic and surgical challenge. Skull Base Surg. 1999;9:87–94.
85. Crovetto-Martínez R, Vargas C, Lecumberri I, Bilbao A, Crovetto-De la Torre M, Whyte-Orozco J. Radiological correlation between the thickness of the roof of the glenoid fossa and

that of the bony covering of the superior semicircular canal. Oral Surg Oral Med Oral Pathol Oral Radiol. 2017;125(4):358–63. https://doi.org/10.1016/j.oooo.2017.12.008.
86. Fraile Rodrigo JJ, Cisneros AI, Obón J, Yus C, Crovetto R, Crovetto MA, Whyte J. Ontogenetic explanation for tegmen tympani dehiscence and superior semicircular canal dehiscence association. Acta Otorrinolaringol Esp. 2016;67(4):226–32.
87. Rodríguez-Vázquez JF, Murakami G, Verdugo-López S, Abe S, Fujimiya M. Closure of the middle ear with special reference to the development of the tegmen tympani of the temporal bone. J Anat. 2011;218(6):690–8.
88. Zayas JO, Feliciano YZ, Hadley CR, Gomez AA, Vidal JA. Temporal bone trauma and the role of multidetector CT in the emergency department. Radiographics. 2011;31:1741–55.
89. Brodie HA, Thompson TC. Management of complications from 820 temporal bone fractures. Am J Otol. 1997;18:188–97.
90. Dahiya R, Keller JD, Litofsky NS, Bankey PE, Bonassar LJ, Megerian CA. Temporal bone fractures: otic capsule sparing versus otic capsule violating clinical and radiographic considerations. J Trauma. 1999;47:1079–83.
91. Little SC, Kesser BW. Radiographic classification of temporal bone fractures: clinical predictability using a new system. Arch Otolaryngol Head Neck Surg. 2006;132:1300–4.
92. Nadol JB, Eavey RD. Acute and chronic mastoiditis: clinical presentation, diagnosis, and management. Curr Clin Top Infect Dis. 1995;15:204–9.
93. Hoberman A, Paradise JL. Acute otitis media: diagnosis and management in the year 2000. Pediatr Ann. 2000;29:609–19.
94. Trojanowska A, Drop A, Trojanowski P, Rosińska-Bogusiewicz K, Klatka J, Bobek-Billewicz B. External and middle ear diseases: radiological diagnosis based on clinical signs and symptoms. Insights Imaging. 2012;3:33–48.
95. Arnold W, Ganzer U. Otorhinolaryngology, head and neck surgery. Berlin: Springer; 2010.
96. Juliano AF, Ting EY, Mingkwansook V, Hamberg LM, Curtin HD. Vestibular aqueduct measurements in the 45° oblique (Pöschl) plane. Am J Neuroradiol. 2016;37(7):1331–7. A4735v1-0.
97. Bianchini C, Aimoni C, Ceruti S, Grasso DL, Martini A. Lateral sinus thrombosis as a complication of acute mastoiditis. ACTA Otorhinolaryngologica Italica. 2008;28:30–3.
98. Hadlock TA, Ferraro NF, Rahbar R. Acute mastoiditis with temporomandibular joint effusion. Otolaryngol Head Neck Surg. 2001;125:111–2.
99. Weissman JL, Hirsch BE, Chan K, Tabor EK, Curtin HD. Dehiscent temporomandibular joint. Radiology. 1991;180:211–3.
100. Bonjardim LR, Gaviao MB, Carmagnani FG, Pereira LJ, Castelo PM. Signs and symptoms of temporomandibular joint dysfunction in children with primary dentition. J Clin Pediatr Dent. 2003;28:53–8.
101. Castelo PM, Gaviao MB, Pereira LJ, Bonjardim LR. Relationship between oral parafunctional/nutritive sucking habits and temporomandibular joint dysfunction in primary dentition. Int J Paediatr Dent. 2005;15:29–36.
102. Ash CM, Pinto OF. The TMJ and the middle ear: structural and functional correlates for aural symptoms associated with temporomandibular joint dysfunction. Int J Prosthodont. 1991;4:51–7.
103. Bernal M, Tsamtsouris A. Signs and symptoms of temporomandibular joint dysfunction in 3 to 5 year old children. J Pedod. 1986;10:127–40.
104. Somers T, de Foer B, Pauw RJ, Van Havenbergh T, Offeciers EF, Casselman JW. Petrous bone cholesteatoma: the value of MR non-EPI-DW imaging for follow-up after surgery. J Neurol Surg. 2014;75:228.
105. Chung R, Dorros S, Mafee MF, et al. Oper Tech Otolaryngol. 2014;25:58–65.
106. Fruauff K, Coffey K, Chazen JL, Phillips CD. Temporal bone imaging. Top Magn Reson Imaging. 2015;24(1):39–55.
107. Vaid S, Kamble Y, Vaid N, Bhatti S, Rawat S, Nanivadekar A, Karmarkar S. Role of magnetic resonance imaging in cholesteatoma: the Indian experience. Indian J Otolaryngol Head Neck Surg. 2013;65(Suppl 3):485–92.

108. De Foer B, Vercruysse JP, Pilet B, et al. Technical report: single-shot turbo spin echo diffusion-weighted MR imaging versus spin echo planar diffusion-weighted MR imaging in the detection of acquired middle ear cholesteatoma: case report. Am J Neuroradiol. 2006;27:1480–2.
109. Vercruysse JP, De Foer B, Pouillon M, et al. The value of diffusion weighted MR imaging in the diagnosis of primary acquired and residual cholesteatoma: a surgical verified study of 100 patients. Eur Radiol. 2006;16:1461Y7.
110. Lincot J, Veillon F, Riehm S, Babay N, Matern JF, Rock B, Dallaudière B, Meyer N. Middle ear cholesteatoma: compared diagnostic performances of two incremental MRI protocols including non-echo planar diffusion-weighted imaging acquired on 3T and 1.5T scanners. J Neuroradiol. 2015 Jul;42(4):193–201.

Benign and Malignant Tumours of the Ear and Temporal Bone

18

Franciszek Burdan

Neoplasms of the temporal bone, especially malignant ones, are rare. Their occurrence is estimated on 0.2% of all tumours of the head and neck, including lesions of the skin of the pinna that spread to the temporal bone, primary tumours of the external auditory meatus, middle ear and various parts to the temporal bone. Among benign neoplasms, the most common are adenoma, chordoma, lipoma, neurofibroma and schwannoma. Malignancies are usually represented by acinic cell carcinoma, adenocarcinoma, adenoid cystic carcinoma, basal cell carcinoma, squamous cell carcinoma, chondrosarcoma, osteosarcoma, haemato-lymphoid tumours (including lymphomas), rhabdomyosarcoma, melanoma, malignant neuroma and paraganglioma as well as metastatic lesions and infiltration by pharyngeal, parotid and CNS tumours [1, 2]. The lymphatic drainage is typically exclusive for structures of external and middle ear (membranes labyrinth does not have lymph vessels), and their primary lymph nodes are retroauricular, paraauricular and upper deep cervical ones (radiological group II) that drain the lymph from both previous groups. Lymph from the auditory tube is also drained into retropharyngeal nodes but finally is collected by deep cervical ones—group II and III [3–5].

18.1 Primary and Secondary Tumours

In case of pinna and external acoustic meatus, pathologies are usually well-visible as polypoid or ulcerated lesions. Patients with middle ear abnormalities usually suffered from hearing loss, ear fullness, discharge and tinnitus. Less commonly headache and dizziness are pointed out. The concomitant pain, facial weakness,

F. Burdan
Department of Radiology, St. John's Cancer Centre, 7 Jaczewskiego Str. PL-20-090, Lublin, Poland

Department of Human Anatomy, Medical University of Lublin, 4 Jaczewskiego Str. PL-20-090, Lublin, Poland

I. Rozylo-Kalinowska, K. Orhan (eds.), *Imaging of the Temporomandibular Joint*, https://doi.org/10.1007/978-3-319-99468-0_18

swelling in the region (asymmetry) and lesion of CN VII (Bell's palsy) and bleeding are typical for malignant tumours. During otoscopy an intact tympanic membrane with a pathological lesion on its inter side, usually without light reflex, are usually visible [6]. The most common tumours of the external ear derive from the skin. It contains basal and squamous cell carcinomas and melanoma. Higher incidence was noted in age 34–85 years, mostly in males for squamous cell cancer due to higher exposure to actinic, frostbite and radiation. A rare transformation from the squamous papilloma was also reported. In case of the middle ear, the carcinomas arise from the cuboidal and/or pseudostratified epithelium, but never from epidermoid formation—an embryonic epithelial rest associated with a congenital cholesteatoma. A chronic inflammation was also pointed as a risk factor, while sun overexposure was confined for melanoma [2, 7, 8]. Lesions are usually evaluated clinically, and radiological procedures are introduced only in advanced local spread (infiltration of the surrounding cartilages, bones, muscles, parotid gland, vessels), presence of abnormal lymph nodes or to evaluate distant metastases. They present similar radiological shape like in other localization, but more commonly a polypoid structure, rather than plaque-like ones, could be found. In CT, they are visible as isodense or hypodense lesions with a contrast-enhanced (ring shape in case of internal degenerative changes). Bone erosion is visible mostly for malignancies, while a benign lesion usually modulated skeleton structures. In MRI, a characteristic high signal in T1-weighted images was only proved for the melanotic melanoma. Other neoplasms are isodense on T1-weighted images and hyperintense on T2-weighted, with a contrast-enhanced and restricted diffusion on DWI sequence. However, restriction of diffusion and perfusion depends on mitotic activity, degenerative changes and size of the tumour [9–11]. It has to be pointed out the although squamous cell carcinoma and melanoma are aggressive tumours as far as local grow and recurrence are concerned, but lymphatic spread was almost exclusively revealed for melanoma [2, 12]. The perineuronal spreading that may complicate squamous cell carcinoma should be evaluated in MRI and requires a small field of view. Typically, enhancement along chorda tympani, facial, caroticotympanic, deep and lesser petrosal nerves may be visible. It is also important to see potential infiltration of meninges, cerebrum, into auditory tube and in external acoustic meatus, including destruction of their cartilage and infiltration on carotid, parapharyngeal, parotid and masticatory spaces, including TMJ. In case of skeleton destruction, the final diagnosis requires HRCT to evaluate bone lytic lesions [10, 11, 13]. Similar procedures should be done for middle ear meningiomas that arise from pia-arachnoid cells but may be present in a tympanic or mastoid cavity and auditory tube [14]. Meningiomas more commonly arise outside from meninges that surround pyramid and in internal acoustic meatus [15–17]. The proper internal tumours are located inside and at least at the beginning are encapsulated by bony elements. The secondary meningiomas of the internal ear may grow into pneumatic structures of the temporal bone from pericerebral space or are considered as intraosseous variant. Both types are more often in females, mainly in age 10–80 years, in mean age in females 52 and 44.8 in males [1, 2]. The clinical symptoms are typical for other benign tumour of the middle ear while radiological one for meningioma of the classic paracerebral localization.

In non-contrast CT, tumours are usually slightly hyperdense or isodense to normal brain. In some cases, a calcification and hyperostosis may be found. Similar features are reported in MRI (Fig. 18.1).

The tumour is usually homogeneous and well-circumscribed, isointense to grey matter on both T1- and T2-weighted images. Lower signal may be seen in fibrous and psammomatous variants. Hyperintense loci in T2-weighted are secondary to cystic lesion and soft or cartilage tissue, choroid deposits and angiomatous variant. In both modalities, a homogeneous post-contrast enhancement of the tumour and surrounding meninges (dural tail sign) is typical. In cystic or malignant variations, the enhancement could be heterogenic. The tumour may present restriction diffusion on DWI [18]. Spectroscopic abnormalities, such as an increase in alanine, glutamine/glutamate and choline (Cho) and absent or significantly reduced N-acetylaspartate (NAA) and creatine (Cr), were reported [19]. It should be noted that radiologically calculated apparent diffusion coefficient (ADC) value and volume transfer constant (k-trans) are helpful to evaluate aggressiveness, since both correlate with histological grade [20, 21]. In suspicion of brain invasion, the surrounding cerebrospinal fluid level and enhancement of the attached part of the brain should be checked. An interventional angiography is currently limited to preoperative embolization to reduce intraoperative blood loss, but even such procedure is rarely used.

Neoplasms, limited exclusively to the external ear, are rare and arise from ceruminous glands. The adenoma (ceruminoma) and syringocystadenoma papilliferum are typical benign tumours, while an adenoid cystic carcinoma is the most common among malignant ones. They are observed in mature persons (mean 49 years; age 26–89) without any sex prediction, in exception to syringocystadenoma papilliferum that is typical for children and young adults. Cylindroma, a benign tumour that develops from the epidermal adnexa, may be found in such localization as well. In some cases, the lesions are multiple and seen in various loci in external ear and scalp as a part of so-called turban tumour [1, 2]. A primary malignant tumour of such localization is a ceruminous adenocarcinoma accounting less than 2.5% of tumours of external auditory meatus, which is characterized by a t(6:9) chromosomal translocation, resulting in *MYB-NFIB* gene fusion [22]. The aural polyp in the external acoustic meatus could be visible in young children [23, 24]. It is formed by embryonal rhabdomyosarcoma that usually develops in the tympanic cavity and extends to the meatus. Their radiological signs are similar to those presented above, but since they are evaluated at an early stage, some of them are not visible due to small size.

A higher contrast enhancement should be seen in tumours with a large amount of blood vessels as angiolymphoid hyperplasia with eosinophilia and soft tissue haemangiomas. The first disease is seen mostly in females in age over 50. Patients usually connect the lesion with an ear trauma, followed by chronic inflammation. Macroscopically and radiologically, the tumour looks similar to inflammatory lesion typical for Kimura disease that has to be differentiated on histological level. Moreover, the disease is endemic and found mostly among man in the Far East [25]. Soft tissue haemangiomas, presently known as slow-flow venous malformations,

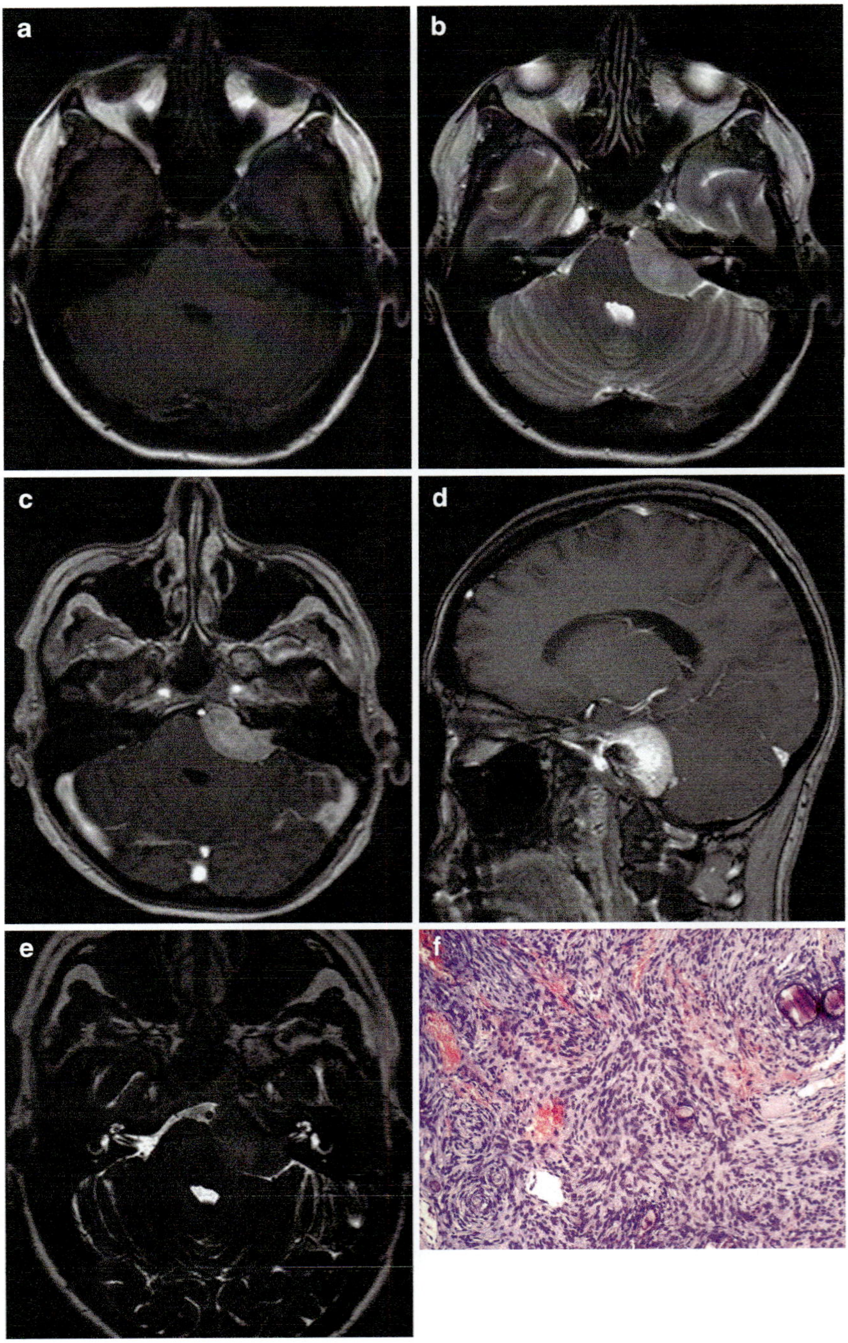

Fig. 18.1 MRI images showing the meningioma of the left pontocerebellar angle with an extension to the internal acoustic meatus. T1-weighted (**a**), T2-weighted (**b**) and T1-weighted post-contrast (**c**) axial images. Sagittal T1-weighted post-contrast (**d**). *3D T2-weighted* isovoxel *sequence* (**e**). Haematoxylin- and eosin-stained specimen of the tumour (**f**)

are lesions with a high female predilection, commonly seen in all age groups, especially in children. Histologically, they are classified into five types: capillary, cavernous, arteriovenous, venous and mixed. In case of skin location, they are well-visible, but muscular, synovial or other ones can be observed on a classic radiogram exclusively in case of large size with a secondary local swelling, which will be concomitant with phleboliths. The method of choice in their primary evaluation is still a colour Doppler ultrasound. In complicated cases, a CT or, better, MR with a contrast enhancement is recommended. In CT, an isodense, lobulated and heterogeneous structures without local invasion but with phleboliths could be seen. Similar features may be observed in T1-weighted sequence in MRI, but the signal could be from intermediate to slightly high in comparing to surrounding muscles. In T2-weighted images, the lesion has high signal. The contrast enhancement is spectacular in both CT and MRI [26].

Adenoma of the middle ear is a benign neoplasm with a differentiation along neuroendocrine and mucin-secreting pathways [1, 13]. It is an uncommon disease that occurs mostly in age of 20–80 years, without any sex privilege. A chronic local inflammation was selected as a precursor lesion. The first symptom is a muffled hearing with a pressure sensation, but in advanced stage after auricular ossicles are involved, a conductive hearing loss may be present. In most cases, the tumour is connected with a tympanic membrane, but it was also reported in other parts of middle ear, including the mastoid cavity and auditory tube. CT is slightly helpful and shows a nonspecific mass, with possible extension to the middle ear and/or the mastoid. The abnormal structure may obliterate auricular ossicles but without any bony destruction. In MRI, the lesion is isointense to hyperintense in the T1-weighted images, with a contrast enhancement. In the T2-weighted images, its signal is comparable to intensity of the grey matter. The lesion has to be differentiated from glomus tympanicum (paraganglioma) that is characterized by pulsatile tinnitus, due to a close relationship between the tumour and tympanic nerve (Jacobson's nerve) or its branches, and flushing vascular angiography [13]. Similar tumours—jugulotympanic paragangliomas (Fig. 18.2)—arise on the level of jugular bulb and damage jugular (inferior) tympanic wall. They are visible mostly in female in age over 50 years. A high coexistence with chondromatosis, pheochromocytoma and other paragangliomas as well as familial settings indicates genetic susceptibility that includes mutation in selected genes: *NF1*, *ATRS*, *HRAS*, *VHL*, *EPAS1*, EGLN1/EGLN2, *CDKN2A*, *RET*, *TP53*, *MET*, *BRAF*, *MAX*, *IDH1*, *KIF1B*, *SDHA/SDHB/SDHC/SDHD/AF2*, *TMEM127*, *FH* and *MEN1* [2]. In case paraganglioma is found, based on radiological observation, it has to be classified according to Fisch-Mattox (Table 18.1) and Glasscock-Jackson system (Table 18.2), applied for the tympanic/middle and tympano-jugular paragangliomas, respectively [27, 28].

Papillary tumour of the middle ear is a rare, aggressive form of adenoma that was reported more often in females with age range 16–55 years, but most patients suffered from various symptoms for many years before surgical treatment [1, 2]. It must be mentioned that some of them were described as a low-grade adenocarcinoma of possible endolymphatic sac origin. The localization is typical, mostly limited to tympanic and mastoid cavity, but cases involving apical part of tympanic pyramid with bone destruction and penetration into the pontocerebellar angle and

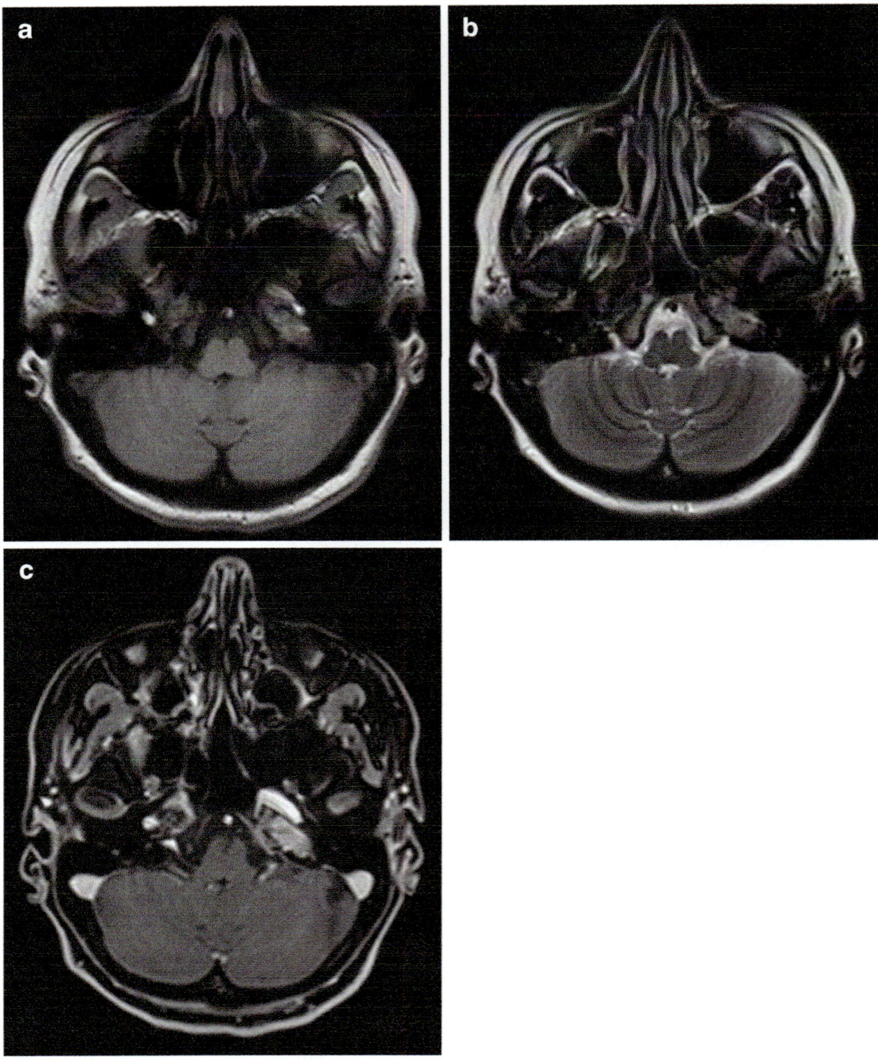

Fig. 18.2 MRI images showing jugulotympanic paraganglioma of the left jugular bulb and apex of the petrous part of the left temporal bone. T1-weighted (**a**), T2-weighted (**b**) and T1-weighted post-contrast (**c**) axial images

cerebellum were found. It is also suggested that the neoplasm coexists and/or is related to the apical petrous bone neoplasia, since they often coexist, share histological similarity and are part of von Hippel-Lindau disease [29]. Clinical features at the beginning are similar to the adenoma, but perforation of tympanic membrane and penetration to the external acoustic meatus were also reported. In CT, a concomitant lytic bone lesion could be seen.

Table 18.1 The Fisch-Mattox classification of tympanic/middle ear paragangliomas [27]

Type	Tumour characteristic
A	Limited to the tympanic cavity
B	Limited to the tympanomastoid area with no infralabyrinthine compartment involvement
C	Involving the infralabyrinthine compartment of the temporal bone and extending into the petrous apex
C1	Limited involvement of the vertical portion of the carotid canal
C2	Invading the vertical portion of the carotid canal
C3	Invasion of the horizontal portion of the carotid canal
D	Intracranial extension
De1	Intracranial but extradural extension less than 2 cm in diameter
De2	Intracranial but extradural extension greater than 2 cm in diameter
Di1	Intracranial and dural extension less than 2 cm in diameter
Di2	Intracranial and dural extension between 2–4 cm in diameter
Di3	Intracranial and dural extension greater than 4 cm in diameter

Table 18.2 The Glasscock-Jackson classification of the tympanic and jugular paragangliomas [28]

	Tumour characteristic	
Type	Tympanic	Jugular
I	Limited to the promontory	Involves jugular bulb, middle ear and mastoid
II	Completely fills the middle ear space	Extends underneath internal auditory canal with or without intracranial extension
III	Fills the middle ear and extends to mastoid	Extends into pyramidal apex with or without intracranial extension
IV	Extend into external auditory canal and may extend anterior to internal carotid artery	Extends into clivus and infratemporal fossa with or without intracranial extension

Similar clinical and radiological features may be shared by other rare neoplasms such as Schneiderian-type and inverted papilloma, originally derived from respiratory epithelium. Hamartoma are rare in temporal bone and its region. Furthermore, a few cases of choristoma (formed by tissues which are not present in the area) were revealed. Hinni and Beatty [30] as well as Kamerer and Caparosa [31] reported salivary gland and glial choristoma in the middle ear, respectively.

Temporal bone is also related to neuronal pathologies. One of them is a vestibular/acoustic schwannoma that derives from glial-neurilemmal junction of nerve sheath, mostly vestibular division of the CN VIII. It is visible in the internal auditory meatus or cerebellopontine/pontine angle [32]. Its occurrence is relatively high and rich 7–8% of all intracranial tumours, with a highest frequency among people in age 50–60 or in younger with neurofibromatosis type 2—an autosomal dominant disorder with schwannomas located bilaterally and involving other cranial and peripheral nerves [2, 33]. Besides typical symptoms such as tinnitus and sensorineural hearing loss, patients also complain on headache, vertigo, facial pain and weakness; even big lesions may often be incidental and asymptomatic findings. Large tumours may develop mass effect with cerebellar and brainstem symptoms, e.g. hydrocephalus and cranial nerve dysfunction other than CNVIII. Radiologically, the tumour presents as a solid nodular mass with a typical intracanalicular component that often widening of the internal porus acoustics. However, the extracanalicular lesions also exist. The tumour may also grow laterally through the cochlea (transmodiolar) or vestibule (transmacular) into the middle ear. Lesions limited exclusively to the vestibule (intravestibular), cochlea (intracochlear) or both structures (vestibulocochlear) were also described [34]. Tumours, especially small ones, may not be seen in non-contrast CT. But large lesions are well-visible as isodense mass with a widening of the internal acoustic canal. The signal of the tumour is slightly hypo- or isointense in T1- or heterogeneously hyperintense to adjacent brain in T2-weighted images (Fig. 18.3). Cystic areas show signal typical for fluid (Fig. 18.4). In both modalities, most tumours show intense contrast enhancement with or without cystic degeneration and haemorrhagic areas. The differential diagnosis includes especially meningioma that is more homogeneous, with calcification and enhancement of the attached dura mater. On the level of cerebellopontine angle, also an epidermoid may be visible, but it has components with restricted diffusion and ones without contrast enhancement. Ependymoma of the IV ventricle and metastases have to be mentioned as well, but they usually never extend into the internal acoustic meatus. On the base of the meatus, microneuromas may be found. They are small non-neoplastic tumours formed by intertwined bundles of neuronal fibres and Schwann cells, forming structure similar to posttraumatic neuromas noted almost exclusively in Paget's disease (see below). However, they are relatively small and seldom observed in any visualization methods. Rare lipoma has to be also mentioned, but it has a high signal on T1-weighted image that is low in fat-saturation sequences. Vascular networks around geniculate and cochlear ganglion are the origin of rare observed haemangiomas of the internal acoustic meatus—their radiological features were explained above [32, 34].

Endolymphatic sac tumour is a rare non-metastatic adenocarcinoma of the endolymphatic sac found only in adults with a higher coexistence with von Hippel-Lindau disease [35, 36]. Its pathognomonic, radiological sign is a destruction of the posterior wall of the pyramid behind the internal acoustic meatus. However, the tumour may infiltrate the middle ear and cerebellopontine angle. Symptoms of Ménière's disease (tinnitus, hearing loss and dizziness) may be reported initially as a result of pathological enlargement of membranous labyrinth, secondary to endolymphatic duct and/or sac obstruction. In a later stage, a lesion of CNVII is common.

In the temporal squama or its junction with a tegmentum tympani and external acoustic meatus, a Langerhans cell histiocytosis (solitary eosinophilic granuloma) may be located. It is a rare disease seen mostly in Caucasian children with 2:1 male/female ratio [2]. Clinically, pain, swelling and tenderness around the lesion are reported. On radiogram or CT, a solitary or lytic area (cortical erosion) without sclerotic rim is noted. In case of flat bone (like temporal squama), a double contour or bevelled edge appearance may be seen, due to greater involvement of the inner layer. In MRI a low signal in T1-, iso- to hyperintense in T2-weighted, hyperintense on STIR (short T1 inversion recovery) and contrast enhancement are visible. Similar characteristic may be seen for solitary plasmacytoma of the bone, but in case of the skull, it was found only in the mandible

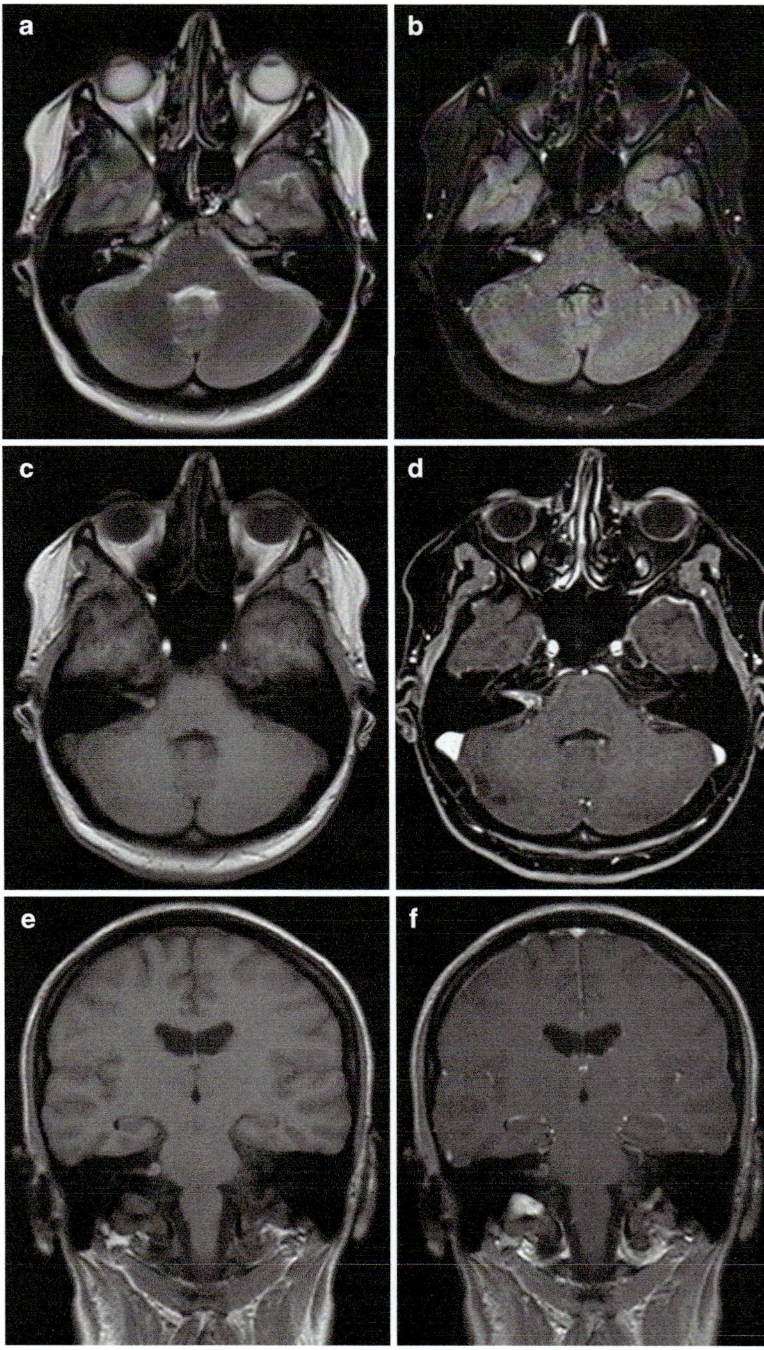

Fig. 18.3 MRI images of small schwannoma of the right vestibulocochlear nerve. T2-weighted (**a**), T2-fluid-attenuated inversion recovery (**b**), T1-weighted (**c**) and T1-weighted post-contrast (**d**) axial images. T1-weighted (**e**) and T1-weighted post-contrast (**f**) coronal images

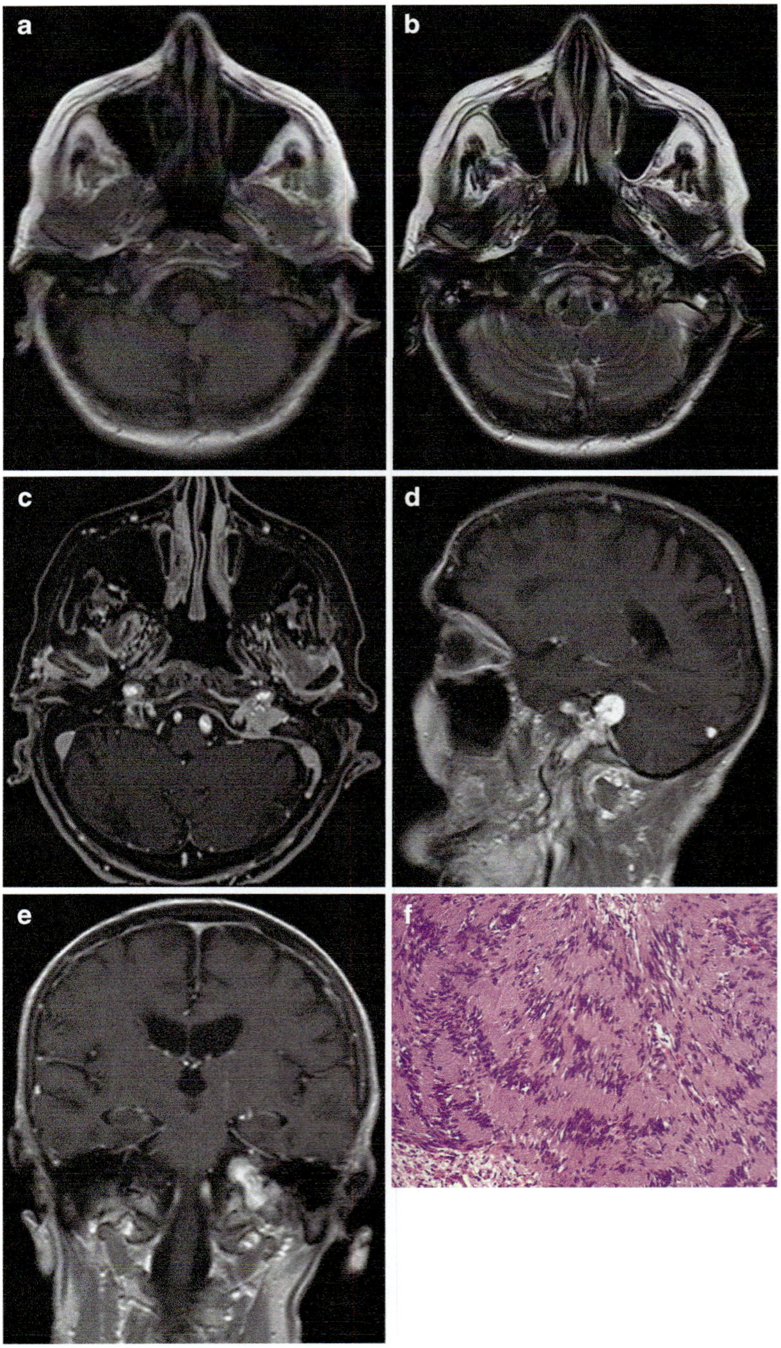

Fig. 18.4 MRI images of giant schwannoma of the left vestibulocochlear nerve with cystic degeneration. T1-weighted (**a**), T2-weighted (**b**) and T1-weighted post-contrast (**c**) axial images. Sagittal (**d**) and coronal (**e**) T1-weighted post-contrast (**d**) images. Haematoxylin- and eosin-stained specimen of the tumour (**f**)

and maxilla [9]. On the other hand, the squamal localization is typical for extremely rare chondroblastoma that arise almost exclusively in the temporal squama. Its high predilection for *H3F3B* point mutation was reported [2]. Other cartilage derivative lesions such as chondroma, idiopathic pseudocystic chondromalacia and chondrodermatitis nodularis chronica helicis are radiolucent and usually too small for radiological evaluation, but in debatable cases, an MRI is recommended to evaluated local advance. They are usually found in cartilage of auditory tube, external acoustic meatus and pinna. Chondrosarcoma and mesenchymal chondrosarcoma develop almost exclusively in facial skeleton, particularly in the maxilla, nasal septum and mandible, but are seldom in patients with Ollier disease and Maffucci syndrome [37, 38]. The first can be seen in any age while the mesenchymal type only in person over 40 years old. A genetic predisposition for chondrosarcoma (mutation in *IDH1/IDH2*) and mesenchymal chondrosarcoma (*HEY1-NCOA2* fusion, absence of *IDH1/IDH2* mutation) was found [2]. Single cases of chondromyxoid fibroma were also described in TMJ region but rarely involving temporal bone [39].

The ear may be also related to bone-related tumours. Osteoma is a benign, slowly growing and, usually, asymptomatic bony tumour, seen in membranaceus derivative bones (e.g. temporal squama). It may be single or multiple (Gardner syndrome—mutation in *APC* gene) [2]. Osteoma has similar radiological features to exostosis (osteochondroma) of the external acoustic meatus, which are trauma-related (chronic exposure to cold water, chronic inflammation or use ear plagues/stethoscope, etc.). Traditionally, lesions are divided into ivory (compact bone without Haversian canals), mature (trabecular bone with canals and marrow) and mixed osteoma. They are usually well-visible during various radiological procedures as radiodense lesions with a density similar to the normal cortex, whereas mature osteomas may present marrow spaces. Surgical excision is recommended only in functional or cosmetic impairment [40, 41].

Osteoid osteoma with typical radiological nidus was only found in the mandible not in the temporal bone. The mandible location is also typical of osteoblastoma and desmoplastic fibroma; while ossifying fibroma (cemento-ossifying fibroma) and familial gigantiform cementoma are limited to alveolar structures of mandible and maxilla [1, 2, 42].

Primary malignant bone tumours have not been reported in temporal bone. Osteosarcoma is rare in TMJ region, but in case it is present, it usually develops from the mandible or maxilla. Osteosarcoma, unlike the peripherally located neoplasm that is typical for children and adolescents in jaw, is seen in person in age around 20–30 years, with a low connection to previous radiotherapy. Higher risk was reported for persons with amplification of *MDM2* gene, retinoblastoma, Li-Fraumeni, Werner and Rothmund-Thomson syndrome [1, 2, 42]. However, the metastatic changes spread by blood and lymphatic canals without direct infiltration from primary lesions occur more commonly. According to various authors, their most typical origins are carcinomas of the breast, head and neck region, lung and prostate and melanoma. They are usually observed in the pyramidal apex, mastoid process, internal acoustic meatus and middle ear, followed by other structures. On the other hand, a direct infiltration is typical for advanced nasopharyngeal and parotid neoplasms [1, 40].

18.2 Tumour-Like Disease

A different characteristic has been reported of tumour-like disease such as fibrous dysplasia, Paget's disease and exostosis [40, 43].

Fibrous dysplasia is a non-neoplastic tumour-like defect in osteoblastic differentiation and maturation, in which the normal bone is replace by fibrous structures and islands of immature woven bone. Cranial monostotic forms—limited to the temporal bone or mandible—are rare. Genreally, the cranial localization has been proved in 10–25 and 50% in monostotic (70–80%) and polyostotic cases (20–30%) that are typical for McCune-Albright syndrome. The disease is related to postzygotic activating missense mutation of *GNAS* that codes the alpha subunit of the stimulatory G protein. The secondary overexpression of cAMP activates bone osteoprogenitor cells that are responsible for an abnormal bone formation. However, different forms such as a craniofacial fibrous dysplasia and cherubism (not true fibrous dysplasia of mandible and maxilla) also exist [2]. The disease is usually asymptomatic and does not require any treatment. Clinical symptoms may arise due to bony expansion or remodelling and secondary compression of vessels and nerves and displacement of adjacent structures. Radiologically, different signs are seen, e.g. ground-glass matrix and cystic, sclerotic or well-circumscribed lesions but without the periosteal reaction. A so-called rind sign—a lesion surrounded by a layer of thick, sclerotic reactive bone—has been also described, but it is well-visible mostly in the femur. The diagnosis is easier in polyostotic form, since bubbly cystic lesions, fusiform enlargement of long bones (especially ribs), limb length discrepancy, bowing deformities, shepherd crook deformity of the femoral neck and protrusio acetabuli helped in the final diagnosis. However, in an early stage, the lesion(s) may be radiolucent. In CT, the ground-glass opacities and homogeneously sclerotic lesions with well-defined borders are seen. Less commonly, cystic lesion, expansion of the bone with intact overlying and endosteal scalloping could be found. CT is more useful than MRI, since heterogeneous signal is typically visible in T2 and T1-weighted images and after gadolinium injection. However, it is helpful in differential diagnosis that includes Paget's disease (similar radiological signs but appears in people over 40 years), neurofibromatosis type I (rare bone changes, mostly in vertebrae and ribs) or, less possible due to location, osteofibrous dysplasia and adamantinoma (mostly tibia) or rarely visible non-ossifying fibroma, simple bone cyst, giant cell tumour and enchondromatosis. A café au lait skin pigmentation and endocrine abnormalities are helpful for the primary diagnosis of McCune-Albright syndrome [40, 44].

Paget's disease is another non-neoplastic tumour-like defect characterized by excessive abnormal remodelling of the skull, bones of pelvis, spine and long bones with an increase blood activity of serum alkaline phosphatase and urine level of hydroxyproline. It appears in personas over 40 with a slight male predilection. Patients complain usually on well-localized pain and tenderness, increased focal temperature (due to hypervascularity) and bone size, bowing deformities, pathological kyphosis of the spine and decreased in the range of motion. The nonspecific treatments (bisphosphonates, non-steroidal anti-inflammatory drugs, etc.) are usually needed, especially in the case of complications that include bone deformity and fractures; damage of nearby located nerves, vessels and structures; and increased risk of osteoarthritis, hyperparathyroidism, extramedullary haematopoiesis, congestive cardiac failure, giant cell tumour and osteosarcoma that in the skull usually occupies the maxilla and mandible. In case of temporal bone involvement, a conductive and sensorineural hearing loss may appear due to fixation of the middle ear ossicles, compression of the CNVIII in the internal acoustic meatus and/or secondary damage of bony labyrinth due to the mineral density loss [1, 2, 42]. The radiological features mostly depend on the form of the diseases (lytic, incipient active; sclerotic, late inactive; mixed, active). However, initially osteolytic changes always occur that later are replaced by coarsened trabeculae and bony enlargement. In the case of the skull, in advance stage, lytic lesions may unit together (osteoporosis circumscripta) or mixed with sclerotic lesions (cotton wool appearance). A diploic widening and frontal bone enlargement (tam-o'-shanter sign) are noted. Cortical thickening could be also observed, but it is more typical for vertebrae and pelvis. All signs could be found on classic radiographs and CT. In MRI, the lytic lesions have relatively low signal in T1- and high on T2-weighted pictures, especially in active process due to granulation tissue, hypervascularity and oedema. Low single in T2 may appear in presence of compact bone or fibrous tissue. All modalities, particularly CT, are helpful in the differential diagnosis that in the case of the skull includes fibrous dysplasia (see above) and hyperostosis frontalis interna (thickening of the internal periosteum limited only to frontal squama) [40, 42].

Tumour-like bone structure could be also seen in otosclerosis that is more typical for Caucasian than for African or Asian population. It is more commonly visible in females, patients with conductive hearing loss in particularly in age over 30–50 with a high familial link. The proper—histologically proved—incidence is even higher as it was found in autopsy studies. The disease is characterized by progressive remodelling of bone labyrinth, secondary to abnormal collagen synthesis. Sclerotic plaques on microscopic level may mimic low-grade neoplasm, and they are observed usually on the level or close to stapes of footplate and cochlea. In advance stages, a thickness of the bony labyrinth with a concomitant decrease of internal space is visible. However, no typical features were reported for an early form [1, 2, 42].

18.3 Summary

Benign and malignant tumours of the temporal bone are rare but may involve a morphology and function of the temporomandibular joint. Among benign neoplasms, the most common are adenoma, chordoma, lipoma, meningioma, neurofibroma and schwannoma. Malignancies are usually represented by acinic cell carcinoma, adenocarcinoma, adenoid cystic carcinoma, basal cell carcinoma, squamous cell carcinoma, chondrosarcoma, osteosarcoma, haemato-lymphoid tumours (including lymphoma), rhabdomyosarcoma, melanoma, malignant neuroma and paraganglioma as well as metastatic lesions and infiltration by pharyngeal, parotid and central nervous system tumours. Tumour-like disease such as fibrous dysplasia, Paget's disease and exostosis may also be visible in such localization.

Acknowledgements I would like to thank Professor Justyna Szumilo and Professor Robert Klepacz (Clinical Pathomorphology Department, Medical University of Lublin), Dr. Luiza Grzycka-Kowalczyk (Radiology and Nuclear Medicine Department, Medical University of Lublin), and Dr. Marzena Janczarek (Interventional Radiology Department, Medical University of Lublin), as well as Dr. Maciej Siczek (Radiology Department, Hospital of Ministry of Interior and Administration in Lublin) for their critical comments on the manuscript and/or photo documentation.

References

1. Barnes L, Eveson JW, Reichart P, Sidransky D. World Health Organization classification of tumours. Pathology & genetics of head and neck tumours. Lyon: International Agency for Research on Cancer; 2005.
2. El-Naggar AK, Chan JKC, Rubin GJ, Takata T, Slootweg PJ. WHO classification of head and neck tumours. Lyon: International Agency for Research on Cancer; 2017.
3. Bochenek A, Raicher M. Human anatomy. Warszawa: PZWL; 2007.
4. Kurlej WL, Gworys B, Burdan F. Anatomy for dentists. Wroclaw: Elsevier; 2011.
5. Standring S. Gray's anatomy, the anatomical basis of clinical practice. 40th ed. New York: Elsevier; 2008. p. 615–34.
6. Trojanowska A, Drop A, Trojanowski P, Rosińska-Bogusiewicz K, Klatka J, Bobek-Billewicz B. External and middle ear diseases: radiological diagnosis based on clinical signs and symptoms. Insights Imaging. 2012;3:33–48.
7. Chen KT, Dehner LP. Primary tumors of the external and middle ear. I. Introduction and clinicopathologic study of squamous cell carcinoma. Arch Otolaryngol. 1978;104:247–52.
8. Testa JR, Fukuda Y, Kowalski LP. Prognostic factors in carcinoma of the external auditory canal. Arch Otolaryngol Head Neck Surg. 1997;123:720–4.
9. Becker M, Stefanelli S, Rougemont AL, Poletti PA, Merlini L. Non-odontogenic tumors of the facial bones in children and adolescents: role of multiparametric imaging. Neuroradiology. 2017;59:327–42.
10. Trojanowska A, Czekajska-Chehab E, Trojanowski P, Olszanski W, Klatka J, Drop A, Golabek W. Comparison of multidetector row CT cross-sectional source images with multiplanar 2D-, 3D- reconstructions and virtual endoscopy in assessment of the middle ear. J Neuroradiol. 2006;33:277–8.
11. Trojanowska A, Trojanowski P, Olszanski W, Klatka J, Drop A. How to reliably evaluate middle ear diseases? Comparison of different methods of post-processing based on multislice computed tomography examination. Acta Otolaryngol. 2007;127:258–64.
12. Patel TD, Chin OY, Baredes S, Eloy JA, Ying YM. A population based analysis of melanoma of the external ear. Otol Neurotol. 2018;39(2):e137–42.
13. Cardoso FA, Monteiro EMR, Lopes LB, Avila MNDC, Scarioli BO. Adenomatous tumors of the middle ear: a literature review. Int Arch Otorhinolaryngol. 2017;21:308–12.
14. Bruninx L, Govaere F, Van Dorpe J, Forton GE. Isolated synchronous meningioma of the external ear canal and the temporal lobe. B-ENT. 2013;9:157–60.
15. Bassiouni H, Hunold A, Asgari S, Stolke D. Meningiomas of the posterior petrous bone: functional outcome after microsurgery. J Neurosurg. 2004;100:1014–24.
16. Carney AS, Ward V, Malluci CL, O'Donoghue GM, Robertson I, Baldwin DL, Maw AR, Coakham HB. Meningiomas involving the internal auditory canal: a diagnostic and surgical challenge. Skull Base Surg. 1999;9:87–94.

17. Moura da Silva LF Jr, Buffon VA, Coelho Neto M, Ramina R. Non-schwannomatosis lesions of the internal acoustic meatus-a diagnostic challenge and management: a series report of nine cases. Neurosurg Rev. 2015;38:641–8.
18. Matsushima N, Maeda M, Takamura M, Matsubara T, Taki W, Takeda K. MRI findings of atypical meningioma with microcystic changes. J Neuro-Oncol. 2007;82:319–21.
19. Fountas KN, Kapsalaki EZ, Gotsis SD, Kapsalakis JZ, Smisson HF 3rd, Johnston KW, Robinson JS Jr, Papadakis N. In vivo proton magnetic resonance spectroscopy of brain tumors. Stereotact Funct Neurosurg. 2000;74:83–94.
20. Chu JP, Mak HK, Yau KK, Zhang L, Tsang J, Chan Q, Leung GK. Pilot study on evaluation of any correlation between MR perfusion (Ktrans) and diffusion (apparent diffusion coefficient) parameters in brain tumors at 3 Tesla. Cancer Imaging. 2012;12:1–6.
21. Santelli L, Ramondo G, Della Puppa A, Ermani M, Scienza R, d'Avella D, Manara R. Diffusion-weighted imaging does not predict histological grading in meningiomas. Acta Neurochir. 2010;152:1315–9.
22. Ruhl DS, Tolisano AM, Swiss TP, Littlefield PD, Golden JB. Ceruminous adenocarcinoma: an analysis of the Surveillance Epidemiology and End Results (SEER) database. Am J Otolaryngol. 2016;37:70–3.
23. Shew M, Bush J, Tawfik O, Ator G. Middle ear aural polyp mimicking glomus tympanicum in a male adolescent. Otol Neurotol. 2017;38:e211–3.
24. Vasiwala R, Burud I, Lum SK, Saren RS. Embryonal rhabdomyosarcoma of the middle ear presenting with aural polyp and facial nerve palsy. Med J Malaysia. 2015;70:314–5.
25. Dokania V, Patil D, Agarwal K, Thakur P, Prajapati P. Kimura's disease without peripheral eosinophilia: an unusual and challenging case simulating venous malformation on imaging studies - case report and review of literature. J Clin Diagn Res. 2017;11:ME01–4.
26. Wu JS, Hochman MG. Soft-tissue tumours and tumorlike lesions: a systematic imaging approach. Radiology. 2009;253:297–316.
27. Fisch U, Mattox DE. Microsurgery of the skull bone. Sttutgart: Thieme Medical Publisher; 1988.
28. Jackson CG, Glasscock ME, Harris PF. Glomus tumours: diagnosis, classification and management of large lesions. Otolaryngology. 1982;8:401–6.
29. Duderstadt M, Förster C, Welkoborsky HJ, Ostertag H. Adenomatous tumors of the middle ear and temporal bone: clinical, morphological and tumor biological characteristics of challenging neoplastic lesions. Eur Arch Otorhinolaryngol. 2012;269:823–31.
30. Hinni ML, Beatty CW. Salivary gland choristoma of the middle ear: report of a case and review of the literature. Ear Nose Throat J. 1996;75:422–4.
31. Kamerer DB, Caparosa RJ. Temporal bone encephalocele – diagnosis and treatment. Laryngoscope. 1982;92(8 Pt 1):878–82.
32. Wiggins RH 3rd, Harnsberger HR, Salzman KL, Shelton C, Kertesz TR, Glastonbury CM. The many faces of facial nerve schwannoma. AJNR Am J Neuroradiol. 2006;27:694–9.
33. Sarolia SP, Danner CJ, Erdem E. Facial nerve schwannoma presenting as a tympanic mass. Ear Nose Throat J. 2006;85:366–8.
34. Bittencourt AG, Alves RD, Ikari LS, Burke PR, Gebrim EM, Bento RF. Intracochlear schwannoma: diagnosis and management. Int Arch Otorhinolaryngol. 2014;18:322–4.
35. Bausch B, Wellner U, Peyre M, Boedeker CC, Hes FJ, Anglani M, de Campos JM, Kanno H, Maher ER, Krauss T, Sansó G, Barontini M, Letizia C, Hader C, Schiavi F, Zanoletti E, Suárez C, Offergeld C, Malinoc A, Zschiedrich S, Glasker S, Bobin S, Sterkers O, Ba Huy PT, Giraud S, Links T, Eng C, Opocher G, Richard S, Neumann HP, International Endolymphatic Sac Tumor (ELST) Consortium. Characterization of endolymphatic sac tumors and von Hippel-Lindau disease in the International Endolymphatic Sac Tumor Registry. Head Neck. 2016;38(Suppl 1):E673–9.
36. Zanoletti E, Girasoli L, Borsetto D, Opocher G, Mazzoni A, Martini A. Endolymphatic sac tumour in von Hippel-Lindau disease: management strategies. Acta Otorhinolaryngol Ital. 2017;37:423–9.

37. Noël G, Feuvret L, Calugaru V, Hadadi K, Baillet F, Mazeron JJ, Habrand JL. Chondrosarcomas of the base of the skull in Ollier's disease or Maffucci's syndrome--three case reports and review of the literature. Acta Oncol. 2004;43:705–10.
38. Sun GH, Myer CM 3rd. Otolaryngologic manifestations of Maffucci's syndrome. Int J Pediatr Otorhinolaryngol. 2009;73:1015–8.
39. Oh N, Khorsandi AS, Scherl S, Wang B, Wenig BM, Manolidis S, Jacobson A. Chondromyxoid fibroma of the mastoid portion of the temporal bone: MRI and PET/CT findings and their correlation with histology. Ear Nose Throat J. 2013;92:201–3.
40. Kunimatsu A, Kunimatsu N. Skull base tumors and tumor-like lesions: a pictorial review. Pol J Radiol. 2017;82:398–409.
41. Vérillaud B, Guilleré L, Williams MT, El Bakkouri W, Ayache D. Middle ear osteoma: a rare cause of conductive hearing loss with normal tympanic membrane. Rev Laryngol Otol Rhinol (Bord). 2011;132:159–61.
42. Scutellari PN, Giorgi A, De Sario V, Campanati P. Correlation of multimodality imaging in Paget's disease of bone. Radiol Med. 2005;110:603–15.
43. Unni KK, Dahlin DC. Premalignant tumors and conditions of bone. Am J Surg Pathol. 1979;3:47–60.
44. Bulakbaşi N, Bozlar U, Karademir I, Kocaoğlu M, Somuncu I. CT and MRI in the evaluation of craniospinal involvement with polyostotic fibrous dysplasia in McCune-Albright syndrome. Diagn Interv Radiol. 2008;14:177–81.

Micro-CT Applications in TMJ Research

19

Kaan Orhan, Mert Ocak, and Burak Bilecenoglu

19.1 Micro-computed Tomography (Micro-CT)

Just like tomography, micro-computed tomography (micro-CT) has the ability to create cross-sectional images of a physical object by making use of X-rays. Cross-sectional images created this way are then processed by relevant software in the computer environment, and a three-dimensional model of the scanned object is hence created in the digital environment. Since the pixels forming the 2D cross-sectional images obtained by micro-tomography are in terms of micro- (μ) units, scientific and processable information on internal structures and geometries of tiny objects or appropriately sized pieces of larger objects can be attained. Research on the use of micro-CT and 3D printer technologies for medical and industrial prototyping processes are becoming ever widespread both in our country and throughout the world. Processing of CT or micro-CT scanning data of a biological structure and subsequent modeling of its three-dimensional model in the digital environment create its own application areas in numerous fields. Having the ability to produce structures by using 3D printers, such as cranial models, skeletal models, bones, organs, etc. to be utilized as educational materials in medical faculties or life sciences departments, results in benefits such as more efficient training regarding the field of education. Another application is the modeling and consequent 3D printing of the body part that is to undertake surgery prior to the surgical operation, which allows attaining more efficient results both for patients and surgeons by shortening the duration of surgery and allowing the surgeon to work with a material similar to the patient's own.

K. Orhan (✉)
Department of Dentomaxillofacial Radiology, Ankara University, Faculty of Dentistry, Ankara, Turkey

M. Ocak
Hacettepe University, Faculty of Medicine, Department of Anatomy, Ankara, Turkey

B. Bilecenoglu
Ankara University, Faculty of Dentistry, Department of Anatomy, Ankara, Turkey

I. Rozylo-Kalinowska, K. Orhan (eds.), *Imaging of the Temporomandibular Joint*, https://doi.org/10.1007/978-3-319-99468-0_19

Hounsfield created the very first full-body computed tomography device back in 1975, and Hounsfield and Cormack received the Nobel Prize for physiology and medicine with this device in 1979. Main components of the micro-tomography device are the X-ray tube, a computer-driven step motor that intermittently rotates the sample mounted on its body, an image intensifier which focuses the X-rays in the medium onto the camera sensor, a CCD camera which converts X-rays received into image data, an image collector, and a computer that controls all these components. Better spatial resolution is attained by 5–10 μm^3 voxel size scan provided by micro-computerized tomography, compared to 1 mm^3 voxel size scan provided by computerized tomography. This makes viewing areas 1,000,000 times smaller than that could be viewed by computerized tomography possible, which in turn allows conducting more detailed investigations. This was regarded as a revolutionary development [1, 2] (Fig. 19.1).

Micro-CT scanners are mostly utilized in academic and industrial research laboratories. Micro-CT scanners are used in such institutions usually for the examination of mineralized tissues such as the teeth and bones, ceramics, polymers, and biomaterials. Different fields of views (FOV) could be selected by micro-CT devices relevant to the dimensions of the area to be examined, and hence, higher-resolution images can be obtained by working on smaller areas. In vitro and in vivo micro-CT devices are currently available, and varying FOV ratios applied in these devices determine the area to be examined and the resolution to be attained [3, 4]. Similar to the cone beam computed tomography devices, micro-CT systems utilize microfocal X-ray sources and high-resolution detectors to create 3D reconstructions of the samples. Main components of the micro-tomography device are the X-ray tube, a computer-driven step motor that intermittently rotates the sample mounted on its body, an image intensifier which focuses the X-rays present in the environment onto the camera sensor, a CCD camera which converts X-rays received into image data, an image collector, and a computer that controls all these components [5].

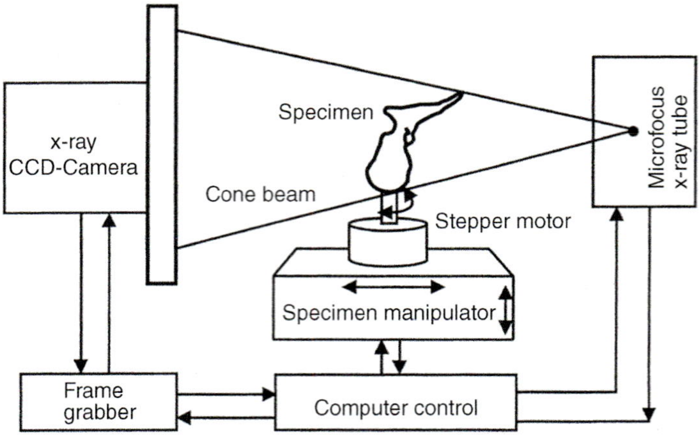

Fig. 19.1 Schematic diagram of micro-computed tomography workflow

19.2 Fundamentals of Micro-computed Tomography (Micro-CT)

From a technical point of view, micro-computed tomography (micro-CT) indeed is a CBCT technique which utilizes geometrically cone-shaped beams for reconstruction and back-projection processes. In contrast to the fan-shaped beams and multiple rotations used in spiral and conventional CT techniques, this technique utilizes a conical X-ray beam, whereas the scanning process is performed by a rotation of 180° or 360° around the field to be scanned, just as it is for CBCT. Having the same operating principle with CBCT, computerized micro-tomography's operating principle is a micro-focus tube that generates X-rays and high-resolution detectors that rotate around the object that is to be scanned, in order to obtain a three-dimensional image of the object. Digital data created by these projections are then converted into images through certain reconstruction algorithms [6–11]. These images can be uploaded to computer environment and if necessary can be modeled in 3D, by using relevant software [1, 2, 9]. These images can be uploaded to computer environment, and if necessary, 3D analyses can be conducted by using relevant software [9]. Micro-tomography (micro-CT) can be used for volumetric and surface measurements of bone tissue whose images were scanned beforehand through cone beam computed tomography. These images are considered equivalent since both CBCT and micro-CT operate on the same working principles. Research cases that evaluate CBCT images by micro-CT software can be found in literature. Reliability of this technique was speculated by researchers. However, they did not come up with a statistically significant difference resulting from analyses of images obtained by two separate devices through micro-CT software [12–15] (Fig. 19.2).

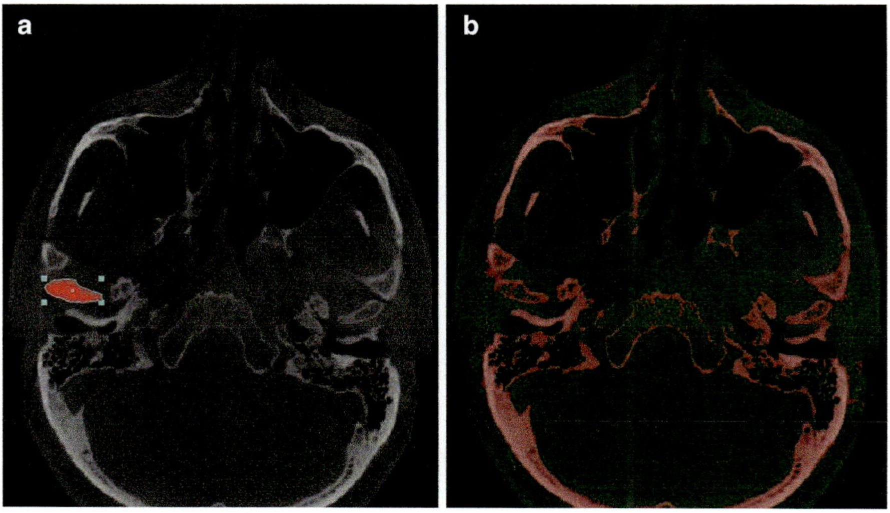

Fig. 19.2 (**a**) ROI selection for mandibular condyle boundaries for quantitative bone measurements. (**b**) The filtered mask of the CBCT image for bone analysis using micro-CT software

19.3 Analysis of Bone Micro-architecture via Micro-computed Tomography (Micro-CT)

The term "bone quality" is commonly used in literature to describe the structural formation and boundaries of the bones. The bone quality is definitely associated with trabecular bone structure. Trabecular bone is the primary anatomical and functional structure of the cancellous bone [16] (Fig. 19.3).

Histomorphometric analyses are destructive, long-term, and costly methods. It is impossible to reuse the same sample for another measurement. Moreover, various artifacts might occur due to slices used for sample preparation, which makes an accurate interpretation of analyses even more tedious. Due to these disadvantages, three-dimensional micro-tomography techniques have been put into use as nondestructive, rapid, and reliable methods for analyzing micro-architecture of the cortical and trabecular bones [17].

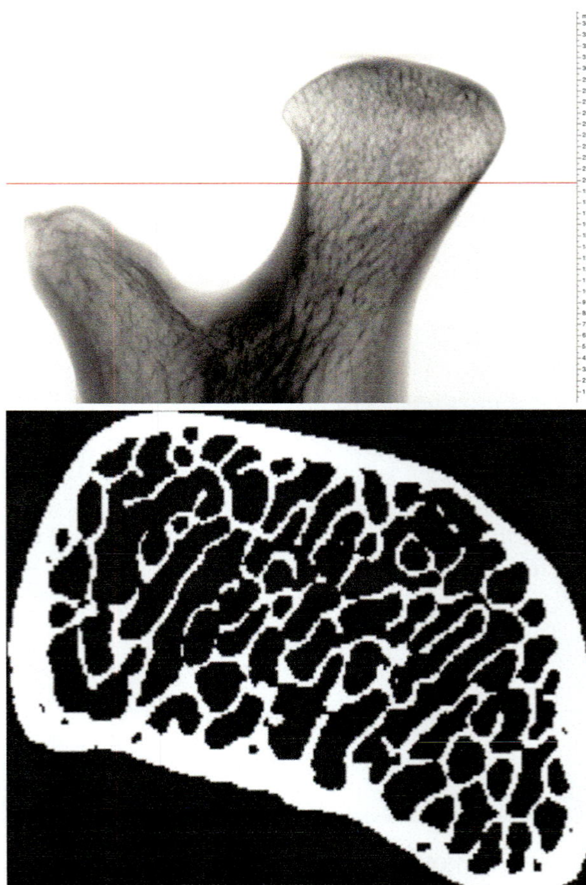

Fig. 19.3 Black and white binarization of ROI after global thresholding procedure

This can be achieved via the use of certain parameters such as trabecular thickness (Tb.Th), trabeculation number (Tb.N), trabecular separation (Tb.Sp), bone volume (BV), total tissue volume (TV), trabecular bone ratio (BV/ TV), structural model index (SMI) that demonstrates numeric features of trabeculation in 3D, trabecular bone junctions, number of trabecular nodes in each tissue volume (N.Nd/ TV), and bone density determined with respect to hydroxyapatite count [18].

Tissue volume (TV), bone volume (BV), percent bone volume (BV/TV) are major parameters that can be calculated in Micro-CT evaluations. BV/TV refers to the total amount of bone present in relation to the analyzed bone volume. It is a parameter widely used in pathologies that alter bone turnover as it reflects perfectly bone gain/loss. It indicates the fraction of a given volume of interest occupied by mineralized tissue.

- Bone surface (BS), the surface area of all the solid objects (bone tissue) within the tissue volume (TV), measured in 3D marching cube method. Bone surface (BS) of the sample and bone surface density (BS/BV) is the relationship between the overall trabecular bone surface and the bone volume of the mineralized bone. But a trabecular bone region does not, for example, extend into or beyond the boundary of the object—such as the cortical boundary of a bone sample. The meaningfulness of measured percent volume depends on the criteria applied in selecting the volume of interest. If the ROI or VOI boundaries are loosely drawn in the surrounding space around an object, for instance, then % object volume has no meaning [18].
- Bone-specific surface (BS/TV) analyzes the relation between the trabecular bone surface and the mineralized bone. In a 3D image, it directly measures distance in space.
- Trabecular thickness determines bone fill as well as the mean thickness of the osseous structures. With 3D image analysis by micro-CT, a true 3D thickness can be measured which is model independent.
- Trabecular separation (Tb.Sp) detects marrow spaces and thus should be correlated to BV/TV: The more BV/TV, the less Tb.Sp. This parameter determines inverse bone density. Histomorphometrists typically measure a single mean value of bone Tb.Th from a trabecular bone site. However a trabecular bone volume—or any complex biphasic object region—can also be characterized by a distribution of thicknesses. Micro-CT outputs a histogram of thickness (and separation also) with an interval of two pixels. Thickness distribution is a powerful method for characterizing the shape of a complex structure [19].
- The trabecular number implies the number of times a trabecular structure is crossed per unit length in a randomly selected way.
- Bone quality is determined by direct nonmetric parameters. Trabecular pattern factor (Tb.Pf) describes quantitatively trabecular connectivity. It is an inverse connectivity index. Therefore, the concavity of the trabecular surfaces implies connectivity, whereas convexity means isolated and misconnected structures. This is an inverse index of connectivity, which was developed and defined by Hahn et al. [16] for application to the trabecular bone. Tb.Pf is calculated in 3D, by comparing volume and surface of binarized solid before and after a single voxel image dilation [16].

- The structural model index determines the relative presence of either plate-like or rod-like trabeculae. It is defined in a range of 0–3, where closer to 0 corresponds to an ideal plate and 3 to an ideal cylinder. Normally, plate-like trabeculae are associated with a higher osseous stiffness. SMI involves a measurement of surface convexity. This parameter is of importance in osteoporotic degradation of the trabecular bone which is characterized by a transition from plate-like to rod-like architecture. An ideal plate, cylinder, and sphere have SMI values of 0, 3, and 4, respectively [20].
- The fractal dimension (FD) fractal analysis is a statistical texture analysis that is based on fractal mathematics for describing complex shapes and structural patterns. It is expressed numerically as "fractal dimension" (FD), which measures self-similarity and indicates a figure's complexity. For the 3D calculation of FD, the volume is divided into an array of equal cubes, and the number of cubes containing part of the object surface is counted.
- Bone mineral density compares between the attenuation coefficients of two hydroxyapatite patterns of known density (250 and 750 mg/cm^3). This is an area of density and not a true volume density as it has a dependency on bone size [21, 22] (Figs. 19.4 and 19.5).

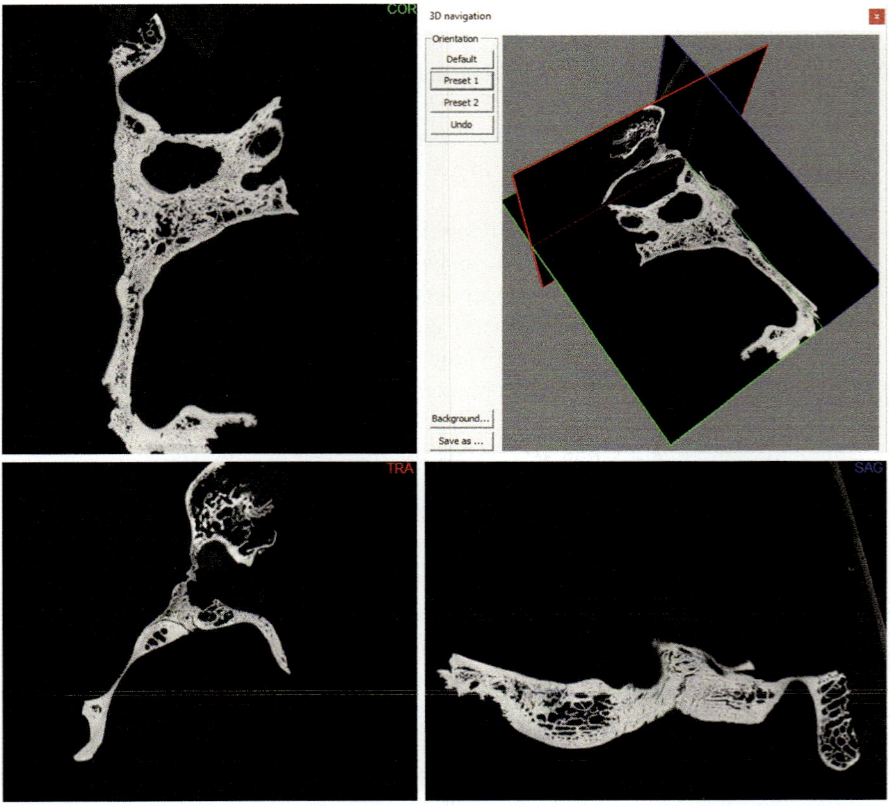

Fig. 19.4 Images of axial, transverse, and coronal sections of the temporal bone and fossa mandibularis

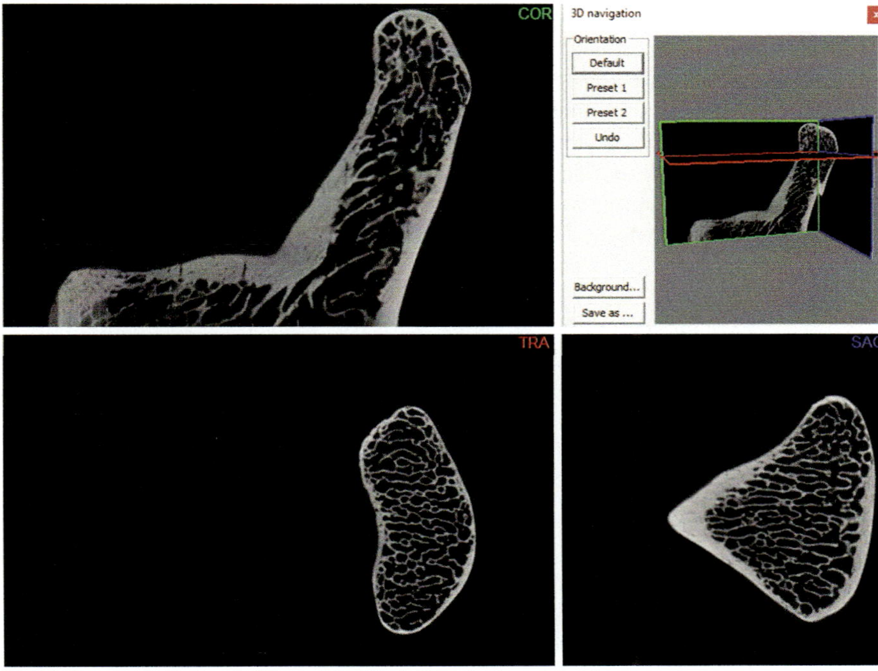

Fig. 19.5 Images of axial, transverse and coronal sections of the mandibular condyle

Dessel et al. [15] worked on determining the accuracy of cone beam CT (CBCT) measurement of trabecular bone microstructure in mandibulae, compared to that measured by micro-CT. They hydrostatically scanned eight mandibulae using three different CBCT protocols and consequently scanned with micro-CT. No statistically significant difference was found for the resulting images.

19.4 Micro-computed Tomography (Micro-CT) in TMJ Bone Research

Images are automatically converted to 8-bit axial images through relevant software for TMJ research. Bone components related to joints are identified in axial images, along with the determination of upper and lower limits required for the realization of analyses. ROIs (regions of interest) are selected by determining bone regions in axial images that lie within these limits. Black and white pixel ranges are determined by setting semiautomatic histogram settings, and global thresholding procedure is applied for realization of automatic analyses within these reference ranges. To make things clear, the gray image that belongs to ROIs within the corresponding range is pixelated as black and white dots. Total tissue volume, total bone volume, bone surface area, percentage rate of bone tissue, and aforementioned detailed trabeculae structure analyses can be measured along the selected ROI regions by the help of relevant software.

The percentage rate of bone tissue reflects the total bone amount that is associated with the analyzed bone volume. It is a parameter used for cases with bone replacement, and it perfectly reflects bone gain and bone loss. It shows the fraction of the volume occupied by the mineralized tissue. Bone surface indicates the total trabecular bone surface [9] (Figs. 19.6, 19.7 and 19.8).

Mulder et al. [23] examined the structure, mineralization, and trabecular bone development of pig condyle by using micro-computed tomography. They found out that the remodeling patterns of anterior and posterior mandibular condyle were

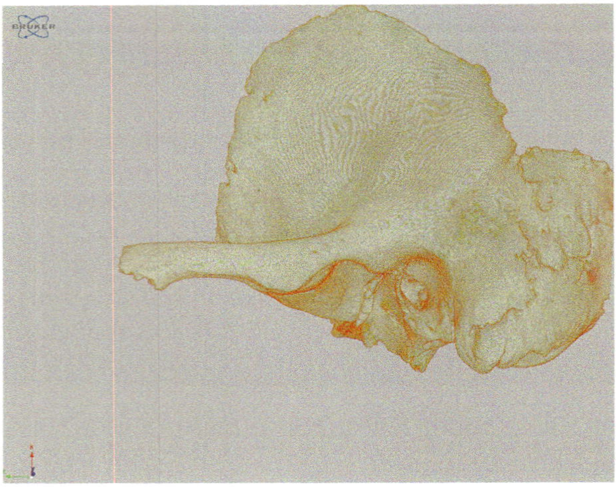

Fig. 19.6 3D reconstruction of the temporal bone

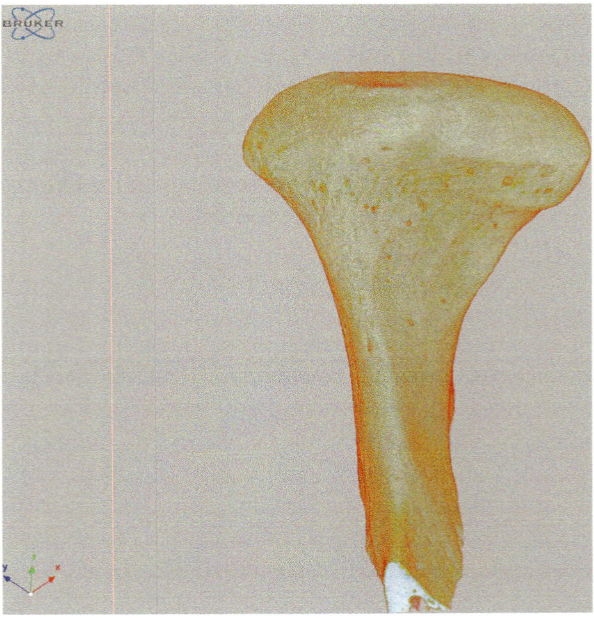

Fig. 19.7 3D reconstruction of the mandibular condyle from coronal view

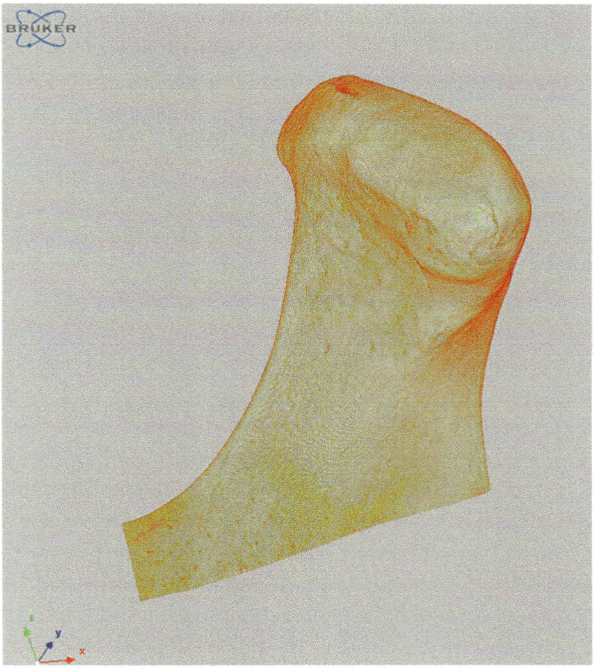

Fig. 19.8 3D reconstruction of the mandibular condyle from sagittal view

different from each other and that the condyle grew more in posterior direction, as a result of this study. They also demonstrated that the trabecular bone volume and thickness were higher in the corpus and that the mineralization value was the same for both the anterior and posterior of the condyle, with the corpus having a higher mineralization value.

Suomalainen et al. [10] scanned the TMJ samples obtained from postsurgical biopsy materials by using micro-CT. They declared that the micro-CT device visualized bone anatomical structures in a precise manner, making it a reliable tool—for instance—with respect to planning of joint prosthesis and treatment, as a result of this study. They also concluded that the device was pretty convenient to be used for diagnosing dental infections.

Kim et al. [24] performed micro-CT analyses in healthy mandibular condyle obtained from nine male cadavers. They succeeded in both imaging the condyle's bone micro-architecture thoroughly and conducting clinically important analyses by creating 3D models of these structures.

In their research conducted with mice, Zhang et al. [25] investigated the effect of platelet-rich plasma treatment (PRP) for bone replacement resulting from loss of the teeth. They defined condylar cartilage and related regions of subcondylar region as their ROI and utilized a total of five consecutive images of ROI for three-dimensional reconstruction and analyses during their research. By analyzing these images, they calculated total volume (BV), trabecular number (Tb.N), trabecular separation (Tb. Sp.), and trabecular bone volume (Tb.Th) per trabecular thickness.

Kaur et al. [26], in their study conducted with 54 Sprague–Dawley rats for studying bone structural parameters, calculated the bone volume to tissue volume ratio (bone volume fraction), trabecular thickness, trabecular number, trabecular separation, and bone mineral density. They compared other imaging techniques through these values by taking micro-CT values as the gold standard.

In another study investigating the effects of chewing muscle atrophy on TMJ, Kün-Darbois et al. [27] used micro-CT to calculate the amount of resorption in alveolar bone and mandibular condyle in adult mice that had been subjected to botox application on the masseter muscle.

Variants of these analyses that can easily be conducted by using micro-CT software can also be performed by using numerous 3D software. Either micro-CT scan images or images obtained from other imaging techniques that work on similar principles can be processed through the software. Gomes et al. [28] scanned 169 TMJ condyles that exhibited osteoarthritis variations (69 subjects with long-term TMJ osteoarthritis (OA), 15 subjects at initial diagnosis of OA, and 7 healthy controls) with CBCT. They consequently created three-dimensional surface models of these condyles through using a special software. As a result of their study, they identified a preliminary diagnostic index for 3D osteoarthritic changes. Cevidanes et al. [29] also conducted a research in order to evaluate the registry of 3D models obtained from CBCT images taken pre- and post-orthognathic surgeries for the assessment of mandibular anatomy and position of mandibulae. CBCT scans were obtained during pre- and post-orthognathic surgery for ten patients that have various malocclusions. These pre- and postsurgery images were reconstructed in 3D and superimposed on each other, and the regions where changes were observed were shown in different colors. Cevidanes et al. [30] reused this method of superimposing 3D models on each other, in order to observe growth-related maxillofacial changes. Researchers obtained pre- and posttreatment CBCT images of three Class III malocclusion patients that are to be orthopedically treated with miniplates. They observed the course of treatment for these patients throughout 1 year, creating 18 pieces of 3D virtual surface models, and then superimposed these images on one another, coloring the growth-related changes. Numerous studies based on 3D reconstruction of bone micro-architecture such as these can be found in literature [31–33]. Three-dimensional (3D) imaging techniques can provide valuable information for clinicians and researchers. However, considering that we recently moved from traditional two-dimensional (2D) cephalometric analyses to novel 3D techniques, we should thus be comparing data obtained by 2D and 3D methods. Regarding a study based on this problem [34], it was proven that CBCT images could effectively be used along with 3D modeling methods.

Micro-CT is used not only in adult TMJ imaging but also in experimental growth studies. In a study conducted with Sprague–Dawley rats that were exposed to effects of various hormones, Khan et al. [35] observed the growth of mandibulae, and they scanned the rats' mandibulae after dissecting them when they were 21 days old. They consequently calculated the bone volume and bone surface area of corresponding mandibulae as well as their bone mineral densities (Figs. 19.9, 19.10, and 19.11).

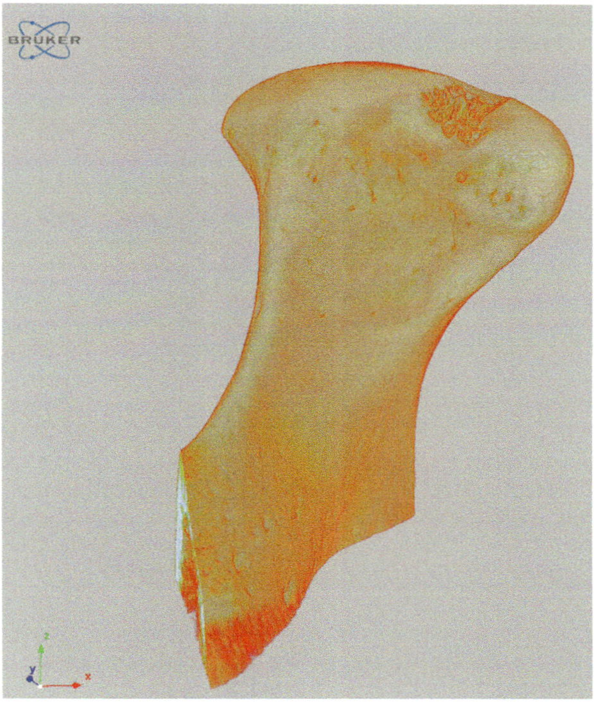

Fig. 19.9 3D reconstruction of osteoarthritis mandibular condyle

19.5 Micro-computed Tomography and TMJ Bone Histopathology

The bone is a highly mineralized and multifunctional tissue, which plays the roles in mechanical support and protection, mineral homeostasis, and hematopoiesis. In recent years, it has become clear that the bone also serves an essential endocrine function. To achieve these functional goals, the bone is organized hierarchically, from nanometer- to millimeter-sized structures. This contributes not only to its mechanical role in support and movement of the body but also to its other functions. At the nanostructural level, the bone is composed of organic and mineral components, mainly consisting of a matrix of cross-linked type I collagen mineralized with nanocrystalline, carbonated apatite. Due to its high mineral content, the bone tissue is extremely resilient, but its organic part also provides a certain degree of flexibility and elasticity improving its behavior under mechanical forces [36, 37].

The "quality" of the bone, as well as its quantity, contributes to the biomechanical performance of the skeleton and encompasses aspects of both macromolecular composition and micro-architectural arrangement [38].

Bone histomorphometry is an essential tool for understanding tissue-level mechanisms of bone physiology and assessing the mechanisms by which bone diseases occur, the mechanisms by which therapeutic agents affect the skeleton, and the

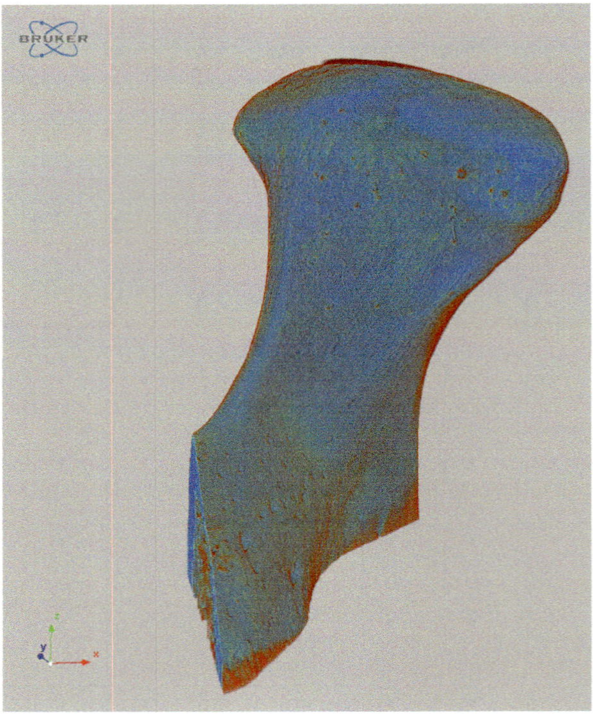

Fig. 19.10 3D reconstruction of normal mandibular condyle

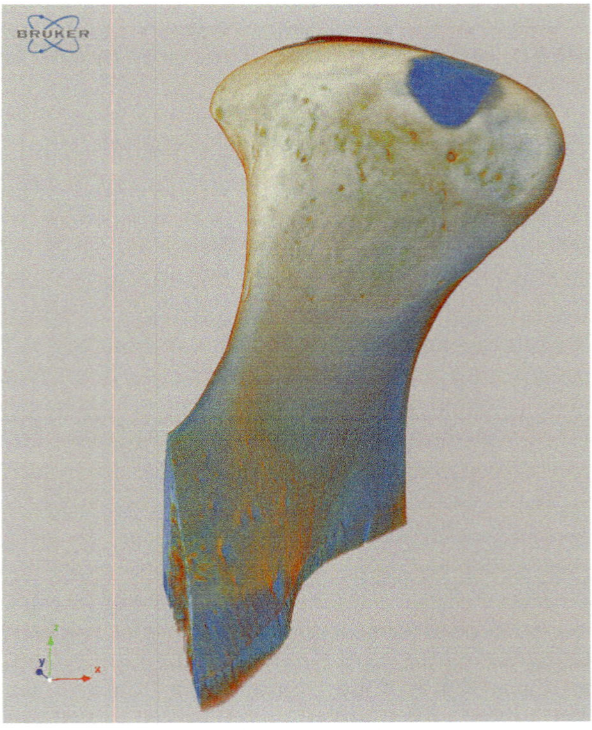

Fig. 19.11 3D registration of normal and osteoarthritic mandibular condyle

skeletal safety of therapeutic agents. It is the gold standard for tissue-level bone activity. It can yield a wealth of information about the bone structure, bone formation, bone resorption, bone mineralization, as well as bone modeling and remodeling activity [39].

Cancellous bone volume can be measured on histologic sections. A more detailed evaluation of trabecular architecture, such as thickness, number, and separation, can be calculated from the primary measures of bone area and surface. Cortical geometry, such as bone area and periosteal and endosteal perimeters can be directly measured [37].

Discriminating between woven and lamellar bone tissue can be valuable for determining whether the bone formation is occurring in a normal fashion. Evaluating lamellar and woven bone is accomplished using polarized light microscopy on unstained sections, although some stains allow collagen orientation to be visualized. In pathologic conditions such as Paget's disease of the bone, the presence of woven bone provides key diagnostic criteria. Lamellar bone, viewed under polarized light, can be assessed in more detail to elucidate features such as the number of lamellae within a given basic multicellular unit (BMU), the thickness of lamellae, or the type of lamellar organization (alternating or homogeneous) [37].

Using stains for osteoid, the examination of mineralized versus nonmineralized bone can provide information about changes in the mineralization process. Analysis of osteoid involves measuring the extent of the bone surface covered by osteoid (and then normalizing it by the total bone surface examined) and either the width or volume of osteoid. Although called osteoid volume in the literature, this is actually an area (given that it is a 2D assessment). If osteoid width is normal, increased osteoid surface is indicative of higher bone formation. Increased width of osteoid is indicative of a mineralization defect [37].

The extent of surfaces covered with osteoblasts and osteoclasts provides a primary index of how bone formation and/or resorption is altered under various conditions. Osteoblasts can be identified using morphological characteristics on sections stained with Goldner's trichrome, von Kossa and McNeal's, or even hematoxylin and eosin. Primary outcomes related to osteoblasts include osteoblast surface and their number, both typically normalized to bone surface. The most commonly employed technique for assessing activity of resorption is to measure eroded (or resorption) surfaces or erosion depth. A variable related to erosion depth from previous remodeling activity is average wall width (W.Wi), a measure of the amount of the bone formed at a given BMU. The balance between W.Wi and erosion depth determines BMU balance [37].

Although osteoblast function can be inferred through measures of osteoid, the most commonly used method is the assessment of fluorochrome labels (dynamic histomorphometry), because it allows the calculation of rates of modeling and remodeling. Mineralizing surface is reported per unit bone surface (MS/BS, %) by dividing the mineralizing surface by the total bone surface measured. MS/BS is often considered an index of osteoblast activity such that interventions that impact osteoblast proliferation and/or differentiation would be expected to change MS/BS [37].

The mineral apposition rate (MAR) is a commonly used parameter for the characterization of bone formation and is often determined to test for experimental effects on the cortical bone.

During histomorphometric analysis, different staining methods can be used which highlight certain features. During histomorphometric analysis, different staining methods can be used which highlight certain features. Toluidine blue is used to identify cavities under polarized light by looking at the presence of cutoff collagen fibers (disruption of the lamellar system) at the edge of the cavity. The polarized light allows visualization of the orientation of collagen lamellae along the mineralized bone surface. The identification of scalloped surfaces can, however, be subjective. Tartrate-resistant acid phosphatase can be used to mark active osteoclasts and thus "active" cavities. Von Kossa/van Gieson staining allows discriminating osteoid from mineralized bone [37, 38].

Before histomorphometric analyses take place, study specimens are subjected to a complex preparation protocol, from sample collection to microscopical observation of the prepared slide: sample collection, fixation and dehydration, infiltration and embedding, orientation/plane of section, and staining.

Using the histologic sections for quantification, the paraffin-embedded sections can distort and shrink up to 15%. This can make a big difference in histologic measurements and potentially obscure real differences between groups. Another limitation of paraffin embedding is that decalcification is usually incomplete. Thus, tissue sectioning is very challenging, resulting in suboptimal sections for analysis. Also, measurement variance associated with bone histomorphometry arises from some factors including intraobserver, interobserver, intermethod, and sample variation. Observer variation is mainly due to the subjective criteria used for identification of features such as osteoid seams, bone structural units, and resorption cavities. The protocol complexity, costs, required time, and high level of expertise and training are limitations of bone histomorphometry. It is also a two-dimensional and invasive technique [37, 38, 40, 41].

More recently micro-computed tomography appeared. It is capable of forming both 2D and 3D images with applications in bone formation quantification, as well as in bone modeling in bone grafts. It is also fast and allows nondestructive analysis without a specific preparation protocol.

The excellent reproducibility and accuracy of micro-CT measurements of bone morphology have been established in several studies [42, 43]. The accuracy of micro-CT morphology measurements has been evaluated by comparing them with traditional measures from 2D histomorphometry both in animal and in human specimens [42, 44, 45]. These studies show that 2D and 3D morphologic measurements by micro-CT generally are highly correlated with those from 2D histomorphometry [46].

Ex vivo micro-CT scanners typically produce scans with pixel sizes in the range of 1–30 μm. This provides sufficient resolution to accurately detect individual trabecular structures in small rodents, such as rats and mice, as well as in larger species. Higher-resolution scans, on a nanometer scale, can be obtained with nano-CT and synchrotron-CT machines [37].

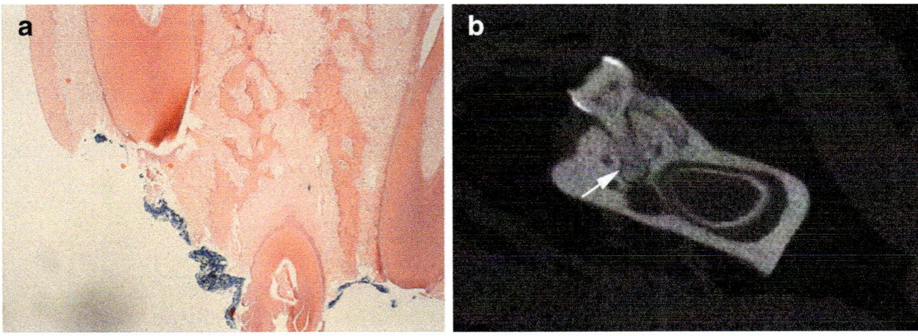

Fig. 19.12 (**a**) Histopathological image of a rat mandible. (**b**) Corresponding micro-CT slice showing destruction of the mandibular bone (arrow)

There are numerous advantages to using micro-CT for assessment of bone mass and morphology in excised specimens: (1) It allows for direct 3D measurement of trabecular morphology, such as trabecular thickness and separation, rather than inferring these values based on 2D stereologic models, as is done with standard histologic evaluations; (2) compared with 2D histology, a significantly larger volume of interest is analyzed; (3) measurements can be performed with a much faster throughput than typical histologic analyses of histomorphometric parameters using undecalcified bone specimens; and (4) assessment of bone morphology by micro-CT scanning is nondestructive; thus samples can be used subsequently for other assays, such as histology or mechanical testing [43, 47].

Micro-CT presents advantages over histomorphometry, but only the latter one can make cellular-level observation [48]. The additional value of micro-CT imaging is that it allows to provide details on the morphology of the cancellous network (avoiding assumptions of trabecular morphology) and more detailed data on cortical bone geometry. It is, therefore, beneficial to use a combination of both histomorphometry and micro-CT to increase the obtained information (Fig. 19.12).

Acknowledgments The authors would like to thank Dr. Umut Aksoy for the preparation of micro-computed tomography and TMJ bone histopathology section and providing histopathology and corresponding rat mandibular micro-CT image.

All specimens in this chapter were scanned with Skyscan 1275 (Skyscan, Kontich, Belgium) which were taken from the Ankara University Research Fund (Project No:17A0234001).

References

1. Feldkamp LA, Goldstein SA, Parfitt AM, Jesion G, Kleerekoper M. The direct examination of three- dimensional bone architecture in vitro by computed tomography. J Bone Miner Res. 1989;4(1):3–11.
2. Kuhn J, Goldstein S, Feldkamp L, Goulet R, Jesion G. Evaluation of a microcomputed tomography system to study trabecular bone structure. J Orthop Res. 1990;8(6):833–42.

3. Guldberg RE, Ballock RT, Boyan BD, Duvall CL, Lin AS, Nagaraja S, Oest M, Phillips J, Porter BD, Robertson G, Taylor WR. Analyzing bone, blood vessels, and biomaterials with microcomputed tomography. IEEE Eng Med Biol Mag. 2003;22(5):77–83.
4. Guldberg RE, Lin AS, Coleman R, Robertson G, Duvall C. Microcomputed tomography imaging of skeletal development and growth. Birth Defects Res C Embryo Today. 2004;72(3):250–9.
5. Rhodes JS, Ford TR, Lynch JA, Liepins PJ, Curtis RV. Micro-computed tomography: a new tool for experimental endodontology. Int Endod J. 1999;32(3):165–70.
6. Arai Y, Tammisalo E, Iwai K, Hashimoto K, Shinoda K. Development of a compact computed tomographic apparatus for dental use. Practice. 1999;12:15.
7. Araki K, Maki K, Seki K, Sakamaki K, Harata Y, Sakaino R, et al. Characteristics of a newly developed dentomaxillofacial X-ray cone beam CT scanner (CB MercuRay™): system configuration and physical properties. Dentomaxillofac Radiol. 2014;33(1):51–9.
8. Mozzo P, Procacci C, Tacconi A, Martini PT, Andreis IB. A new volumetric CT machine for dental imaging based on the cone-beam technique: preliminary results. Eur Radiol. 1998;8(9):1558–64.
9. Orhan K, Ocak M. Use of micro-computerized tomography (micro-CT) in dentistry (Diş hekimliğinde mikro-bilgisayarlı tomografi (Mikro-BT) kullanımı) (Turkish). In: Yakıncı ME, Polat S, editors. Ulusal mikro-ct yaz okulu ders notları. Ankara: 72 Tasarım Ltd; 2016.
10. Suomalainen A, Vehmas T, Kortesniemi M, Robinson S, Peltola J. Accuracy of linear measurements using dental cone beam and conventional multislice computed tomography. Dentomaxillofac Radiol. 2014;37(1):10–7.
11. Weber AL. History of head and neck radiology: past, present, and future 1. Radiology. 2001;218(1):15–24.
12. Ho J-T, Wu J, Huang H-L, Chen MY, Fuh L-J, Hsu J-T. Trabecular bone structural parameters evaluated using dental cone-beam computed tomography: cellular synthetic bones. Biomed Eng Online. 2013;12(1):115.
13. Ordinola-Zapata R, Bramante C, Versiani M, Moldauer B, Topham G, Gutmann J, et al. Comparative accuracy of the Clearing Technique, CBCT and Micro-CT methods in studying the mesial root canal configuration of mandibular first molars. Int Endod J. 2017;50(1):90–6.
14. Parsa A, Ibrahim N, Hassan B, Stelt P, Wismeijer D. Bone quality evaluation at dental implant site using multislice CT, micro-CT, and cone beam CT. Clin Oral Implants Res. 2015;26(1):e1–7.
15. Van Dessel J, Huang Y, Depypere M, Rubira-Bullen I, Maes F, Jacobs R. A comparative evaluation of cone beam CT and micro-CT on trabecular bone structures in the human mandible. Dentomaxillofac Radiol. 2013;42(8):20130145.
16. Hahn M, Vogel M, Pompesius-Kempa M, Delling G. Trabecular bone pattern factor – a new parameter for simple quantification of bone microarchitecture. Bone. 1992;13:327–30.
17. Parfitt AM. Bone histomorphometry: proposed system for standardization of nomenclature, symbols, and units. Calcif Tissue Int. 1988;42:284–6.
18. Currey JD. The many adaptations of bone. J Biomech. 2003;36:1487–95.
19. Odgaard A, Gundersen HJ. Quantification of connectivity cancellous bone, with special emphasis on 3-D reconstructions. Bone. 1993;14:173–82.
20. Hildebrand T, Ruegsegger P. Quantification of bone microarchitecture with the structure model index. Comput Methods Biomech Biomed Engin. 1997;1:15–23.
21. Southard TE, Southard KA, Krizan KE, Hillis SL, Haller JW, Keller J, et al. Mandibular bone density and fractal dimension in rabbits with induced osteoporosis. Oral Surg Oral Med Oral Pathol Oral Radiol Endod. 2000;89:244–9.
22. Tosoni GM, Lurie AG, Cowan AE, Burleson JA. Pixel intensity band fractal analyses: detecting osteoporosis in perimenopausal and postmenopausal women by using digital panoramic images. Oral Surg Oral Med Oral Pathol Oral Radiol Endod. 2006;102:235–41.
23. Mulder L, Koolstra JH, Weijs WA, van Eijden TM. Architecture and mineralization of developing trabecular bone in the pig mandibular condyle. Anat Rec A Discov Mol Cell Evol Biol. 2005;285(1):659–66.

24. Kim JE, Yi WJ, Heo MS, Lee SS, Choi SC, Huh KH. Three-dimensional evaluation of human jaw bone microarchitecture: correlation between the microarchitectural parameters of cone beam computed tomography and micro-computer tomography. Oral Surg Oral Med Oral Pathol Oral Radiol. 2015;120(6):762–70.
25. Zhang YT, Niu J, Wang Z, Liu S, Wu J, Yu B. Repair of osteochondral defects in a rabbit model using bilayer Poly(Lactide-co-Glycolide) scaffolds loaded with autologous platelet-rich plasma. Med Sci Monit. 2017;23:5189–201.
26. Kaur H, Uludağ H, Dederich DN, El-Bialy T. Effect of increasing low-intensity pulsed ultrasound and a functional appliance on the mandibular condyle in growing rats. J Ultrasound Med. 2017;36(1):109–20.
27. Kün-Darbois JD, Libouban H, Chappard D. Botulinum toxin in masticatory muscles of the adult rat induces bone loss at the condyle and alveolar regions of the mandible associated with a bone proliferation at a muscle enthesis. Bone. 2015;77:75–82. https://doi.org/10.1016/j.bone.2015.03.023.
28. Gomes LR, Gomes MR, Jung B, Paniagua B, Ruellas AC, Gonçalves JR, et al. Diagnostic index of three-dimensional osteoarthritic changes in temporomandibular joint condylar morphology. J Med Imaging. 2015;2(3):034501.
29. Cevidanes LH, Bailey L, Tucker G Jr, Styner M, Mol A, Phillips C, et al. Superimposition of 3D cone-beam CT models of orthognathic surgery patients. Dentomaxillofac Radiol. 2005;34(6):369–75.
30. Cevidanes LH, Heymann G, Cornelis MA, DeClerck HJ, Tulloch JC. Superimposition of 3-dimensional cone-beam computed tomography models of growing patients. Am J Orthod Dentofac Orthop. 2009;136(1):94–9.
31. Cevidanes LH, L'Tanya JB, Tucker SF, Styner MA, Mol A, Phillips CL, et al. Three-dimensional cone-beam computed tomography for assessment of mandibular changes after orthognathic surgery. Am J Orthod Dentofac Orthop. 2007;131(1):44–50.
32. De Clerck H, Nguyen T, De Paula LK, Cevidanes L. Three-dimensional assessment of mandibular and glenoid fossa changes after bone-anchored class III intermaxillary traction. Am J Orthod Dentofac Orthop. 2012;142(1):25–31.
33. Goncalves JR, Wolford LM, Cassano DS, Da Porciuncula G, Paniagua B, Cevidanes LH. Temporomandibular joint condylar changes following maxillomandibular advancement and articular disc repositioning. J Oral Maxillofac Surg. 2013;71(10):1759.e1–e15.
34. Cevidanes LH, Styner MA, Proffit WR. Image analysis and superimposition of 3-dimensional cone-beam computed tomography models. Am J Orthod Dentofac Orthop. 2006;129(5):611–8.
35. Khan I, El-Kadı A, El-Bialy T. Effects of growth hormone and ultrasound on mandibular growth in rats: microCT and toxicity analyses. Arch Oral Biol. 2013;58(9):1217–24.
36. Clarke B. Normal bone anatomy and physiology. Clin J Am Soc Nephrol. 2003;3(3):131–9.
37. Allen MR, Burr DB. Techniques in histomorphometry. In: Basic and applied bone biology. London: Academic Press; 2014. p. 131–48.
38. Aaron JE, Shore PA. Bone histomorphometry. In: Handbook of histology methods for bone and cartilage. New York: Humana; 2003. p. 331–51.
39. Erben RG, Glösmann M. Histomorphometry in rodents. In: Bone research protocols. New York: Humana; 2012. p. 279–303.
40. Vandeweghe S, Coelho PG, Vanhove C, Wennerberg A, Jimbo R. Utilizing micro-computed tomography to evaluate bone structure surrounding dental implants: a comparison with histomorphometry. J Biomed Mater Res B Appl Biomater. 2013;101(7):1259–66.
41. Vedi S, Compston J. Bone histomorphometry. In: Bone research protocols. New York: Humana; 2003. p. 283–98.
42. Bouxsein ML, Boyd SK, Christiansen BA, Guldberg RE, Jepsen KJ, Müller R. Guidelines for assessment of bone microstructure in rodents using micro–computed tomography. J Bone Miner Res. 2010;25(7):1468–86.
43. Chappard D, Retailleau-Gaborit N, Legrand E, Baslé MF, Audran M. Comparison insight bone measurements by histomorphometry and μCT. J Bone Miner Res. 2005;20(7):1177–84.

44. Bonnet N, Laroche N, Vico L, Dolleans E, Courteix D, Benhamou CL. Assessment of trabecular bone microarchitecture by two different x-ray microcomputed tomographs: a comparative study of the rat distal tibia using Skyscan and Scanco devices. Med Phys. 2009;36(4):1286–97.
45. Müller R, Van Campenhout H, Van Damme B, Van Der Perre G, Dequeker J, Hildebrand T, Rüegsegger P. Morphometric analysis of human bone biopsies: a quantitative structural comparison of histological sections and micro-computed tomography. Bone. 1998;23(1):59–66.
46. Matthew AR, Burr DB. Techniques in histomorphometry. In: Basic and applied bone biology. New York: Elsevier; 2014. p. 131–48.
47. Swain MV, Xue J. State of the art of micro-CT applications in dental research. Int J Oral Sci. 2009;1(4):177–88.
48. Compston JE. Bone density: BMC, BMD, or corrected BMD? Bone. 1995;16:5–7.

Genetic Studies and Approaches on TMJ Pathologies

20

Didem Ozdemir-Ozenen, Derya Tabakcilar, and Meltem Ozdemir-Karatas

20.1 Introduction

Orofacial pain constitutes an important part of approximately 10% of Americans with chronic pain. The causes of this pain can be dental, neurological, muscular, or skeletal. Pain in the facial area is an important sign for temporomandibular joint diseases (TMD) and besides includes a corresponding proportion of TMD total cases among orofacial pain disorders. According to reports from the National Dental Craniofacial Research Institute (NIDCR), National Institutes of Health (NIH), approximately ten million people are suffering from TMD pain at any time in the United States [1]. According to Magnusson et al., TMD complaints are not seen only in adults but also in children and are increasing with age [2]. Numerous studies (stress, family studies, animal experiments, and genetic studies) have been conducted to find out the causes of TMD [1].

The American Academy of Orofacial Pain guidelines (2008) introduced genetic factors in the section dedicated to the etiology of TMD. In this chapter, gene polymorphism has been shown to be the evidence of pain sensitivity and an effect on the development of myogenic TMD [3, 4].

In this book chapter, the genes that are effective in the causes of pain and pathologies in the development of temporomandibular joint (TMJ) are classified according to the topic and contributed to the health workers in order to get information on this subject and to shed light on future studies.

D. Ozdemir-Ozenen (✉) · D. Tabakcilar
Yeditepe University, Faculty of Dentistry, Department of Pediatric Dentistry, Istanbul, Turkey

M. Ozdemir-Karatas
Istanbul University, Faculty of Dentistry, Department of Maxillofacial Prosthodontics, Istanbul, Turkey

I. Rozylo-Kalinowska, K. Orhan (eds.), *Imaging of the Temporomandibular Joint*, https://doi.org/10.1007/978-3-319-99468-0_20

Table 20.1 TMJ morphogenesis genes (OMIM: www.omim.org) [58]

TMJ part	Gene code	Gene symbol	Cytogenetic location
Condylar cartilage	*RUNX2*	Runt-related transcription factor 2	6p21.1
	SOX9	Sry-Box9	17q24.3
	SPRY1	Sprouty 1	4q28.1
	SPRY2	Sprouty 2	13q31.1
Articular disc and joint cavities	*IHH*	Indian hedgehog homolog	q35
	SMO	Smoothened	7q32.1
	GLI (family)	Glioma-associated oncogene homolog	12q13.3
	TRPS1	Zinc-finger transcription factor	8q23.3
	SHOX2	Short stature homeobox gene	3q25.32

20.2 Genetic Influences on TMJ's Growth and Development

TMJ's growth and development is different from the other organs. The secondary cartilage in TMJ and other tissues within the joint develop later than the joints of the other organs. Therefore, the genetic effect of TMJ's growth differs from that of the other joints. In Table 20.1, genes affecting different tissues of TMJ are shown.

20.2.1 Genes Affecting Mandibular Condylar Cartilage

RUNX2 (Runt-related transcription factor 2) is required for bone tissue production, tooth development, and differentiation and regulates hypertrophic chondrocyte differentiation [5, 6]. *RUNX2*, which is effective in bone formation, and *SOX9* (SRY-box 9), which is effective in the formation of cartilage form, are expressed in mesenchymal condensation, which is needed at the beginning of the mandibular condyle formation. When there is local variation in the MCC (Mandibular Condylar Cartilage) at the E15 phase, both genes can be extracted from the preconditioning region [7].

In a study conducted by Shibata et al. on rats, *RUNX2* (−/−) rats did not form any bone, and no abnormality was observed in primary cartilage formation. However, agenesis has been seen in secondary cartilage (such as MCC) [5].

Fukuoka et al. showed that when exogen *Bone morphogenic protein-2 (BMP2)* is added, *RUNX2* (−/−) condyle explants may cause chondrogenic differentiation. This shows that the products resulting from the operation of osteoblasts can help in forming secondary cartilage [8].

When the *Sox9* gene was inactivated, the researchers concluded that agenesis of the condylar cartilage and deficiency in fossa mandibularis and articular disc formation occurs when the *SOX9* gene was inactivated. However, RUNX2 gene could still be expressed from the mandibular ramus and mandibular fossa where no Meckel's cartilage was found [6, 9, 10].

20.2.2 Genes Affecting Mandibular Fossa

Wang et al. have investigated the development of mandibular fossa in cases where mandibular condyle is not available. Their research has exploited the mandibular fossa structure to be initiated from neural crest cells and lack of *SOX9*. In the fossa, mesenchymal condensation was delayed in ossification and began to regress (normally occurring at E14.5); eventually only a small bone fragment was found laterally at E18.5. As a result, there was no fossa formation, and the fossa could not complete its development and even started to drop back [10].

Also as a result of the experiments made in mice, when Sprouty1 (*SPRY1*) and Sprouty2 (*SPRY2*) were deficient together, the development of the mandibular fossa was observed to be inadequate. These genes encode intracellular inhibitors of the receptor tyrosine kinase signaling pathways [11]. They are expressed in muscles of pterygoid and temporalis where the fibroblast growth factor receptors *FGFR1*, *FGFR2*, and *FGFR3* were expressed in the periosteum, perichondrium, and MCC. Temporalis and pterygoid muscles are mostly expanded although Meckel's cartilage, articular disc and condyle were unaffected when *SPRY* genes were deleted. However, mandibular fossa agenesis was observed, and only a very small side was formed. Sprouty RTK signaling antagonist 1 or 2 (*SPRY1* or *SPRY2*) inactivation alone does not cause any changes on TMJ. The authors suggested that the enlarged temporalis muscle may have impeded the condensations of the temporal bone from fusing to form the mandibular fossa in the mutant animals [6, 11].

20.2.3 Genes Affecting Articular Disc Formation and TMJ Cavities

The first studies of joint disc agenesis or anomalies founded have a link with the Indian hedgehog homolog (*IHH*) gene, Smoothened (*SMO*), and Glioma-associated (*GLI*) family [12, 13]. *IHH* is a regulatory gene of bone growth, chondrocyte maturation, and endochondral ossification [14]. Artificial disc formation in mice failed in *IHH*-inactivated studies. The authors hypothesized that *IHH* signaling is required for the later stages of the development for articular disc cavitation, morphogenesis, and maturation [13].

Researchers reported that articular disc formation was delayed or not started when *TRPS1* gene interacted with *IHH*. Ttranscriptional repressor GATA binding 1 (*TRPS1*) gene encodes mutated tricho-rhino-phalangeal syndrome transcription factor. It was observed that the articular disc and articular cavity were not completely formed in mice lacking *TRPS1*. These mice have the same phenotype as the *IHH* (−/−) mutant [15]. *TRPS1* regulates growth plate proliferation and maturation and ossification of the perichondrium [16]. Besides, *TRPS1* exerts a suppressive effect on *RUNX2* and is excreted from MCC at E15.5 [15, 16].

Inactivation of the *SHOX2* (short stature homeobox gene) that is located in cranial neural crest cells causes slow development of articular disc and all TMJ parts. Articular disc had taken shape in wild-type mice, although the articular disc inception was missing in the *SHOX2* (−/−) mice. Eventually, a disc had finally occurred in the newborn *SHOX2* (−/−) mice, but mandibular fossa and condyle were attached to each other [17]. In summary, *SHOX2* (−/−) mice showed decreased expression of both *RUNX2* and *SOX9*. In addition, they exhibited different expression types, decrease in the MCC, and ectopic in the fossa. According to Hinton, it is hypothesized that in condyle, decreased *IHH* may contribute to delayed and malformed disc and joint cavities [6].

20.3 TMJ Pain

20.3.1 Studies in Family/Twins

In a family study, Raphael et al. investigated the presence of orofacial pain and myofascial TMD in first-degree relatives. As a result of this study, they found that the relationship between orofacial pain and TMD symptoms in the first-degree relatives between the case group and the control group was not significantly different to produce a familial outcome [18].

In a study conducted on twins in the 1980s, 75 monozygotic (MZ) and 19 dizygotic (DZ) twins are compared about myofascial pain. The severity of pain between the MZ and DZ twins did not differ significantly. In this study, no evidence has been obtained for such a genetic predisposition [19].

In another twin study in 2000, Michalowicz et al. compared 146 MZ and 96 DZ twins about TMJ-related signs and symptoms. No significant difference in pain between the MZ and DZ twins were determined according to the results of this twin study [20].

Plesh et al. emphasized that TMD pain is inherited by 27% according to the results of their twin studies [15]. There were a large number of samples in their work (1236 MZ, 570 DZ same gender). They reported that hereditary risk factors associated with TMD pain were partially associated with migraine headache seen in women.

There is little evidence of inheritance from family studies of TMD pain [21]. However, these studies provide convenience in the determination of the method of genetic studies to be performed in the future.

20.3.2 OPPERA (Orofacial Pain Prospective Evaluation Risk and Assessment) Study

OPPERA is a project to investigate the etiological causes of TMD: to evaluate and determine biopsychosocial, environmental, and genetic factors. For this purpose, a group of researchers planned a prospective cohort study for 7 years, and they evaluated the results of this study.

The first OPPERA study was a case-control study. Candidate pain-related 358 genes were assessed on 348 chronic TMD patients and 1612 control group patients. They found that there was a link between TMD pain and seven candidate genes: *HTR2A*, *COMT*, *NR3C1* (glucocorticoid receptor), *CAMK4* (calcium-/calmodulin-dependent protein kinase type IV), *CHRM2* (muscarinic cholinergic receptor), *IFRD1* (interferon-related developmental regulator 1), and *GRK5* (G protein-coupled receptor kinase 5) [22, 23].

NR3C1 (glucocorticoid receptor) gene's three polymorphisms were associated with lower possibility of occurrence of TMJ diseases. *NR3C1* integrates with cortisol. This steroid hormone is the most important element of the hypothalamic-pituitary-adrenal system which has been correlated with the pathophysiology of TMD [22].

It may be difficult to discover the relationship between gene activities and TMJ pathologies because of insufficient data. Also in some cases, environmental factors may cause acute pain, and chronic TMD pain may be confused by the individual [24].

20.3.3 * Sexual Dimorphism of TMJ Pathologies/*Gender Differences/Estrogen Activity[1]

In the literature, there are controversial results of studies on gender differences in the prevalence of TMJ disorders. There are both human and animal studies in the literature that demonstrate gender differences in the perception of pain [18].

TMJ diseases are more common in women, about four times more prevalent [25]. The prevalence of TMJ pain in the preadolescent period was found to be 2–4%. There is no significant difference for males and females [26]. Besides, the incidence of pain in adult female is higher than male, and the rate starts to decrease when women reach postmenopausal period [27]. These results suggest that female hormonal axis, especially estrogen hormone, may contribute to the development of TMJ pathogenesis.

According to LeResche and Macfarlane, oral contraceptive medicaments and hormone replacement therapy are associated with higher prevalence of TMD complaints by women [27, 28]. Serum estradiol ratio (in luteal phase) was significantly higher in men and women with TMJ dysfunction and pain than in the healthy control group without TMJ complaints [29].

The estrogen receptor has two types: alpha (α) and beta (β). The α-receptor resides in intra-articular cartilage, osteocytes, and many other cells. Besides it regulates intracellular mediators [25, 30]. In the *PVUII* and *XBAI* regions, the estrogen receptor-alpha gene has two most common polymorphisms, and these regions are defined as polymorphisms of the restriction fragment length of *PVUII* and *XBAI* [25, 31, 32]. These polymorphisms have already been implicated in conditions alone or combined type such as decreased bone density, rheumatoid arthritis, osteoarthritis, and TMJ disorders [23].

Besides, the GC haplotype's presence in the polymorphic region *XBAI* has been shown to increase the possibility of TMD displacement and arthralgia [31, 32].

According to Ribeiro-DaSilva, such a genotype can affect the level or the function of the estrogen receptor-alpha or the activity of estrogen on inflammatory mediators [31]. On the other hand, another study conducted by Kim et al. [25] has no association between any risks of TMD correlated to different polymorphisms of the regions *PVUII* and *XBAI* of the estrogen receptor-alpha gene.

[1] Asterisk denotes gender differences in TMJ pathologies.

20.3.4 Serotonin Activity and Metabolism/Serotonin Transporter Gene Polymorphism

Serotonin (5-hydroxytryptamine, *5-HT*) is a neurotransmitter that acts an important role in enhancing endogenous analgesic mechanisms [23, 33]. The human serotonin transporter gene (*5-HTT*) is located on chromosome 17q11.1–q12. This gene is a candidate for painful disorders, such as TMD.

The serotonin transporter gene regulates the activity of serotonin. This gene has two polymorphic regions: the variable number tandem repeat (*VNTR*) and the gene-linked polymorphic region (*LPR*) [23].

According to Herken [34], subjects homozygous for allele STin 2.10 in the polymorphic region *VNTR* had increased predisposition of TMD pain and dysfunction; on the other hand, the alleles STin 2.12 in the same region could reduce such risk.

The *5-HTT* gene has a 44-bp insertion/deletion polymorphic region and two allelic forms: the long and short. According to in vitro studies, the short alleles have higher transcriptional activity than long alleles. Thereby, this higher transcriptional activity could give rise to an increased uptake of serotonin, which leads to lower extracellular concentration of serotonin [23]. Long allele form increases the risk of TMD pain; conversely the presence of a short allele form reduces [35]. But this hypothesis has not been confirmed by any *in-vitro* or *in-vivo* study. No significant difference was recorded between TMD patients and control groups regarding the presence of long and short allele forms for *5-HTT* gene [34, 36].

Another gene polymorphism (serotonin 2A receptor gene) is related to the action of serotonin in the literature. In the *T102C* region can change the possibility of TMD pain and dysfunction. The homozygous subjects in the C allele have higher risk while in the T alleles have lower risk [37, 38].

Besides the same gene in the rs9316233 region, the presence of the allele minor G showed a protective effect against the TMD pain risk [22]. Slade et al. [39] showed that combined six SNPs genes involved in serotonin receptor pathway were predictors of localized TMD.

Tryptophan is an α-amino acid that is used in the biosynthesis of proteins. This amino acid is a serotonin precursor and is transformed into serotonin by tryptophan hydroxylase enzyme. Tryptophan hydroxylase gene alleles C/C in the polymorphic region A218C were shown to raise the risk of TMD [40].

Kopp has shown that the role of serotonin in the genesis of TMJ symptoms, specifically TMJ pain on mandibular movement, restricted mandibular mobility, TMJ hyperalgesia, and allodynia. These results were in agreement with the two studies that Kopp did in 1998 and 2001 [41, 42].

20.3.5 Catecholamine Activity

COMT (catecholamine-O-methyltransferase) is the enzyme that metabolizes catecholamines (epinephrine, noradrenaline, and dopamine), L-dopa, catechol estrogens, ascorbic acid, and melanin [23, 43]. The differences in catecholamine physiology are associated with altered, in particular reduced, COMT activity, resulting in higher levels of catecholamines that increase the duration of pain [23, 44].

The relationship between the six single nucleotide polymorphisms (SNPs) in the *COMT* gene was found in more than 40% of the human population, and the pain sensation in TMD was investigated [23].

The gene coding for the enzyme COMT has three types of haplotypes according to the severity of the experimental pain: lower (LPS), average (APS), and high pain sensitivity (HPS). The presence of at least one LPS allele has been determined to greatly reduce (as much as 2.3 times) the myogenic TMD risk. This enzyme appears to play a role in the pathogenesis of TMD, as the LPS allele can produce more COMT [4, 22]. APS and HPS were observed to have a higher risk of higher TMD pathogenesis. At the same time, in rat experiments, *COMT* inhibition caused a great increase in pain sensitivity. It was later stated that the three major haplotypes direct COMT activity in humans and that myogenesis is inversely proportional to the risk of developing TMD [45]. These haplotypes in the genomic promoter region may play a regulatory role in the *COMT* gene and are more susceptible to TMJ diseases by affecting DNA transcription, RNA insertion, mRNA stability, and mRNA transport and translation [46].

Slade et al. investigated the psychological relationship (e.g., depression and anxiety), which was an important factor in the development of *COMT* and TMD, but no such interaction was observed. This suggests that there are different etiological situations in psychological characteristics and genetic variants of the *COMT* gene change the risk of a person developing TMD [47].

20.3.6 Folate Metabolism

Folate (vitamin B9, folic acid) metabolism is involved in nucleic acid synthesis and regulates DNA and protein methylation. This is why it has an important influence on the formation of growing tissues. Myofascial pain and impairment of TMD movements are often caused by insufficient intake of folic acid [36].

Four polymorphic variants of three genes (serine hydroxymethyltransferase 1 gene, methylenetetrahydrofolate dehydrogenase 1, methionine synthase reductase) involved in folate metabolism were found to be more associated with TMD risk. Serine hydroxymethyltransferase 1 gene encodes an enzyme which intervenes in the folate synthesis. The presence of the allele G in the polymorphic region rs1979277 and the presence of the allele C in the polymorphic region rs638416 of this gene have been related to a higher risk of TMD. Another gene is the methylenetetrahydrofolate dehydrogenase 1, which encodes another different enzyme involved in folate synthesis. The polymorphism of the gene of another enzyme, the methionine synthase reductase, has been related to higher risk of TMD. The presence of an allele A in the polymorphic region rs1801394 of this gene raises the affinity of the enzyme for the substrate [36, 48].

20.3.7 Glutathione Activity

Oxidative stress is produced by the production of nitric oxide and peroxynitrite. The overloaded DNA may be damaged, and this may play a role in the formation of synovial hyperplasia of TMJ [49]. Oxidative stress is closely related to TMJ infection [49, 50]. This suggests that a reduced detoxification capacity may increase the risk factor in TMD. Enzyme mu-class glutathione S-transferase's function is the detoxification of electrophilic compounds (such as carcinogens, drugs, toxins, and oxidative stress products). This result is accomplished by the conjugation with glutathione. A deletion in the related gene has been associated with higher risk of TMD, because of decreased detoxification capacity [36, 48].

20.3.8 ANKH Gene

Huang et al. in their research conducted in 2011 observed that the *ANKH* gene was among the causes of ankylosing spondylitis in humans and the formation of arthritis in mice. Two alleles were identified in the ANKH-OR polymorphic region: the 1-allele and the 2-allele. The homozygote genotypes both of 1/1 and 2/2 were associated with disc displacement without reduction of TMJ. Since fibrous ankylosis of the TMJ of *ANKH* mutant mice was detected in the same study, it can be hypothesized that the formation of fibrous adhesions and ankylosis has the possibility of the disc displacement without reduction in humans [36, 51].

20.3.9 Extracellular Matrix Breakdown

MMPs (matrix metalloproteinases) are a family of enzymes (this family consists a minimum of 19 members) that degrades the components of the extracellular matrix, such as collagen, fibronectin, and proteoglycans. Collagen type II extracellular matrix exhibits resistance to force, and proteoglycans provide elasticity in joint surface tissues [52, 53]. Fibroblasts and chondrocytes produce MMPs. Aggrecanases and MMPs are responsible for TMJ degeneration process [1, 54]. If there will be an imbalance between the synthesis and the destruction of diverse types of extracellular matrix, the outcome of this situation will be degenerative changes in the TMJ [53].

According to the two previous studies of Yoshida et al. with *MMP2*, *MMP9*, and aggrecanase, the aggrecanase expression in the TMJ of patients with internal derangement may be indicative of a disturbance caused by the joint [54, 55].

MMP1 gene's two polymorphisms have been identified in the rs1799750 region: the 1G and 2G variants. Homozygous 2G alleles are associated with TMD risk. Furthermore, the presence of the allele 1G and the heterozygous 1G/2G genotype showed opposite effect. The presence of the 2G allele is associated with higher levels of the MMPs, intensifying degradation of the extracellular matrix in the TMJ [36, 53].

20.3.10 Cytokine Activity and Metabolism

Cytokines do destructive missions of the pathology of rheumatoid arthritis and connective tissue [56]. IL-lj3 and IL-lja subtypes of IL-1 are found in synovial fluid from patients with RA. In rats, IL-lj3 has been found to be inclined to chronic inflammation and to cause hyperalgesia. Because of the potent inducing effect of IL-lj3 on the bone and cartilage resorption, IL-l also can be highly suspected to be involved in the joint destruction, pannus formation, and development of fibrous or ankylosis in the TMJ [42].

Slade et al. studied *TGFB1* (transforming growth factor beta 1) gene and *IL-8* (interleukin-8 polymorphic gene) that interact with each other and showed different movements. The minor T variant of the *TGFB1* increased the risk of TMD when associated with the homozygous allele major A of the *IL-8*, but such risk was reduced when it was associated with at least one minor A allele of the *IL-8* [57]. Polymorphisms of genes could change the synthesis and release of cytokines. Pro-inflammatory cytokines may be due to the transformation from acute to chronic TMD pain by activating transcription of genes.

20.4 *Syndromic Forms of TMJ

In the OMIM (Online Mendelian Inheritance in Man) archive, seven syndromes affecting TMD had been seen [1]:

Auriculocondylar syndrome
Ehler-Danlos syndrome type III
Fibrodysplasia ossificans progressiva
Schwartz-Jampel syndrome type I
Ophtalmomandibulomelic dysplasia
Tight skin contracture syndrome
FGFR3 achondroplasia

20.5 Conclusion

Temporomandibular system is a compaction mechanism consisting of muscles, bones, and joints, and any disorder seen in any one affects the entire system. Because of the high prevalence in society, scientists have done a lot of research to investigate the etiology. Each individual could perceive environmental factors that cause TMD risk differently. Even if the pain perception stimulus is the same, the body's response to pain varies according to the person. Because each individual has a unique genetic structure, the risk stimuli vary according to the individual.

For this reason, it is necessary to understand the genetic structure of TMJ. When genetic factors of TMD are well known, it can be predicted that the measures to be taken during the growth and development period can reduce the future damage to a minimum. However, future studies are needed to find new treatments.

References

1. Oakley M, Vieira AR. The many faces of the genetics contribution to temporomandibular joint disorder. Orthod Craniofacial Res. 2008;11(3):125–35.
2. Magnusson T, Egermark I, Carlsson GE. A prospective investigation over two decades on signs and symptoms of temporomandibular disorders and associated variables. A final summary. Acta Odontol Scand. 2005;63(2):99–109.
3. De Leeuw R. Orofacial pain: guidelines for assessment, diagnosis, and management. In: Klasser GD, editor. Orofacial pain. 5th ed. Chicago: Quintessence Publishing Co; 2013. p. 129–204.
4. Diatchenko L, Slade GD, Nackley AG, Bhalang K, Sigurdsson A, Belfer I, et al. Genetic basis for individual variations in pain perception and the development of a chronic pain condition. Hum Mol Genet. 2005;14(1):135–43.
5. Shibata S, Suda N, Yoda S, Fukuoka H, Ohyama K, Yamashita Y, et al. Runx2-deficient mice lack mandibular condylar cartilage and have deformed Meckel?s cartilage. Anat Embryol. 2004;208(4):273–80.
6. Hinton RJ. Genes that regulate morphogenesis and growth of the temporomandibular joint: a review. Dev Dyn. 2014;243(7):864–74.
7. Shibata S, Suda N, Suzuki S, Fukuoka H, Yamashita Y. An in situ hybridization study of Runx2, Osterix, and Sox9 at the onset of condylar cartilage formation in fetal mouse mandible. J Anat. 2006;208(2):169–77.
8. Fukuoka H, Shibata S, Suda N, Yamashita Y, Komori T. Bone morphogenetic protein rescues the lack of secondary cartilage in Runx2-deficient mice. J Anat. 2007;211(1):8–15.
9. Mori-Akiyama Y, Akiyama H, Rowitch DH, de Crombrugghe B. Sox9 is required for determination of the chondrogenic cell lineage in the cranial neural crest. Proc Natl Acad Sci. 2003;100(16):9360–5. Available from: http://www.pnas.org/cgi/doi/10.1073/pnas.1631288100.
10. Wang Y, Liu C, Rohr J, Liu H, He F, Yu J, et al. Tissue interaction is required for glenoid fossa development during temporomandibular joint formation. Dev Dyn. 2011;240(11):2466–73.
11. Purcell P, Jheon A, Vivero MP, Rahimi H, Joo A, Klein OD. Spry1 and Spry2 are essential for development of the temporomandibular joint. J Dent Res. 2012;91(4):387–93.
12. Shibukawa Y, Young B, Wu C, Yamada S, Long F, Pacifici M, et al. Temporomandibular joint formation and condyle growth require Indian hedgehog signaling. Dev Dyn. 2007;236(2):426–34.
13. Purcell P, Joo BW, Hu JK, et al. Temporomandibular joint formation requires two distinct hedgehogdependent steps. Proc Natl Acad Sci. 2010;107(8):18297–302.
14. Koyama E, Ochiai T, Rountree RB, Kingsley DM, Enomoto-Iwamoto M, Iwamoto M, et al. Synovial joint formation during mouse limb skeletogenesis: roles of Indian hedgehog signaling. Ann N Y Acad Sci. 2007;1116:100–12.
15. Michikami I, Fukushi T, Honma S, Yoshioka S, Itoh S, Muragaki Y, et al. Trps1 is necessary for normal temporomandibular joint development. Cell Tissue Res. 2012;348(1):131–40.
16. Napierala D, Sam K, Morello R, Zheng Q, Munivez E, Shivdasani RA, et al. Uncoupling of chondrocyte differentiation and perichondrial mineralization underlies the skeletal dysplasia in tricho-rhino-phalangeal syndrome. Hum Mol Genet. 2008;17(14):2244–54.
17. Gu S, Wei N, Yu L, Fei J, Chen YP. Shox2-deficiency leads to dysplasia and ankylosis of the temporomandibular joint in mice. Mech Dev. 2008;125(8):729–42.
18. Raphael KG, Marbach JJ, Gallagher RM, Dohrenwend BP. Myofascial TMD does not run in families. Pain. 1999;80(1–2):15–22.
19. Heiberg A, Helöe B, Heiberg AN, Helöe LA, Magnus P, Berg K, et al. Myofascial pain dysfunction (MPD) syndrome in twins. Community Dent Oral Epidemiol. 1980;8(8):434–6.
20. Michalowicz BS, Pihlstrom BL, Hodges J, Bouchard TJ Jr. No heritability of temporomandibular joint signs and symptoms. J Dent Res. 2000;79:1573–8.
21. Visscher CM, Lobbezoo F. TMD pain is partly heritable. A systematic review of family studies and genetic association studies. J Oral Rehabil. 2015;42(5):386–99.

22. Smith SB, Maixner DW, Greenspan JD, Dubner R, Fillingim RB, Ohrbach R, et al. Potential genetic risk factors for chronic TMD: genetic associations from the OPPERA case control study. J Pain. 2011;12(11 SUPPL):T92–101.
23. Meloto CB, Serrano PO, Ribeiro-Dasilva MC, Rizzatti-Barbosa CM. Genomics and the new perspectives for temporomandibular disorders. Arch Oral Biol. 2011;56(11):1181–91.
24. Smith SB, Mir E, Bair E, Slade GD, Dubner R, Fillingim RB, et al. Genetic variants associated with development of TMD and its intermediate phenotypes: the genetic architecture of TMD in the OPPERA prospective cohort study. J Pain. 2013;14(12 Suppl):T91–T101.e3.
25. Kim BS, Kim YK, Yun PY, Lee E, Bae J. The effects of estrogen receptor α polymorphism on the prevalence of symptomatic temporomandibular disorders. J Oral Maxillofac Surg. 2010;68(12):2975–9.
26. Leresche L. Epidemiology of temporomandibular disorders: implications for the investigation. Crit Rev Oral Biol Med. 1997;8(3):291–305.
27. LeResche L, Mancl L, Sherman JJ, Gandara B, Dworkin SF. Changes in temporomandibular pain and other symptoms across the menstrual cycle. Pain. 2003;106(3):253–61.
28. Macfarlane TV, Blinkhorn AS, Davies RM, Kincey J, Worthington HV. Association between female hormonal factors and oro-facial pain: study in the community. Pain. 2002;97(1–2):5–10.
29. Landi N, Lombardi I, Manfredini D, Casarosa E, Biondi K, Gabbanini M, et al. Sexual hormone serum levels and temporomandibular disorders. A preliminary study. Gynecol Endocrinol. 2005;20(2):99–103.
30. Omar Abubaker A, Raslan WF, Sotereanos GC. Estrogen and progesterone receptors in temporomandibular joint discs of symptomatic and asymptomatic persons: A preliminary study. J Oral Maxillofac Surg. 1993;51(10):1096–100.
31. Ribeiro-Dasilva MC, Peres Line SR, Leme Godoy dos Santos MC, Arthuri MT, Hou W, Fillingim RB, et al. Estrogen receptor-α polymorphisms and predisposition to TMJ disorder. J Pain. 2009;10(5):527–33.
32. Kang SC, Lee DG, Choi JH, Kim ST, Kim YK, Ahn HJ. Association between estrogen receptor polymorphism and pain susceptibility in female temporomandibular joint osteoarthritis patients. Int J Oral Maxillofac Surg. 2007;36(5):391–4.
33. Hranilovic D, Stefulj J, Schwab S, Borrmann-hassenbach M, Albus M, Jernej B, et al. Serotonin transporter promoter and intron 2 polymorphisms: relationship between allelic variants and gene expression. Biol Psychiatry. 2004;55:1090–4.
34. Herken H, Erdal E, Mutlu N, Barlas Ö, Cataloluk O, Oz F, et al. Possible association of temporomandibular joint pain and dysfunction with a polymorphism in the serotonin transporter gene. Am J Orthod Dentofac Orthop. 2001;120(3):308–13.
35. Ojima K, Watanabe N, Narita N, Narita M. Temporomandibular disorder is associated with a serotonin transporter gene polymorphism in the Japanese population. BioPsychoSoc Med. 2007;1:1–4.
36. Melis M, Di Giosia M. The role of genetic factors in the etiology of temporomandibular disorders: a review. Cranio. 2016;34(1):43–51.
37. Mutlu N, Erdal M, Herken H, Oz G, Bayazıt Y. T102C polymorphism of the 5-HT2A receptor gene may be associated with temporomandibular dysfunction. Oral Dis. 2004;10(6):349–52.
38. De Freitas LVS, Lopes ACP, Piatto VB, Maniglia JV. Association of temporomandibular dysfunction with the 102T-C polymorphism in the serotonin receptor gene in Brazilian patients. Arch Med Sci. 2013;9(6):1013–8.
39. Slade GD, Smith SB, Zaykin DV, Tchivileva IE, Gibson DG, Yuryev A, et al. Facial pain with localized and widespread manifestations: separate pathways of vulnerability. Pain. 2013;154(11):2335–43.
40. Etoz OA, Ataoglu H, Erdal ME. Association between tryptophan hydroxylase gene polymorphism and painful non- osseous temporomandibular disorders. Saudi Med J. 2008;29(9):1352–4.
41. Kopp S. Neuroendocrine, immune, and local responses related to temporomandibular disorders. J Orofac Pain. 2001;15:9–28.
42. Kopp S. The influence of neuropeptides, serotonin, and interleukin 1beta on temporomandibular joint pain and inflammation. J Oral Maxillofac Surg. 1998;56(2):189–91.

43. Männistö PT, Kaakkola S. Catechol-O-methyltransferase (COMT): biochemistry, molecular biology, pharmacology, and clinical efficacy of the new selective COMT inhibitors. Pharmacol Rev. 1999;51(4):593–628.
44. Nackley AG, Tan KS, Fecho K, Flood P, Diatchenko L, Maixner W. Catechol-O-methyltransferase inhibition increases pain sensitivity through activation of both β2- and β3-adrenergic receptors. Pain. 2007;128(3):199–208.
45. Diatchenko L, Anderson AD, Slade GD, Fillingim RB, Shabalina SA, Higgins TJ, et al. Three major haplotypes of the β2 adrenergic receptor define psychological profile, blood pressure, and the risk for development of a common musculoskeletal pain disorder. Am J Med Genet B Neuropsychiatr Genet. 2006;141(5):449–62.
46. Michelotti A, Liguori R, Toriello M, Sacchetti L, et al. Clin J Pain. 2014;30(2):129–33.
47. Slade GD, Diatchenko L, Bhalang K, Sigurdsson A, Fillingim RB, Belfer I, et al. Influence of psychological factors on risk of temporomandibular disorders. J Dent Res. 2007;86(11):1120–5.
48. Aneiros-Guerrero A, Lendinez AM, Palomares AR, Perez-Nevot B, Aguado L, Mayor-Olea A, et al. Genetic polymorphisms in folate pathway enzymes, DRD4 and GSTM1 are related to temporomandibular disorder. BMC Med Genet. 2011;12:1–9.
49. Yamaza T, Masuda KF, Atsuta I, Nishijima N, Kido MA, Tanaka T. Oxidative stress-induced DNA damage in the synovial cells of the Temporomandibular joint in the rat. J Dent Res. 2004;83(8):619–24.
50. Ueno T, Yamada M, Sugita Y, Ogawa T. N-acetyl cysteine protects TMJ chondrocytes from oxidative stress. J Dent Res. 2011;90(3):353–9.
51. Huang B, Takahashi K, Sakata T, Kiso H, Sugai M, Fujimura K, et al. Increased risk of temporomandibular joint closed lock: a case-control study of ANKH polymorphisms. PLoS One. 2011;6(10):2–8.
52. Lark MW, Bayne EK, Flanagan J, Harper CF, Hoerrner LA, Hutchinson NI, et al. Aggrecan degradation in human cartilage: evidence for both matrix metalloproteinase and aggrecanase activity in normal, osteoarthritic, and rheumatoid joints. J Clin Investig. 1997;100(1):93–106.
53. Planello AC, Campos MIG, Meloto CB, Secolin R, Rizatti-Barbosa CM, Line SRP, et al. Association of matrix metalloproteinase gene polymorphism with temporomandibular joint degeneration. Eur J Oral Sci. 2011;119(1):1–6.
54. Yoshida K, Takatsuka S, Tanaka A, Hatada E, Nakamura H, Nakagawa K, et al. Aggrecanase analysis of synovial fluid of temporomandibular joint disorders. Oral Dis. 2005;11(5):299–302.
55. Yoshida K, Takatsuka S, Hatada E, Nakamura H, Tanaka A, Ueki K, et al. Expression of matrix metalloproteinases and aggrecanase in the synovial fluids of patients with symptomatic temporomandibular disorders. Oral Surg Oral Med Oral Pathol Oral Radiol Endod. 2006;102(1):22–7.
56. Duff GW. Cytokines and acute phase proteins in rheumatoid arthritis. Stand J Rheumatol. 1994;100(9):20.
57. Slade GD, Conrad MS, Diatchenko L, Rashid NU, Zhong S, Smith S, et al. Cytokine biomarkers and chronic pain: association of genes, transcription, and circulating proteins with temporomandibular disorders and widespread palpation tenderness. Pain. 2011;152(12):2802–12.
58. OMIM (Online Mendelian Inheritance in Man®):An Online Catalog of Human Genes and Genetic Disorders [Internet]. [cited 2018 Apr 1]. Available from: www.omim.org.

Printed by Printforce, the Netherlands